TREATING CANCER WITH
INSULIN POTENTIATION THERAPY

Learn How Insulin Can Help Target Chemotherapy and Be Used as Part of a Comprehensive Natural Medicine Approach to Reverse Cancer and Cancer Physiology

Dear family, friends, colleagues, those with cancer and the people that love them:

We did our best to share with you the personal experiences we went through during the loss of someone we loved very much. Yes, cancer took the life of Pastor Peter, but through the grace of God and some special teachers, we learned what it takes to successfully treat cancer. In the end we are confident that like us, you will say that for someone to beat cancer they must reverse cancer physiology and once having considered everything, treat their cancer with Insulin Potentiation Therapy!

Sincerely with warm regards,

Ross + Marion

CANCER

TREATING CANCER
WITH
INSULIN
POTENTIATION
THERAPY

Learn How Insulin Can Help Target
Chemotherapy and Be Used as
Part of a Comprehensive Natural
Medicine Approach to Reverse
Cancer and Cancer Physiology

Ross A. Hauser, M.D.
Caring Cancer and Interventional Natural Medicine Center

Marion A. Hauser, M.S., R.D.
Caring Medical and Rehabilitation Services, S.C.

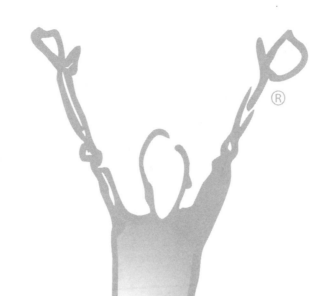

TREATING CANCER WITH INSULIN POTENTIATION THERAPY
LEARN HOW INSULIN CAN HELP TARGET CHEMOTHERAPY AND BE USED AS PART OF A COMPREHENSIVE NATURAL MEDICINE APPROACH TO REVERSE CANCER AND CANCER PHYSIOLOGY

ISBN 0-9661010-6-5

Text and illustrations copyright © 2002, Beulah Land Press
Cover and page design copyright © 2002
Illustrations and Charts by Thomas Penna and M. Hurley

Published by Beulah Land Press
715 Lake Street, Suite 600, Oak Park, Illinois 60301

Printed in the United States of America

Design by Teknigrammaton Graphics
773-973-1614 • Teknigram@worldnet.att.net
7312 N. Hamilton • Chicago, Illinois 60645

Scripture quotations are from: **Holy Bible, New International Version®, NIV®**
Copyrights © 1973, 1978, 1984, International Bible Society. Used by permission of Zondervan Publishing House. All rights reserved.

TABLE OF CONTENTS

The information presented in this book is based on the experiences of the authors and is intended for informational and educational purposes only. **In no way should this book be used as a substitute for your own physician's advice.**

Because medicine and particularly oncology (the medical field that specializes in cancer and cancer therapy) is an ever-changing science, readers are encouraged to confirm the information contained herein with other sources, including their own personal oncologist (a doctor who specializes in cancer). The authors of this book have used sources they believe to be reliable to substantiate the information provided. However, because of the possibility of human error or changes in medical sciences, neither the authors, publisher, editors, nor any other party who has been involved in the preparation or publication of this work warrants that the information contained herein is in every respect accurate or complete; they are not responsible for any errors or omissions or for the results obtained from the use of such information. This is especially true when a person with cancer receives Insulin Potentiation Therapy or any of the therapies described in this book and a bad result occurs. The authors, publisher, and editors of this book do not warrant that Insulin Potentiation Therapy or any of the therapies described in this book will be effective in any medical condition, including cancer, and cannot guarantee or endorse any type of cancer therapy or practitioner who treats cancer patients.

No major therapy is 100% effective. This includes surgery, radiation, chemotherapy (with or without Insulin Potentiation Therapy), or any other therapies described in this book. Thus, this book guarantees no particular results for the cancer patient or any other person reading it.

It is the responsibility of the individual cancer patient to thoroughly research the various cancer treatment options and discuss these options with their families, friends, and other confidants, as well as their health care providers, including their oncologists, before deciding on a particular treatment course. If the consensus is that Insulin Potentiation Therapy is to be given, it is still up to the individual cancer patient and the above individuals to choose a physician who is competent in this particular treatment modality. As of yet, there is no certification available in Insulin Potentiation Therapy to ensure competency in this treatment. Any licensed medical or osteopathic doctor in the United States can perform Insulin Potentiation Therapy according to the law.

Physicians should use and apply Insulin Potentiation Therapy and the other therapies described in this book only after they have received extensive training and demonstrated the ability to administer the treatment safely. The authors, publisher, editors, and any other person involved in this work are not responsible if physicians who are unqualified in the use of Insulin Potentiation Therapy **1.** administer the treatment based solely on the contents of this book or **2.** if they receive training but do not administer it safely and a bad result occurs.

If Insulin Potentiation Therapy or any other treatment regime described in this book appears to apply to your condition, the authors, publisher, and editors recommend that a formal evaluation be performed by a physician who is competent in treating cancer patients with these various treatments. Those desiring Insulin Potentiation Therapy or any other treatment modality described in this book should make medical decisions with the aid of a personal physician. No medical decisions should be made solely on the contents or recommendations made in this book. ∎

The people in this book are real and their stories are true. Some of their names, identifying characteristics, and facts have been altered to protect their privacy.

This book is dedicated to four people who had a tremendous impact in our zealousness to treat cancer patients.

To our first cancer patient, Flora D'Apice: thank you for your trust in us and showing us the tremendous need that cancer patients have to find physicians who will listen and administer alternative medical treatments.

To our pastor, friend, counselor, and confidant, Peter Blakemore: thank you for making us part of God's family and yours. You were the finest person we have ever known. You had no idea how much we loved you and now miss you. We knew that your cancer could be cured; we just found the cure too late.

To Steven G. Ayre, M.D.: Thank you for decades of zealousness in Insulin Potentiation Therapy and teaching us the technique. It was because of you that the treatment came to the United States. Because of you, the world is a better place.

To Donato Pérez García, Jr., M.D.: Your care for patients and humble demeanor is an inspiration to us. You are a godly man, and anyone around you can see and sense this. It is no wonder your patients love you. You are a role model for us. Thank you for taking us under your wing and giving the world a treatment that is sure to change the way cancer therapy is done. Thank you for passing on what your grandfather discovered and your father taught. As the Bible says in 1 Timothy 5:17: "Let the elders who rule well be considered worthy of double honor, especially those who labor in preaching and teaching." We hope that you feel this book honors you and your family, for it is written with this intention.

The influence of these four people permeates the pages of this book. For their influence on this project and on our lives, we will forever be indebted. ∎

Marion A. Hauser, MS, RD
Ross A. Hauser M.D.

THE WORLD'S DEDICATION...

The world owes five men a great deal of gratitude for their sacrifice to the cause of IPT... We gratefully acknowledge the pioneering effort and dedication of Donato Pérez García, Sr. M.D. (1896-1971), who first conceived of and developed the treatment protocol called "Insulin Potentiation Therapy" (IPT). Dr. Donato's son and grandson (Drs. Donato Pérez García y Bellón, and Donato Pérez García, Jr.) also are owed a debt of acknowledgement for the many years of effort they have invested in this work under the most trying of circumstances that are the lot of most innovators in medicine.

We thank Steven G. Ayre, M.D., for his scientific interpretations and publications on IPT that have served to make this valuable medical therapy accessible to the larger medical community.

Finally, the efforts of Chris Duffield, Ph.D., are truly inspiring. His unselfish devotion to help educate professional and lay people about IPT by creating and supporting the web site (www.IPTQ.org) has helped bring the message of IPT to the world. ∎

ACKNOWLEDGEMENTS

The Bible says in Proverbs 3:5-6: "Trust in the Lord with all your heart and lean not on your own understanding; in all your ways acknowledge him, and he will make your paths straight." Acknowledgments should always start with God. In 1985, we both decided to use the Bible as our guide. In that same year, we volitionally dedicated our lives to Jesus Christ who died for our sins and through which we have eternal life. We acknowledge God as our guide and source of strength. We hope that the words we say and write and the activities that we engage in will always bring Him honor and glory. For the person who is sick or those who are trying to help the sick, it is the truth that must be followed. John 1:17 states, "For the law was given through Moses; grace and truth came through Jesus Christ." Truth begins with God, His word, and His grace that came through Jesus Christ. We believe it is God who leads us; the events that have happened to us had a purpose, one of which was to allow us to write this book. If this book is God ordained, then it will surely be a blessing to the world.

Numerous people in our lives have influenced us to be people that love helping other people. Most notably these people include our parents, siblings, friends, and the church families at Harrison Street Bible Church and Calvary Memorial Church, both in Oak Park, Illinois.

We were both heavily into healing disease with natural medicine prior to learning about Insulin Potentiation Therapy. This was only possible because of our teachers and mentors, Gustav A. Hemwall, M.D., who taught us Prolotherapy, and Steven Elsasser, M.D., who taught us everything else. Much of what we know and do is because of these two godly men.

We are grateful for our "book writing/publishing team" that includes

- **Tommy Penna, master illustrator who did the majority of the drawings**
- **Molly Hurley of Teknigrammaton Graphics who put the text and illustrations into a book form**
- **The editing team, including Candace, Laurie, and Caryl**
- **Evic Loutfy of Imagicom, "printer extraordinaire"**

We would not be able to write any books unless we had a research team, which includes Nicole Baird who worked endlessly and tirelessly, always with a smile on her face. The staff of Caring Medical in Oak Park have each helped in their own way to give us the knowledge to write this book. A special thank you to Doug Skinkis, human relations director, who sidelines as an illustrator. Doug, you are a man of many talents. However, we still do not understand your fetish with Montana.

There would be no book writing if it were not for Barry Weiner of Media for Doctors. He technically is our publicity director but functions more as our friend and neutral third party when we disagree. Harry S. Truman once said, "The buck stops here!" Well for us, "The buck stops with Barry!" Barry was successful in helping us change the way pain management is done throughout the world by the success of our various books on Prolotherapy, including *Prolo Your Pain Away!* and *Prolo Your Sports Injuries Away!* We hope Barry helps us have as much success in the way cancer patients are treated. If anyone can do it, Barry can.

We would not have written this book if it were not for all of the cancer patients who saw us prior to us doing Insulin Potentiation Therapy. We, of course, are indebted to our first cancer patient, Flora D'Apice, and our friend, Pastor Peter Blakemore. Pastor Peter's bout with cancer made cancer very personal to us. We acknowledge the fact that almost every cancer patient we have served has somehow influenced us and is reflected in this book.

To Chris Duffield, Ph.D., and Aimé Ricci for your hard work to bring IPT to the masses—we say a heart-felt "Thank you!" To our teachers, Steven G. Ayre, M.D., and Donato Pérez García, Jr., we acknowledge your willingness to share your expertise with us, which allowed us to learn Insulin Potentiation Therapy. Thank you both for your fortitude in your pursuit to help get this therapy accepted into the mainstream of oncology. It is only because of your willingness to teach other doctors that this therapy continues to grow each year. We hope that this book will help educate the masses with cancer that there is a way to treat cancer without all of the side effects of traditional high-dose chemotherapy, and that way is Insulin Potentiation Therapy. ■

by Ross A. Hauser, M.D., and Marion A. Hauser, M.S., R.D.

Our environment has been described as a "sea of carcinogens," awash with a variety of chemicals and, to a lesser extent, oncogenic viruses and high-energy radiations, all of which may contribute significantly to cancer incidence in humans. Most chemicals used in industry and even in the foods we eat have not been adequately tested for their long-term carcinogenic potential. Simply stated, a carcinogen is any substance or agent that significantly increases tumor incidence.

In 1996, the Advisory Committee on Diet, Nutrition, and Cancer Prevention of the American Cancer Society made the following statement:

> The evidence suggests that about one third of the 500,000 cancer deaths that occur in the United States each year is due to dietary factors. Another third is due to cigarette smoking. Therefore, for the large majority of Americans who do not smoke cigarettes, dietary choices and physical activity become the most important modifiable determinants of cancer risk.

About 1.4 million Americans will be diagnosed with cancer this year alone. There is a phenomenon occurring in the United States in regard to the interest and use of natural remedies. Because of this, physicians and health care clinicians who use natural remedies (called natural medicine specialists) are being inundated with patients. For the person who is a true natural medicine specialist, it is only a matter of time before cancer patients start coming. This started occurring in the early 1990s at Caring Medical and Rehabilitation Services, the natural medicine clinic that we founded. Now after 10 years of treating cancer patients, it seems appropriate that we write a book on one specific type of cancer therapy, Insulin Potentiation Therapy (IPT).

IPT has been around for more than 60 years, but, like many more holistic or natural therapies, was suppressed by the medical establishment.

Her breast cancer metastases in her neck and lungs vanished in a matter of weeks. ...She had no side effects from the treatment.

The treatment was founded by Donato Pérez García, Sr., M.D., in Mexico and was first utilized to successfully treat neurosyphilis. He, along with his son, Donato Pérez García y Bellón, M.D., and grandson, Donato Pérez García, Jr., M.D., continued to improve the technique and apply it to other diseases, including cancer. Steven G. Ayre, M.D., an American family physician, tried for over 25 years to get the treatment accepted in the United States. He finally received an audience before the NIH Cancer Advisory Panel for Complementary and Alternative Medicine in Bethesda, M.D., in September 2000. He was joined at this presentation by Donato Pérez García, Jr., and myself (Ross). Dr. Ayre and Dr. García also taught the first comprehensive course on IPT at a medical convention in February 2001.

I (Ross) became involved with IPT because two of my patients had cancer recurrences while on aggressive natural medicine regimes, including the Gerson program and Laetrile. Dr. Ayre performed IPT on one of the patients. Her breast cancer metastases in her neck and lungs vanished in a matter of weeks. As amazing as this was, she had absolutely no side effects from the treatment. It was clear that this treatment was safe enough to be done in a doctor's office (as it was done in our office) and could be done by the person's family physician. This is remarkable because normally cancer treatments are reserved for specialists in cancer therapy, oncologists.

Since that initial patient, we have treated numerous cancer patients with IPT. It is not the panacea for cancer therapy, but it is a major step in the right direction. IPT is a safe technique that is powerful and effective and can be done safely in a doctor's office. We utilize IPT as part of a comprehensive natural medicine approach to cancer. **Note, however, that the primary modality that we use in the treatment of cancer is Insulin Potentiation Therapy.** No longer does a physician, like myself, who specializes in natural medicine, have to be relegated to only supporting the immune system; such physicians can be the cancer patient's primary physician. Let's be honest: Cancer patients hate high-dose chemotherapy and often do not like the doctors who administer it.

The *American Cancer Society's Guide to Complementary Alternative Cancer Methods,* published in 2000, downplays nearly all of the natural cancer remedies. However, they do recommend the following:

★ Educate yourself first.
★ Be nonconfrontational.
★ Ask questions.
★ Bring someone with you to the physician's office.
★ If taking dietary supplements, review usage.
★ Follow up.
★ Be open to change.

They recommend all of the above in regard to alternative remedies and to discuss this with your oncologist. Well, when patients do all of the above and try to discuss it with their oncologists, they may as well be speaking Chinese. **The traditional oncologist does not have a clue about natural medicine and thus pooh-poohs it!** Even if a patient tells an oncologist that the natural medicine treatments are helping him or her feel better, they are often "thrown" out of the office and humiliated. We have seen it happen far too often.

Patients are becoming their own doctors. They are researching treatments on the Internet. They are doing this not only for alternative remedies, but also with *conventional* treatments. Patients are realizing that the benefits from high-dose chemotherapy do not warrant all the risk that the treatment poses. Most people know someone who became bald, emaciated, and horribly sick and in pain, eventually dying of his or her cancer after high-dose chemotherapy. For us and our friends, this was Pastor Peter Blakemore.

Pastor Peter was the kindest man we ever knew. He emulated the attributes of Jesus in that he was humble, kind, and loving. He would do anything for us. He loved us unconditionally. It was because of him and his wife Marla that Marion and I have a strong marriage today.

In 1993, 40-year-old Pastor Peter started limping. Soon cancer was diagnosed. He endured surgery, radiation, high-dose chemotherapy, more radiation, and then more high-dose chemotherapy. He went through the whole gamut of traditional cancer remedies and then sought out alternatives. We saw him suffer excruciating pain, suffocation, and eventual death. He died in our presence. We tried to revive him but to no avail. The emotional scars from his death are still imprinted on our hearts. At a moment's notice, we could both break down and cry, and it has been seven years since his death.

Thus we started our crusade. When a cancer patient comes to our clinic, it is personal not only for the patient but also us. We see a little bit of Pastor Peter in every cancer patient. Patients with cancer generally love to come to Caring Medical. To accommodate all of the cancer patients, we renovated a floor in the Medical Arts Building in which we are located and formed the Caring Cancer and Interventional Natural Medicine Center (CCINMC). This is where IPT is administered in our office.

To further improve the odds of survival or at least the quality of life of our cancer patients, the staff at Caring Medical started helping me with my cancer research. We would go to Loyola Medical Center for hours, reading cancer articles and formulating innovative therapies.

We utilize IPT as our main cancer treatment therapy, combining it with diet, natural medicine techniques, and supplements to reverse cancer physiology. Half of this book is on IPT; the other half describes cancer physiology and how to reverse it.

We hope that this book will explain the principles of IPT to the layperson and doctor. The book details the history of IPT, the remarkable physiology of insulin, how insulin potentiates medications such as chemotherapy, the technique itself, and some of the results. Some case studies are given, both successful and unsuccessful. This book is by no means comprehensive in its explanations. We were told by Barry Weiner, our publicity director, that there will be no more 900+ page books. Our last book, *Prolo Your Sports Injuries Away!*

> When a cancer patient comes to our office, it's personal—not only for the patient—but for us. We see a little bit of Pastor Peter in every cancer patient.

> While you have been reading this foreword, about five more people have died of cancer. We are confident that IPT can save many of these people.

weighs seven pounds, is 901 pages, and retails for $99. It is not easy to get athletes to pay $99 for a book, let alone read a 901-page book. He wanted this book to be 200-300 pages, so we compromised at around 414 pages.

The reader should also realize that this is not a comprehensive book on cancer or even the natural medicine approach to cancer. One is not going to see pages and pages on ozone therapy or Laetrile. Mention will be made about various natural medicine treatments, but the primary focus is on therapies that potentiate the effects of chemotherapy and natural remedies to reverse cancer physiology.

We are often asked by cancer patients if there is a book they could read to describe the therapies they are receiving at CCINMC, including IPT. Unfortunately until now, the answer was always no. While there are some good books on the natural approach to cancer, most of them discuss natural remedies but not interventional natural medicine techniques. This book specifically involves IPT and its treatment of cancer, though we also provide a section on using IPT to treat rheumatologic disorders and various infections.

This book is not an anthology of cancer physiology. That book has yet to be written. We hope to write that book at a later date. It would not be right to wait several more years to write about IPT because this book is needed right now!

Each day, about 1,400 people in the United States die of cancer, or about one person per minute. While you have been reading this foreword, about five more people have died of cancer. We are confident that IPT can save many of these people.

The theory behind IPT, like many natural type remedies, is very simple. Cancer cells have more insulin receptors than normal cells. When a cancer cell is stimulated by insulin, it "wakes up" and starts replicating. Insulin tells the cancer cell that food is coming, but instead of food, low-dose chemotherapy is given. The insulin potentiates the cancer-killing effects of the chemotherapy. Thus, IPT is a treatment that helps target low-dose chemotherapy to the cancer site.

The reader may cringe at the mention of the word chemotherapy, so part of this book is to show the reader that unless some cancer-killing agent is given to a cancer patient, death is the most likely result. If a cancer is no longer localized, then a cancer-killing agent (chemotherapy) must be used for a person to be cured of cancer. Since chemotherapy means a substance that kills cancer cells, a patient who says "I don't want chemotherapy" is basically saying that he or she does not want something that kills cancer cells. What they mean to say is, "I don't want traditional chemotherapy that is going to make me feel terrible, suppress my immune system, and decrease my odds of survival."

IPT uses about 10-25 percent of the typical chemotherapy dose given by oncologists, so it is magnitudes safer than high-dose chemotherapy. Though IPT uses insulin as its primary agent to potentiate medications, other substances can also be utilized, including DMSO (dimethyl sulfoxide), oxidizing agents, and various nutrients. Other natural medicine treatments, such as hyperthermia, ozone therapy, and specific nutritional regimes are discussed because they apply to a science-based approach to cancer.

The main problem with proving that natural remedies prolong life or increase survival is the fact that people wait too long to seek out a natural medicine specialist. This book tells of some of the patients seen at Caring Medical, who were intelligent, successful people in their careers, but naive and downright stupid with regard to their health. You will hear of women who monkeyed with some herbal potions and allowed their breast cancers to take over their lives by metastasizing to their lungs, liver, and brain and then expected some natural medicine specialist to cure them. We could have easily discussed various male cancer patients who have done the same thing in relation to their cancers.

Cure is easy with cancer if the tumor load is not great. Hopefully, people and their loved ones who read this book will get the message: **See an IPT physician as soon as you don't feel good or at least as soon as cancer is diagnosed.** In many respects, the natural medicine specialist (especially one who performs IPT) is *more valuable* than the oncologist because only the natural medicine specialist has the knowledge and available remedies to reverse cancer physiology and utilize treatments such as IPT that can kill cancer cells safely. It is also the natural medicine specialist who knows what remedies decrease the side effects of high-dose chemotherapy and radiation therapy. The oncologist of the future will have to be a natural medicine specialist because cancer patients will insist on it.

The natural medicine cancer specialists of the future will give treatments that not only support the immune system but also reverse cancer physiology. Apoptosis (cancer cell death) will be induced and differentiation (helping cancer cells turn into normal cells) started. Tumor site acidosis, blood alkalosis, and systemic toxicity will be reversed. The cancer patient will undergo therapies, such as IPT, that cause tumor

shrinkage and are virtually free of side effects. The above is not a dream, as it is occurring everyday because of a revolutionary treatment called "Insulin Potentiation Therapy." By targeting cancer-killing remedies, people are becoming free of cancer and side effects. People are taking

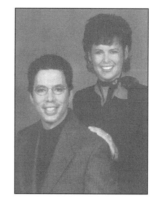

charge of their own health care. Those with cancer are leading the way. They desire natural and safe remedies that rival the traditional counterparts. It is for this reason that they are realizing that IPT is the cancer treatment of the new millennium. ∎

Marion A. Hauser, MS, RD
Ross A. Hauser, M.D.

Ross and Marion Hauser

PETER BLAKEMORE—OUR PASTOR, BIBLE TEACHER, AND FRIEND...

...AND MUCH, MUCH MORE...

To the right is Pastor Peter Blakemore. He was a phenomenal preacher, bringing the Bible alive.

In the lower right picture: Peter and his wife, Marla with the Thursday night bible study. As a Ph.D. in Church History, Pastor Peter taught the bible with the depth of a scholar—but with the love of Messiah.

In the upper right: Peter and Marla celebrate with us at Dr. Hauser's graduation from Medical School..

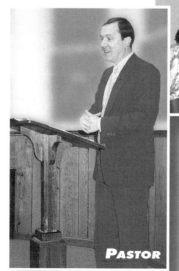

PASTOR

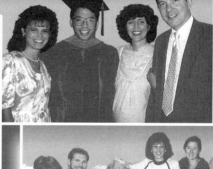

FRIEND

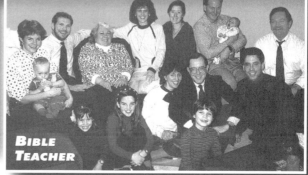

BIBLE TEACHER

Insulin Potentation Therapy—The Passion

According to a biblical principle, God is to receive the "first fruits" of our labors. God should get our best. God should be paid first with our tithes, offerings, and talents. Well, regarding this book, surely the "first fruits" is in the very beginning. Therefore, we are dedicating this section of the book to the five men who have worked so diligently to discover, research, and promote Insulin Potentiation Therapy, so people like us can use this powerful weapon in our practices. The very lives of people all over the world that have been saved through Insulin Potentiation Therapy are owed because of these men. People all over the world owe these five men a great debt.

The passion of IPT began with Donato Pérez García, M.D., the man who discovered Insulin Potentiation Therapy. We will refer to Insulin Potentiation Therapy as "IPT." Donato Pérez García, M.D., will be called "Donato 1," because the first three doctors of IPT were all from the same family, with the first name "Donato." The grandfather, Donato 1, taught IPT to his son Donato Pérez García y Bellón, M.D. (denoted Donato 2), who subsequently taught it to his son Donato Pérez García, Jr., M.D., who is "Donato 3." As you will see, it is because of the efforts of these three men that the therapy of IPT wasn't lost. They did their best to train other doctors and to achieve acceptance in other countries—but even in their native country, Mexico, the medical profession did not accept this therapy.

Recently, Donato 3 stated "My number one goal with IPT is for it to become available to people around the world in its purest and most effective form, through highest quality teaching and practice. . .My number two goal with IPT is that the original developer, my grandfather, gets credit for his work. My father deserves credit as well, because without him no one would have learned the procedure." We hope that this book will aid in the fulfillment of the above goals.

Part of the fascination with the history of IPT comes from the fact that the two men who became most excited about IPT from the above three men, were a family practice doctor from the Chicagoland area, and a visiting scholar from Stanford University. Steven G. Ayre, M.D., is the Medical Director of the Contemporary Medicine Center in Burr Ridge, Illinois. Dr. Ayre is a conscientious and compassionate human being, who also has a great sense of humor. He combines his role as an innovative medical practitioner with that of medical teacher in his capacity as Clinical Assistant Professor in the Chicago Medical School's Department of Family Medicine. In addition, over the last twenty-five years, Dr. Ayre has worked with an uncommon passion on a scientific research project to validate Insulin Potentiation Therapy. The history of IPT is full of references to him, as it should be. He continues to this day to be the premier physician giving scientific presentations on IPT, soliciting government bodies to devote research dollars into validating IPT, as well as teaching physicians the technique.

Chris Duffield, Ph.D., is a visiting scholar with the Center for Latin American Studies at Stanford University. After hearing the passionate Dr. Ayre speak on IPT in 1986, Chris was hooked. He has devoted countless volunteer hours to IPT which is obvious by the web site he hosts on IPT at www.IPTQ.org. He notes on his home page that one of his personal quests is "to help develop radically new technologies and scientific understandings." He is doing just this by his work with IPT. We can think of no better place for *Treating Cancer with Insulin Potentiation Therapy* to start than for Donato 3 to introduce the therapy and Chris to give us his reasons for his passionate involvement in IPT and why he calls IPT the "Medicine of Dreams." ■

INTRODUCTION

by Dr. Donato Pérez García

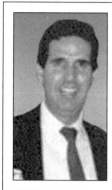

Dr. Donato Pérez García is the most experienced IPT doctor now living. He learned IPT from his father, Dr. Pérez García y Bellon (Donato 2) in 1983 and practiced alongside him in Mexico City for five years, until moving his practice to Tijuana, Mexico. He specializes in the treatment of cancer with IPT. He has been very active in IPT education and research, including managing the IPT doctors-only web site and email group. Besides being fluent in both Spanish and English, the authors of this book consider him to be one of the most distinguished, kindest people they have ever met.

Contact Donato García at: **DONATO PÉREZ GARCÍA, M.D.**
Blvd. Agua Caliente #4558-1503A.
Tijuana, B.C. 22420 Mexico
PHONE: *011-52 664-686-5473*
FAX: *801-459-9928*
www.IPTQ.com
donatopg3@yahoo.com

IPT is a wonderful medical procedure. It has taken more than 70 years to gather the attention it has now. During those years, I believe my grandfather, my father and I learned how to give the treatment in a manner to maximize results and minimize side effects. In other words, we learned what not to do. I am quite aware that soon there will be doctors doing IPT who will modify the technique somewhat to enhance its results even further.

My number one goal with IPT is for it to become available to people around the world in its purest and most effective form, through the highest quality teaching and practice. My second goal is that my grandfather, Dr. Donato Pérez García (Donato 1), the originator of the technique, receives the credit that he deserves. He called the therapy *Cellular Therapy to Change the Bio Physical Constraints of the Blood and then Donatian Therapy*. My father, who learned the technique from him, also should be acknowledged for continuing to use the technique for some 44 years—despite no support from the established medical profession. As I think about the tremendous numbers of patients that were successfully treated by these two men, it makes my eyes fill with tears of emotion and pride. To help understand the sentiment about my father, (Donato 2) consider the following quote from a friend,

> I'm not sure how long before the cancer research conference in Houston (1989) I first met your father on his travels to Texas. I do remember that your father was referred to me on one of his visits when he called upon Dr. Charles A. LeMaistre (who was president of M.D. Anderson at the time). I can say without hesitation that your father was always very kind and thoughtful. Anytime he visited Texas, he would call, usually from San Antonio or sometimes Houston, and ask if I had time to drop by. Of course, I remember very vividly the last time he visited (December of 1999) and we sat in the lobby of the clinic building in the early evening talking about his latest studies as well as his family and my planned retirement. I promised to let him know of my plans that I might be contacted. I will always remember your father with foundness.

> –*Tony Mastromarino October 8, 2001*

Without my father's perserverance and love for the treatment, no one would have learned about Insulin Potentiation Therapy—or, as he like to call it—IPT. He taught me the technique and I have been using it in my practice in the treatment of cancer and general medicine conditions for the past 19 years. My role has been to be the one to start to teach IPT accurately to more doctors. As of today (February 21, 2002) the number of doctors using the treatment with similar good results has increased rapidly since 2000. There are now **43 physicians, representing eight countries** including Mexico, U.S.A., Canada, Argentina, Ecuador, France, Brazil, and Switzerland. The National Cancer Institute of the U.S. National

Institutes of Health has acknowledged this model for treating cancer patients.

All my life I have heard about IPT, formulas, ways of injecting, vaginal inserts, hair formulas, topical dressings, and so forth, all involving the use of insulin with some specific drugs. Even my father developed formulas of his own for skin care products that work. The IPT treatment has its limits, such as its availability, type of disease IPT can effectively treat, and a patient's body condition. For some diseases, like end-stage cancer, the improvement in the patient's quality of life is incredible. It is remarkable when a dying patient recovers energy, has an appetite, does not have to take potent analgesics every four hours, and is able to talk to family and loved ones freely. It makes me very happy to think of the many patients that have been treated by any of the Donatos that are disease-free today. We have had many patients thank us and God for what we were able to do for them. I believe that all human disease can be cured, but not all patients can be cured, not all patients can be treated with IPT and not all patients can be cured with IPT.

I have read Ross and Marion's description of the IPT treatment. I am confident they understand it well—so much so that they wrote the first book in English. I believe this book will make an important contribution to help make people aware of the treatment of IPT. I am happy to be part of this project, and it has become part of my life. It is a project that God dropped into the front door of my professional life—and I now share it with you. It has not been easy. Ever since I remember, on the one hand, I have faced grateful patients, (some poor, some wealthy and powerful). On the other end, I faced comments about the treatment made by medical doctors who did not understood the magnitude of this medical procedure. These facts are now history; the letters, the rejection by doctors' associations, some friends and family too were ashamed of us. Nevertheless, *time is always on the side of truth.* Unfortunately, as is the case of my grandfather and father, they did not live long enough to see their dream of doctors listening to their theories and practicing the treatment come true.

I have worked on what my grandfather and my father started and built. Constructing new theories, new knowledge, all contributing to preserve the human body to its fullest and most productive health. It is a life task that means hard work, perseverance, and love for what you are and what you do. Every occasion I have to learn of my patient's full recovery is an amazing event.

This year (2002) started differently. In the first week, I trained Dr. Doug Brodie, a U.S. doctor who is considered one of the top authorities in the field of alternative therapies. The second week of January, I trained the first doctor from Europe: Dr. Jean R. Lepan and Dr. Nelson Modesto from Brazil, who both made this comment: "Your patients, Donato, come smiling for their treatment and leave smiling to go home." Last week, I treated Michelle Dixon, a 12 year-old girl with a brain tumor, and she had a very good improvement noticed the next morning. She was capable of drawing pictures and she made one for me (**See drawing.**) and today I finished reading the book from Ross and Marion Hauser.

Finally, these people whose contributions to bring IPT to your attention deserve a big "thank you" for their efforts and dedication. God knows how hard we have worked to be here: Steven G. Ayre, M.D., Anthony Mastromarino, Ph.D., Mary Ann Richardson, M.D., Jeff White, M.D., Robert Rowen, M.D., Ross Hauser, M.D., Marion Hauser, R.D., and Chris Duffield, Ph.D. ∎

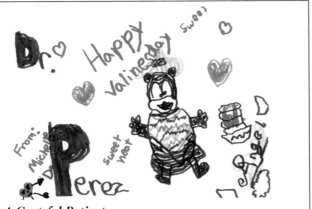

A Grateful Patient
Above is Michelle Dixon's drawing, given in gratitude to Dr. Donato Pérez García.

Donato Pérez García

CHAPTER 1

Medicine of Dreams, by Chris Duffield, Ph.D.

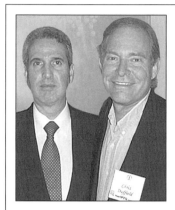

Chris Duffield *(on the right side of this picture, next to Dr. Donato Pérez García on the left)*, though not trained in the medical field, has a passion for innovation and science. He is a Visiting Scholar in the Center for Latin American Studies at Stanford University. He has done more than any other lay person for IPT. After hearing about IPT and the potential possible benefits to humanity, Chris made IPT, its acceptance, and world wide availability one of his life missions. He founded and hosts www.IPTQ.org, (the most comprehensive web site on IPT) with help from Donato Pérez García, M.D., (Donato 3). He believes that IPT is the "Medicine of Dreams" and we hope that with help from this book the reader will be convinced of that fact.

Contact Chris Duffield at: **E-MAIL: *chris@IPTQ.org***
CHRIS DUFFIELD • P.O. BOX 19652
STANFORD, CA 94309-9652
PHONE: 650-723-6144 • FAX: 413-702-9849

PASSION

I am grateful to Dr. Hauser for inviting me to write an essay for this book, and asking me the seed question, "Why are you so passionate about IPT?"

First, his question helped me admit that indeed I am passionate about Insulin Potentiation Therapy. Very passionate. Without passion, I would not have devoted thousands of hours to IPT over 15 years, made personal and financial sacrifices, incurred the incredulity of family members, written thousands of letters and emails, made hundreds of phone calls, traveled thousands of miles by air and car, done research in medical libraries, helped write patents, attended technical conferences, and crafted and hosted a large web site about IPT at www.IPTQ.org… Yes, passionate indeed.

INDUCTION

Actually, I have been passionate about IPT since I first heard about it from Dr. Steven G. Ayre, one summer night in 1986. We had both just attended a large and wonderful formal dinner in the Miami Beach Convention Center, and out in the lobby I overheard him talking enthusiastically about IPT to another man. I interrupted, and the other guy fled, while I absorbed. Dr. Ayre had talked with hundreds, probably thousands of other people about IPT, since he first ran into it in 1975. And only a few had been moved to partici-

pate. For some reason, I was among them. IPT made complete sense to me, I felt excited, got stars in my eyes, and instantly recognized that I wanted to be involved.

What attracted me? I think it was many of the elements of IPT. A simple and easy to understand secret of great worth and power. A great genius, Dr. Donato Pérez García 1, now dead, who was ahead of his time (and even ahead of our time) and who, along with his son and grandson, had been ignored. A Nobel Prize that should have been awarded. The powerful elegance and simplicity of IPT, and its broad spectrum of uses, including treatment of cancer and AIDS. The chance to do tremendous good, without harm, for suffering and dying people, worldwide. The chance to work with doctors and contribute to medicine without going to medical school. The chance to help right the injustice of a great medical discovery being ignored by powerful interests, to their profit and humanity's loss. And there was even the possibility (laughable in retrospect, at least so far) of making a lot of money. In short, it was a great cause, and it needed help. And I was hooked.

FRUSTRATION

Dr. Ayre called an organizational meeting in San Antonio, Texas, in the summer of 1987, which I attended. Three attendees—Dr. Ayre, a patent attorney named Mel Silverman, and I—soon formed a for-profit corporation (Sana

11

Institute) to develop IPT, in cooperation with Drs. Pérez García 2 and 3. With visions of quick and easy success, we embarked on a disastrous three year journey. We applied for and got patents, and knocked on many doors, but attracted no investors. Later, the five of us idealistically formed a nonprofit corporation (Medical Renaissance Foundation), but we found that it was even difficult to give IPT away for free. I brought in the only outside donation, which was just a drop in the bucket of our expenses, which included, at various times, an ad in the LA Times, two 800 numbers at my home, and a high-rise office in San Diego. We all lost a lot of money, and split up with some bitterness, each in our own direction.

And so ended another frustrating chapter in IPT's long book. Another cycle of hope, excitement, action, and disappointment. Just one of many for the three generations of Drs. Pérez García, and a real learning experience for me.

RESURRECTION

I stayed in touch with Dr. Pérez García 3 over the years, visiting him in San Diego and Tijuana from time to time. The Internet grew, and in 1996 or 1997, he put up a simple web page about IPT. In 1998 we came up with the idea for a larger web site. We both had a lot of IPT material to share with the world, and we were tired of having to photocopy, collate, and fax or mail stacks of material every time we met someone new who might be interested. With a web site, people everywhere in the world would be able to read all the wonderful historical and scientific IPT documents for free any time they wanted, following their own pace and interests. And such a web site could serve as a meeting place and catalyst for the growing IPT community that we dreamed of.

The name I came up with for the IPT web site was "IPTQ.com," standing for "The IPT Question." The site began to take shape from my Visiting Scholar office here at Stanford University, and its scope grew into huge proportions as we dug deeper into our archives. It became obvious to me that IPTQ needed to be independent, and it needed to be not-for-profit, in order to have the greatest credibility and impact. So I changed its name to "IPTQ.org," and also registered "IPTQ.net"—just to be sure.

This web site has worked. Patients, doctors, researchers, writers, and philanthropists have learned about IPT through it. And, still growing, it now stands ready for whoever wants to know more about IPT, especially as the word gets out to a larger public through published articles, talks, and books like this one.

PROLIFERATION

Then something new happened that no web site could accomplish: More doctors learned to practice IPT. The first two were Dr. Eduardo A. Katsiyannis of Buenos Aires, Argentina, who started getting trained by correspondence with Dr. Pérez García 3 in November, 1999, and Dr. Ross Hauser, who learned the basics from Dr. Ayre in December 1999, with further training from Dr. Pérez García 3 in late February/early March 2000.

I was excited, and encouraged Drs. Pérez and Ayre to teach even more doctors. It had always been clear that having more IPT doctors was the only way that IPT could grow and become available to more patients—with or without governmental, corporate, or philanthropic support. And now, from the grass roots, it was finally happening!

The rest is an accelerating and exhilarating history, which is still just beginning. In June 2000 Drs. Frank W. George and Hayle T. Aldren of Sun City, Arizona, were trained in Tijuana by Dr. Pérez.

On September 18, 2000, Drs. Ayre, Pérez 3, and Hauser presented a series of best cancer cases to an advisory panel of the National Institutes of Health (NIH). Unfortunately, no significant public actions have resulted, to date.

On November 23, 2000, we were all deeply saddened by the death of the real master of IPT, Dr. Donato Pérez García y Bellón. I was chatting by computer with his son, Dr. Pérez García 3, at the moment when it happened, and I felt crushed by this devastating and unexpected loss. We have to carry on without him, and one day I hope we will reconstruct what knowledge we can from his notes and papers.

The next great milestone was when Dr. Robert J. Rowen, a nationally known holistic doctor from Anchorage, Alaska, learned IPT from Dr. Ayre in September and Dr. Pérez in October 2000. Largely through Dr. Rowen's influence and connections, the first large IPT training seminar was held in Las Vegas, Nevada on February 21-22,

2001. To Drs. Pérez García 1 and 2, this would have been truly amazing, the almost miraculous fulfillment of their decades of dreams. They taught IPT to one and three doctors, respectively. But in those two days in Las Vegas, twenty doctors, two nurses, and one veterinarian learned IPT. And I was pleased to be there to witness this great event.

I have been continually impressed with the very high personal, creative, and professional qualities of the doctors who are attracted to IPT, and the openness and heartfelt qualities of the patients who have been seeking this treatment. It has been a great pleasure to meet and work with all these people.

As I write this, IPT is beginning to blossom. Almost 40 doctors have learned IPT, and more are signing up, including the first from Europe. I think we have achieved critical mass to assure IPT's success. More doctors are sharing information on an IPT doctors email group, and more are joining a secure doctors-only web site, IPTQMD.com, that I run for Dr. Pérez. More IPT-related web sites and web pages are showing up on search engines. More patients are e-mailing me and contacting doctors for IPT treatment. More wonderful IPT results are being recorded and published. A senior research oncologist has decided to make sure that IPT-boosted chemotherapy will get the clinical trials it deserves. A national foundation I contacted is investigating IPT. And some books, including this one, are being prepared for publication.

For someone who is passionate about IPT, this is a very exciting time!

OBSTRUCTION

Dr. Hauser's seed question to me implies another question: "Why isn't everyone so passionate about IPT?" Indeed most people haven't been, since Dr. Donato Pérez García 1 discovered IPT 75 years ago. This has always puzzled me and others, as well.

Why did nothing happen after Dr. Pérez's triumphant demonstration of IPT treatment of neurosyphilis in the US, and his appearance in Time Magazine in April, 1944? Why do the surgeons in the audience at his 1950 presentation about treatment of appendicitis and ulcers without surgery look so uncomfortable in the old photo, and

why didn't they ever try it? Why were his reversal of polio paralysis in children, and his successful treatment of cancer with non-toxic insulin-potentiated chemotherapy, ignored in the 1940s and 1950s? Why was his son, Dr. Pérez García 2, also ignored, despite his scientific investigations, his unceasing efforts to communicate with doctors, researchers, and pharmaceutical companies, and his continued stunningly successful practice of IPT?

Even in the last 20% of IPT's history, in which I have been involved, I have often run into skepticism, and sometimes arrogance and antagonism, towards IPT. And mostly I have run into ignorance of IPT. There are two types of ignorance. The first is passive ignorance, where people have never heard about IPT. This type is easy to understand and excuse. The second type is active ignorance, where people are exposed to IPT, but don't acknowledge or do anything about it. I have run into plenty of both types.

In my efforts to seek interest, involvement, support, and even just acknowledgment of IPT, I have been ignored or turned down by many rich and powerful people and organizations, by millionaires and billionaires, by famous actors, by some of the biggest names in medical research, by drug companies, by some of the best known foundations. I have been sneered at in person by the head of the National Institutes of Health (NIH), and given bureaucratic redirection (or no answer at all) by administrators of other regional, national, and international health organizations.

This has been a source of continuous amazement for me, for years. Again and again I have gotten excited about a new contact, only to find that yet another famous, powerful, high-level person or organization that states publicly their desire to help patients and humanity, and to advance science and medicine, will simply ignore or politely reject the IPT information. I have persistently (and passionately) tried many different approaches, but usually with frustrating results.

I have collected numerous polite rejection letters from philanthropists and foundations, wishing us good luck. A researcher who specializes in the molecular system of insulin receptors congratulated me for thinking way outside of the box, and then said he wasn't interested. Some doctors have violently reacted to the idea of giving insulin to a non-diabetic patient, saying it would be unethical, and likely to result in malpractice lawsuits. Drug companies have been more terse and opaque in their rejections; it is clear that IPT, not being a patentable new drug, and reducing the dose of existing drugs, does not fit into their business models. Probably for similar reasons, venture capitalists and other financial people quickly lose their smiles and change the subject or move away when they hear the details of the IPT innovation. News reporters have not yet been interested because IPT clinical trials have not yet been done, and it has not appeared in mainstream journals.

It seems to me as though many people and organizations want to keep looking for solutions, without actually finding one. Or at least not this one. Somehow IPT is not yet politically correct, probably because for some special interests, it is not yet economically correct. And because these are the very people and organizations that doctors and patients look up to and trust, very little has happened in the IPT world, for three generations. It is a classical new paradigm, with diffusion problems. Most doctors are still very skeptical about IPT because it hasn't appeared in the journals or the news. Most patients are reluctant to try IPT because their doctors don't know about it. And so it seems that, at least in the case of IPT, humanity has not been well served.

But why? Rejection and ignorance of IPT have been so widespread for so long that a conspiracy seems unlikely. I have come to the conclusion that IPT has been rejected and ignored by one person or organization at a time, for 75 years, for one of three main reasons:

Some reject or ignore IPT because it doesn't fit in with their strategies and self interest. This probably applies most specifically to drug and device companies, and some health agencies, researchers, and surgeons.

Others reject or ignore IPT because it is essentially invisible to them; it doesn't fit in with their habitual concepts and does not come from the usual authoritative sources. This probably applies to most doctors and the media.

And most people and organizations reject or ignore IPT (if they even hear about it) because they trust and depend on people and organizations that fall into the first two categories.

The health system is a huge worldwide industry, with many entrenched special interests. And so IPT, by its very nature, has a geopolitical dimension. The cumulative cost to humanity of ignoring and rejecting the findings and promise of IPT for three generations, in terms of lives, suffering, and wealth, has been staggering, although until now basically invisible. This is a story that will certainly be more widely investigated and retold in future years.

TRANSMUTATION

Finally, though, the tide of IPT is turning. We have more doctors and more patients, and more information is buzzing around. This is a revolution in the making, which we have been predicting and awaiting for years. And now it appears that IPT's time has finally come.

It's an explosion waiting to happen. More fuel is being added, and the ignition sequence has begun. IPT is a simple medical procedure, and is easy for any doctor to learn in a few days of training. It uses standard supplies and equipment available everywhere. It is just a slight modification of standard medical techniques. It promises better results for patients, at lower cost for providers. It appears to be a better treatment not only for cancer, but for serious infections, and many other diseases. And, most unusual, it uses standard drugs, only in much smaller doses, and without toxic side effects. It makes regular drugs act like super drugs, without having to wait for government approval. It acts like alternative and holistic medicine, while still using standard medications. So the only thing alternative about IPT is that it is not yet well known.

In short, IPT is better software for using the medical hardware that we already have. And the computer industry has shown us how fast and easily software can blanket the world, once the word gets out.

When this story finally breaks, it will be a big one. Look at all the press attention that new drugs get. Imagine the effect of the much bigger story that the hormone insulin has a second and probably greater use (what I have trademarked as "The second discovery of insulin"), and that it has been known and ignored for 75 years. The IPT idea, history, and reality are so powerful that many people may need help to deal with the shock, denial, anger, and guilt that they may feel.

There will come a time, I am convinced, when IPT will be a widespread, standard treatment. It could come quickly. Look at how the antibiotic treatment of ulcers (which Dr. Pérez García 1 was doing better with IPT in the 1940s) went from heresy in the 1980s to orthodoxy in the late 1990s. And I believe that we will look back at today's medicine, especially today's oncology, as part of an ignorant and barbaric time, when patients were administered highly toxic doses of expensive drugs, while a gentle technique using insulin potentiation was being widely ignored.

I don't think the drug companies, the oncologists, and the research community can ignore IPT much longer, either passively or actively. Ignaz Semmelweiss, who discovered in the 1847 that hand washing by doctors could prevent infection, was ridiculed and obstructed in his lifetime, but was later recognized, and his innovation widely (but still not universally) adopted. Drs. Pérez García 1 and 2 experienced similar humiliation and exclusion in their lifetimes for their even greater discovery. But with the number of IPT doctors and patients now growing exponentially, the time for the public justification and honor of the Drs. Pérez will soon be upon us.

And I suspect that IPT is just one of many such long-ignored innovations that have been hidden away and that will finally be widely recognized.

PROGNOSTICATION

Where will IPT go in the years to come? To me, it is a fundamental medical discovery, on a level comparable to the discoveries of antibiotics and anesthesia, and it will probably go in many directions. Here are some future future visions I'm having today.

Most likely, IPT will have its first worldwide impact in oncology. Who would have guessed that the very same chemotherapy drugs that devastate the health of patients in the effort to cure them, could be given more safely, effectively, and efficiently with just the addition of the IPT protocol? IPT chemotherapy without surgery, radiation, or side effects could become the first treatment of choice for many cancers.

IPT could also become the first cancer treatment that is available to, and affordable by millions of low-income people in developing countries. This would be possible because IPT is chemotherapy at one-tenth the normal dose, a simple procedure using simple equipment, and low-tech medicine with high-tech results.

Pharmaceutical companies are now developing chemo drugs that specifically target tumors and spare normal cells. But IPT has been targeting tumors since 1947. And IPT could probably help these targeted drugs work even better.

I think it is likely that insulin receptor assays will become a standard part of pathology lab analysis of tumor biopsy samples. If the insulin receptor count is high, IPT probably has a higher chance of success. If low, other strategies may also be needed.

The second major impact of IPT is likely to be in the area of infectious diseases. This was the first use of IPT in the 1920s, and could be the most far-reaching application today. By making antibiotic and anti-viral drugs more effective, and by delivering them better throughout the body, IPT could offer a way to clear resistant infections like herpes from the body, or to keep infections like HIV/AIDS more tightly under immune control. By treating patients faster and more effectively, treatment compliance might be increased for global scourges like malaria, tuberculosis, and HIV/AIDS, and today's growing problem of drug resistance could be addressed.

There are also likely to be major impacts of IPT, and its future derivatives, in treatment of respiratory, cardiovascular, digestive and liver/gallbladder, dental, neurological, and other diseases and conditions.

Insulin is a known growth factor for many types of cells, including stem cells. We may find that IPT works in part by stimulating stem cell proliferation and differentiation, making it a less expensive way to give or enhance stem cell therapy for healing and regeneration in all parts of the body.

Insulin is also a known promoter for angiogenesis (new blood vessel growth). This could explain some of the benefits of IPT, and especially in regard to cardiovascular diseases.

Dr. Pérez García 3 has been telling me for years that he thinks pharmaceutical companies will eventually develop new drugs specifically to work better with IPT. And certainly, as IPT finally gets the laboratory research that it deserves, and as we begin to understand it better, new modifications of IPT, new treatment strategies, and even new drugs may result.

IPT is likely to become popular for treatment of dogs and cats, racehorses and breeding stock, animals in zoos, and perhaps even whales and dolphins. Insulin has similar actions in all mammalian species, and can be traced back into older life forms, so IPT may find many applications throughout the animal kingdom.

IPT also seems ideal for use in remote locations where intensive medical care and even doctors may not be available. The simple cancer therapy that IPT offers, along with Dr. Pérez García 1's demonstrated non-surgical treatment for appendicitis, would seem ideal for use at outposts in Antarctica, the far north, or on the moon. IPT could even go interplanetary as a simple, safe, and effective nonsurgical treatment on manned missions to Mars.

For people who are only interested in money, IPT still shows great promise. Based on the analysis methods published in 1998 by University of Chicago economists Kevin Murphy and Robert Topel, I conservatively estimated (on www.IPTQ.org) that the total value of making IPT available to humanity, including life extension and reduction of pain, fear, and suffering, could be on the order of fifty trillion dollars. This is about five years of today's US gross domestic product (GDP), and 14 months of world GDP. The true value could very well be more.

Thus introduction of IPT, while perhaps temporarily impacting short-term profits for a few major companies, could bring a huge windfall to humanity as a species. I think it is only a matter of time before a major foundation or philanthropist jumps at the chance to invest in IPT research and proliferation for a benefit to cost ratio of about a million to one.

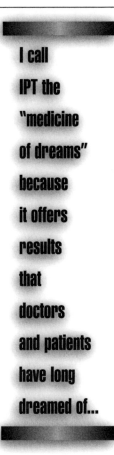

I call IPT the "medicine of dreams" because it offers results that doctors and patients have long dreamed of...

CONCLUSION

One of the great medical discoveries of all time has been ignored for three generations, and is just now being born on the world stage. More doctors are learning it, more patients are receiving it, the word is getting out, and the long-neglected research is about to be done. Everyone who wants to can participate in this birth, even if it is just by telling someone about it.

I call IPT the "medicine of dreams" because it offers results that doctors and patients have long dreamed of, but didn't dare to expect in reality. In the movie "Field of Dreams," a cosmic voice says, "Build it and they will come." Like the baseball field in that film, IPT was discovered by one individual, and has been lovingly cultivated by a handful of others. And now they, the people of this world, are coming. This is truly a great time to be passionate about IPT. ■

CHAPTER 2

Insulin Potentiation Therapy: A Renaissance in Cancer Chemotherapy
by Steven G. Ayre, M.D.

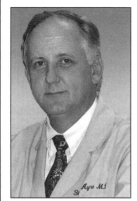

Steven G. Ayre, M.D., is the Medical Director of the Contemporary Medicine Center in Burr Ridge, Illinois. Dr. Ayre has thirty years' experience with what he calls "Integrative Medicine." Integrative Medicine is a combination of all the best in traditional medical care and exciting variety of treatment options in the growing field of Complementary and Alternative Medicine. He was the first American physician trained in IPT and brought the therapy to the United States. He has been instrumental in providing the scientific rationale for the treatment. He is also very active in training other physicians to do IPT. He is currently working on several large research studies to validate the therapy.

Contact Dr. Steven G. Ayre: E-MAIL: *steven303@aol.com*
WEB SITE: *www.contemporarymedicine.net*
CONTEMPORARY MEDICINE • STEVEN G. AYRE, M.D.
322 BURR RIDGE PARKWAY • BURR RIDGE, ILLINOIS 60521
PHONE: 630-321-9010

Insulin Potentiation Therapy (IPT) manipulates the mechanisms of malignancy to therapeutic advantage by employing insulin as a biologic response modifier of cancer cells' endogenous molecular biology. The autonomous proliferation of malignancy is supported by autocrine secretion of insulin for glucose/energy uptake by cancer cells, and a similar autocrine and/or paracrine elaboration of cellular factors to stimulate cancer growth. Amongst these, the insulin-like growth factors (IGF) has been identified as the most potent mitogens for cancer cells. Of primary importance for IPT, cancer cell membranes also have six times more insulin receptors and ten times more IGF receptors per cell than the membranes of host normal tissues. Further insulin can cross-react with and activate cancer cell IGF receptors.

Thus, per cell, cancer has sixteen times more insulin-sensitive receptors than normal tissues. As ligand effect is a function of receptor concentration, these facts serve to differentiate cancer from normal cells—a vital consideration for the safety of cancer chemotherapy.

In light of these revelations, exogenous insulin acts to enhance anti-cancer drug cytotoxicity, and safety, via:

1. A membrane permeability effect to increase the intracellular dose intensity of the drugs,

2. An effect of metabolic modification to increase the S-phase fraction in cancer cells, enhancing their susceptibility to cell-cycle phase-specific agents, and

3. An effect of biochemical differentiation based on insulin receptor concentration that focuses the first two insulin effects predominantly on cancer cells, sparing host normal tissues.

Significantly less drug can thus be targeted more precisely and more effectively to cancer cell populations that are more susceptible to the chemotherapy drug effects—all this occurring with a virtual elimination of the dose-related side effects of these powerful drugs.

Because of this favorable side effect profile, cycles of low-dose chemotherapy with IPT may be done more frequently. There is good patient acceptance of the hypoglycemic side effect of insulin in this protocol and the "rescue phenomenon" occasioned by the timely administration of hypertonic glucose actually serves to provide patients with an experiential metaphor for the rapid recovery of their well being. It is acknowledged that cancer treatment can often be debilitating for patients. In those undergoing treatment with IPT, an overall gentler experience promotes their concurrent use of other important elements in a program of comprehensive cancer care, which includes nutrition for immune system support and mind-body medicine to encourage a healing consciousness.

A BRIEF HISTORY OF INSULIN POTENTIATION THERAPY

Insulin Potentiation Therapy (IPT) was developed for the treatment of human disease by Donato Pérez García, Sr., M.D. (1896-1971) in 1932. A surgeon lieutenant in the Mexican military establishment, this man's preliminary work with insulin involved an innovative course of self-treatment for an emaciating gastrointestinal problem he had suffered from for years. All previous treatments had failed to resolve it. When he first learned of the then newly-discovered hormone insulin for treating diabetes, he noted that in addition to diabetes it was also indicated for the treatment of non-diabetic malnutrition. So he decided to try it on himself. The treatment was completely successful, his symptoms disappeared and his weight became normal. Reflecting on his experience here, Dr. Pérez García considered that the insulin had helped his body tissues assimilate the food he had eaten. He then went on to reason that perhaps insulin might have a similar effect to help tissues assimilate medications.

He first used IPT in the treatment of tertiary neurosyphilis, the standard treatment which was relatively ineffective for advanced cases with brain involvement. Dr. Pérez García reasoned that treatment might be improved with the addition of insulin to help the brain assimilate the anti-syphilis medications. An animal study using this concept showed an increased brain uptake of Salvarsan—the agent used to treat syphilis—and this data was published in *Revista Medica Militar* (1938). Applied to his patients, Dr. Pérez García's treatment was completely successful. In many patients, the spinal fluid Wasserman and Lange's colloidal gold reactions (tests for syphilis) got reversed, and there was a concomitant clearing of the symptoms and physical findings in these patients. In 1937 Dr. Pérez García was invited to the United States to demonstrate his therapy at the Austin State Hospital in Austin, Texas, and at St. Elizabeth's Hospital in Washington, D.C. In 1944 he was again invited to treat some patients at the San Diego Naval Hospital, producing the same positive results in patients with neurosyphilis, malaria, rheumatic fever, and chole-

cystitis. This 1944 visit to San Diego led to a *Time Magazine* write-up of Dr. Pérez García and what they called his "insulin shock treatment."

The first successful treatment of cancer with the therapy happened in 1947 when Dr. Pérez García treated a patient with a squamous cell carcinoma of the tongue. This patient subsequently survived—disease free—for another thirty years. Numerous other cancer cases followed, with many startling responses—particularly in patients with newly diagnosed, and previously untreated disease. There had always been much criticism and controversy surrounding Dr. Pérez García and his treatment—fed no doubt by some professional jealousy. The addition of the issue of cancer only served to harden the feelings of many Mexican physicians against him. In 1955, Dr. Pérez García's son—Donato Pérez García y Bellón, M.D., graduated from medical school, and joined in working with his father at his clinic in central Mexico City. Together father and son continued to expand the applications of IPT to more and more different diseases and, as before, continued to produce remarkable clinical results. And, as with so many medical innovators before them—the likes of Ignacz Semmelweis and Louis Pasteur—the excellence and unorthodoxy of the Drs. Pérez García earned them nothing but rejection from their peers. In one instance this censure came to an extreme. A senior medical student who had been told by his professors of the evils of the Drs. Pérez García came to confront the two in their clinic, brandishing a pistol with the intention of killing them both for the disgrace he believed they were bringing down on the Mexican medical profession. There were some dramatic moments that night, a grappling struggle for the gun, it went off—leaving a hole in the ceiling. After subduing him, the Drs. Pérez García explained and clarified their position. The young man listened and then left, bemoaning that darker side of human motivation that could create such falsehood.

In 1971 Dr. Pérez García, Sr. died of a stroke. The younger physician then continued on his own—more alone now than before, and more resolved than ever to bring credit and credibility to his father's pioneering work. He himself fared no better with the local medical community, but his many grateful patients continued to thrive, and to refer others, who thrived, etc. In the fall of

1975, a Canadian Family Physician—Steven G. Ayre, M.D. (myself)—came to hear of the insulin treatment, and visited Dr. Pérez García's Mexico City clinic. Dr. Ayre studied along side Dr. Pérez García during the month of November of that year, and returned to his native Montreal filled with an enthusiasm and an urgency to communicate with others concerning this amazing Insulin Potentiation Therapy. He also met with only suspicion and ridicule, and thereafter he too resolved to carry the fight to bring this truth to light.

Dr. Pérez García y Bellón had a son himself, Donato Pérez García, Jr., who earned his M.D. degree in 1983. In his turn, this youngest of the family namesake undertook the practice of IPT and continued the family heritage of producing remarkable clinical successes with his practice of the therapy. Dr. Pérez García, Jr. took himself and his family north to Tijuana after several years of partnership with his father and, is practicing there to the present.

After his visit to Mexico, Dr. Ayre set about trying to develop an appropriate scientific basis for what was empirically being observed with his friends' practice of IPT in Mexico. He realized that trying to create some credibility for a cancer cure from Mexico was like trying to make a silk purse out of a sow's ear—which everyone knows is impossible. He sustained himself by personally adopting the credo that things which are impossible take just a bit longer to accomplish than those which are simply difficult. Here in 2001, it has turned out to be quite a bit longer.

Another Canadian Family Physician—Jean-Claude Paquette, M.D.—had heard about IPT back in 1978. This jovial francophone was far more adventurous and forthright than Dr. Ayre with his penchant for doing things "by the book," scientifically speaking. Dr. Paquette just went ahead and practiced IPT—first in his home Canadian Province of Quebec, and then at a clinic he set up in Haiti, and then back in Quebec again after the political intrigues that beset Haiti.

Dr. Paquette brought a clinical expertise born of thirty years of medical practice to the struggle to establish the worth of IPT. Like the Drs. Pérez García, Dr. Paquette did well by his practice of IPT—as far as his patients' welfare was concerned. As far as his local medical college was concerned, the outcome was tragically different. Returning from Haiti, unable to even consider returning to a conventional practice of medicine, Dr. Paquette did what he had to do. He practiced IPT and he tried to show the medical world what IPT could do via his numerous and remarkable anecdotes. For his pains, Dr. Paquette was stripped of his license to practice medicine. A few short years later in the summer of 1996, Dr. Jean-Claude Paquette died—literally broken-hearted—of a myocardial infarction.

Meanwhile, Dr. Ayre continued with his efforts to develop a scientific basis for IPT. By 1990, he had four articles published in the peer-reviewed medical literature, he had presented his scientific theories about IPT at a number of national and international conferences, and had even undertaken two animal studies on the unorthodox actions of insulin on biomembranes. Through all this time, Dr. Ayre remained ever cautious, controlling his urge to just go ahead and practice IPT. The precedent of his colleague's fate was enough to dissuade him from going further.

In the summer of 1996, there was a significant development. Some years before in 1989, the Drs. Pérez García and Dr. Ayre had been invited to present IPT at the Forty-Second Annual Symposium on Fundamental Cancer Research at the prestigious M.D. Anderson Institute in Houston, Texas. In response to the winds of change in medicine, M.D. Anderson had set up its own Center for Alternative Medicine Research. Through contacts established at their 1989 meeting, a first hand look at the "Mexican—Insulin Potentiation Therapy" was undertaken. After reviewing what was there to be reviewed, the investigator performing the site visits with the two Drs. Pérez García—one in Mexico City and the other in Tijuana—remarked, "This is incredible! How come nothing has ever been done about this before?"

Next, by virtue of the concerted efforts of the M.D. Anderson people, an invitation was extended to the trio of IPT doctors to present the scientific background on IPT, and some case presentations from the clinical work done in Mexico. This presentation was made at the National Institutes of Health, Office of Alternative Medicine POMES conference in August of 1997. Another invitation was extended to the Drs. Pérez García and Dr. Ayre to make a Best Case Series presentation before the members of the Cancer Advisory Panel of the Center for Complementary and Alternative Medicine at the National Institutes of

Health in Bethesda, Maryland. This presentation was made on September 20, 2000. Also, a program to develop a clinical trial protocol for IPT in the treatment of breast cancer is currently underway in collaboration with one of the Comprehensive Cancer Centers of the National Cancer Institute. During the sixty-five years of history that tells the story of Insulin Potentiation Therapy, all who have had a hand in it have held to the conviction that the therapy is a valuable thing, and that the knowledge of it should be made widely available to the medical profession. Efforts to this end continue. It has become clear that the way to accomplish the desired goals for IPT is to work quietly and diligently, treating those patients who ask for help, documenting all results, and publishing these results in medical journals. As the history of IPT unfolds, so too has the strength and maturity of its proponents. They have come to understand that it does no good to try and push the river, so to speak. The river will flow, ceaselessly, at its own pace. The Drs. Pérez and Dr. Ayre take comfort in knowing that "stronger than all the armies in the world is an idea whose time has come," and it appears that the time for IPT may now be approaching.

IN MEMORIAM

Dr. Donato Pérez García y Bellón died of a heart attack in Mexico City on November 23, 2000. His passing was a great loss for the world medical community as Dr. Pérez García was the acknowledged master of the practice of Insulin Potentiation Therapy. His dedication to completing the work of IPT started by his late father—Dr. Donato Pérez García, Sr.—was total and uncompromising. He accomplished much in this regard. More remains to be done, and will be—by his son, Dr. Donato Pérez García, Jr., and Dr. Steven G. Ayre. This is our common dedication. Dr. Pérez García y Bellón will be greatly missed.

A SUMMARY OF INSULIN POTENTIATION THERAPY

And now, I am pleased for this opportunity to add my own reflections on Insulin Potentiation Therapy (IPT) to this book written by Dr. Ross Hauser. He was the first clinician that I instructed in the principles and practice of this therapy in the fall of 1999. Since that time he has had his own share of clinical successes combining the therapy with his plans of management for patients suffering from cancer. Dr. Hauser has written several other excellent books on a variety of topics in complementary and alternative medicine, and I am glad that he has chosen to offer his writing expertise to popularize the story of IPT in this present book.

IPT has been a personal passion of mine, as well as my dedication to the medical profession, ever since I first learned of it back in September of 1975. During the years between 1975 and 1999, I chose not to proceed with the actual practice of IPT myself, but elected rather to develop something in the way of a scientific basis for it. I understood this to be a most important first step before consideration could be given any novel idea in medicine. IPT was developed empirically in the early 1930s by Donato Pérez García, Sr., M.D. in Mexico City, at a time when the requisite scientific sophistication for clearly describing how insulin worked in his therapy did not exist. The science for this did not develop until the late 1970s. Taking advantage of this evolution in science and acting in the capacity of scientific liaison for the Dr. Pérez García family of physicians (See IPT History), I managed to get five articles on IPT published in recognized medical journals under our combined authorship.

These articles, plus presentations made at major national and international scientific meetings, ultimately led to a Best Case Series presentation on IPT before members of the Cancer Advisory Panel of the National Center for Complementary and Alternative Medicine at the National Institutes of Health in Bethesda, Maryland, in September of 2000. This meeting in turn led to an invitation by a nationally recognized cancer researcher, the director of one of the Comprehensive Cancer Centers affiliated with the National Cancer Institute, to do a proper scientific study of IPT on human subjects. As of this writing (September 2001) plans are under way to produce an appropriate study design for a clinical trial. This work is to be submitted to the FDA and then to the National Cancer Institute for the necessary funding.

My passion and dedication to developing IPT has been sustained over these many years by numerous reports of anecdotal successes by the Drs. Pérez García using the therapy in the treatment of cancer—as well as in many other disease processes. I chose to focus uniquely on the application of IPT in the treatment of cancer because that is where there was the best science—findings associating the molecular biology of cancer with the physiology of the hormone insulin and its related compounds. The story constructed from these scientific findings, coupled with the decades of reported anecdotal results, I believe, provides a compelling intellectual argument for proceeding with a program of clinical study for this medical innovation.

As a physician, my primary concern has always been to provide the highest quality of patient care. Cancer is the condition for which it is said that the treatment is worse than the disease. It is an acknowledged fact that the one factor above all that has driven the rapid growth of interest in alternative medicine in the American patient population is the desire to have improved treatments for cancer. For myself, the importance of IPT is the possibility that it may prove to be of value in providing an improved quality of care for cancer patients. From the years of experience with IPT, both abroad and now here in the United States, there is little question but that the reduced doses of chemotherapy used in the protocol do afford patients side-effect free treatment with these powerful drugs. In this connection, one other very important point about IPT and cancer treatment was emphasized in the following statement from the Cancer Advisory Panel meeting in September, 2000: "If IPT is found to be at least as effective as current conventional treatment, it would be considered an improved therapy." (Note this web site link: http://nccam.nih.gov/nccam/ne/newsletter/fall2000/capcam.htm.) This important question about IPT is to be addressed in forthcoming clinical trials.

All of these developments have taken place over a long period of time in my life. At the beginning, my motive was to try and beat the medical profession into submission to accept what I was certain was a simple and wonderful new idea. I was in a hurry. Many years into the fray, worn out and worn down, I came to realize that IPT would be better offered as a gift rather than a foregone conclusion from my own belief system. I also recognized that for any gift to be received, this must first be made properly acceptable—and so my work proceeded. Through this work, I myself

learned as much from IPT as I thought I might be able to teach others with it. Now I look forward to the day when mainstream specialists in medical oncology will have access to this treatment. I think they would love it—should studies prove its value. I pray that this may be the case—for these physicians, and for the cancer patients they care for as they do.

I am certain that IPT will not cure everybody with cancer. I am hopeful that it will help control cancer in many patients. I believe that IPT will do no harm to patients from chemotherapy drug reactions. As far as proposed clinical studies on IPT are concerned, I remain surrendered to the outcome—come what may. With my work on IPT, this much I have learned: "Thy will, oh Lord, not mine, be done."

PHILOSOPHICAL PERSPECTIVES ON COMPREHENSIVE CANCER CARE AND THE PREVENTION OF CANCER

Prior to my medical education, I received a Bachelor of Arts degree from McGill University in my hometown of Montreal. My major was Philosophy and Comparative Religion. Because of frustrations over many long years with the pace of efforts to interest medical science in IPT, I took a measure of comfort in reflecting on things from my philosophical perspective. I must first say that I am not one to believe those stories of there being some sinister conspiracy between government and industry to interfere with the evolution of new cancer treatments in this country. I do believe, however, that there are processes of evolution at work unwinding things in two important areas related to cancer. One of these has to do with a changing perception about the scientific method itself, and the other involves a new immediacy apropos our common understanding of this disease we call cancer.

Contemporary writings by eminent scientists—many of them Nobel laureates—have characterized compelling evidence for an alternate view of things concerning our scientific methodology. Discoveries in the areas of quantum theory and human conscious awareness have created a new paradigm for science, one that places our own human psychological and spiritual realities on a comparable footing with the classically observed facts of modern science: what science has always regarded as objective truth is now seen to be intimately associated with our own human subjectivity. Surprisingly, this new understanding now makes it rational and acceptable for us to actually want what we want from our scientific investigations through a phenomenon called "top-down causality." We are thus no longer limited by having to accept what truths may simply tumble out from our scientific experiments. To be sure, this new perspective of working purposively with our science represents a tremendous breakthrough—as well as an immense challenge to modern scientific theory, and to the many scientists accustomed to working with this.

Just as immense is the shift in our societal awareness of the meaning that cancer has come to have in all of our lives. Cancer in the United States is definitely on the rise. We represent six% of the world's population, and yet we account for 20% of the world's cases of cancer. More personally, statistics from the Centers for Disease Control tell us that one man in two alive now in America, and one woman in three, may expect to get cancer in their lifetime. And the projection is that by the year 2050, these statistics will become one in one for both men and women. We are thus facing a potential human tragedy of totally unmanageable proportions.

I have heard it said that, "Cancer is not the disease; cancer is the cure. Civilization is the disease." Looking realistically at what we have done on this planet, it seems this may be true. The growth of our Western civilization has proceeded hand in hand with an ever increasing and widespread process of industrialization, all under our "sacred" imperative of a never ending process of economic growth and development. If there is supposed to be some balance between the sacred and the profane within a mature society, we would have to admit that the profane has all but taken over here where we live. We are collective-

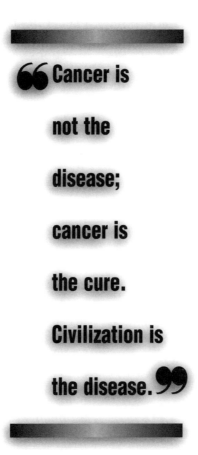

"Cancer is not the disease; cancer is the cure. Civilization is the disease."

ly striving towards a non-sustainable future. The unwanted result of all this is pollution—external and internal: pollution of the air and water in our natural environment, pollution of the quality of our food supply, and a pollution of those natural feelings of compassion and loving kindness for ourselves and for one another as we all compete, individually, to "get ahead." And I believe the bottom line in all this has come to be our burgeoning epidemic of cancer.

These perceptions about our ecology and our social (dis)integration may stand as a critical new focus for our collective attention. A motive to arrest this destruction has to come to the fore—and soon. The power of a new science responsive to conscious human desire, directed by the evident danger and urgency in our current circumstances, can and must lead us to more promising possibilities for our future.

It should be clear from these opinions that dealing effectively with cancer is going to take more than just time, money, and better ways of killing cancer cells. As necessity is the mother of invention, a new and broader approach to cancer management has already made inroads into the existing medical scheme of things. This is called Comprehensive Cancer Care. There are three distinct therapeutic areas in this:

1. Methods for treating the cancer;
2. Nutritional biochemistry to support improved immune function; and
3. Mind-Body medicine for deeper healing.

As a method of treating cancer, IPT may represent the ideal modality for the first approach in this model of Comprehensive Cancer Care. The other therapeutic approaches of Nutrition and Mind-Body medicine demand high levels of patient participation. Because of the non-toxic nature of chemotherapy treatments given with IPT, patients are going to feel much better under

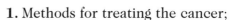

treatment with it as compared to the typical reactions seen with conventional dose chemotherapy. IPT patients will be much more available—physically and emotionally—to participate in making better choices about what they might eat and drink, and how they might think and feel. It is my hope and expectation that this kinder and gentler and more comprehensive approach to cancer management will prove significantly more effective than extant medical practices.

There is a great deal more depth and breadth to Comprehensive Cancer Care than can simply be spelled out here in words. It is difficult to see how medicine, as it is currently structured, could allow physicians to even speak some of these words to their patients, words like love, soul, and God. Some further evolutionary steps—and possibly some revolutionary ones—will have to be taken before we are all free enough to overcome our fears of being who we are with each other, and able to act with genuine power and authenticity.

One of my favorite philosophical thinkers was a man of inspiration by the name of Pere Teilhard de Chardin. He spoke optimistically of Man soon coming of age, and assuming responsibility for participating—together with God—in his own ongoing process of evolution. This one of his quotations below captures much of what I feel to say about where we are going, and where I believe the disease called cancer would have us go: to rise above, to survive, and to positively enjoy our existence together on this good earth. ∎

"SOME DAY, AFTER WE HAVE MASTERED THE WINDS, THE WAVES, THE TIDES, AND GRAVITY, WE SHALL HARNESS FOR GOD THE ENERGIES OF LOVE. THEN FOR THE SECOND TIME IN THE HISTORY OF THE WORLD, MAN WILL HAVE DISCOVERED FIRE."
-Pere Teilhard de Chardin

CHAPTER 3

The Medical Pioneers of Insulin Potentiation Therapy

It wasn't until this book was just about completely done that I (Ross) read the book by Donato Pérez García, M.D. (Donato 1) and Donato Pérez García y Bellón, M.D. (Donato 2) entitled *Cellular Cancer Therapy Through Modification of Blood Physico-Chemical Constants (Donatian Therapy)*. This book was translated from Spanish to English by Mike Dillinger and scanned and edited for www.IPTQ.org by Chris Duffield. (The entire book is available at that web site.) For purposes of this chapter, the term, "Donatian Therapy" will be used to denote IPT. Originally, the technique was called "Donatian Therapy" after its originator.

Treating Cancer with Insulin Potentiation Therapy would make one think the entire book is on IPT, which it is not, so we added a subheading. It goes like this: *Learn How Insulin Can Help Target Chemotherapy and Be Used as Part of a Comprehensive Natural Medicine Approach to Reverse Cancer and Cancer Physiology,* which indicates that the book will also discuss comprehensive natural medicine and how it can help reverse cancer and cancer physiology. It would be possible for someone to read this book and think the authors are very smart. To some extent, this may be true for Marion—but, for me—I am just good at looking at other people's research, and applying it clinically to my patients.

As you will come to realize, Donatos 1 and 2 were truly medical pioneers and way ahead of their time. Most of what is described in *Cellular Cancer Therapy* is the work of Donato 1. He was truly a medical pioneer. He was clearly way ahead of his time, as evidenced by the fact that he knew most likely by the 1920s that:

- Insulin could be used for other conditions besides diabetes.
- Insulin could give a person his or her appetite back.
- Insulin was an anabolic hormone.
- Insulin increased the permeability of cell membranes.
- Insulin crossed the blood-brain barrier.
- Insulin could be used to increase the efficacy of medications.

- Insulin could be used with medications to cure many incurable diseases.

By the early 1940s he knew that:
- Cancers recurred despite surgery, radiation and chemotherapy.
- Cancer occurred because of the person's cancer milieu.
- The cancer milieu could be tested and measured.
- Donatian Therapy helped reverse this cancerous terrain.
- Donatian Therapy could cure many different cancers.

So you see, when you read this book and I (Ross) am talking about cancer physiology, Donato 1 knew about it long ago. He could reverse cancer physiology with Donatian Therapy 60 years ago and my writing about it just validates that what he found and wrote about was true.

He first injected himself with insulin in 1926 and was treating patients with IPT in 1928. He started out with a traditional M.D. education with specialized training in surgery, dental surgery, urology, and gynecology/obstetrics. He became the Medical Director of the Civil Hospital M.A. Camacho and the Director of the Military College Hospital. He was the personal doctor to Mexican presidents Manuel A. Camacho and Lazaro Cardenas. He was very active and honored as a military doctor during the Mexican Revolution, retiring with the rank of Brigadier General. Though he made many discoveries about insulin and IPT, perhaps his greatest gift was teaching the technique to his son, Donato Pérez García y Bellón, M.D. (Donato 2).

Though I had only one conversation with him (he died unexpectedly in November of 2000), it was clear to me that he was a very passionate man. He had more experience with IPT than any other doctor in history: 44 years. He practiced medicine from 1956 to 2000 in Mexico City and contributed to IPT education and research. He successfully treated a wide range of cancers, infectious diseases, arthritis, and many other conditions. He was fluent in Spanish, English, and French. He also taught his son about IPT, Donato Pérez García, M.D. (Donato 3). Donato 3, along with Dr. Ayre, are the physicians who taught us the technique of IPT. In this book, "Donato 1" means the grandfather; "Donato 2" designates the son; and "Donato 3" designates the grandson who is in active practice today in Tijuana, Mexico and referred to throughout the book.

DONATIAN THERAPY CURES MANY DIFFERENT TYPES OF CANCERS

By the mid 1940s, Donato 1 was successfully treating cancer with Donatian Therapy. Over the subsequent years and decades, there were numerous types of cancers that he and his son successfully treated, including the following:

BILIARY CANCER	LIVER CANCER	SKIN CANCER
BLOOD CANCERS	LUNG CANCER	SMALL INTESTINE CANCER
BONE CANCER	LYMPH CANCER	STOMACH CANCER
BREAST CANCER	MOUTH CANCER	TESTICULAR CANCER
CERVICAL CANCER	NECK CANCER	THROAT CANCER
COLON CANCER	OVARIAN CANCER	THYROID CANCER
ESOPHAGUS CANCER	PROSTATE CANCER	UTERINE CANCER
LIP CANCER	RECTAL CANCER	VULVA AND VAGINAL CANCER

The above information is in their book, *Cellular Cancer Therapy*. They wrote that Donatian Therapy is effective for many different types of cancers, including the following:

ADENOCARCINOMA	FIBROSARCOMA	OSTEOSARCOMA
CARCINOID TUMORS	HODGKIN'S DISEASE	RHABDOMYOSARCOMA
CARCINOMAS	KAPOSI'S SARCOMA	SEMINOMAS
CHONDROSARCOMA	LEIOMYOSARCOMAS	SEROUS TUMORS
DIFFERENTIATED CARCINOMAS	MELANOMA	SMALL CELL CARCINOMA
LYMPHOMA	MUCINOUS TUMORS	SQUAMOUS CELL CARCINOMA
EPIDERMOID CARCINOMA	MULTIPLE MYELOMA	TERATOMAS
EWING'S SARCOMA	MYCOSIS FUNGOIDES	UNDIFFERENTIATED CARCINOMAS
	NON-HODGKIN'S DISEASE	

It should be evident to the person with cancer, or for those taking care of someone with cancer, that Donatian Therapy is power-medicine. As it was in the 1940s and still applies today, a person with cancer should consider Donatian Therapy as a treatment option. Besides helping reverse cancer physiology, and cause tumors to shrink and go into remission, it is virtually free of side effects.

DONATIAN THERAPY REVERSES CANCER MILIEU

"Milieu" is another term for environment. Donato 1 and 2 knew that for a cancer to form, a certain cancerous milieu must be present in the person's body. The title of their book even signifies this: *Cellular Cancer Therapy Through Modification of Blood Physico-Chemical Constants.* They wrote:

> Cancer is a general bio-physico-chemical dis-equilibrium of the whole organism that is inherited and which constitutes the terrain in which neoplasias may arise… . Metastases are not distributed randomly in the organism, for all of the types and sites of malignancy have patterns and characteristic routes that the metastasis most probably will take. These routes are determined by the physical and chemical compounds that are present in the tissue or organ, the degree of surface tension and intracellular pH, as well as the concentration of the different chemical elements that make up the tissue or organ…

The origin of cancer could be expressed by the following equation:

External factor + adequate dose + internal susceptibility + time = Cancer

They wrote that "any process that enters into a cause-effect relationship with the production of malignant neoplasias is called a *carcinogenic factor.* This implies the action of an external agent (virus, inhibited immunological reaction), adequate doses of this agent, internal susceptibility (immunological or hormonal deficiency, genetic anomalies, etc.), and the passing of relatively large periods of time." They also noted that the above was not, in general, reversible with surgery, radiation therapy, and chemotherapy.

Donato 1 and 2 correctly noted that the Donatian Therapy was not only killing the cancer cells, but also normalizing the cancerous terrain that allowed it to grow. They noted:

> In patients with cancer who were treated with Donatian Therapy, blood alkalosis becomes

acidosis, an important curative factor, since that in itself alters the neoplastic terrain, which doctors have not been able to do thus far with any therapeutic procedure, and this is why treatments that were thought to be possible cures for cancer did not succeed.

Based on the equation: cancerizable terrain plus cancerogenic agent equals cancer, we proceeded in therapy to attack both the cancerogens and the terrain. **In this way we have achieved total cures of cancer in a large percentage of patients, even in those who had undergone classical therapy, i.e., surgical removal of tumors and radiation therapy with the subsequent intensification of the disease. We have managed, with Donatian Therapy, to really alter significantly the cancerizable terrain.**

It is obvious that insulin is not the medication that cures the patient of cancer. This hormone simply constitutes the means of sensibilizing and modifying the organism to make the therapeutic action of specific medications efficient. In the almost fifty years we have used Donatian Therapy, we have never encountered any symptoms that might rule out its use as we have described it.

The reason why surgery and classical treatments (alkalinizing substances, oncolytic antibiotics, radiation) do not cure patients with malignant neoplasias is rooted in the cancer equation we cited above from Thomas and Roffo. After surgical treatment or treatment with classical medications, it is either forgotten or unknown that the biochemical terrain remains exactly the same, and that the patient will produce other tumors, or more metastasis, as a consequence of the other part of the equation: the cancerogenic agent.

Donato 2 noted that cancer can be defined as "an absolute and total disorder of the chemical reactions and the physical laws that govern the normal functioning of each of the organs and systems of the human body, with the concomitant loss of the functional harmony among them." He noted, "If in the treatment of other diseases, we attack the cause(s) and not the effects, so then, why not do the same with cancer? Donatian Therapy is one way of proceeding in this direction."

Donatian Therapy is the treatment of the cell by changing the bio-physico-chemical constants

and parameters of the blood, attacking first the cancerous cell itself, through its intracellular environment, as well as the extracellular one, by permeabilizing the membrane with insulin. Donatian Therapy involved the injection of insulin along with many other substances that helped reverse cancer physiology. They stated "Insulin, by permeabilizing the cell membrane, permits the introduction of specific medications (the recognizably most efficient and best-known) that can therefore combat the disease directly. The external environment is also

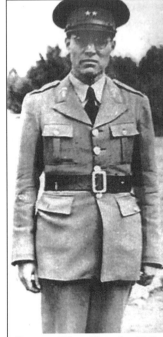

Donato Pérez García, M.D. (Donato 1)
He is the discoverer of "Donation Therapy," now called "Insulin Potentiation Therapy" (IPT).

therefore attacked by way of the physicochemical modifications… ." The effects were very profound and reproducible. They wrote, "We then saw that the application of insulin invariably changes the blood pH and in at least 95% of the patients, it went down after treatment and became acid."

As noted above, Donatian Therapy involved the introduction of specific medications. In the book *Cellular Cancer Therapy,* it is clear that in addition to chemotherapy medications, Donatian Therapy also involved the injection or taking of natural hormones, vitamins, minerals, as well as natural and synthetic agents to help with swelling and detoxification. In other words, various aspects of cancer physiology that were known and could be corrected were corrected.

SUMMARY

The medical pioneers, Donato Pérez García, M.D. (Donato 1), and Donato Pérez García y Bellón, M.D. (Donato 2), discovered, modified, and utilized a technique termed Donatian Therapy, which they used to treat many different

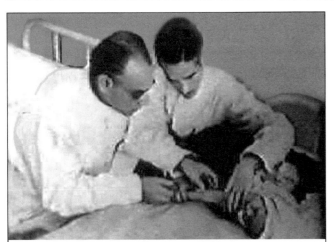

Drs. Pérez García 1 and 2, Late 1950s
The medical pioneers in action.

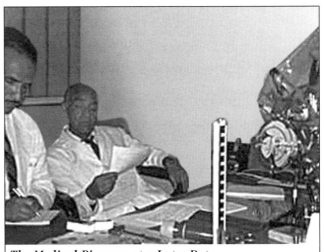

The Medical Pioneers at a Later Date...
Donato 2 (shown on the left) practiced *Donatian Therapy* for 44 years and passed his knowledge down to his son, Donato Pérez García, M.D. (Donato 3). Donato 3 now continues his legacy of curing cancers with IPT at his medical clinic in Tijuana, Mexico.

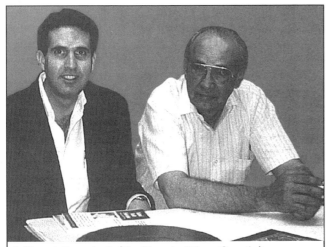

A Young Donato 3 (Dr. Donato Pérez García)
With his father, Donato 2, he practiced Insulin Potentiation Therapy in Mexico City. Later, Donato 3 moved his practice to Tijuana, Mexico.

types of cancers successfully. Donatian Therapy involved the injection of insulin, along with other substances, and was able to modify the blood's physicochemical constants. They noted that the high failure rates with conventional therapies such as surgery and radiation were because they had no effect on the cancerizable terrain in the individual. Donatian Therapy gave cancer a two-fold attack by **1.** Using insulin's ability to increase cell membrane permeability and get the cancer-killing agents to the cancer cells themselves, as well as, **2.** Using insulin's ability (along with the other substances used) to modify the cancer cell terrain, for instance, changing the blood pH from alkaline to acid. Donatian Therapy could profoundly and reliably change the biochemical properties of the individual, so a large percentage of cancer patients were cured of their disease—even those who had previous surgery, radiation therapy, and recurrences. ∎

CHAPTER 4

The Cancer Patient's Dilemma: What to Do?

It must have been two months ago when the call came in. "Would you talk to him?" I said, "Of course, but only if he wants to." There was a well-known Chicago celebrity who had cancer, and his agent (as well as his clients) who had experienced the life-changing natural medicine therapies of Caring Medical knew this particular individual needed our help. Shortly after talking with the agent, the person called our office. It was clear from the outset that it was primarily the agent's idea to call because the person with cancer was not yet ready for natural medicine or to have an alternative or complementary therapy to what he was already doing. I (Ross) spoke in a language the celebrity could understand. "Why did the White Sox do so well this past year (2000)?" "I do not know," the person answered. "Because they had a good offense. Joe (name changed), this is what you need. To fight cancer, you need a good offense. It is your immune system that fights the cancer. As of yet, you have nobody on your cancer-fighting team (I call them oncobusters) helping you get on a good, scientifically sound, nutritional program geared at stimulating your immune system... ." I explained that he needed to reverse his cancer physiology. I talked to him briefly about ozone therapy and Insulin Potentiation Therapy (IPT). He just was not ready. We were cordial to each other, but I had that sickening feeling that another person was going to die.

About seven weeks after the above conversation, this person's agent called and asked if we (Marion and I) would be willing to do a house visit to talk in person to the individual. We agreed, and a few days later we were sitting in his living room. The situation was like other homes and families we had met, where someone was loved and struggling for his or her life with cancer. People were coming in and out of the house. There were books everywhere on how to fight cancer. There was a vast array of medications and some herbal products that looked as if they were bought at a department store. In regard to the latter—think about it. The medications are prescribed by some "cancer expert," and in this person's situation this included Zofran for nausea; Decadron to decrease swelling; and procarbazine, an oral (taken by mouth) chemotherapeutic agent. In contrast, the herbal product was bought on the recommendation of a clerk earning $6/hour at a department store. Do you see the difference? *Why do people with cancer and other serious conditions not have a natural medicine specialist on their team to help them decide which nutritional products are needed, and at what potency required to fight their condition?* Why rely on an expert for medications and not one for herbal remedies that you are taking to have a similar pharmacological effect? Is one more important than the other? The answer to this is a resounding no! **The science behind nutriceutical compounds is just as sound, and in many instances sounder, than for the medications people take.**

We had a very cordial visit with this family, and it was clear from the beginning that the major item bothering them was *mass confusion.* They had already seen several oncologists; the person already had two major surgeries and one round of intravenous chemotherapy. He was now on oral chemotherapy, seeing a Chinese medicine specialist, and being bombarded by friends with various herbal products and books and tapes that touted the cure for his particular cancer. Interestingly, one of the products sent to them cost $500 for one month, and the "friend" expected them to pay for it. Do you now see why, when a person has cancer, a natural medicine specialist is someone who *must be on his or her oncobuster (cancer-fighting)* team? Someone who is a specialist in natural remedies should be the person in charge of this aspect of care or else mass confusion will result. As a side note, **confidence in what a person is using to cure his or her condition is vital to getting better.** A person with cancer who is not sure the treatment regime is going to work or if it is the right regime is doomed to failure. In other words, *a person with cancer needs to have confidence in who is recommending what and respect the person.* It will be difficult for a person wracked with cancer to have confidence in an herbal product bought at a large department store that costs $6.99 for a big bottle and is full of green and yellow dyes.

The nutritional and herbal part of a person's care should be done by a specialist in using these products and preferably by someone who has success in treating cancer patients.

In regard to this patient, it was clear that the patient and his immediate family were confused and had no idea what to do. In this particular instance, the primary concern of the cancer patient was that he was not sleeping and felt bad. Well, who would sleep with all this confusion, and once you miss even one night's sleep, you feel terrible. We gave him some simple recommendations:

1. Stay on your oncologist's medications.

2. Take a particular medication for sleep tonight. It will work.

3. Throw out these junky herbal products and take these other herbal products.

4. Start vegetable juicing and taking a green drink (Superfood).

5. Get Insulin Potentiation Therapy.

That was all of our advice. Very simple. We explained IPT as the only modality available to help target the various therapies to the cancer site. This person's particular cancer involved the brain, and besides insulin, he needed DMSO (dimethyl sulfoxide) to help transport substances across the blood-brain barrier. In addition to the chemotherapeutic agents that we would give him, IPT and DMSO would help increase the efficacy of the chemotherapy he was already on, procarbazine. They seemed somewhat interested but wanted me (Ross) to speak to his oncologist (not one of my favorite pastimes). We also spoke to him about getting on some natural chemotherapy, which included high-dose vitamin D and water-soluble vitamin A. In addition, we wanted him on a testosterone cream and DHEA (dehydroepiandrosterone) to help decrease the muscle wasting that occurs with advanced cancers.

On the following Monday, I spoke with the person's oncologist. Because of the celebrity status of this particular individual, I received much better service than normal when calling oncologists. My phone call was answered promptly. This particular oncologist seemed open to the idea of IPT, which was somewhat of a shock. This got my hopes up somewhat that the person would actually come in for treatment. I was confident the treatment was going to help the person, so I excit-

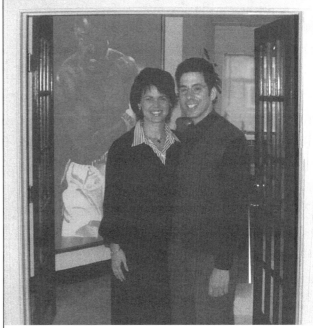

Figure 4-1: The Caring Cancer and Interventional National Medicine Center

The center is located in Oak Park, Illinois. It is run by the authors of this book, Ross A. Hauser, M.D. and Marion A. Hauser, M.S., R.D.

edly called the family. Miracle of miracles, they came in the next day for his first treatment.

This person's cancer treatment regime was given at the Caring Cancer and Interventional Natural Medicine Center (CCINMC). (See **Figure 4-1**.) It started with him being given major autochemotherapy, which is a type of ozone therapy. About 100-200 cc of blood are withdrawn into a glass bottle and then mixed with a similar amount of ozone gas. This blood-ozone mixture is then transfused back into the person. This has several effects, including oxygenating the blood, stimulating tumor necrosis factor, enhancing interferon production, and perhaps most importantly oxidizing the blood. The immune system and chemotherapy **kill cancer cells primarily by oxidizing them.** After the ozone therapy, the person was taken to his own room for the IPT. The room is equipped with a hospital bed and wonderful decorations (each room has a different theme). Throughout the time the person is receiving the IPT, a registered nurse is with the person. At various times during the procedure, one of the natural medicine specialists of Caring Medical visits with the person to see how he or she is feeling and to make sure the procedure is being well tolerated.

Before the first IPT treatment, the person is instructed on the whole procedure and its risks. A consent form is signed. The person is told that during the first IPT session, the blood sugar is generally lowered to between 25 and 35, causing a hypoglycemic reaction. In regard to the celebrity, the procedure went great. His blood sugar went down to 32, and he left the office on his own accord. The only side effect was being ravenous and tired, but who would not be ravenous after fasting all night and having your blood sugar dropped to 32? Because of the aggressiveness of his cancer, I recommended that he receive another treatment a few days later.

On the day of the appointment, I received a call from the patient. I was shocked. He was having trouble articulating why he would not come in, a side effect of one of the drugs he was taking. It was the very reason why he needed IPT. His wife then came to the phone at his request, stating that another oncologist (one who does integrative medicine) was concerned that IPT would open up the blood-brain barrier and potentially cause metastases to form. I could not believe it! We talked for a few more minutes; and it was clear he was not going to get additional IPT, but she wanted me to speak to her after I spoke with this oncologist. What a great way for me to start a Friday morning. I knew this was another example of the nocebo effect, something that frequently happens to cancer patients. The nocebo effect occurs when a physician says something negative to the patient that is not true but still has a profound negative effect on them. In other words, this other oncologist said IPT could enhance metastases, which was untrue, but yet it was having a profound negative effect on the person because he no longer trusted the therapy and was not going to receive

> It is not until the person decides to take full responsibility for his or her complete health care that he or she will truly get comprehensive care, including natural medicine therapies.

it anymore. Another example of the nocebo effect is when the physician says you have a tumor. He then explains the aggressiveness of this type of tumor and that most likely you will dead within six months. The tumor turns out to be benign, but you are already of the mind-set that you have cancer and live in fear that you have cancer. You know what then occurs: You either develop cancer or die in six months.

About a half hour after the conversation with the person's wife, I was talking with this integrative oncologist.

"Ross, you have it all wrong. I can tell from your voice that you are upset." (You bet I was upset. Someone telling my patient untrue things about a therapy I am giving him without talking to me first or knowing very little about the therapy.) I did not tell them that it would increase metastases. It was that the patient was not feeling good. They did not want to do the therapy because he was tired after it... ."

We had a nice, respectful conversation. We both came to the conclusion that he had a very aggressive cancer, and if something was not done now, it soon would not matter. The other factor that we both agreed on was that *no one was taking charge of his care and that he was in no shape to be the one making the decisions!* Because of his brain cancer and the high-dose Decadron, he was not in a position to make informed decisions, and his wife would have to take the role. In the end, it was clear that this oncologist as well as the person's other oncologist were supportive of him getting IPT; at worst, they were not against it. I have tried to reach the patient's wife but have not as of this writing.

We tell this story because it is a common one. It shows many of the struggles that the cancer patient and his or her family face, as well as the natural medicine physician, in trying to decide which treatment regime is best for the person. Also, it shows just how difficult it is for the person to get IPT or natural medicine therapies. It is not until the person decides to take full responsibility for his or her complete health care that he or she will truly get comprehensive care, including natural medicine therapies. Relying on traditional oncology opinions about herbal supplements, natural therapies, or IPT is ludicrous, since most oncologists know nothing or very little about it. For such opinions, a "true expert" is needed.

We suspected that without IPT, the patient would soon die. This is another reason that this book was written. It is hoped that many of the questions about natural medicine therapies for cancer will be answered and in the end you will agree that IPT can help target chemotherapy and be used as part of a comprehensive natural medicine program to reverse cancer and cancer physiology.

And now the rest of the story. On June 6, 2001, the patient's son called me. This occurred after a couple of months of not hearing anything. He and his sister desperately wanted their father to continue the IPT treatment. He notified me that after the IPT treatment (the one that he had), an MRI (magnetic resonance imaging) scan revealed that the tumor had shrunk. He stated that his dad was not thinking clearly because of the steroids and other medications. He was a different person. He was now on antipsychotic medications. I reiterated the fact that it was my opinion now, as it was before, that without IPT the chances of any therapy working were negligible. Even the best chemotherapy agent has little chance of killing his specific tumor because the drug cannot concentrate enough in the brain. My opinion was that IPT with insulin and DMSO would allow the chemotherapy drugs to get to the tumor site and kill it. I also explained the fact that IPT would not interfere with the other therapies his oncologist was giving him, including the oral chemotherapy. I told him that his father cannot make an informed decision—the family has to make it. If they want him to get IPT, then they will need to bring him in for treatment.

Like many cancer stories, this one did not have a happy ending. The family never brought him in for more IPT. About two weeks after the conversation, the person died.

Getting better from cancer is not an easy task. Because cancer affects the whole family, the appropriate treatment regime should involve the whole family, but ultimately someone has to be the decision maker. Generally, this is the cancer patient, and **once the decision is made as to which therapy will be used, we say "Go for it!" Nothing will help a cancer patient's survival more than doing a therapy that he or she believes in and having people around who love the patient and give their support.** For the patients of the future, this will mean treating their cancer with Insulin Potentiation Therapy. ∎

CHAPTER 5

The Purpose of Being a Natural Medicine Physician
by Ross A. Hauser, M.D.

One of my father's famous quotes about me is, "Son, you walk to the beat of a different drummer." He is also known to have told my wife, "Marion, you and I do not agree on how a person gets to heaven, but one thing I am sure of...you're in." He usually repeats the latter after I have broken, spilled, ripped, or otherwise damaged something. To say the least, to do what I do, you have be different—different in thought, perspective, and especially motivation. One thing for sure, is that I love my dad. I think what scares him the most is that I take after him.

The purpose of my being a natural medicine physician is to give patients at least the opportunity to be **cured** of their condition. Whether cancer, diabetes, hypertension, obesity, chronic pain, autoimmune disease, or even diseases we have never heard of, the overwhelming motivation is to find some way to help them become cured of their condition. For a majority of the people who come to Caring Medical and Rehabilitation Services in Oak Park, Illinois this is exactly what happens. They come for a consultation, have some natural medicine tests run, undergo natural medicine treatments, and generally experience a change in their biochemistry within a year. They become totally different people. Once their health is restored, they are generally never seen again, though we wish they would come in for their yearly checkups. In the words of one of the Mayo brothers, founders of the Mayo Clinic, "The physician's job is to keep the patient out of the physician's office."

Each time patients undergo a treatment that is not designed to cure them, even when such a treatment is available, a healthy life could be lost forever. **Figure 5-1** lists some common ailments and the various treatment options available for each.

One could go on and on; it is neverending. One of the most common consults we do is the ol' second opinion. A person has a surgery scheduled or is contemplating one and wonders if there are other options. You bet there are options besides

FIGURE 5-1: COMMON AILMENTS AND TREATMENTS

AILMENT	CONVENTIONAL THERAPY	NATURAL MEDICINE THERAPY
ATHEROSCLEROSIS	MEDICATIONS, BYPASS SURGERY	DIET, EXERCISE, CHELATION THERAPY
CANCER	SURGERY, RADIATION, HIGH-DOSE CHEMOTHERAPY	INSULIN POTENTIATION THERAPY
CELLULITE	LIPOSUCTION	DIET, EXERCISE, MESOTHERAPY
CHRONIC PAIN	NARCOTICS, SURGERY	NUTRICEUTICALS, PROLOTHERAPY
DIABETES	INSULIN SHOTS	DIET, EXERCISE, HERBS
ENDOMETRIOSIS	LAPAROSCOPY	NEURAL THERAPY, DIET
FATIGUE	ANTIDEPRESSANTS, COUNSELING	OZONE THERAPY, DIET, PHOTOLUMINESCENCE
FIBROMYALGIA	ANTIDEPRESSANTS, NARCOTICS	ALLERGY ELIMINATION, FUNGAL TREATMENT
HYPERTENSION	MEDICATIONS	DIET, EXERCISE, HERBS
MENSTRUAL IRREGULARITY	BIRTH CONTROL PILLS	DIET, HERBS
SPORTS INJURY	R.I.C.E., NSAIDs	M.E.A.T. PROTOCOL ENZYMES, PROLOTHERAPY

surgery. At Caring Medical, we believe we have never seen a woman need a laparoscopy or a hysterectomy for endometriosis, fibroid tumor, or other menstrual problems, as these can all be taken care of by various natural medicine protocols. In regard to chronic pain, various traumas, and sports injuries, the verdict is similar. Natural medicine treatments, such as Prolotherapy, can stimulate the body to repair the area, and thus there is no need for anti-inflammatories, cortisone shots, arthroscopies, or surgeries. If you do not believe us, at least consider reading some of the books we have written, including *Prolo Your Pain Away!* and *Prolo Your Sports Injuries Away!* These books have thousands of references that show it is possible to get rid of sports injuries and chronic pain, but the way to do it is not by anti-inflammatories or cortisone shots. Since when is a chronic pain caused by an ibuprofen deficiency? Pain is almost always caused by weakness. Correct the weakness in the structure with exercise or Prolotherapy, and the chronic pain disappears. The average person has no idea just how far modern medicine has strayed from its roots. The job of the physician is supposed to be teacher. The very word *physician* means "teacher"—teaching people how to stay healthy and how to get healthy again once a disease sets in. This is not what is being done in our medical institutions and universities. There must be mavericks spreading the word about effective natural medicine treatments, even if they might rattle some of the more "learned" clinicians.

Perhaps in no other field of medicine has the public been sold a set of goods more than in oncology or cancer therapy. The average oncologist does what he or she has been taught and knows deep down that in many situations the therapy simply does not work. In a recent conversation I had with a local oncologist who did his internship with me (we had shared some meals together at that time), he confessed, "Many of the chemotherapy regimes increase life just two to four months, but this is all we have to offer." As sad as this fact is, oncologists are paid by insurance companies tens of thousands of dollars for a treatment that often robs the person of his or her dignity and hastens death. Sure, it may not hasten death because the therapy prolonged life as compared to doing nothing, but it surely decreased the quality and duration of life as compared to if they would have done natural medicine and/or IPT.

One of the purposes of this book is to show people and doctors a new way of thinking about chemotherapy and helping people realize that they have a choice about the health care that they receive. The person with cancer who blindly follows an oncologist's advice without considering options is, at best, not wise and, at worse, a fool. It is another sad fact that people will spend more time shopping for new clothes than they do on a doctor who is control of their cancer therapy. They are like cattle. Whoever the insurance company pays for, this is who they will go to. Well, we are here to tell you that oncologists may not be so good, and the treatment they are going to give you may only have a 5% chance of inducing a remission and a 90% chance of making you sick as h*ll!

This book includes some of our own personal interactions with patients. We try to tell their stories. Not all of them are success stories, but in each of them we sure learned something and hope you will as well. At best, we hope that after reading this book you will be the one who decides your destiny and not an overbearing "I am God" doctor or insurance company. We also hope that you will follow the principles laid down in this book and will seek a physician who does IPT before your immune system is wrecked by traditional high-dose chemotherapy.

This book is not an anthology in cancer care. We are in the research phase of such a book. We wrote such an anthology in regard to sports medicine—*Prolo Your Sports Injuries Away!*—in which almost every aspect of sports medicine care was shown to be incorrect. This was supported by scientific literature. Such a book needs to be written in regard to cancer care, and with the grace of God and time, we hope to write such a book. This book is not that. In this book, an old concept in cancer therapy is revisited: Chemotherapeutic agents that kill cancer cells *can be directed* at the tumor site. Because it is an old concept, modern oncology will not embrace it anytime soon. The other item that will not excite modern pharmacotherapeutics is the fact that the target-inducing substance is insulin. Insulin is a natural hormone in the human body that can be bought inexpensively in many different forms. Nobody is going to make a lot of money with insulin.

Insulin has been around for over 75 years. It has been studied perhaps more than any other hormone in the human body. Its discovery has changed the lives of millions of people with diabetes and continues to do so. In this book, you will learn of its remarkable abilities and how its unique physiology can be used to potentiate the effects of certain drugs, including chemotherapeutics. As we often tell patients, "If what we tell you is true—that chemotherapy can be targeted and its cancer-killing effects enhanced—then truly this is a tremendous advance in cancer therapy." After reading the information in this book, we are confident that you, along with others with cancer, will say with us emphatically that Insulin Potentiation Therapy helps target chemotherapy and should be used as part of a comprehensive natural medicine approach to reversing cancer and cancer physiology. ∎

> **The person with cancer who blindly follows an oncologist's advice without considering options is, at best, not wise, and at worst, a fool.**

CHAPTER 6

Ross Hauser's Story

"DOCTOR, I HAVE NOWHERE ELSE TO GO. YOU HAVE TO TRY."
–Flora D'Apice

It is difficult for me to know where to begin. If you told me in medical school, residency, or even a few years ago that I would be writing a book on cancer, I would say that you were nuts. I am a physiatrist, not an oncologist. In case you missed it, let me make it clear from the start: I am not an oncologist but a physiatrist. A physiatrist is a Physical Medicine and Rehabilitation Specialist. I received my undergraduate degree in biochemistry at the University of Illinois in Champaign and my medical degree at the University of Illinois in Chicago in 1988. I did my internship at Hines VA Hospital and subsequently a three-year residency training program at Hines VA Hospital, Marionjoy Hospital, and Loyola Hospital. I received my Physical Medicine and Rehabilitation residency degree from Loyola Hospital in Maywood, Illinois.

Upon completion of my formal training, I worked with the world expert in Prolotherapy, Gustav Hemwall, M.D. He taught me old-fashioned medicine, as he was 83 years old when I started working with him. We treated patients from all over the world who came to the center in Oak Park, Illinois. They primarily came with chronic pain complaints and needed the Prolotherapy treatments. I was convinced that I would spend my career doing what Dr. Hemwall was training me to be…a specialist in chronic pain. Prolotherapy is a treatment that stimulates the body to repair painful areas. It involves injecting the painful areas with a solution that induces the proliferation of the injured structure. Prolotherapy is successful at helping heal muscles, ligaments, tendons, menisci, joints, and cartilage. It can help cure pain from such conditions as sports injuries, degenerative joint disease, arthritis, ligament sprains, meniscal tears, degenerative disc disease, herniated disks, myofascial pain syndrome, fibromyalgia, and many others. My wife and I have written eight books on the subject. One of our books, *Prolo Your Pain Away!* is printed in both softcover and hardcover editions and has been translated into Spanish and Korean.

There are now Prolotherapy clinics in Korea, as the treatment modality is flourishing over there.

In seeing chronic pain patients everyday, it became clear that a good portion of them had chronic pain because they had lost the ability to heal. For me to help get them well, they would have to regain this ability. All Prolotherapy could do is start the process, but the person's immune system needs to be able to repair the area. So here was the start of my own quest to learn natural medicine. This was combined with my own health concerns, as I was wracked with chronic fatigue. My wife, being a dietitian, literally threw out all of the "canned goods" I had bought and started feeding me green and orange things. Do you know since I have been married (15 years now), I have not had Spaghetti O's? Such sacrifices! Soon, I started to feel better and so did my patients. I was eating less simple carbohydrates and getting myself and my patients on vitamin, herbal, and natural hormonal supplementation, and quickly we were all feeling better.

It did not take long before my patients were saying that not only were their pains gone but also as a consequence of the change in their diets and nutritional supplementation, their skin looked better, their fatigue was vanishing, their menstrual cycles regulated, and a whole host of other benefits. I soon was no longer a physiatrist treating pain but a natural medicine family physician seeing every human disease.

I started attending natural medicine conferences around the world. I learned ozone therapy from Gerd Wasser, M.D., then president of the German Ozone Therapy Society, and worked in the offices of Jurgen Huneke, M.D., of Germany and Lorenz Fisher, M.D., of Switzerland, both considered the tops in the field of Neural Therapy. Thus it went; whoever was the best in a particular field, I met, befriended, and learned from them. (See the color section of this book.) I should also state that because of my expertise in Prolotherapy, I supplied some reciprocal training.

Soon people with more and more serious conditions started coming to Caring Medical. Chronic fatigue syndrome, diabetic peripheral neuropathy, herpes, hepatitis infection, autoimmune diseases, and cancer patients eventually found their way to the office. Amazingly, the majority of people had their lives completely changed by the natural medicine therapies that they were put on. Of course, not everybody improved, but even those who did not improve were glad that somebody was willing to try and help them.

The first patient with cancer who asked for my help was Flora D'Apice. Flora was frantic. She had been diagnosed with colon cancer with metastases to the liver. She knew there was no hope with traditional medicine. She blamed traditional medicine for her cancer because back in the 1960s and 1970s, people with Crohn's disease or ulcerative colitis would continually receive barium enemas to assess their disease. She felt the continual radiation exposure from the barium was the reason for her current cancerous condition. She did not trust conventional doctors. Surgery was not an option for her condition, and she just did not feel strong enough for chemotherapy. She also was all alone. The debilitation that would occur with high-dose chemotherapy was something she felt she could not handle alone.

We talked about her options. She did not want to go the home nursing route and was convinced that she should not do high-dose chemotherapy. She explained that she had been in the health care field for many years and was very informed about her various options. She wanted to try 714X and Carnivora. I had not heard these terms before. Because of her insistence, I agreed to look into these particular therapies.

I talked to the people who sold these products, and soon she was started on them. She was a true natural medicine zealot and wanted to do intravenous Carnivora. I had compassion on her; so with the help of the church, my wife and I attended, Harrison Street Bible Church, we found an apartment near my office for her to use (she lived about an hour from the office, which was too far to drive alone) while she received the treatments. It should be noted that friends of ours, Joe and K. J. LoDico, donated the apartment she used, and many parishioners of the church helped take care of Flora.

Like most cancer patients, Flora needed a lot of help. She needed help cooking, juicing, and cleaning; eventually even driving an automobile and walking were difficult. She tolerated the new treatments well, but her cancer continued to

progress. I eventually hospitalized her. I started an around-the-clock hydrogen peroxide drip. Yes, you read right, I started the drip in the hospital. I made the bags in my office and started the drip during the evening of her first day in the hospital. By early the next morning, I was called into the chief of staff's office or some other yuckity yuk who explained that experimental procedures could not be done in the hospital. I explained that her condition was much improved since starting the drip, and it would be more dangerous for the hospital and especially the patient to stop the treatment. Flora had also agreed to sign whatever the hospital wanted to free the hospital from any legal responsibility. The hospital refused, and soon the treatment was stopped. The hospital would not even let me administer high-dose intravenous vitamin C. It was shortly after this that I had to tell Flora that I could not keep her in Oak Park. She would have to be transferred to a hospital closer to her home. She cried; she knew it was a death sentence.

I still remember quite vividly the drive that Marion and I had with her to the hospital by her home. We had her on oxygen in our car while transporting her. We were not even sure we could get her there in time. At the hospital, she talked to me alone, stating that she wanted me to have all her books on natural medicine. I had not charged her for much of the therapy that she received at our office. I made sure she wanted me to have them, so I recorded our conversation. That recording is one of my most precious possessions. She gave me the keys to her apartment, and Marion and I loaded the books in our car. She had many of the classic books on natural medicine that are now out of print. I will always remember Flora D'Apice because she was responsible for starting my involvement in cancer therapy and offering patients alternatives. She died shortly after we left her, but she died on her own terms, and she died trying.

One might consider the above story and say "oh that's nice," but it deserves much more than that. It took a whole church to help Flora. It takes tremendous effort to help a cancer patient get better. Harrison Street Bible Church is a small, independent Bible Church in Oak Park. It was lead by John Blakemore for over 30 years until his son, Peter Blakemore (Ph.D. from Bob Jones

University), took over when his father died in the early 1990s. Pastor Peter was much more than our pastor to Marion and I. He was our spiritual mentor and had a tremendous love and respect for God's word, the Bible. He passed on this love for God and the Bible to those in his church. He taught that the Bible should be read every day and that it was one of the key tenets to keep one on the straight and narrow path to following God's ways. In simplistic terms, this meant how to love God, your spouse, and fellow man and to live in a modern secular society but obey the Ten Commandments and do the types of things that Jesus did and taught.

Marion and I started attending Harrison Street Bible Church shortly after our marriage. The church befriended us, and we became very close to our church family, especially Pastor Peter and his family. When Marion and I were having marital trouble, it was Pastor Peter and Marla (his wife) who would counsel us and make us realize our mutual selfishness. We always thought we would write a book called *Why the First Two Years of Marriage Were Like Hell But the Rest Are Like Heaven.* We had some major battles, but Marla and Pastor Peter were there for us. They both taught us what love meant, and we owe them a great debt.

I would often leave my office in the early days of practice when I was not too busy to have serious, deep discussions with Pastor Peter. He did everything he could to make sure that I excelled in my faith and not let worldly success ruin the more important matters in life. He taught Marion and me what it meant to have true success in life. He made us realize that true joy comes from God through faith in Jesus Christ. He was the person we most admired in the world. Just that one statement alone could say volumes; he was our pastor, but he was also our friend, confidant, teacher, and brother.

In 1993, Pastor Peter started limping. Everyone felt it was just a groin pull, but when it would not go away, he had it x-rayed. The x-ray showed that the pelvic bone had been eaten away, so a biopsy of the area was needed. The biopsy was done, and I called the physician. Pastor Peter knew immediately the news was going to be bad— immunoblastic lymphoma. The slides had to be sent to California and were reviewed by a couple of medical centers, and before we all knew what

was going on, Pastor Peter was in the hospital getting radiation therapy to the area, as well as high-dose chemotherapy. Marion and I, along with our fellow attendees of Harrison Street Bible Church, were there every step of the way. Like most friends and family of cancer patients, we just assumed everything was going to be okay. Pastor Peter went through his course of radiation therapy to the pelvis

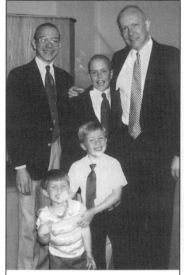

Figure 6-1:
Pastor Blakemore is seen with his "bald" sons.

and chemotherapy, and everybody felt everything was going to be okay.

By this time, the congregation was going through a metamorphosis in which we all started eating better and taking nutritional supplements. Pastor Peter had some side effects from the radiation therapy and chemotherapy, including going bald, but his sons shaved their heads, so it lessened the blow. (See **Figure 6-1**.) One Tuesday morning, he called me saying he was short of breath. When I went to his house, he could barely breathe. I insisted he go to the hospital. He insisted we pray. He never did anything before praying. I thought he had a blood clot in his lung, but he did not want to go because he was to marry his older sister at the church on Saturday. With my urging he went to the hospital, where a blood clot in the lungs was diagnosed.

As the week progressed, it was clear that he was not going to be able to marry his sister in the church, so plans were made to do it in the intensive care unit. He still was not doing well. Even on Saturday morning when we saw him, he was short of breath and coughing up blood. On the day of the wedding, Elizabeth (bride) and David (groom) looked beautiful as they walked through the intensive care unit. Pastor Peter began the service, but it was clear he could not do it; he was just too sick. He could barely breathe, let alone speak. Just as he started to put the book he was going to use to

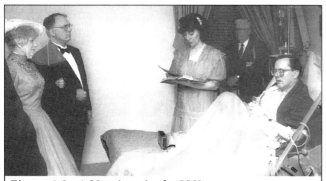

Figure 6-2: A Marriage in the ICU
Paul Blakemore, Elizabeth's brother, stands with her during the marriage ceremony while Marla conducts the service. Yes, David and Elizabeth Tye were married in the Intensive Care Unit at West Suburban Hospital in Oak Park.

do the marriage ceremony down, his wife Marla took it from his hand. "Dearly Beloved, We are gathered together today..." Soon there was not a dry eye in the place. Marla did the whole service without losing it with tears. (See **Figure 6-2**.)

The night before the marriage ceremony in the intensive care unit, Pastor Peter was able to write the sermon for the marriage on a paper from which Marla read. It was, I'm sure, one of the most beautiful and meaningful marriage ceremonies of all time. Marion and I were privileged, along with a few close friends, to have witnessed the marriage of Elizabeth and David Tye in that intensive care unit.

During the chemotherapy, like most patients, Pastor Peter would get fevers. So every time this would happen, he would be put in the intensive care unit again. They would run a bunch of cultures and never find anything. Because of this, he was pumped full of I.V. antibiotics each time for no reason. It finally dawned on us that the fever was the body's response to his low blood counts. One Friday night around 10 pm, we were at the lab at the hospital, his white blood cell counts were real low again, and he had a fever. His oncologist was insisting that he be hospitalized. Pastor Peter asked him, "Why?" The oncologist quickly said, "You need to be watched by trained medical personnel around the clock." Pastor Peter said, "What if I am watched at home?" "Who's going to do that?" his oncologist pecked. I was soon on the phone, and Pastor Peter was sleeping soundly in his own bed. By early the next day, he was fine.

The above is only a small sampling of what transpired during the 18 months that Pastor Peter battled cancer. When the cancer continued to

grow, Pastor Peter did not want to go through more chemotherapy, as the first round had failed. We, the church, he, and friends around the country went on a search to get Pastor Peter healthy. Marion and I took him down to Texas to see Doug Kaufmann, a nutritionist, and other natural healers. Shortly thereafter he started on intravenous treatments with physicians who use a more holistic approach to healthcare. On many of the visits, we went with him. Marion and I, to a large measure, put our lives on hold to help save the life of our friend. We did not function as his doctor during most of this time, just informed friends. Many others at Harrison Street Bible Church did the same thing.

During the 18 months Pastor Peter was sick, there was not a second that I thought he was going to die. Marion and I thought: He is a man of God. He has served God ever since his youth. We had started Beulah Land Natural Medicine Clinic, a Christian charity natural medicine clinic in rural Illinois only because of the influence Pastor Peter had on our lives. No, God would lead us to the right person or else he would miraculously heal his body.

The church prayed. Friends prayed. Even during his illness, Pastor Peter encouraged us.

The cancer continued to spread. It caused a large bony overgrowth in one of his ribs that was excruciatingly painful. Pastor Peter had to be on very high-dose narcotics intravenously. They made him sleepy and dopey, and he hated it. He desperately desired to get off of them. We prayed about it and agreed to get him off the high-dose morphine in only one night. It was the longest night I have ever experienced. Several men of the church assisted me, as we prayed and stayed by him all night and much of the next day. Miraculously, God granted our wish, and when he awoke in the morning, he was off the morphine pump and in no pain. The pain would not recur either.

Pastor Peter's cancer soon caused his blood counts to go low, so he was needing blood transfusions at home. We saw him grow weaker and weaker. We prayed, the church prayed, the family prayed. One day after church, Marion and I went to Pastor's house. We were not there but a few minutes when someone screamed. I went into the room. Pastor Peter was not breathing. We put him on the floor. Marion, I, and the friends who were there, including his son Peter, tried to resuscitate him, but he was gone. Pastor Peter was dead. Even at his funeral, we and others thought Pastor Peter was going to come back to life, but he never did. Pastor Peter went to see his Savior on August 25, 1995.

Shortly after his death, Marla gave us a grand-father clock that she and Pastor Peter had picked out for us, for all the help we had been to them. The clock sits in the middle of our home in Oak Park. (See **Figure 6-3**.) The inscription has the names of Marla and Peter Blakemore on it, as well as the date of Pastor Peter's death. It is a constant reminder of the best friend we ever had. We have shed many tears since that day, and a cancer patient and his or her family could never accuse us of not caring or understanding. Marion and I have been there. We know what it is like to be scared and not be sure of how to approach the cancer of a loved one. We have been in the inten-sive care units; we have been in the home; we have watched someone we loved more than life itself die.

When someone asks me why I, a physiatrist, am treating cancer patients, I just do not have the time to tell them the whole story. The story is actually much longer than what I have alluded to here, but I believe you have enough information to understand. I believe everything happens for a reason, even the death of my best friend, some-one who loved me unconditionally. Perhaps part of my own healing after his death is helping can-cer patients get well with IPT and writing this book, but this I do know: Pastor Peter would sure-ly have died if it meant the saving of another. Perhaps his favorite word from the Bible was *hupomone* which he clearly explained was not a heap of money. *Hupomone* is a Greek word that means "enduring" or "patience." During his can-cer, one of the verses he used to get him through it was 2 Timothy 2:10: "Therefore I endure (*hupomone*) everything for the sake of the elect, so that they may also obtain the salvation that is in Christ Jesus with eternal glory."

Throughout his illness, Pastor Peter honored God. It was like seeing Job in the flesh (the Job from the Bible). For the reader of this book, you will not meet Pastor Peter unless you make it to heaven. Pastor Peter taught from the Bible, which says in 1 John 5:11-12: "And this is the testimo-ny: God gave us eternal life, and this life is in his Son. Whoever has the Son has life; whoever does not have the Son of God does not have life."

For the person who accepts Jesus Christ as his or her Savior, eternal life with God awaits. For the person who rejects God's forgiveness, then his or her sin remains. As the Bible says about heaven in Revelation 21:27: "But nothing unclean will enter it, nor anyone who prac-tices abomination or false-hood, but only those who are written in the Lamb's book of life."

The real question to answer about the purpose of life is, "Are you in the Lamb's book of life?" Have you asked God for forgive-ness when you do wrong? Have you asked him to for-give you all of your sins? Have you asked Jesus Christ into your life, to be your personal Lord and savior? The only way to have the whole slate clean

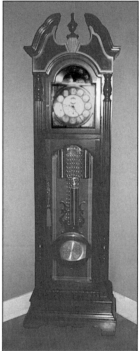

Figure 6-3: The Grandfather Clock
The grandfather clock given to us by Marla, reminds us of the impact that this one man's life has had—and will have—on ours and many other lives.

before God is to ask Jesus Christ into your life. God came down in the form of a man to show us the way. He lived the perfect life, but we condemned him. He was willing to die because the penalty for man's sin is death—eternal separation from God. Someone had to die. God chose it to be himself. Imagine someone taking your cancer and dying from it instead of you. Would you appreciate that person? Would you thank him or her? Would you reciprocate? Would you love the person? Well, God has done even more for you because he has taken away all of your sin and allows you to live with him in paradise forever. As Revelation 21:4 puts it: "I (God) will wipe every tear from their eyes. Death will be no more; mourning and crying and pain will be no more, for the first things have passed away."

Everything happens for a reason. It could be that you or a loved one has an illness to get you to come to God for the first time. It may be that you need to rededicate your ways to him. Why not do it right now?

Dear God, I accept your love and forgiveness. I know I am a sinner and have strayed from your ways. I do not know what is going to happen to me even tomorrow, but right now I commit my life to you. My salvation is in your hands. I accept Jesus' atoning sacrifice for my sins. Thank you Lord. Thank you for your love. Help me to serve you and be faithful to you. Amen and Amen.

PASTOR PETER TAPES

We know Pastor Peter would love to speak with you. We have some of his sermons on tape available to give to you at no charge. Several of these sermons were recorded when he was wracked with cancer. They have been an encouragement to us, and we are sure they will be to you. If you desire them, please give us a call at Caring Medical at 1-708-848-7789 or just e-mail the request to drhauser@caringmedical.com. If you are not a Christian or are not sure of the beliefs of Christianity and would like a Bible or a book that explains what it means to be a Christian, we would be happy to send them to you. The book was written by our current pastor, Ray Pritchard. Both of these will be sent free of charge. If any of these items encourages you, we would love to hear from you. May God bless you as you seek His will and guidance. ∎

CHAPTER 7

Natural Medicine Is Not "Alternative."

"LEAVE YOUR DRUGS IN THE CHEMIST'S POT IF YOU CAN HEAL THE PATIENT WITH FOOD."
—Hippocrates, Father of Medicine

The list of necessary nutrients is the same for every human being, but the relative amounts needed by each individual are as distinctly different as fingerprints. Why is this so? Because the kind of food we eat; the physical, mental, and emotional stresses we experience; the environment in which we live and work; our unique, individually determined biochemical heredity pattern; the type of soil in which the food is grown; the type of water we drink; and the amount of exercise we have all add up to determine the fact that our bodies are not a conglomeration of cells needing a "one for all and all for one" minimum daily requirement. You are a unique individual with unique biochemical needs. If the body cells are ailing, as they do in any form of human disease, the chances are good that it is because they are not being adequately provided with the optimum nutrients they need to sustain and propagate healthy tissues, organs, and life in general (See **Figure 7-1**). In other words, cellular health is not based on a minimum daily requirement but on an *optimum daily need* determined by the person's own biochemical uniqueness. This is precisely where natural medicine comes to the front lines in the battle against and the prevention of disease.

Natural medicine, in many respects, is the practice of medicine as it was originally intended (See **Figure 7-2**). For the average person, the above paragraph makes *complete* sense. If the body's cells are missing some essential nutrient for health, then they cannot be healthy. In other words, disease starts with cellular malnutrition. Correct this and many diseases will be cured. On a simplistic scale, **Figure 7-3** explains various conditions and symptoms that can often be alleviated just with nutritional supplementation.

Two thousand five hundred years ago, Hippocrates, the "father of medicine," said to his students, "Let thy food be thy medicine and thy medicine be thy food." Disease prevention and, even more so, disease cure starts with a proper

FIGURE 7-1: ESSENTIAL NUTRITIONAL REQUIREMENTS

AMINO ACIDS	HISTIDINE,[1] ISOLEUCINE, LEUCINE, LYSINE, METHIONINE (CYSTEINE[2]), PHENYLALANINE (TYROSINE[3]), THREONINE, TRYPTOPHAN, VALINE
FATTY ACIDS	LINOLEIC ACID (ARACHIDONIC ACID[3]), α-LINOLEIC ACID[4]
VITAMINS WATER-SOLUBLE	ASCORBIC ACID (C), BIOTIN,[5] COBALAMIN (B_{12}), FOLIC ACID, NIACIN, PANTOTHENIC ACID, PYRIDOXINE (B_6), RIBOFLAVIN (B_2), THIAMIN (B_1)
FAT-SOLUBLE	VITAMINS A, D,[6] E, K[5]
MACROMINERALS	CALCIUM, CHLORIDE, MAGNESIUM, PHOSPHORUS, POTASSIUM, SODIUM
MICROMINERALS (TRACE ELEMENTS)	CHROMIUM, COPPER, IODINE, IRON, MANGANESE, MOLYBDENUM, SELENIUM, ZINC
FIBER	REQUIRED FOR OPTIMAL HEALTH
WATER	THE MOST CRITICAL COMPONENT OF THE DIET
ENERGY	UTILIZATION OF CARBOHYDRATES, FATS, AND PROTEIN IN VARIABLE PROPORTIONS

[1] Required in infants and probably in children and adults.

[2] May be partly essential in infants.

[3] Cysteine, tyrosine, and arachidonic acid spare the requirement for methionine, phenylalanine, and linoleic acid, respectively.

[4] Researchers disagree whether α-linoleic acid is essential in the human diet.

[5] Synthesized by intestinal microorganisms; therefore, dietary requirement uncertain.

[6] Exposure of the skin to sunlight reduces dietary requirement.

Figure 7-1: Essential Nutritional Requirements
The amount of essential nutrients required depends upon the health or illness of the individual.

Adapted from Harper's Biochemistry, 24th Edition. Robert K. Murray, M.D., Ph.D., Daryle K. Granner, M.D., Peter A. Mayes, Ph.D., D.Sc., and Victor W. Rodwell, Ph.D.

A SHORT HISTORY OF MEDICINE

A patient tells a doctor, "I have an earache." The doctor replies:

2000 B.C.	"Here—eat this root!"
1000 A.D.	"That root is heathen. Here, say this prayer."
1850 A.D.	"That prayer is superstition. Here, drink this potion."
1940 A.D.	"That potion is snake oil. Here, swallow this pill."
1985 A.D.	"That pill is ineffective. Here, take this antibiotic."
2000 A.D.	"That antibiotic is artificial. Here, eat this root."

Figure 7-2: A Short History of Medicine

diet and nutritional supplementation. Linus Pauling, Ph.D., twice a Nobel Prize winner, coined the term *orthomolecular,* which literally means "pertaining to the right molecule." Orthomolecular physicians (natural medicine physicians) believe that the treatment of infectious and degenerative disease should be a matter of varying the concentration of "right molecules" (vitamins, minerals, trace elements, amino acids, enzymes, hormones, etc) that are normally present in the human body. This belief is based on the idea that the nutritional microenvironment of every cell in our body is extremely important to optimum health, and deficiencies in this environment constitute the major cause of disease (for example, See **Figure 7-4**).

The substrates for this microenvironment come from the food that we eat and assimilate. It has been said that "one man's food is another man's poison." This is especially true for the person with a lot of food allergies. In this scenario, a person's immune system is making antibodies against cer-

tain foods that are eaten, so instead of receiving nutrients for the cellular microenvironment from the food, the food is causing resources to be taken away. This is especially important for the person with an autoimmune disease, such as rheumatoid arthritis, lupus, or scleroderma. At Caring Medical in Oak Park, Illinois, it is this production of antibodies by the immune system against various allergens that is often found as the source for the production of autoantibodies. **Thus, the allergic reaction is the key to curing some people with autoimmune diseases.**

Natural medicine physicians find all kinds of allergens as the cause of chronic diseases. An allergy is defined as the exaggerated reactivity of a living organism to a foreign substance that sometimes occurs following exposure to the substance, often even in a very small amount. Allergens, the substances that cause allergies, can be in the form of foods, chemicals, and inhalants in the environment. For someone with a chronic condition, an evaluation for allergies is key to obtaining optimum health.

Any person should know that taking ibuprofen for chronic pain or Pepcid AC for chronic stomach upset does nothing to cure the underlying problem. A person's chronic pain is not an ibuprofen deficiency, and chronic heartburn is not a Pepcid AC deficiency. If the latter is due to an excessive amount of acid secretion in the stomach, a better approach than prescribing an antacid is to find the cause of the problem. Excessive acid secretion can be caused by food allergies, stress, bacterial infec-

FIGURE 7-3: NUTRIENTS AND HUMAN DISEASE

Nutritional supplementation can alleviate the symptoms of many common conditions.

CONDITION	NUTRIENT SUPPLEMENTATION
Acne	Zinc, vitamin A
Allergies	Vitamins C, B_6, B_{12}
Carpal tunnel syndrome	Vitamin B_6
Fatigue	Carnitine, glutamine
Hypertension	Calcium, magnesium
Hypoglycemia	Vanadium, manganese, chromium
Muscle spasms	Malic acid, magnesium
Neuropathy	Vitamins B_1, B complex
Psoriasis	Vitamin D
Restless leg syndrome	Potassium, magnesium, vitamin E

tion, improper digestion, and enzyme deficiency, among others. Natural medicine clinicians seek out the cause of the heartburn and then correct it. We have almost no stomach, gastrointestinal, or heartburn patients on antacids because antacids do not correct the underlying problem and often make it worse because they impede digestion. So by definition, antacids make the person sicker in the long run because they *stop* acid secretion, which is vital to digesting and assimilating food and nutrients.

Another principle of natural medicine is to rid the body of anything that it does not need, such as heavy metals or infections. Heavy metal poisoning and chronic low-level infections are becoming more and more common. Caring Medical now takes care of many children who have heavy metal poisoning. Researchers are now discovering that many childhood illnesses, including autism, have as part of their etiology heavy metal poisoning. Some of that poisoning is from the mercury preservative that was in the child's vaccine shots! Most commonly, natural medicine providers instruct the person to undergo chelation therapy, which involves taking an agent that can bind the metal in the tissues and excrete it in urine. This can be something that is taken by mouth or given intravenously.

People are oblivious to the parasites, bacteria, fungi, and other varmins that are lurking about

ROLE OF VITAMINS IN HEALTH AND DISEASE

Vitamin	Biochemical Function	Deficiency Results	Prevents/Treats
B_6	Transamination cofactor	Convulsions	Carpal tunnel syndrome
B_{12}	Transmethylation cofactor	Anemias	Cognitive dysfunction
C	Hydroxylation cofactor	Scurvy	Oxidative stress
D	Calcium transport	Rickets	Osteoporosis
E	Antioxidant	Hemolytic anemia	Immune deficiency
Folic acid	Single carbon transport	Megaloblastic anemia	Hyperhomocysteinemia
Niacin	NAD, NADP component	Pellagra	Hypercholesterolemia

ROLE OF MINERALS IN HEALTH AND DISEASE

Mineral	Biochemical Function	Deficiency Results	Prevents/Treats
Calcium	Cell signaling	Osteoporosis	Colorectal cancer
Chromium	Insulin cofactor	Impaired glucose tolerance	Diabetes
Iron	Electron transfer	Hypochromic anemia	Cognitive impairment
Magnesium	ATPase cofactor	Tetany	Eclamptic convulsions
Potassium	Cell membrane potential	Muscle weakness	Hypertension
Selenium	Glutathione peroxidase cofactor	Cardiomyopathy	Cancer
Zinc	Metalloenzyme cofactor	Growth retardation	Immune deficiency

Figure 7-4: Role of Minerals in Health and Disease
Minerals are essential to metalloenzymes, acid-base balance, muscle contraction, and neurotransmission, and function as well in other roles. Consumption of several minerals beyond the dose necessary for prevention of deficiency symptoms may play a role in health promotion. Generous intakes of calcium, potassium, and magnesium are associated with antihypertensive actions, each via different mechanisms. Iron deficiency anemia in children impairs intellectual ability, but supplemental iron can improve cognitive performance in some children without anemia. Zinc deficiency induces hypogonadism in young men, but increasing zinc status in older adults is associated with improved taste acuity and immune response. Selenium deficiency results in cardiomyopathy, but intakes greater than that needed for glutathione peroxidase activity are associated with chemopreventive actions. Calcium deficiency results in osteomalacia, but high intakes reduce the risk of lead poisoning in children, premenstrual syndrome in women, and colonic neoplasia in older adults.
Adapted from The Atlas of Endocrinology. ©2000, Current Medicine, Inc., Philadelphia.

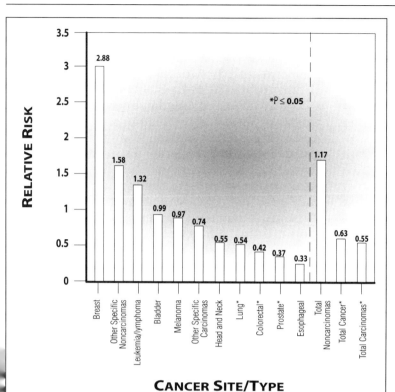

Figure 7-5: Selenium Levels and the Relative Risk of Cancer Development

Selenium in chemoprevention: Epidemiologic investigations reveal an inverse correlation between selenium status and cancer incidence. The higher the selenium intake in the diet, the lower the risk of most types of cancer.

Adapted from The Atlas of Endocrinology. ©2000, Current Medicine, Inc., Philadelphia.

NATURAL MEDICINE AS IT APPLIES TO CANCER THERAPY

Cancer, in many respects, can be thought of as the complete breakdown of cellular physiology. As such, it is of utmost importance to do as much as possible to reverse this degenerative cellular makeup. The above principle applies to all diseases and conditions, but especially to cancer. In other words, the person with cancer should ideally have an assessment of diet, nutritional supplementation, psychological/emotional status, heavy metal levels, concomitant infections, and any other factors that would affect biochemistry. For a cancer to form, one can imagine that *many* bodily homeostatic mechanisms had to break down. It is up to the patient and the natural medicine specialist to correct as many as possible, and in doing so, increase the likelihood for successful treatment. So even in cancer therapy, natural medicine is not the alternative; it is the place to start regaining health.

Much of this book will discuss cancer physiology. Cancer physiology is the cellular makeup in a person with cancer. When a person has cancer, there is typically a certain type of physiology that has occurred that allowed the cancer to start and continue to grow. Reversing this cancer physiology is one of the means to assist in the success of treatment. Consider, for example, the relative risk of a person getting cancer who has a selenium deficiency. As can be seen in **Figure 7-5,** the risk of developing the majority of cancers is inversely proportional to a person's selenium status. The proposed chemopreventive mechanisms of selenium include enhanced antioxidant protection by selenium-dependent glutathione peroxidase, alterations in carcinogen metabolism to decrease mutagenicity, endocrine-mediated alterations in carcinogen metabolism to less potent compounds, stimulation of immune responses, production of cytotoxic selenium metabolites, inhibition of protein synthesis and

and ready to cause disease. Because the body fights these infections by producing antibodies against them, these can also be a cause of autoimmune disease. It is now possible to diagnose low-level infections in people's blood. Natural medicine clinicians have long known that infections can infest a person without causing overt signs of fever but more indolent symptoms such as malaise and fatigue. When the infectious agent is identified and then treated appropriately, the underlying condition abates. Interestingly, for more serious conditions and infections, Insulin Potentiation Therapy with various anti-infectious agents is a treatment to consider (See **Chapter 21**).

cell proliferation, and/or stimulation of apoptosis (cancer cell death). If one studies the biochemical effects of selenium, one can see why it would be a good idea for a cancer patient to take it.

Studies will be described later that show that selenium, like insulin, potentiates the effects of chemotherapy. This means that when selenium is given with certain chemotherapy drugs, a greater kill ratio is seen than when the chemotherapy drug is given alone. Selenium also helps prevent some of the side effects of chemotherapy drugs such as Cisplatin. Selenium also has some independent cancer-killing effects.

Giving selenium to a cancer patient is done because it has been shown scientifically to be warranted. I do not like the term *alternative medicine* because it makes it seem second rate. I use the term *natural medicine* to signify the safest, most natural treatment that is available for a given condition that will, in all likelihood, be as effective for the condition as a much more toxic regime. **Natural medicine treatments for cancer are science based.** In many respects, they are more science based than traditional high-dose chemotherapy. It is probable that in the not too distant future, high-dose chemotherapy will fall by the wayside and only be used in the most desperate of situations. Traditional chemotherapy studies are already starting to show that individualized, lower-dose chemotherapy regimes are as efficacious and much safer than high-dose protocols. This is something that the founders of IPT knew over 55 years ago. This is why I can say that the natural medicine treatment that we use for cancer is Insulin Potentiation Therapy. It uses insulin as a guide to help target the chemotherapy to the cancer. In this way, it potentiates the effects of the chemotherapy, so substantially lower amounts of the chemotherapy are needed at each visit. This makes the treatment magnitudes safer for the patient. ■

CHAPTER 8

Natural Medicine Principles in Cancer Therapy

"WHILE GREAT ADVANCES HAVE BEEN MADE IN TREATING A MINORITY OF CANCERS, THE MAJORITY OF PEOPLE WHO GET CANCER TODAY STILL DIE OF THEIR DISEASE... . BEHIND THESE FIGURES LURKS A HUMAN TRAGEDY OF ALMOST UNIMAGINABLE PROPORTIONS. EVERY ONE OF THOSE MILLIONS OF DEATHS IS A HUMAN LIFE WASTED AND OFTEN A FAMILY RUINED."
—Ralph W. Moss, Ph.D., Cancer Therapy

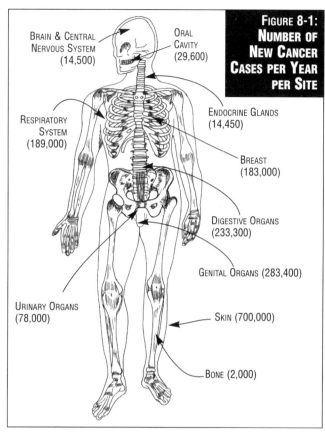

FIGURE 8-1: NUMBER OF NEW CANCER CASES PER YEAR PER SITE

BRAIN & CENTRAL NERVOUS SYSTEM (14,500)
ORAL CAVITY (29,600)
RESPIRATORY SYSTEM (189,000)
ENDOCRINE GLANDS (14,450)
BREAST (183,000)
DIGESTIVE ORGANS (233,300)
GENITAL ORGANS (283,400)
URINARY ORGANS (78,000)
SKIN (700,000)
BONE (2,000)

This book would not be necessary if conventional cancer therapies were generally successful. But we all know it is not. On December 26, 1990, the United Press International news wire carried the following headline:

CANCER NOW LEADING KILLER OF MIDDLE-AGED

The article reported that for people ages 35 to 64, cancer had overtaken heart disease as the leading cause of death.[1] Cancer kills more women in the United States than any other illness, and it is estimated that soon it will be the leading cause of death among all Americans.[2] This year, more than one million Americans will be diagnosed with cancer. Roughly two out of three cancer patients will die of the illness (or related therapy) within five years of diagnosis.[3] Despite the government spending billions of dollars in the "war on cancer" that was launched in December 1971 by then president Richard Nixon, cancer death rates continue to rise even among US children.[4]

The more one learns about the trends in regard to cancer, the more frightening the disease becomes. Cancer now claims about 600,000 lives each year in the United States alone. When one considers the over one million new cases per year, the numbers are astounding (See **Figure 8-1**). While some cancers have declined slightly, many of them are on the rise, sometimes dramatically:

- Lung cancer among women: 548.7% increase
- Malignant melanoma: 346.7% increase
- Multiple myeloma: 205.4% increase
- Prostate cancer: 189.9% increase[5, 6]

To mainstream doctors, cancer is a localized disease, to be treated in a localized manner. By cutting the tumor out, irradiating it, or flooding the body with chemotherapy drugs, the allopathic physician hopes to destroy the tumor and thus save the patient. But all too often, even after all of these measures are done, the cancer is still present and has metastasized elsewhere.

In contrast, the natural medicine specialist regards cancer as a *systemic disease,* one that involves the whole body. In this view, the tumor is merely a *symptom,* and the therapy aims to correct the root cause. Instead of aggressively attacking the tumor, many natural medicine specialists focus on rebuilding the body's natural immunity and strengthening its inherent ability to destroy cancer cells. A number of natural medicine therapies also include treatments that directly attack and destroy tumors, such as Insulin Potentiation Therapy, which is the primary focus of this book.

Unfortunately, most people do not seek out a natural medicine approach until it is too late. You would be amazed how many times Caring Medical is contacted by family members calling about their loved ones when they only have a few weeks to live. The time to call is when the diagnosis is first made or, even better yet, when cancer is trying to be prevented. The following case study will illustrate this point.

BEAUTY QUEEN WITH BREAST CANCER

In the early 1990s, a beautiful, young black woman came in with her significant other. She said she had a breast mass. When she unveiled her blouse, she had a mass all right; the mass had obliterated one breast. The mass was probably six inches by six inches. By the time testing was complete in the next few days, it was clear that she had widespread cancer. We spent the next three weeks speaking with her and her family. It soon became clear that she was a well-known national figure (though we did not know this at first). She was extremely intelligent, but we soon learned from her mother that she had this "significant other" who had been giving her herbal remedies and wraps on the breast for the good part of a year. We have no doubt this person loved her deeply, and both were very religious Muslims, but this particular person had a completely curable disease at the initial stages of her diagnosis. This was a case of a cancer patient completely trusting a loved one who had no medical or natural medicine training. Within a few weeks of meeting her, this young lady died. While contemplating the praying we had done together and the many conversations we had with her and her family I heard from the television in the doctor's lounge of the hospital where I was sitting, an announcement on CNN that "the first black beauty queen…had died of cancer…" It was a one minute blurb on CNN…probably 99.9% of the people hearing it would forget it almost immediately— but she was a life and had a family; most importantly, *she should still be alive.*

If there is one principle that we would like people to learn in reading this book, it is that natural medicine should be the *first* treatment considered. When we say that **natural medicine should be the first treatment option considered**

> Hopefully, after reading this book and researching the various cancer treatment options, IPT will be the first choice of many cancer patients.

when a person has cancer, this assumes the person giving the natural medicine advice is familiar with both traditional and non-traditional approaches to cancer including IPT. If one uses this definition of a competent health care provider for the cancer patient, then it must be a physician. There are many good herbalists and chiropractors, but they do not have sufficient training to know when IPT versus high-dose chemotherapy, surgery, radiation therapy, or a combination of the above should be recommended. There are times when cancer patients come to the office already under the care of a natural medicine practitioner and are coming to us for IPT. In such a case, we review their diet and nutritional list and then test their cancer physiology. You could be on the greatest vitamins in the world and still have cancer physiology. This is another reason why it is essential for a cancer patient to be under the care of a physician who treats cancer patients holistically. There are plenty of times when a cancer patient needs to have surgery for his or her particular cancer, and there are even instances when we demand it. Sometimes natural medicine can do only so much by itself.

BEE VENOM THERAPIST AND CERVICAL CANCER

About five years ago, a well-known bee venom therapist in the Chicagoland area came to see me because she was recently diagnosed with cervical cancer. Her gynecologist recommended a hysterectomy, but she wanted a second opinion. We listened to her story and were amazed when she insisted that bee venom therapy was going to make her well. She had recently become acquainted with this therapy and knew that we had done a study on it and used it in our practice. She was, in essence, willing to risk her life on bee venom shots. We agreed to continue to see her as a patient, as long as she was willing to do an aggressive natural medicine program with herbs, along with the bee venom, but she would have to do another pap smear in three months. She saw us after the pap smear still showed the cervical cancer. We vividly remember discussing her care with her. "Maggie, you know that we are the last people to recommend conventional therapy. But the likelihood of a cure for you with a hysterectomy and nutritional support is almost 100%. If you were our sister or friend, we would vehemently insist that you get a hysterectomy. If you do not, we cannot be your physicians any longer." I had known Maggie for awhile, as the natural medicine community in the Chicagoland area is not that large. We were sure she knew that we had said these words in love because we cared for her. We also knew the only chance to get her to have a hysterectomy was to give her a chance to use bee venom therapy for the cancer. We were not sure what she was going to do when she left the office. But we were relieved when she showed up in our office two years later completely healthy. She had the hysterectomy and some radiation therapy and was just coming in to get her hormones checked. We truly believe no one else could have said the above words to her, let alone made her listen.

Why did we not offer IPT to Maggie? We did not know about it then. The difficulty with Maggie and others with cancer is that they are sometimes so against allopathic medicine because of all the harm that it does that they do not see the good that allopathic medicine can provide. If natural medicine can heal one of our patients, we say "go for it," but if allopathic medicine is needed, we have no qualms about using it or referring someone to a caring allopathic physician. A natural medicine specialist's primary focus is the patient—to always do what is in the best interests of the patient.

For the treatment of cancer, we have utilized the whole gamut of natural therapies. We have witnessed patients with a 105° fever from Coley toxin injections (called shake and bake) and have injected ozone therapy directly into tumors. We have had people call us in cancer remission from something as simple as live cell therapy that was very inexpensive. We have heard of people doing all of the above and spending $140,000—and still saw their loved one die. There are some things that money cannot buy.

The person with cancer has many alternative therapy options. Caring Medical has experience with just about all of them, and sometimes they are used along with IPT or by themselves. The fol-lowing list is the more common alternative cancer therapy options available to patients:

COMMON ALTERNATIVE CANCER THERAPY OPTIONS

714X	Hydrazine Sulfate
Antineoplastin Therapy	Immuno-Augmentative Therapy
Carnivora	Issel Therapy
Chelation Therapy	Kelly Metabolic Therapy
Coley's Toxin	Live Cell Therapy
DMSO Therapy	Livingston Therapy
Enzyme Therapy	Macrobiotic Diet
Essiac Tea	Mistletoe
Germanium 132	Ozone Therapy
Gerson Therapy	Revici Therapy
Herbal Therapy	Vaccine Therapy
Hoxsey Formula	*...And a host of others!*

People often ask us, "Do they work?" Do the above therapies work? They all work to varying degrees. But for the person who has an aggressive cancer, using the above treatments alone is like shooting a BB gun at a charging grizzly bear. Occasionally, you will hit a vital organ and live, but most of the time, you are going to be the bear's dinner. The natural medicine specialist often does not do just a single natural therapy but multiple therapies for the person with cancer. For the person who wants to do the most aggressive natural medicine cancer therapy available, then IPT is utilized along with one or several of the therapies above. Most of these alternative cancer therapies have been adequately explained in other books, so only those that pertain to IPT will be discussed in this book. For the person desiring information on the above therapies, please refer to the bibliography for this chapter.[7,8,9]

IPT CAN STAND ALONE

Recently, I (Ross) was at a natural medicine conference and talking to Garrett Swetlikoff, a naturopathic doctor practicing in Kelowna, British Columbia. He is like my twin on earth. We attend the same conferences, have similar practices, have TMJ, and have many of the same mannerisms. We have met numerous natural medicine practitioners and have used many of the modalities available in the natural realm to treat cancer. We concur that we have never had a person with a Stage Four (adenocarcinoma) cancer ever go into complete remission and never saw a documented case, where the person just used natural remedies (without IPT). This is an incredible statement. Having traveled to many parts of the world and utilized some of the most innovative natural medicine treatments, I have never had or seen a documented case of a metastatic cancer go into complete remission without the use of some type of chemotherapy.

We (Garrett and Ross) have cases where we saw metastatic cancer patients get better with the combination of traditional and natural medicine but never with natural medicine alone. This was before learning IPT.

We (Caring Medical) can now say with confidence and boldness that we have documented cases of patients with Stage Four (adenocarcinoma and many others) that are completely clear of cancer because of IPT. Donato Pérez García, Jr., M.D., of Tijuana, Mexico, the world expert in the technique, has many patients who have been clear of cancer for over a decade after having been treated with just IPT.

IPT can stand alone. Dr. García (Donato 3) and other IPT physicians do not do many of the natural medicine treatments described in this book, nor do they have to do them. They know the power of IPT in reversing cancer and cancer physiology. Dr. García's grandfather and father knew for decades that IPT can stand alone as a sole cancer treatment.

TERESA MILLER, LUNG CANCER TREATED BY DR. GARCÍA

Teresa Miller is a 55-year-old woman who was diagnosed with cancer in her left lung at the age of 46 in May 1992. Her original doctor whom she saw when she was diagnosed told her that she had six months to live. Her doctor said that she could extend her life to two years if she underwent surgery to remove half her lung. But when the doctor ordered a biopsy, her lung was punctured in the process, and she decided to find a different doctor. One of Teresa's daughters told her about a treatment—Insulin Potentiation Therapy—that she knew had recently cured a cancer patient. In October 1992, Teresa decided not to have surgery but instead try IPT with Donato 3 at Tijuana Mexico office. Teresa received eight IPT treatments, one treatment every eight days; then eight treatments once every two weeks; then one treatment per month. By the following May, eight months after her first treatment in October, Teresa's CT (computed

tomography) scans showed no cancer. The doctors were so stunned that they scanned her under several machines, thinking the machines were not working properly. But sure enough, Teresa was cured!

Teresa experienced no side effects from the IPT. She "felt relief after just the first treatment" and more relief with each subsequent treatment. She was able to conduct her normal activities and, in fact, has not had so much as a cold or cough since she got IPT in 1992. Teresa tells anyone she meets

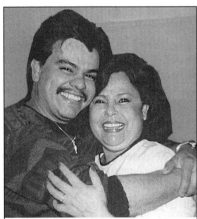

Teresa Miller with Her Son
Teresa Miller is one of the many cancer patients who are very grateful that they found out about IPT.

with cancer about IPT. She referred a man who had prostate cancer who was cured by IPT in three months. Teresa feels very strongly about IPT and its abilities to cure cancer.

CANCER FOLLOW-UP IS CRUCIAL

IPT is a very successful cancer therapy, but all too often cancer patients, even those healed with treatments such as IPT, do not get enough professional monitoring of their condition. When cancer patients start feeling better, they are prone to thinking everything is ok, when it is not. A good example of this is a patient whom we took care of at Caring Medical.

JUDY, BREAST CANCER RECURRENCE

Judy was in her mid-20s when we first met her. She recently had a lumpectomy with clear margins. It appeared to be a case where the surgeon "got it all," but we insisted she start an aggressive natural medicine treatment regime, have cancer markers drawn, and receive close follow-up. She had an AMAS test (cancer marker—antimalignin antibody screen) that was initially positive. This indicated that she was at risk of still having some cancer cells in her body. We followed her until her blood breast cancer markers were negative as well as her AMAS test. Like many people, as soon as her cancer markers were normal, she stopped treatment. Bad mistake. She showed up a few years later with elevated cancer markers. She admitted she was involved with a much older man, had started smoking, was not taking her nutritional supplements any more, and the diet—well, what diet? Anyone with cancer who thinks the battle is over as soon as the tests are clear is delusional. About half of all cancer patients who survive after five years and are felt to be cured of their disease die between their fifth and tenth year after diagnosis.[7] Cancer monitoring and follow-up is for life.

Basic Principles

In seeking out natural medicine therapies for cancer, there are some basic principles that need to be followed by all patients.

1: **Make sure your cancer is either being followed by an oncologist or a natural medicine physician who is familiar with monitoring cancer patients.**

The person with cancer needs an osteopathic physician or a medical doctor following his or her case. The physician needs to be able to monitor the cancer closely by x-rays, CT scans, PET scans, and blood tests. People often ask their oncologist to do these tests because the tests are often covered by insurance. There are many qualified nutritionists, chiropractic physicians, and other natural medicine clinicians, but ultimately the primary care physician should be familiar with cancer markers and physiology, both allopathic and alternative medicine techniques, and nutritional supplementation. If a person can get all of the natural medicine aspects covered by someone who is a nutritionist, for example, then at least have an oncologist do the cancer monitoring. It is imperative a person know exactly his/her health status, as this will determine the therapy needed. For the person whose cancer is regressing, the treatment being received is continued; if the cancer is arrested (neither growing or regressing), the treatment options are to continue with the current regime or change to a stronger regime. If the person's cancer is progressing, then a more powerful regime such as IPT is in order.

As a side note, the person with cancer must not use the way he or she feels as a barometer for how he or she is doing. Almost any cancer patient who takes a few herbs and makes dietary changes will feel better. To know the status of a particular cancer therapy, whether it is working or not, requires that cancer markers and CT scans be done periodically.

2: **Evaluate the success of the therapy chosen in the shortest amount of time.**

Most cancer therapies can be evaluated in about six weeks. So if a person with cancer is starting a new therapy today, then he or she needs to know how progress will be monitored in six weeks. The main ways of monitoring cancer patients are seen in **Figure 8-2**. One would like to see tumor regression via x-ray, but often x-ray studies change much slower than patient symptomatology and blood tests. If the CT scan is the same but a person feels better, has less pain and nausea, is gaining weight, and has more energy, then surely the treatment will be continued because at least it is helping the quality of the person's life and may be reversing the cancer physi-

---

Ways of Monitoring Cancer Therapy Progress

Blood Cancer Marker Numbers
Blood Cancer Physiology Markers
Blood Immune System Analysis
Blood Nutrition Markers
CT Scans of Tumor Size
Patient Symptoms
Patient Weight
PET Scans
X-rays of Tumor Size

Figure 8-2: The method of treatment will, in large measure, be determined by the results of one or more of the above tests.

---

ology and starting to cause tumor regression. It may be that enough time has not passed for the x-ray studies to show the regression.

A person with cancer needs to know after an appointment when the next evaluation will be for the progress of therapy. For a person who has recently had a cancerous tumor removed and desires to use natural medicine or IPT instead of high-dose chemotherapy or radiation therapy, the person and his or her blood tests are typically reviewed every six weeks until a clear response is shown. If the person is free of cancer then evaluations are done once every three months for a year or so, then once every six months for a couple of years, then once a year indefinitely. The person who has experienced cancer go into remission still needs to be seen at least yearly to check cancer markers and cancer physiology.

3: Get a second opinion.

Recently, a 15-year-old was brought in by her mother because she had a breast mass that a surgeon wanted to take out because it "may be" cancerous. Slice open the breast of a 15-year-old? Within a week, we had done an MRI of the breast and some cancer markers. What was the final diagnosis? Puberty. She is fine. She is taking some herbal remedies, and the breast cysts are no longer present. Always get a second opinion about the diagnosis and the therapy. Even traditional doctors differ in their opinions about various therapies for cancer.

Now with the known availability of a safe alternative to high-dose chemotherapy, it is even more prudent than ever to get a second opinion. IPT can help not only prevent the side effects of chemotherapy (or at least minimize them) but also in many instances provide an alternative to surgery for cancer. IPT has the power to treat cancer safely but aggressively. For the newly diagnosed cancer patient, an evaluation by a physician who utilizes IPT is a must.

4: Always get a natural medicine opinion.

Modern cancer therapy does not include a natural medicine consultant in its lists of "musts". This is unfortunate because this is what could save the person's life. Do not be fooled that the answer to cancer lies in the big walls and white coats of academia, for many more people have died, in such institutions, which is a far greater percentage than in any natural medicine specialist's office. Also, if the person does not get a competent natural medicine evaluation, he or she may end up drinking some herbal juice and believe this is the cure because a friend of a friend read a book given by another friend that this stuff

cures cancer. Unfortunately, people spend more time researching which stock or mutual fund they are going to buy than the care they are to receive for cancer. We do not remember a person with cancer being disappointed about getting a natural medicine consultation. A natural medicine consultation is only a telephone call away.*

5: Always have a natural medicine specialist on your cancer care team.

John came in with newly diagnosed Hodgkin's lymphoma. He was young and strong and looked in perfect health. He was following all the rules. He had his traditional oncology consultation and knew his odds were good with traditional chemotherapy. He came to see us for a second opinion. We quickly could tell the likelihood of a cure for him was excellent regardless of the care he received. In other words, the odds were in his favor to be cured with either high-dose chemotherapy or IPT. We said to him:

> John, Caring Medical can be your primary clinician giving you the various cancer therapies, including IPT. During IPT, you would get similar medications that the oncologist would give except at much lower doses. You know that we are a comprehensive natural medicine clinic, so you would also receive natural treatments, including ozone therapy and many others. If you decide to undergo high-dose chemotherapy, then we would still advise you to be an active patient of Caring Medical because we could decrease the amount of side effects experienced from the high-dose chemotherapy. By using nutritional supplementation, there is also a good chance we could increase the efficacy of the traditional therapies you receive.

About a week later, John told us that he and his wife decided that he should undergo high-dose chemotherapy but would like to reverse the cancer physiology and start a comprehensive natural medicine regime. He was placed on about 10 nutriceutical items** and was told to follow up every six weeks while undergoing

---

* Natural medicine consultations by a natural medicine specialist at Caring Medical can be done over the phone if a person is not able to come to Oak Park, Illinois, or feels it is best to first do so over the phone. Phone consultations can be made by calling our number, 1-708-848-7789 or via our web site at www.caringmedical.com.

** The nutriceuticals John used are from Beulah Land Nutritionals. These are some of the same ones that are recommended for the patients at Caring Medical. The complete line of nutriceuticals from Beulah Land Nutritionals is available on the Internet at www.benuts.com, or by calling 1-877-RX-BEULAH (877-792-3852). Dr. Hauser works as a consultant for Beulah Land Nutritionals, giving advice on which supplements to carry and helps to formulate some of them.

chemotherapy. John did extremely well. He did not have any of the typical side effects from chemotherapy because of the nutritional supplements he was taking—no hair loss, nausea, fatigue, vomiting, or immunosuppression. In contrast, he told us of someone he knew with the same diagnosis who underwent the same regime except with no natural medicine. This particular individual lost all his hair, was in and out of the hospital, lost a lot of weight, and had a terrible time with the chemotherapy. John is still an active patient of Caring Medical, though his cancer is quite inactive. He is cancer-free according to all of his tests, but still undergoes close follow-up by his oncologist and by us using natural medicine testing procedures.

Natural medicine has many potential benefits for the cancer patient, including the following:

- Strengthening the immune system
- Decreasing the side effects of chemotherapy
- Helping the body detoxify
- Potentiating the effects of chemotherapy
- Enhancing one's nutritional status
- Getting a person ready to handle surgery
- Potentiating the effects of radiation therapy
- Providing emotional and spiritual support
- Decreasing the tumor load directly
- Reversing cancer physiology
- Improving one's quality of life

Natural medicine, at minimum, will give the body a good offense. Cancer is a battle between the person's immune system and some rogue cells. Either the rogue cells are going to win or the immune system will win.

6: Make sure someone is looking at your nutritional status.

A person's nutritional status directly correlates with survival for many serious conditions, including cancer. Some of the markers used to analyze a person's nutritional status include weight; lean body mass; and levels of serum albumin, globulin, hemoglobin, vitamins, minerals, hormones, and cholesterol. When a person is put on a metabolically correct diet during natural medicine cancer care, he or she will sometimes lose some weight, but nutritional blood markers such as albumin improve.

To give an example of what the person with cancer is up against, consider **Figure 8-3**. Cancer physiology causes the person to lose their appetite and starts breaking down muscle and fat. The net result is that the person becomes weaker and weaker. One of the ways to reverse this is to give the person with cancer Growth Hormone shots, testosterone cream, or

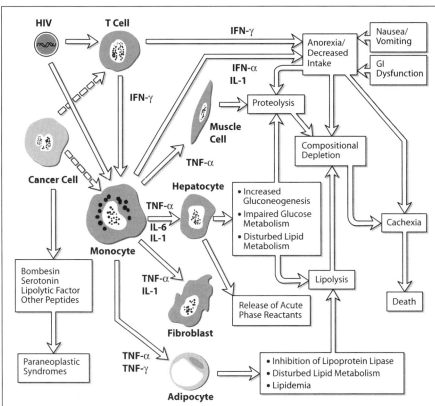

Figure 8-3: The Multiple Metabolic Effects of Tumors on Host Metabolism
Cancer physiology often involves muscle catabolism (breakdown), liver lipogenesis, fat cell lipolysis, anorexia, and reduced food intake. The net result is that the person gets weaker and weaker. Natural medicine intervention can reverse this trend.

Adapted from The Atlas of Clinical Endocrinology. ©2000, Stanley G. Korenman, M.D., Series Editor, and David Heber, M.D., Ph.D., Volume Editor. Current Medicine, Inc., Philadelphia, PA.

FIGURE 8-4:	DIFFERENCES BETWEEN A POTENT NUTRICEUTICAL PRODUCT AND THE WORTHLESS COUNTERFEIT	
	POTENT PRODUCT	COUNTERFEIT
Dyes in Product?	No	Yes
Fillers in Product?	No	Yes
Good For?	Health	Little
Hypoallergenic?	Yes	No
Ingredients Tested?	Yes	No
Manufacturing Process?	Expensive	Cheap
Pharmaceutical Grade?	Yes	No
Potency Standardized?	Yes	No
Quality Tested?	Yes	No
Where Bought?	Natural Medicine Specialist's Office	Grocery Store

DHEA capsules. These methods are discussed in further detail in **Chapter 25**.

7: Supplements, like medications, should be prescribed.

Not all supplements are created equal. It is common for a cancer patient on a first visit to Caring Medical to bring in a bunch of vitamin and supplement bottles that are clearly junk. There is a big difference between a "potent" nutriceutical product and a "worthless" counterfeit (See **Figure 8-4**).

May God bless Wal-Mart, Walgreens, and other national chains and grocery stores. It is amazing how many nutritional products they now carry when just a decade ago they refused to carry them. What changed their minds? Are you surprised they now carry a bunch of vitamin supplements? No, not when one considers all of the money they are making on the items. Vitamins and supplements are big business, and big business is making sure they get their share. It is sad to think of all the money that is being wasted on these products. In our opinion, vitamins bought at these kinds of places are not recommended for people with serious conditions, such as cancers. A vitamin and herbal product that is made with dyes and is nonstandardized (no guarantee of active ingredients) does not have the consumer's

best interests at heart, no matter how good the marketing. These "generic" brands that are two bottles of 250 pills for $3.99 are worth exactly $3.99. Cancer patients who come to our office with these types of vitamins are told to leave them with us so they can be disposed of properly.

It was for these reasons that we began selling vitamins at Caring Medical. When I (Ross) first started a natural medicine practice, I had patients buy their own vitamins. When no improvement was seen, it became clear that it was the vitamin products themselves. I would prescribe milk thistle, chitosan, and licorice root at appropriate doses for, say, a liver condition, yet the liver function tests would not improve. When I would prescribe the same regime and patients would take the herbal products that I carried in the office with a known potency and made of pharmaceutical grade ingredients, then the condition would improve. I no longer have the products in the office. Instead, they are sold through an internet supplement company, Beulah Land Nutritionals. I am a paid consultant to that company. Beulah Land Nutritionals is physically located in the same building where Caring Medical is located in Oak Park, so the nutriceutical products are available to Caring Medical patients. To view the complete line of nutriceuticals for purchase from Beulah Land Nutritionals, go to www.benuts.com. The nutritional products that I use for my cancer patients can be purchased at that site (www.benuts.com). If you have a question concerning any of the products, just e-mail me at drhauser@caringmedical.com. All a person has to do is click on "cancer" at the site, and the complete line of supplements used will appear, including the products for cancer that I personally formulated. All of the products that I have developed to reverse cancer physiology are available at that site. The cancer line is designed to reverse the cancer physiology discussed in this book. These products are not a substitute for close follow-up by a physician and active treatments such as IPT.

It is fine to start using potent nutriceutical products, but it is always best to have them prescribed by a natural medicine specialist. The danger for a person with a serious condition just buying products from a friend of a friend after reading something on the Internet is that the person will not get the appropriate natural medicine care needed. This is why phone consultations are available by the natural medicine specialists at Caring Medical. Caring Medical understands that some people are either too sick to come to the office or live too far away, although we have serviced people from Canada, the Caribbean, Europe, and Australia, as well as all over the U.S.A. Phone consultations also provide a means for a person to see if he or she is an appropriate IPT patient. A patient fills out a new patient packet and sends it back to us, along with x-ray reports, biopsy reports, previous hospitalization discharge summaries, and cancer marker results. This information is then discussed via a phone consultation, where recommendations are made with regard to further care, including nutritional supplementation, IPT, and any other form of therapy that may be needed.

8: It is not what you take in—it is what you *absorb*.

If someone eats the best kinds of foods and takes the most potent supplements but they are not absorbed, they will not have a pharmacological effect. This is because absorption is more important than what you ingest.

The enzyme content of food is rapidly declining. We no longer go into our backyards and grab an apple out of the tree and eat it. Such a "live" food is full of enzymes that help us absorb the food and assimilate it. Enzymes are vital for life. Because fruit is picked months before we eat it, we are becoming enzyme deficient. That is why any good natural medicine program necessitates an evaluation of the ability of a person to assimilate the food that he or she is eating and a determination if enzyme supplementation is warranted. Many of the nutritional products used at Caring Medical (via Beulah Land Nutritionals) contain enzymes for easy digestion and absorption.

Enzymes have added benefits for the cancer patient in addition to absorption properties. Enzymes are known to help decrease pain and swelling and to help thin the blood. All of these properties are needed to help the cancer patient fight the condition.

9: Don't stop any prescribed nutritional products unless the natural medicine specialist advises it.

When John (previous case study) decided to do traditional high-dose chemotherapy, the goal of the natural medicine care was initially to help him get through the chemotherapy. When this was accomplished, We didn't see John for about six months. When he showed up, he admitted that he was not eating as well as he should and had stopped taking some supplements without permission to stop. When we tested John's blood, urine, and saliva at the office that day, he got a rude awakening. His previous cancer physiology was far from corrected. The test results got his attention, and he quickly went back on a strict dietary and herbal regime and is now reversing his cancer physiology.

We don't want to belabor this point too long, but cancer patients need to realize that cancers do not go into remission easily. Just because an oncologist said you are free of cancer does not mean that you are. We have tested many patients in such a scenario and showed them that some of their cancer markers were still elevated. Even when a biopsy report shows that the margins are clear and the mammogram or CT scan is clear, this does not mean some cancer cells are not still present in the person's system or that all cancer physiology has been eliminated. The person with cancer needs to get advice from a natural medicine specialist and do what he or she says. Don't stop because you feel good. Stop only on the advice of the physician who is monitoring your cancer.

10: Know the goal of the natural medicine care.

The examining room was packed. It was clear that the problem was serious because there were so many people in the room. We met Donna (daughter), Jessica (granddaughter), James (son-in-law), Frank (husband), Scott (brother), and several other relatives. Elissa had a fast-growing sarcoma of the femur. The doctors wanted to perform surgery to remove the tumor, but it would necessitate some type of prosthesis in the leg. The whole family wanted a second opinion.

Because of the aggressiveness of the tumor, we agreed with the recommendation of Elissa's other doctors that she needed surgery, except in her current disease state, she was not ready for surgery. She agreed. She was not adverse to surgery, but she felt that she could not handle it. This brings up another important point: Often, **the natural medicine specialist's job is to get the person** ready for or able to tolerate traditional medicine's **armamentarium of weapons, including** surgery, radiation, and high-dose chemotherapy. One can never say that these therapies are not warranted. Used correctly, they can have a life-saving effect.

Elissa started in our office with intravenous nutritional support, as well as an aggressive natural medicine regime that included some easily absorbable soy protein powders to help her protein status. She was placed on some natural hormone replacement to give her some strength. Within a month, she underwent successful surgery. She is continuing to do extremely well and is followed up closely by her oncologist. We see her for her natural medicine care.

The goal of natural medicine for cancer is not usually direct tumor kill. **A person receives IPT for direct tumor kill.** A person does not take a protein supplement for direct tumor kill but for direct nutritional enhancement.

Natural medicine has many possible applications for the cancer patient. It is important for the family, the natural medicine specialist, and especially the patient to realize from the beginning the exact goals of the care. Some of the goals of natural medicine care can be seen in **Figure 8-5**.

11: The whole family should agree on the care.

Megan came in with her mother and sister. Megan had a large breast mass. By now, the tumor had spread to her lymph nodes and liver. They were referred from another natural medicine specialist for an IPT evaluation. On the initial visit, she was so short of breath that we were convinced she was on death's door and most likely had lung metastases. She was severely malnourished. She had an extremely high tumor load, and it was quite obvious that her tumors were progressing despite the other therapy she was receiving. We urged the family to let us give her some intravenous fluids and nutritional supplements and that IPT should be started the next day. They were not convinced, so they left. We made it clear to the mother, however, that Megan would soon be only a memory if she waited long.

Megan was brought in the next week to start therapy. She was to come for IPT twice per week. It took about eight sessions before the tumor started to shrink; by the fourteenth session, the tumor appeared to be about half its original size.

SOME OF THE GOALS OF NATURAL MEDICINE FOR THE CANCER PATIENT

★ enhance immune system
★ improve nutritional status
★ pain control
★ relieve nausea
★ reverse muscle wasting
★ decrease side effects of chemotherapy
★ potentiate chemotherapy's cancer-killing effects
★ direct tumor kill (apoptosis)
★ induce differentiation (cancer cells to be more normal)
★ prescribe appropriate standardized nutriceuticals
★ give emotional, psychological, and spiritual support to the patient and family
★ make the person laugh (and keep a positive outlook)

Figure 8-5: Some of the Goals of Natural Medicine Care for the Cancer Patient
The natural medicine specialist can have many roles in the care of the cancer patient.

Within six weeks of starting therapy, the patient had gained 12 pounds, had color in her face, and had even gone to a church function and ate some steak. This is an example of the power of IPT. Megan was on death's door, yet six weeks later, there was no indication she was even sick.

She was doing great, but then she missed a week of therapy and her mother called, "Steve's kidnapped her." She then relayed this story about how bad Megan's husband Steve was, and soon Steve was calling and telling us about the mother. When Ross eventually talked with Steve, he told how the mother was convinced that Steve was bad because he didn't follow the Jehovah Witness faith and that prayer and coffee enemas were going to save her daughter. Steve was relieved to find out that Ross was an actual medical doctor because Steve was concerned Ross was another coffee enema guy. Well, Megan didn't do well being in the middle of this family feud. We even had yelling between the various parties in the office while the patient was receiving IPT. It was a mess. Megan hung on for about eight months, but surely her life was cut short, not only because of the tumor, but because of a loss of love.

The above story is not against a particular religion or coffee enemas but to show that **when a family member has cancer, the family** must come together for the patient's sake.

Not doing so could and does cause the early demise of some people. We have seen this, and so has every other natural health practitioner who sees cancer patients. Do not underestimate the power of love, worth, and self-esteem or the lack thereof.

We urge families to agree on the therapy to be given, *prior to* the therapy being started. We do not care if it is high-dose chemotherapy, herbs, IPT, surgery, or another treatment. It is more important for the family to agree that the therapy is worthwhile and should be given, than which therapy it is. Do not underestimate the power of unity. In other words, if a particular therapy is to be done, then do it with all the gusto *the whole family* has to give. This experience can bring the family together, not split it apart. A family that is fully together is a powerful weapon against anything, including cancer.

12: The Hauser Principle

Something that is often quoted in the office is the Hauser principle: **A positive thought has a positive effect on the body, while a negative thought has a negative effect.**

A natural medicine specialist often finds himself or herself taking care of people with chronic medical problems. As such, there are a lot of issues involved, including bad medical care in the past, a horrific trauma, money constraints, divorce, medication side effects, lost jobs, terrible pain, no emotional support, loneliness, anger toward God, and a host of others. One can imagine the stories that are told. One does not need to watch soap operas when one works with people who are hurting. It is amazing how some people survive.

We like to tell people that any experience will do one of two things: **1.** give you a disability or **2.** give you an ability. We are now equipped to treat cancer patients with a natural medicine, holistic perspective because we have experienced someone we love go through the undignified process by allopathic physicians and health care providers and suffer a bad outcome after spending $140,000. We know what it is like to be unsure; cry; watch your loved one in pain, cough up blood, and being short of breath; going to the intensive care unit day after day; going to bed at night not knowing if he or she will be alive in the morning; watching blood transfusion after blood transfusion keep him or her alive; as well as the other side of watching family and friends come together for support, prayer, and love. We have used that experience with our friend and pastor to help strengthen us in our quest to be a better person, doctor, dietitian, manager, writer, neighbor, brother, and friend. One could say that it is only because of the experience that we had, the most painful and impressionable experience we ever had, that this book is even being written. You are benefiting from the cancer that Pastor Peter was afflicted with and ultimately died from, as well as the passion it left in us. We do not know why God does the things he does. Why do some people get cancer and survive while others die? But we are convinced that if we knew what God knew, then we would do as God does—a little wisdom we learned from Pastor Peter while going through his illness.

Some people harbor and hang onto bitterness, anger, and resentment. The Hauser principle says that a negative thought has a negative effect on the body. People with such feelings are only hurting themselves. The Bible says in Philippians 4:6-7: "Do not be anxious about anything, but in everything, by prayer and petition, with thanksgiving, present your requests to God. And the peace of God, which transcends all understanding, will guard your hearts and minds in Christ Jesus."

Anxiety does nothing about tomorrow's troubles but does take away today's joy. Every day is a gift from God to be lived with appreciation and gratitude. Is there someone today who needs a smile or a hug? Don't be afraid to tell someone that you love them. For Hauser's principle says that a positive thought has a positive effect on the body. ■

CHAPTER 9

Cancer Prevention Is NOT Cancer Treatment

About every month or so, some newscaster or reporter will tell of a new compound, food or food group, genetic finding, or supplement (vitamin, mineral, or nutritional) that decreases one's cancer risk. These findings are great and play a role in natural medicine care, especially if someone who has a high cancer risk is trying to prevent cancer. There is nothing better than preventing cancer from forming, but **cancer prevention is not cancer treatment.**

Ben came in with all of his supplements. He had lycopene supplements, modified citrus pectin, Echinacea, selenium, saw palmetto, and a host of others. Any supplement that he read about that supposedly helped the prostate gland he bought and used. He must have been taking 200 pills a day from about 20 different bottles. He was also eating healthy foods and drinking distilled water. His PSAs (prostate-specific antigens) were not climbing as quickly, but they were still going up and were now hovering about 28. A biopsy confirmed prostate cancer.

Ben, God love him, was slowing the progression of his disease, but it was still progressing. Most of the items that he was taking were great for prostate health, and I (Ross) should take them now while my prostate still has some juice left in it, but they were not likely to give him tumor remission, which was the ultimate goal. I (Ross) explained the possibilities with natural medicine, IPT, surgery, and the differences in nutritional supplements. We agreed that some of the supplements were of good potency, while others were filed under t-r-a-s-h. Some of the latter ones were replaced by appropriately potent nutriceuticals from Beulah Land Nutritionals, supplements designed to reverse cancer physiology. He underwent a comprehensive prostate cancer profile that looked at various hormone levels. We agreed that he needed to get his dihydrotestosterone levels down, which was one of the factors involved in feeding his cancer. He was started on a nutritional supplement for this. I also felt that he may have some heavy metal toxicity that might be related to his cancer, but he choose to just go ahead with prostate removal. He has done well and remains cancer free. He continues to take his nutritional supplements and eat a healthy diet.

Ben had read a lot about prostate cancer prevention and felt that he must take gobs of selenium. Well, that is great if you want to get selenium poisoning. As already discussed, selenium is a good mineral for a cancer patient to take, but what is the goal of therapy? If it is tumor regression, a cancer patient then needs to be under the care of a physician, preferably one who does IPT. Just because a vitamin, mineral, or nutritional product has some cancer prevention properties does not mean that it will cause a tumor to shrink. One can almost assume the opposite; it will be great for tumor prevention but not nearly strong enough for tumor regression. This is why when picking an appropriate cancer treatment or therapy, or even a supplement for that matter, it is important to know what its purpose is. Taking a little selenium is fine if you have prostate cancer; just don't put your hopes in it to shrink your tumor.

For a cancer therapy to be effective for tumor remission, it has to have powerful and effective direct tumor-killing effects. If a particular agent is able to kill 99.9% of cancer cells, there will still be a million of them around to start growing again. In other words, to induce tumor regression, the therapy or substance has to be an effective chemotherapeutic agent. The word *chemotherapy* essentially means the use of chemicals in the treatment of disease. With increasing frequency, the term *chemotherapy,* or as it is popularly abbreviated, *chemo,* has come to refer specifically to the chemical treatment of malignant (cancerous) diseases. Thus a chemotherapeutic agent is one that can kill cancer cells. So chemotherapy by this definition is a good thing. I love using high-tech medical words…*like a good thing.* As a medical student, I once said a patient had a rash in his armpit, and the attending physician almost had a coronary when he heard the word *armpit* instead of *axilla.* The odd thing is that most people have no idea what the axilla is, but everyone knows where the armpit is located.

The primary goal of curative chemotherapy in regard to cancer is to kill every cancer cell lurking in the body. Its method is to shrink and destroy the primary cancer and all measurable metastases and to bring about cancer remission.

You see, it is not generally a matter of whether the chemotherapy will kill the cancer cells; it is just a matter of how much and how many.

At Caring Medical in Oak Park, we have many patients with cancer who look at their cancer as they would any other chronic disease. Sure, everyone hopes that they can find the right combination of treatments to cause the tumor to regress completely, but many times this does not happen. If one thinks about it, nearly 100% of the people who live to be over 80 die with some chronic disease not associated with their death. Most medications ease the pain and suffering of some chronic disease. For instance, I (Ross) have hypoglycemia. If I don't eat every few hours, my blood sugar drops drastically, and I feel very tired. If I eat too many carbohydrates at a meal or snack, I feel exhausted in about 30 minutes. I am generally aware of my hypoglycemia, but I still lead a perfectly fulfilling life. I will die having hypoglycemia but not because of it.

CANCER'S IMMEDIATE NEEDS FOR TREATMENT

There are times when a cancerous growth causes the life-threatening muscle-wasting syndrome called cachexia. At other times, cancer can infiltrate an organ such as the liver, causing the blood to become toxic and fluid to accumulate in the lungs, thus making breathing difficult. In these emergency type situations, the tumor load has to be decreased quickly. In such a situation, one cannot monkey around with only natural medicines; a more aggressive therapy like IPT is needed. There are numerous other situations in which a cancer patient should immediately consider aggressive treatments such as IPT (See **Figure 9-1**).

For the cancer patient who is feeling fine and not having an immediate life-threatening situation, the above concept of cancer being looked at as a chronic disease gives some therapeutic options. In this scenario, we would still recommend a powerful protocol with IPT, along with natural medicine, but there is the option of just doing aggressive natural medicine treatments (besides IPT). This does not mean to go on vitamins and minerals that help prevent the particular cancer you have or doing some "bargain" nutritional shopping at Kmart. It means a consul-

tation with a natural medicine specialist who has experience with cancer, close cancer monitoring, and the utilization of natural chemotherapeutic agents. Even if high-dose chemotherapy or IPT is not utilized, all people with cancer regardless of the type must use some type of chemotherapeutic agent that will help destroy the tumor cells, otherwise the tumor will continue to grow, and eventually the person will be in a situation where an emergency exists.

*When the amount of tumor cells is being destroyed at about the same rate as the tumor is growing, the cancer is said to be **arrested.*** This term makes it seem that the tumor is resting or held captive, but nothing could be further from the truth. The patients at Caring Medical whose cancers are arrested and have been in that situation for years are typically natural medicine fanatics. Sometimes we think they know more about natural medicine than we do. Every time they come to the office, they have a list of questions and the latest information from the Internet. They know that staying well from cancer is a team effort, and the physician is just one member of the team. Their tenacity encourages us to keep up on the latest developments in both traditional and nontraditional cancer therapy. This is why Caring Medical has experience with synthetic drug chemotherapeutic agents, as well as chemotherapy drugs from plants such as Taxol, Vincristine, Poly-MVA, Carnivora, Mistletoe, and Ukraine. We have patients taking items from all over the world and treat patients from all four corners of the globe. We even have an Australian working in the office. What can I say, I like being called "mate." "Good day, mate! How is it going, mate?" Though it is not as much fun as my wife calling me "sugar lips."

FIGURE 9-1: SITUATIONS IN WHICH A CANCER PATIENT NEEDS AGGRESSIVE CANCER THERAPY SUCH AS IPT

AGGRESSIVE TUMOR GROWTH	LOSING HOPE
BRAIN METASTASES	MALNUTRITION
BREATHING TROUBLES	SEVERE PAIN
CACHEXIA	SPINAL CORD INVOLVEMENT
LIVER METASTASES	SYSTEMIC SWELLING

Figure 9-1: IPT, surgery, radiation therapy, and/or high-dose chemotherapy are needed when organ damage is pending or the cancer is threatening life.

On the first visit with the cancer patient and his or her significant others, we make it very clear that getting well from cancer is not much fun. It takes a lot of work on everyone's part, and the person who should put in the least amount of effort is the patient. The person with cancer needs to rest, drink clean water and juice, eat nutritional food, exercise to tolerance, laugh, watch sunsets, and often take a tank full of nutritionals. We generally recommend that the person with cancer have someone else in the household or a very close friend be his or her caregiver. This person is responsible for the cancer patient eating, drinking, and taking his or her supplements correctly. Sometimes we ask the patients to quit their jobs. The person with cancer has enough to worry about, and often it is the job or some other stress that is contributing to the person's cancerous condition. Sometimes when we give this advice, it is not too well received.

PAUL, COLON CANCER, AND HIS JOB

Paul came to the office with an aggressive colon cancer that had affected his gastrointestinal tract and bladder. He had already undergone two surgeries, and it was obvious that he was not doing well by his dehydrated, malnourished body. He told us about his restaurant, one of the premiere places to eat in the suburbs of Chicago. It soon became apparent to us that the restaurant was killing him. He was working horribly long hours, while at the same time undergoing surgeries and radiation therapy treatments. We recommended that he take a leave of absence and enroll in an aggressive natural medicine program. Two days after the consult, his cousin, a traditional pharmacist, was calling us about the testosterone cream we prescribed for him. Testosterone is one of the agents we use to help reverse malnutrition and cachexia in cancer patients. It helps the person regain his or her appetite and start building muscle and retaining protein tissue instead of losing it. We explained to the cousin all of the reasons we had for the supplements and other remedies prescribed for Paul. Paul came back about two months later having used only about one fourth of the items that were prescribed for him because of the recommendations of his cousin. We explained to Paul that he was entrusting his life to a traditional pharmacist who does not have the primary responsibility of taking care of even a single cancer patient. Paul was working as many hours as ever, and we again reiterated the fact that he needed to take a leave of absence from his work, that we needed to see his wife and family in the office with him, and that he needs to take other drastic steps or he would no longer be alive to take care of any restaurant. We never saw him again; the task of getting better from his cancer was too great, and he died about six months later.

HOLLYWOOD SOAP OPERA STAR PICKS JOB VERSUS CANCER CARE

Just as sad a story is when we were called by a local naprapathic physician because he had one of the Hollywood soap opera stars in his office and wanted us to give her an examination. As soon as she walked in, several staff members recognized her. We could see immediately why she was sent over. She had significant lymph nodes in her groin, and she looked very dusky. People who become pale generally have low blood counts, which can be a sign of a cancerous condition. We ordered some blood tests and CT scans. Within a couple of days, we told her that she had metastatic ovarian cancer and that we should start some type of aggressive treatment. We also told her that she immediately needed to take a leave of absence from work. She said this was absolutely impossible. She then explained about the many years it took her to get her current role and that if the studio found out she had cancer, her character would be written off the show. We made it clear to her that if she did not take a leave of absence, they would have to write her character off the show because the actress would not be around to play the role. She humored us by starting on a few supplements and soon was off to Hollywood. About two months later, we heard from the other physician that the actress had passed away.

Cancer is not something to be thought of as an inconvenience to a person's life. **Once the physician says you have cancer, it means cancer is your life.** It is your life until it either takes your life, you arrest it, or it completely goes into remission. This is why a person with cancer needs to have a designated caretaker and have as much supporting staff as he or she feels comfortable with. When a cancer patient is surrounded by love and support, this can be the best medicine. As the Bible says in Proverbs 17:22, "A cheerful heart is good medicine."

It sometimes is difficult for driven people to rest. Marion is like this; she has a difficult time resting. She becomes annoyed at me when I am relaxing. Once she exclaimed "What are you doing?" "I'm resting because you don't—I have to do it for both of us!" She didn't appreciate my humor on this occasion when I was resting while she was doing the laundry. Rest is a necessary part of life. The cancer patient needs a lot of rest. Even if a person has a great caretaker, there is still going to be a lot of shopping for organic foods, preparing them, juicing them, taking supplements, exercising, doing fun activities, attending church or religious services (the more people praying for a sick person the better), going to doctor appointments, getting blood tests and x-rays, and the whole gamut of activities that are necessary for life, such as visiting friends and relatives. Getting better from cancer is more than a full-time job. It is impossible to do all of the above well and get enough rest while a person works a full-time job that in all likelihood is partly responsible for the disease in the first place. Do not underestimate rest as a powerful cancer treatment.

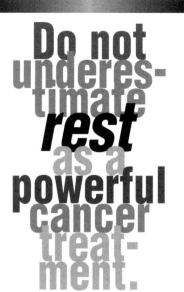

CANCER CAN BE A CHRONIC DISEASE

Some people who undergo aggressive natural medicine treatments will find that initially their tumors regress but then stabilize. In other words, no more shrinkage occurs. The tumor is said to be in the arrested state. In this instance, IPT should be considered. IPT is unique in its ability to help target chemotherapy to the cancer site. Cancer has a remarkable ability to adapt and not be killed completely by the remedies a person is taking. In other words, a cancer can adapt to and quickly become resistant to a particular therapy. This is less likely to happen with IPT because multiple chemotherapeutic agents are used at the same time. If IPT is unable to completely rid a person of cancer and there are no other viable treatment options, the cancer will most likely have to be thought of as a chronic condition like hypertension, diabetes, or heart disease. The latter three conditions are serious and can be life threatening,

but with close follow-up, diet, exercise, nutrition, supplements, and medications, they can be controlled, and the person can have many wonderful years in good health. The key, though, to the many wonderful years of good health is dependent on the person receiving close follow-up and being fanatical about taking all of the recommended nutriceutical agents that are helping the body fight the cancer and keeping it in check. For the person in such a situation, close contact with his or her natural medicine specialist is vital, so that any change in their health condition can immediately be reported.

For the person with cancer, even a mild cold can be life threatening. We have seen people with cancers under very good control who have deteriorated almost overnight because of a simple upper respiratory infection. Caring Medical recently lost such a patient.

Ingrid was a delight. She came in with her mother, and there was obviously a tremendous amount of love between them. She had gastric cancer and was having a difficult time digesting any food because of the growing cancer in her stomach. We wanted to start immediate IPT, but the daughter did not want any chemotherapy medications given to her mother, even the smaller doses used in IPT. We agreed to do aggressive vitamin intravenous drips, ozone therapy, and nutritional supplementation (though we had to use primarily liquid or powdered agents), but only for two weeks. If she was not feeling better by then, IPT would need to be started.

She was definitely better in two weeks; you could tell by the color in her face. After reading the information available on IPT, she decided to start receiving it every two weeks (though we had recommended it once a week). As occurs in many patients, within the first six treatments, she had a remarkable improvement. By the fourth week, she was eating solid foods (she could barely get liquids down when she came in), signifying that the tumor was shrinking. She received a total of eight treatments and then stopped the treatment against our medical advice. She was out of crisis, and the family saw this as a sign that "everything was okay" when it was not. To people on the outside watching her, Ingrid appeared perfectly healthy. She could now tolerate any kind of food, had great energy, and looked great. **But again the point must be made that the way a person feels is not an indication that the tumor is gone or regressing.** For such an assessment, it is best to do an x-ray study or blood cancer marker test. They were going to do intravenous Laetrile at home because the patient's brother was a physician. I continued to see her for ozone therapy but tried to tell them that while a cancer is getting beaten, you need to continue to beat it until it is busted! About four months later, she was having difficulty swallowing again, so she had about six IPT treatments and was able to eat solid foods again. She again stopped coming for care, so we had our staff check up on her about every two weeks. They reported that she was just taking supplements at home. After about another four months, the staff learned that she had died after a bout of cold or pneumonia. I saw the daughter after this, and she was so grateful to the staff for the care that she received. However, what really puzzled us was that the family had their family physician take care of the infection she ultimately died from. I wished they would have consulted Caring Medical.

The reason why an infection is so dangerous to a cancer patient is that the person has so little immunological reserve. The immune system is so busy fighting the cancer that there just is not much left to do anything else. This is why even a mild cold might allow an arrested cancer to become out of control, which can occur in a matter of days. We have had people double and triple their cancer marker numbers from just one relatively "mild" infection, thus undoing months of natural medicine care.

This also brings up a common question, "Why can't my immune system get rid of the cancer when I am the only one in the family who does *not* get sick?" It is a fallacy to assume that all cancer patients have weakened immune systems. At Caring Medical, we often test a person's immune function by measuring the amount of natural killer cells (cells that fight and kill cancer) as well as their function. We have found that most cancer patients have excellent immune systems, perhaps because many of them are using nutritional supplements even before they get to our office. (See **Chapter 27** on the immune system and cancer.)

Checking immune function is important in cancer, because if a person has a strong immune system even though the cancer is getting out of control, it probably means that his or her immune system is *not recognizing* the cancer as something abnormal that needs to be killed. This is much like a pregnant woman's immune system that does not recognize the fetal growth in her uterus as abnormal. The placenta protects the baby from the mother's immune system. Some people's cancers have a tremendously strong ability to hide from the immune system. In such a situation, where a person has good immune function via blood tests and a lack of infections and colds, but yet there is evidence that the cancer is pro-

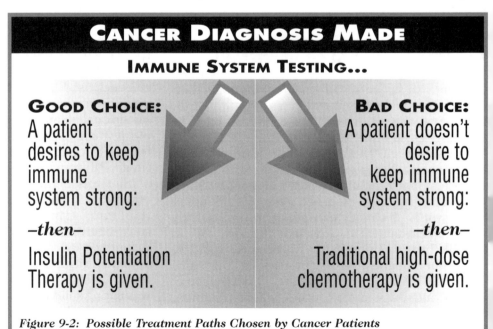

CANCER DIAGNOSIS MADE

IMMUNE SYSTEM TESTING...

GOOD CHOICE:
A patient desires to keep immune system strong:

–then–

Insulin Potentiation Therapy is given.

BAD CHOICE:
A patient doesn't desire to keep immune system strong:

–then–

Traditional high-dose chemotherapy is given.

Figure 9-2: Possible Treatment Paths Chosen by Cancer Patients
The above shows the interactions between immune system and cancer therapy. IPT can be given to cancer patients while keeping their immune systems strong.

gressing, then aggressive therapy like IPT (See **Figure 9-2**) is needed. The person needs to ignite an atomic bomb in the middle of the cancer. The best atomic bomb we know is IPT.

One of our favorite colleagues, Robert Rowen, M.D., a family physician located in Santa Rosa, California, wrote us about his experiences with IPT and his approach to cancer.

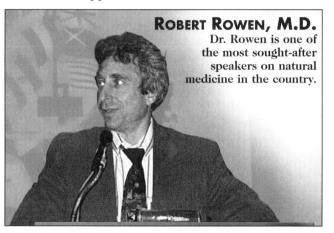

ROBERT ROWEN, M.D.

Dr. Rowen is one of the most sought-after speakers on natural medicine in the country.

R.R., a 76-year-old male developed a rapidly growing mass in his lung on x-ray. He previously had a throat cancer treated with surgery and radiation. This had left him with a serious swallowing problem and it seemed that half his neck had been cut away. Having apparently beaten cancer once, he was eager to beat it again, but the swallowing problem from the radiation was taking its toll.

After three months of intensive alternative therapies for the lung mass, and the mass continued to grow, I (Robert) recommended IPT. We began IPT twice weekly for several weeks. The lung mass stopped growing immediately and became a non-problem. IPT sessions were tapered to less than once a month and the tumor never started growing again. However, the radiation treatment in his neck caught up with him and several months later he developed yet another cancer in his larynx, next to the swallowing mechanism. Radiation may give some relief today, but a high price will be paid by the surrounding tissue tomorrow and a high chance of radiation-induced cancer next year will remain. Most studies show that radiation is not effective yet the practice continues. Mr. R's care was severely limited by the radiation damage to his swallowing mechanism.

D.U. is a 61-year-old male with lung cancer whom I treated in Alaska for six years. Laetrile stopped tumor growth for a year. Then the tumor began regrowing and we would try another alternative therapy. Usually, we saw the tumor growth stop for many months, then start again. After we came across IPT, he reluctantly went ahead with treatment thinking it would not work for a slowly growing tumor. After six weeks, I got an excited call from the radiologist who had been following his lung CT scans for years. He exclaimed, "what are you doing?" He expressed shock that in the first time in all those years he was happy to report not just a stalling of growth, but an actual 40% shrinkage of the tumor. Further treatments shrunk it even further and the tumor had not grown back after many months.

J.O. is a 55 year-old male with through-and-through cancer of the bladder. His urologist wanted to remove his bladder and make a urine-holding bag out of a part of his colon. He refused such mutilating surgery, which would have left him impotent, and possibly incontinent. Instead, he chose six treatments with IPT, and instillation of ozone into his bladder.

Follow up with his urologist was most favorable. The specialist reported no recurrence of tumor that was expected and was impressed with the local healing. Follow up over many months still showed no recurrence of cancer and the patient, of course, was most delighted.

D.E. is a relatively young 46-year-old female who came to me with Stage Four breast cancer. She had metastases to the spine. The cancer was eating out vertebrae and compressing the spinal cord causing significant pain and limping. She refused conventional therapy, knowing it would only be horrific, with no chance of remission. She chose IPT, immune therapy with nutrition and a dendritic cell vaccine. Her results were significant. Over six months of therapy, when we would definitely expect her to significantly suffer progressive neurological impairment, she improved, with less pain, no limp and able to return to work. At the time of this writing, her disease is stable and she bravely is continuing to embark on therapies to provide maximum assistance to her body.

None of these patients experienced any significant toxicity to IPT other than minor hair loss, reversible mild drops in blood counts, or a bit of indigestion.

ROBERT ROWEN'S APPROACH TO CANCER

The most important part is prevention. I believe we should be spending 10 times as much money and attention to prevention rather than to treatment since cancer is largely an environmental, stress and dietary disease. I do not believe any one therapy will ever be a magic bullet for cancer. Nor do I believe all people should be treated the same. Successful strategies for cancer include entering as many pathways into the dysfunction of the body and immune system as possible, to get the greatest net effect. I emphasize treating the person, not the disease. Causes for cancer should be looked for and addressed, such as toxin exposure, dental interference fields, diet, lifestyle, stress, etc. I tell all my patients I take a multifold approach and treat them as a whole, not just as a cancer. Thus, I ask them to address the mind-body connection since the mind and body are *one* and the *same*. This can be done through meditation, guided imagery, and prayer—whatever fits the individual's spiritual makeup. Next is detoxification strategies including dry brush massage, coffee enemas, colon hydrotherapy, far infrared sauna, mercury removal and cavitation removal. Diet is next. Blood pH should be balanced with a diet designed for metabolic type. William Donald Kelley, who is still alive, first pioneered this work in the 1980s. I still see patients of his who once had cancer. Today, they are still cancer free. I also combine oriental philosophies on food (yin-yang) with a modified macrobiotic approach. Vegetables are stressed no matter what.

Next come nutritional supplements, designed for the type of cancer, the individual and the major therapies I might be doing. I use many different kinds of antioxidants, glutathione stimulators, and immune builders. I am now offering angiogenesis inhibition with supplements and COX-2 inhibitors. IPT is an integral part of practice, however, I am more using it to buy time for the other therapies to take hold since most people come to me with advanced cancer when IPT is much less effective.

I am also closely looking into helping the immune system recognize the cancer. Cancer progresses because of the relative inactivity of the immune system and the NK cells to destroy the cancer. New discoveries with dendritic cell vaccines offered by ITL in the Bahamas are seeing weakened immune cells come alive with rejuvenated ability to seek out, recognize and destroy cancer.

In Alaska, I was blessed to be working in a political atmosphere where the patient could come first and not the treatment. Thus, I gained very broad knowledge and experience in a variety of complementary strategies and approaches to the cancer problem.

For bladder cancer specifically, in Alaska, I used intravesical instillation of ozone for early cancers, which have a very high rate of recurrence. I have never seen a recurrence, with regular use of ozone.

DOC, I'M CONVINCED I NEED AGGRESSIVE CARE. WHAT DO I DO NEXT?

Much of the information presented thus far in this book is to explain our experiences of why many cancer patients never get better. Cancer is life or death. It gives us little satisfaction to treat cancer patients at the end of their lives because they already had high-dose chemotherapy destroy their body reserves or they tried useless herbal potions and allowed their cancers to grow unleashed in their body. There are hundreds of other reasons why people do not seek out the advice of a natural medicine specialist.

Hopefully the reader is convinced that such an opinion is needed. It is only the natural medicine specialist who has the knowledge to reverse cancer physiology with diet, lifestyle changes, and nutritional products. But even as good as these recommendations are, they do not have the potency to reverse a high tumor load. For such a task, there is only one treatment that we know of that can do it safely, allowing the person to go on with much of his or her normal daily activities while keeping the immune system strong, and that treatment is IPT. IPT has the power and the ability to help target chemotherapy and can be used as part of a comprehensive natural medicine program to reverse cancer physiology and ultimately the cancer itself. ∎

CHAPTER 10

Insulin Potentiation Therapy: The History
by Ross and Marion Hauser, with Donato Pérez García, M.D.

"IPT...THE SECOND DISCOVERY OF INSULIN..." ™ *
– Chris Duffield, Ph.D., www.IPTQ.org
Creator and Host

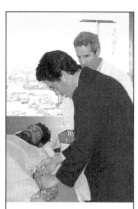

Figure 10-1:
Dr. Hauser receives training in IPT at Dr. Pérez's clinic in Tijuana, Mexico.

In 1999, Steven G. Ayre, M.D., came to Caring Medical and treated several of our cancer patients with IPT. He convinced us and the Caring Medical staff that it was safe and efficacious, and he provided us with documentation that it was *scientifically sound.*

Ross and Marion are not easy "sells." To further our understanding about IPT, we spent a week with Donato Pérez García, M.D., at his clinic in Tijuana, Mexico, (See **Figure 10-1**). During this time, it became evident to us that he was an extremely caring person who was curing cancer patients. It was important for us to meet the most experienced clinician in this therapy and talk with patients under his care. Dr. Pérez clearly treated us as equals and is available to us, even to this day, to answer any questions we might have concerning this treatment. In talking with him, it was clear that he, his father, and his grandfather had been trying during the last 70 years to get this treatment accepted in the United States. It is our hope that by describing the history of Insulin Potentiation Therapy, the Pérez family will get the credit that they deserve and that IPT will be known as The Second Discovery of Insulin.™

For the person who does not want to read this entire chapter, let's look at IPT history in brief:[1]

1896: October 22, Donato Pérez García (Donato 1) was born in Mexico City.

1921: Insulin discovered by Frederick Banting, Best and McLeod.

1923: Nobel Prize in Medicine awarded to Banting and Charles H. Best for insulin discovery and purification.

1924: Donato 1 receives Medical Diploma.

1926: Donato Pérez García, Sr., M.D. a military doctor in Mexico City, first injects himself with insulin at 8:45 A.M. on July 25 for a chronic gastrointestinal condition and malnutrition. He makes a complete recovery. (See **Figure 10-2**.)

1930: November 18, Donato Pérez García y Bellon (Donato 2) is born.

1934: First IPT treatment of patient with syphilis on February 14, 1934.

1935: Donato 1 applies for a U.S. patent for his method of treating syphilis, which is granted in 1939 (U.S. patent 2,145,869 entitled "Intravenous Therapy for the Treatment of Syphilis").

1935: Donato 1 is invited by Harvard University to discuss Insulin Cellular Therapy (later termed Insulin Potentiation Therapy).

1937: The Mexican government sends Donato 1 to San Antonio, Texas, for a year to demonstrate his technique. At Austin State Hospital, Insulin Cellular Therapy caused the rapid and complete return to health in seven patients with tertiary syphilis.

1938: Donato 1 is invited by U.S. Secretary of War Harry H. Wood-ring to demonstrate Insulin Cellular Therapy at Saint Elizabeth Hospital in Washington, D.C.

1939: The Mexican Secretary of Health, Alberto P. Leon, signs a declaration acknowledging the effectiveness of Insulin Cellular Therapy.

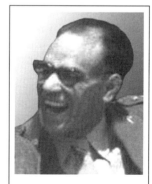

Figure 10-2: Donato Pérez García, M.D. (Donato 1)

The discoverer of Insulin Potentiation Therapy.

---

* *The Second Discovery of Insulin is a trademark of Chris Duffield.*

1939: US patent number 2,145,869 is granted for IPT treatment of syphilis.

1940: An official document recognizing the effectiveness of IPT is signed by J. Agustin Castro, Mexican Secretary of Defense (See **Figure 10-3**).

The Secretary of Defense wrote about Donato 1's cellular therapy "…That the results obtained up to the time I left command of this section of the service greatly exceeded expectations in each case treated, without a single accident. That said therapy was 100% effective… . That because of its economy, ease of application, safety, rapidity, and effectiveness, it is my opinion that this therapy should be officially adopted by all branches of the Armed Forces of the Republic."

1941: Donato 1 sets up a clinic to successfully test IPT in the Mexican military.

1943- Donato 1 is invited to demonstrate IPT
1944: in U.S. at Naval Hospital in San Diego.

1944: The April 10 issue of *Time* magazine ran an article entitled "Insulin for Everything" about Donato 1 and Insulin Cellular Therapy successes in typhoid fever, syphilis, peritonitis, malaria, and rheumatic fever. *Time* reported that Donato 1 had given 11,000 treatments over 15 years without fatal effect. They also reported that Insulin Cellular Therapy reversed a case of paralysis from tertiary syphilis. In one case, the woman walked after four treatments.

1944: Mexican military loses national election in 1944, ending Donato 1's chance to be the Mexican Secretary of Health.

1945: Donato 1 successfully treats a cancer patient with Insulin Cellular Therapy.

1947: Donato 1 demonstrates IPT in the US.

1948: Donato 1 cures ulcers with antibiotics and IPT 49 years before treatment with antibiotics became a standard practice.

1950: Donato 1 presents ulcer results to 9th Cong. of Surgeons in Mexico City.

1953: Donato 1 publishes *Terapia Celular (Cellular Therapy)*, which covers his work in detail.

PROPOSED: That the Department of Health considers that the treatment of neurosyphilis with insulin shock therapy (IPT) is deserving of comprehensive scientific investigation.

MEXICO, D.F., SEPTEMBER 21, 1939
The Senior Official of the Secretary of National Defense.
Calle de la Moneda. C I U D A D

The General Official of the Anti-venereal disease Campaign through memorandum No. 36-11-1198 dated the 11th of this month, has sent to the General Secretary copies of the memorandum No. 36-11-110 dated August 20th of last year, and through these communications has made known in that office the contents of your official notice, no.05844, Exp. F/512.5/11 dated August 3rd, in relation to which it is my pleasure to inform you of the following:

"The Department of Public Health is aware of a number of experiments performed by Dr. Donato P. García, both in this country and in Boston, Washington and Austin, Texas, in the U.S.A. concerning the treatment of neurosyphillis—using a modality called 'insulin shock therapy.' "

"As demonstrated in the above experiments, and as corroborated by the opinions of medical specialists both in the U.S.A. and this country, the treatment of neurosyphilis by the insulin shock therapy is something that is based on rigorous fundamentals of science. The results obtained have revealed that the curing or improvement produced is much more rapid, as indicated both by the clinical evolution of the patients under treatment and the changes in the serologic reactions of their blood and cerebro-spinal fluid."

The reactions observed as a consequence of the insulin shock were at first alarming, however to the degree that the technique of application for the procedure became more perfected, these reactions have become diminished showing the actual innocuousness of the procedure. While the question yet remains whether the curing of syphilis by same is radically effective or not, it will be necessary to have more complete documentation on a larger series of cases and over a longer period of time to permit arriving at any definite conclusions about this illness with its natural evolution particularly after long term treatment.

We think that this treatment has produced good results, particularly in cases of early syphilis, while older more advanced forms of the disease with scarred lesions have not responded as well.

Because of this and other reasons, this Department considers that the treatment of neurosyphilis by insulin shock therapy deserves intensive scientific investigation by virtue of its propositions being of such great theoretical and practical interest.

We consider that it would be well worth our effort to undertake this interesting study on account of its future possibilities and on account of this Mexican doctor who has created this initiative, whose treatment is economical, and which work is already supported by a certain force of scientific investigation.

I offer you my sincerest regards and most distinguished consideration.

THE SECRETARY GENERAL (SIGNED) DR. ALBERTO P. LEON

Figure 10-3: Mexican Department of Health Document
This is an English translation* of a document signed and sealed by the Mexican Secretary General of the Department of Health in 1939, attesting to the success of IPT as practiced by Dr. Donato Pérez García (Donato 1) and recommending further research.

* *Translation done by Chris Duffield*

1955: Drs. Pérez García 1 and 2 reversed paralysis of polio in children with IPT.

1956: Donato 2, joins his father's medical practice Mexico City.

1958: March 30, Donato 3 is born in Mexico City.

1960s: Donato 2 develops and researches a simple medical diagnostic method called "The Oncodiagnosticator."

1971: Donato 1 dies on December 12.

1975: Steven G. Ayre, M.D., a Canadian doctor (now practicing in Burr Ridge, Illinois) meets Donato 2 and starts researching Insulin Cellular Therapy.

1976: Jean-Claude Paquette, M.D., a Canadian doctor in Quebec, receives training from Donato 2 and starts practicing Insulin Cellular Therapy in Canada.

1977: First treatment of multiple sclerosis with IPT by Jean-Claude Paquette M.D.

1983: Donato Pérez García, M.D. (Donato 3), joins the family clinic.

1986: Chris Duffield, Ph.D., meets Steven G. Ayre, M.D., starting his long involvement with IPT.

1986: Dr. Ayre and Donato 2 and 3 publish an article in *Medical Hypothesis* entitled "Insulin Potentiation Therapy: A New Concept for Management of Chronic Degenerative Diseases" (vol. 20, no. 2, pp. 199-210).

1987: "Project 87" is convened by Steven G. Ayre M.D., leading to the founding of SANA Institute, and the Medical Renaissance Foundation, the grant of two IPT patents, and team efforts promote IPT research and treatments.

1987: Donato 2 and 3 successfully treat three patients with HIV/AIDS using IPT.

1988: Donato 3 moves from Mexico City to establish his practice in Tijuana.

1989: Dr. Ayre and Donato 2 and 3 present a poster at the 42nd Annual Symposium on Fundamental Cancer Research, Cellular and Molecular Targets of Cancer Therapy at the M.D. Anderson Cancer Center at the University of Texas in Houston. It is entitled "Breast Carcinoma Treated by a Regime of Low-Dose Chemotherapy and Insulin: Report of Four Cases and Pharmacokinetic Considerations." (See **Figure 10-4**.)

1989: Steven G. Ayre M.D. publish two articles about IPT treatment of HIV/AIDS.

1990: Donato 2 and 3 and Dr. Ayre receive a U.S. patent for IPT treatment of cancer and viral diseases (U.S. patent 4,971,951 entitled "Insulin Potentiation Therapy").

1991: Dr. Ayre and Donato 2 and 3 make a presentation at the Third International Congress on Neo-Adjuvant Chemotherapy in Paris, France, entitled "Insulin Plus Low-Dose CMF as Neo-Adjuvant Chemo-hormonal Therapy for Breast Carcinoma." Because of this presentation, *Oncology News* carries IPT as its lead article in the July-August 1991 issue.

1991: Dr. Ayre begins correspondence with Reps. Patricia Schroeder and Constance Morella, co-chairpersons of the Congressional Caucus on Women's Issues in response to their "Breast Cancer Challenge" which was issued to the medical profession in June, 1991. The "Breast Cancer Challenge" charged American researchers and physicians to come up with an effective treatment for breast cancer by the year 2000.

1991: Dr. Ayre sends a letter to Susan Love, M.D. of the Faulkner Breast Center in Boston, Massachusetts. The letter informs her of IPT and its possible safety and efficacy in the neoadjuvant chemo-hormonal treatment of breast cancer. Dr. Love is

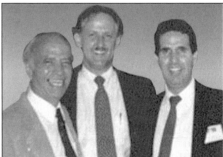

Figure 10-4: Drs. Donato 2 and 3 surround Dr. Ayre in 1989. They made a presentation on the remarkable results of IPT in the treatment of breast cancer.

the chief medical spokesperson for the Breast Cancer Coalition.

1991: As a result of the correspondence with the "Breast Cancer Challenge" Dr. Ayre receives a copy of a letter from Bernadine Healy, M.D., Director, National Institutes of Health, addressed to Rep. Constance Morella (Dated October 23, 1991). This letter discusses IPT and mentions that the matter had been referred to the National Cancer Institute's Division of Cancer Treatment, Cancer Therapy Evaluation Program (CTEP).

1991: Dr. Ayre submits to the FDA a protocol entitled "Neoadjuvant combination chemo-hormonal therapy for the treatment of breast carcinoma using CMF plus insulin." The intent of this protocol is to perform a small pilot study using IPT and low-dose chemotherapy in the treatment of subjects newly diagnosed with breast cancer (Stages I-IIIB). The Principal Investigator for this study was Ira J. Piel, M.D., F.A.C.P., a medical oncologist-hematologist affiliated with the Illinois Masonic Medical Center in Chicago, IL.

1991: Dr. Ayre receives letter from Susan Love. M.D. in her capacity as coordinator of the Breast Cancer Coalition Research Task Force, informing him of the Research Hearings to be held in Washington, D.C. on February 5 & 6, 1992, (Dr. Ayre attends.)

1991: As a result of correspondence between Dr. Ayre and Dr. Bernadine Healy, as well as between Rep. Constance Morella and Dr. Healy, a letter is received from Michael A. Friedman. M.D., Associate Director CTEP, informing Dr. Ayre that Ms. Diane Bronzert would be getting in touch to discuss grant application procedures to fund IPT studies.

1991: Dr. Ayre submits to Kay Dickerson, Ph.D., of the Breast Cancer Coalition Research Hearings, requesting time to offer oral testimony at the Hearings on the use of IPT with low-dose chemotherapy for the neoadjuvant treatment of breast cancer.

1991: December 31, FDA rules on IND submission. Protocol is put on clinical hold. The reasoning behind this decision was that there are safe and effective forms of treatment for early stages of breast cancer already in existence, and that denying subjects the value of these treatments would put them at unreasonable and significant risk of illness or injury. Donato 3 is informed that the only appropriate group of patients for the study of any new therapy would be patients for whom standard appropriate therapy had failed and whose disease had progressed, i.e. patients with Stage IV disease.

1992: Dr.Ayre receives a letter from Charles L. Vogel. M.D., Medical Director of the South Florida Comprehensive Cancer Centers, and Moderator of the Clinical Science Session of the Breast Cancer Coalition Research Hearings. Dr. Vogel states that IPT must still be considered an unorthodox therapy needing scientific corroboration of its effectiveness. Dr. Ayre is invited to attend the Research Hearings as an observer. Dr. Vogel is also informed of the NCI's initiative to evaluate unorthodox or non-conventional medical therapies, and is referred to Michael Hawkins, M.D. of the National Cancer Institute's Cancer Therapy Evaluation Program to discuss the matter further.

1992: Dr. Ayre holds a telephone conversation and subsequent correspondence sent to Michael J. Hawkins, M.D., Chief of Investigational Drug Branch, Cancer Therapy Evaluation Program, Division of Cancer Treatment, National Cancer Institute. Correspondence to Dr. Hawkins includes an informational brochure on IPT, plus a copy of the "on-clinical-hold" breast cancer protocol.

1992: Dr. Ayre receives official written confirmation from Gregory Burke. M.D., Ph.D., Director, Division of Oncology and Pulmonary Drug Products, Office of Drug Evaluation 1, Center for Drug Evaluation and Research concerning the FDA's ruling placing the IPT/Breast Cancer protocol on clinical hold. His letter reiterates the recommendation that the most appropriate group of breast cancer patients to first be studied/treated with IPT would be subjects with Stage IV metastatic breast cancer who had failed primary therapy with standard approved treatment modalities.

1992: Dr. Ayre receives correspondence from Dr. Hawkins at CTEP making a similar recommendation as that from Dr. Burke at the FDA. The best breast cancer population to study would be women with metastatic disease who had not previously received chemotherapy for their metastatic disease (adjuvant therapy would be permitted if they recurred more than six or 12 months after their last chemotherapy treatment). Also included in this mailing is a document prepared by the CTEP entitled, "Preparation of a Best Case Series and the Conduct of Pilot Clinical Trials Using Unconventional Cancer Treatments." Dr. Hawkins also offers generous collaboration and assistance in the design and review of protocols for the proposed clinical studies.

1992: Breast Cancer Coalition Research Hearings are held in Washington, D.C. Comments are made about IPT during Session 3 (Clinical Science) mentioning that the therapy was a novel therapeutic idea in need of clinical confirmation. These comments are entered into the written testimony of the Hearings.

1992: Drs. Ayre and Donato 2 and 3 submit to the Cancer Therapy Evaluation Program (CTEP) a "Best Case Series" of IPT treatment involving a variety of different cancers. The intent of this submission is to introduce the CTEP to the historical context of the practice of IPT abroad, and to demonstrate the kinds of clinical results that have been experienced with this practice over the last several decades.

1992: Dr. Ayre holds a telephone conversation initiated by Michael J. Friedman. M.D., Associate Director of NCI's Cancer Therapy Evaluation Program, with information to the effect that CTEP was proceeding with an investigation of a number of unconventional cancer therapies including IPT, and that a decision on their evaluation would be forthcoming by the end of July 1992.

1992: Dr. Ayre receives correspondence from Charles L. Vogel. M.D. of The Mount Sinai Comprehensive Cancer Center in Miami Beach. Florida. Having reviewed a copy of the Best Case Series on IPT. Dr. Vogel expresses interest in performing a trial of IPT in the treatment of patients with advanced breast cancer. Current plans are to develop a new IND submission to the FDA for treating Stage IV breast cancer patients with IPT. and with Dr. Vogel acting in the capacity of Clinical Investigator for this proposed study.

1992: Dr. Ayre submits response to FDA's letter of 11/28/92 that had put the original IPT protocol submission on clinical hold. In this letter of response. the argument in favor of treating women newly diagnosed with breast cancer is pursued further. The minimal risks of the protocol are emphasized as well as the benefits (breast conservation, quality of life under treatment, etc.). It is argued that theoretical arguments against such a program of study would seem less important than practical observations made over several decades of practice with IPT and that women with newly diagnosed breast cancer should be given the option of breast-preserving treatment for their disease.

1992: Dr. Ayre receives notification from the FDA that the July 29 IND submission had been put on clinical hold for reasons similar to those given for putting the first IND submission on hold.

1992: Donato 2 and 3 and Dr. Ayre receive a U.S. patent for IPT treatment of many diseases (U.S. patent 5,155,096 entitled "Method for Potentiation of a Therapeutic Agent").

1992: Dr. Ayre is notified by Mary McCabe, R.N., Clinical Trials Specialist with CTEP that their agency was interested in insulin potentiation of chemotherapy, and that a process of review was underway to determine the most appropriate way of scientifically evaluating IPT.

1993: Dr. Ayre is notified by Mary McCabe that CTEP had decided not to proceed with any formal investigation of IPT.

1993: Materials on IPT are sent to the newly established Office of Alternative Medicine (OAM) at the National Institutes of Health. In subsequent communications with Dr. Michael Eskinazi at OAM. Dr. Ayre is given the opinion that IPT is more mainstream medicine than alternative therapy, and that it should be evaluated through established channels for evaluating such medical discoveries.

1993: Dr. Ayre receives a telephone call from Dr. Michael Hawkins, formerly with CTEP and now with the Georgetown University Medical Center, Division of Medical Oncology, offering to perform an animal study to investigate the workings of IPT. Dr. Hawkins indicates that should the results of the animal studies be supportive of the IPT concept, there is the possibility that clinical trials of IPT in the management of Stage IV breast cancer might thereafter be undertaken at Georgetown University.

1993: Donato 3 receives a formal written proposal from Dr. Hawkins concerning the animal study, complete with itemized budget for same. Fund raising efforts for this study are begun through a not-for-profit corporation called Medical Renaissance Foundation, an entity that had been established expressly for the purpose of funding IPT-related research.

1993: Dr. Ayre attends the Secretary's Conference to establish a National Action Plan on Breast Cancer at the National Institutes of Health in Bethesda, Maryland. Materials on IPT are accepted and made available for review in the Conference's Reference Room.

1993: Dr. Ayre is notified by a friend and business associate, Mr. Rich Moret of the advertising firm of Moret Worldwide and China West in Tucson, Arizona, that there is a developing interest in studying

and possibly practicing IPT in the Far East.

1993: Donato 2 visits Henry Cisneros at his home in San Antonio Texas.

1994: Dr. Ayre receives a call from Ms. Shirl Thomas at the Office of the Secretary of Housing and Urban Development, in Washington, D.C. The Secretary himself—the Honorable Henry G. Cisneros—is a personal friend of one of the Mexican physicians responsible for pioneering the practice of IPT—Donato Pérez García y Bellon, M.D. Following the Christmas holiday season the two spend much time together in San Antonio, discussing IPT at some length with his friend, Mr. Cisneros. Ms. Thomas is instructed to contact Dr. Ayre on Mr. Cisneros' behalf with the offer of whatever help he and his office might be able to give to help promote the scientific study and development of IPT in the United States.

1994: Dr. Ayre receives a letter from Hassan S. Rifaat, M.D. President of Texas Health Innovators, a private not-for-profit corporation with the following mission statement: **1.** To expedite the objective scientific evaluation of health care innovations, **2.** To promote the public and professional distribution of such scientific evaluations, **3.** To promote and facilitate access to the health care innovations that work. **4.** To achieve our goals in the most time and resource efficient way. Dr. Rifaat states that IPT had been highly recommended to him by Michael J. Friedman, M.D., Associate Director of NCI's Cancer Therapy Evaluation Program. (It was his office that had declined to formally study IPT back in September 1992. I informed Dr. Rifaat of the ongoing initiatives for the study of IPT with the animal study at Georgetown University Medical Center and developments in China. The possibility of funding for research is discussed.

1994: Dr. Ayre makes a presentation to the Cancer Treatment Research Foundation of the Cancer Treatment Centers of America requesting funding for the animal study at Georgetown University Medical Center.

1994: Collaborative efforts for the study of IPT undertaken with medical Personnel at the Xuzhou Medical College Cancer Center in Xuzhou, China.

1994: Acceptance of grant request to the Cancer Treatment Research Foundation to fund an animal study at Georgetown University Medical Center. This study is designed to investigate the effects of insulin on adriamycin cytotoxicity on human breast cancer cell explants in athymic nude mice.

1995: Jean-Claude Paquette, M.D., prints his book about IPT, *Médecine de l'Espoir* (Medicine of Hope).

1996: Completion of the animal study at Georgetown University Medical Center with inconclusive results. Difficulty with the study model—translating the IPT protocol from human subjects to athymic nude mice—is considered to be a contributing factor in the failure to scientifically document IPT effects to enhance tumor cell killing in the human breast cancer cell explants.

1996: First IPT web site (one page) by Donato 3.

1996: Donato 2, visits Tony Mastromarino, Ph.D., Director of Scientific Research, Office of the Vice-President, M.D., Anderson Cancer Center in Houston, Texas. Dr. Mastromarino communicates his interest in IPT to Mary Ann Richardson, Ph.D., from the UT School of Public Health, who is co-PI of the OAM-funded Center for Alternative Research in Cancer. Dr. Mastromarino had been responsible for the 1989 invitation to the Drs. Pérez García and Dr. Ayre to prepare their poster presentation for M.D. Anderson's Forty-second Annual Symposium on Fundamental Cancer Research.

1996: Dr. Mary Ann Richardson conducts a site visit at the office of Donato 1 in Tijuana, Mexico, and subsequently invites the Drs.

Pérez García and Dr. Ayre to come to an OAM meeting to be held in Bethesda in August.

1997: NIH/OAM Conference on "Monitoring and Evaluation Approaches for Integrated Complementary and Alterative Medicine Cancer Practices," is held in Bethesda, MD. The purpose of the Conference is to launch an initiative to facilitate entry of extant cancer protocols into a Phase II clinical trials environment. The name of this initiative is "Practice Outcomes Monitoring Evaluation System" (POMES). Dr. Ayre presents a paper entitled "Best Case Series Approach: Insulin Potentiation of Chemotherapy." Clinical cases were provided by the Drs. Donato Pérez García.

1997: Dr. Ayre visits Donato 3 for 14 days in Tijuana to get trained on current IPT method. Dr. Ayre receives his IPT instructor certificate.

1997: Protocol for a multicenter prospective clinical trial of IPT in the treatment of stage IV cancers of the breast, lung, and ovary is submitted to, and approved by, the Institutional Review Board of the Great Lakes College of Clinical Medicine at their fall meeting.

1997: Steven G. Ayre, M.D. begin to treat cancer with IPT under an IRB-approved protocol.

1998: Chris Duffield, Ph.D., creates the web site www.IPTQ.org to promote Insulin Potentiation Therapy.

1999: Dr. Ayre and Donato 2 and 3, receive an invitation from Jeffrey D. White, M.D., Director, Office of Cancer Complementary and Alterative Medicine to present a Best Case Series on the clinical experience with IPT before the members of the Cancer Advisory Panel of the Center for Cancer Complementary and Alterative Medicine at the National Institutes of Health.

1999: Jean-Claude Paquette's book *Medecine de l'Espoir* (on IPT) *is* made public for the first time, in the original French.

1999: Aimé Ricci translates Dr. Paquette's book, *Medicine of Hope,* from French into English.

2000: Dr. Ross Hauser receives IPT training by Donato 3 in Tijuana, Mexico

2000: IPTQ.org is submitted to all major search engines over the internet.

2000: Drs. Frank George and Hayle Aldren receives IPT training by Dr. Donato Pérez García at his Tijuana office.

2000: On September 18, Drs. Ayre, Donato 3, and Ross Hauser present Insulin Potentiation Therapy to the NIH Cancer Advisory Panel for Complementary and Alternative Medicine in Bethesda, MD (See **Figure 10-5**).

2000: Dr. Robert Rowen receives IPT training by Dr. Donato 3 at his Tijuana office.

2000: Donato 2 dies on November 23 in Mexico City.

2001: In Las Vegas, Nevada the first IPT training seminar was held, bringing a total of 20 doctors plus one veterinarian.

2001: Dr. Ayre, Donato 3, and Robert Rowen give the first comprehensive IPT training seminar in the United States to over 20 physicians. (See **Figure 10-6**.)

2001: Seven more doctors and one nurse receive IPT training at the IPT workshop in Oklahoma City. The total number of practicing IPT doctors is now 37.

2001: Donato 3 starts www.IPTQMD.com, a web site for physicians who utilize IPT in their practices. It is a place to exchange information and protocols on IPT.

2002: Dr. Jean Remy Lepan from France and Dr. Nelson Modesto from Brazil receive IPT training by Dr. Donato 3.

2002: Dr. Philippe-Gaston Besson from Switzerland receives IPT training by Dr. Donato 3. IPT is available now from 44 doctors worldwide, in eight countries: the U.S., Canada, Mexico, Argentina, Brazil, France, Switzerland and Ecuador. Also one veterinarian in Arizona.

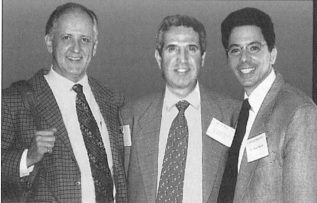

Figure 10-5: Drs. Ayre, Perez, and Hauser Convene before Presenting IPT

Drs. Ayre, Perez, and Hauser are seen before presenting IPT to the NIH Advisory Board for Complimentary and Alternative Medicine, 2000. Dr. Steven G. Ayre was instrumental in setting up this meeting. It was one of the many hundreds of things he and others have done to try to achieve acceptance for Insulin Potentiation Therapy accepted into mainstream oncology.

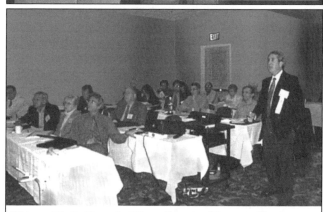

Figure 10-6: Donato Pérez García (Donato 3) at a Physician Training Seminar on IPT

The other teachers included Steven G. Ayre, M.D., and Robert Rowen, M.D.

2002: Third IPT training workshop is held in Dallas Texas.

2002: Ross A. Hauser, M.D., and Marion A. Hauser, M.S., R.D., write and publish the book entitled *Treating Cancer with Insulin Potentiation Therapy.*

In regard to the extensive information on the history of Insulin Potentiation Therapy, we refer the reader to www.IPTQ.org, created and hosted by Chris Duffield. Chris, like Dr. Ayre and Dr. Pérez, has a passion for IPT. These three men are owed a great debt for their dedication and persistence to get this therapy accepted. Chris writes in the IPT web site, "I have invested a lot of my precious time, energy, and resources in this web site. My motivation is philanthropy—the love of fellow human beings. IPT could be of great importance to all of us." Having met Chris, Dr. Ayre, and Dr. Pérez, we can affirm that they all have this same belief and motivation.

As can be seen from the brief synopsis of the history of IPT, shortly after insulin was discovered, Donato 1 started using it to treat conditions other than diabetes. In the late 1920s, he found that insulin could increase a drug's concentration in the central nervous system and surmised that insulin could be given before various medications/chemicals to increase the drugs' concentration into various cavities and cells of the body to treat various neurological conditions that had an infectious etiology. **He was apparently the first physician to reverse the devastating neurological effects of neurosyphilis.** He treated other conditions, including polio, with insulin and medications and then went on to successfully treat cancer by increasing various drug efficacies by first administering insulin. We should note that Donato 1 called his therapy by various names, including cellular therapy or Donatian Therapy. It was Dr. Ayre who changed the name to Insulin Potentiation Therapy.

Donato 1 was way ahead of his time. He surmised that Insulin Cellular Therapy did three things:

1. Balances the biophysical and biochemical systems of the cells and the body.

2. Detoxifies the cells and the body by allowing the transport of toxins from cells.

3. Increases the effectiveness of medications (potentiation) by enhancing their transport into cells.

Donato 1 was convinced that insulin changed the chemistry of the blood and sometimes referred to Donatian Therapy as cellular therapy (or cellular cancer therapy) because of the change of the physiochemical constants of the blood. Later Jean-Claude Paquette called the therapy *Therapie Insulino-Cellulaire* or TIC in French, and Insulin-Cellular Therapy or ICT in English. In the 1970s, Dr. Ayre called the method Insulin Potentiation Therapy, emphasizing the agent used and its action. It should be noted that besides the name,

Dr. Ayre was the first physician to use Humalog, a very fast-acting, human-based insulin that drastically cut the time involved in the procedure. Donato 1, 2, and 3 performed IPT using various insulins that had much longer half-lives.

Donato 2 had the most clinical experience with IPT. He further perfected the technique that his father had developed. He expanded the technique to treat many types of infections, arthritis, neurological conditions, and many other diseases. He was responsible for training his son, Donato 3, as well as Dr. Paquette and Dr. Ayre. It is because of his pioneering spirit and willingness to train others in the technique that IPT is beginning to flourish today.

The skeptic of IPT will surely ask, "How could such a remarkable treatment be done for over 75 years and the medical establishment not recognize it?" We would be quick to point out that many outstanding therapies took just as long to be accepted; the most obvious example is chiropractic care. It took a lawsuit by the chiropractic profession for the AMA (American Medical Association) to finally back down their assault on this therapy. Closer to home for us, it is only recently that Prolotherapy (an injection technique that stimulates the body to repair painful areas because it helps ligaments, tendons, cartilage, and other connective tissues heal) is being considered by major medical organizations as an appropriate treatment for curing chronic pain, though it has been practiced since the 1940s. Not until the 1990s did a branch of the National Institutes of Health (NIH) study alternative medicine, and we are not yet able to say that the AMA wholeheartedly endorses natural or alternative medicine. The battle continues for many effective alternatives to modern allopathic medicine.

It does appear that one of the major blows to IPT was the discovery of penicillin (1928—the same year Donato 1 discovered IPT). When World War II occurred, penicillin was found to be a wonder drug, so the interest in the treatment of various infections, such as syphilis, was more in the antibiotic realm; the need to use insulin to cure the condition was not very great. It should be noted that even with the discovery of penicillin, Donato 1 continued his research into IPT and found that the combination of insulin and penicillin could reverse pyloric stenosis, a severe narrowing or blockage of the opening from the stomach into the small intestine and generally only treatable by surgery. Donato 1 found as far back as 1944 that the condition could be treated by the potentiating effects of insulin on penicillin. Since pyloric stenosis generally starts with gastritis (inflammation of the stomach), which progresses to ulcers and then to the stenosis, Donato 1 believed that the condition must have an infectious etiology. This was proven true in the late 1980s, but it was not until 1995 that the NIH officially recognized the bacterium *Heliobacter pylori* as the cause of most ulcers. The practice of treating ulcers with antibiotics did not become a common practice in the United States until 1997, a full 50 years after Donato 1. Yes, Donato 1 was way ahead of his time.

Here is a summary of the experience of the main proponents of IPT:

- Donato Pérez García, Sr., M.D. (1896-1971, Donato 1), discoverer of IPT, practiced it for 43 years in Mexico City and demonstrated it many times on several tours through the United States.

- Donato Pérez García y Bellón, M.D. (1930-2000, Donato 2), son of Donato 1, practiced IPT for 44 years in Mexico City.

- Donato Pérez García, Jr., M.D. (1958- , Donato 3), son of Donato 2, has practiced IPT for 19 years in Mexico City and Tijuana, Mexico.

- Jean-Claude Paquette, M.D. (1927-1995), met Donato 2 in 1976 and practiced IPT for 16 years in Canada and Haiti.

These four individuals represent 121 years of cumulative experience with IPT, representing tens of thousands of treatment sessions on thou-sands of ill patients. Not a single death has been reported from this procedure. This is a remarkable safety record. In a manuscript sent to me (Ross) in April 2000 by Donato 2, he wrote that "we have treated more than 30,000 patients with all kinds of diseases..." The fact is that no fatalities have occurred from IPT in over 120 years of medical practice was reiterated by Donato 3 at the IPT meeting in 2000.

Any technique will not be accepted by mainstream medicine unless there are some clinicians promoting its acceptance. IPT is fortunate to have the tenacity of Dr. Ayre, who is doing everything within his power to promote the technique. When he taught us and the staff at Caring Medical the technique in 1999, Ross was only the sixth person in the world to be trained in the technique. Because of the new "openness" to more complementary or natural treatments in the United States, medical doctors, patients, and medical organizations are becoming more open to IPT. In the last several years, Dr. Ayre has done presentations on IPT before hundreds of physicians at such prestigious alternative/natural medicine organizations as the American College for the Advancement of Medicine, the International Biooxidative Medicine Association, and the Great Lakes College of Clinical Medicine.

Because more physicians are being exposed to IPT, the number of clinicians practicing IPT is growing tremendously. As more clinicians become proficient at IPT and patients are cured of their cancers and other diseases, it will only be a matter of time before IPT is accepted as a viable alternative to more conventional cancer therapies. ■

CHAPTER 11

Insulin Potentiation Therapy: The Science

In understanding the power of IPT to heal, one must appreciate the magnificent world of insulin. Insulin is a protein hormone secreted by the islets of Langerhans, which are clusters of endocrine cells in the pancreas. The power of insulin can be found in the fact that insulin acts directly or indirectly on most tissues of the body. When insulin is injected, it stimulates anabolic processes that cause the cells to get more energy and the body as a whole to store energy. The cells of the body are provided energy by glucose, body proteins are maintained, and excessive calories (regardless of source) are stored primarily as fat.

Insulin induces in its target cells a large number of changes that fall into two general categories: alteration of either membrane transport or enzyme function (See **Figure 11-1**). The most known effect of insulin is to increase glucose transport into most cells. This causes an immediate increase in energy production in the cells. Insulin also stimulates the active transport of amino acids into most cells, thereby making more amino acids available for protein synthesis.

As glucose and amino acids enter cells, protein, glycogen, and adipose tissue synthesis are enhanced. This net process is termed *anabolism*, which increases the body's net energy stores. In addition, insulin alters the activities or concentrations of many of the intracellular enzymes involved in the anabolic and catabolic (degradation of body energy stores) pathways of the body. It stimulates the enzymes involved in anabolic processes and inhibits those involved in catabolism (See **Figure 11-2**). The main mechanism by which enzyme function is altered by insulin is *phosphorylation* (adding phosphate) or *dephosphorylation*.

Insulin affects carbohydrate metabolism by inhibiting almost all of the critical liver enzymes that catalyze *gluconeogenesis*; the net result is that insulin abolishes glucose release by the liver. In contrast, insulin stimulates glycogen synthesis in the liver by increasing glucose uptake in the cells, increasing the activity of the rate-limiting step in glycogen synthesis, and inhibiting the enzyme that catalyzes glycogen catabolism. Insulin favors glucose transformation into glycogen by many mechanisms.

Insulin's action on fat is analogous. As glucose uptake into adipose tissue increases, it provides the precursors for the synthesis of fatty acid and glycerophosphate and their combination into triacylglycerol (storage form of fat); simultaneously, insulin increases the activity of certain enzymes that accelerate fatty acid synthesis, and, most importantly, inhibits the enzyme triacylglycerol uptake lipase that stimulates triacylglycerol breakdown. Again, insulin stimulates key enzymes

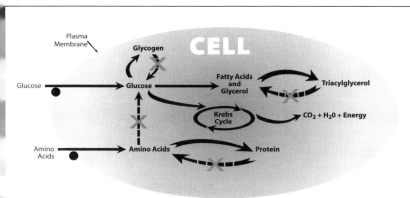

Each solid arrow (——▶) represents a process enhanced by insulin.
✖ denotes a reaction inhibited by insulin.

Figure 11-1: The Major Effects of Insulin upon Metabolism

Insulin stimulates the cells to get more energy—and the body as a whole to store energy.

Adapted from Human Physiology, The Mechanisms of Body Function, 3rd Edition. *Arthur J. Vander, M.D., James H. Sherman, Ph.D., and Dorothy S. Luciano, Ph.D. McGraw-Hill*

FIGURE 11-2: ENZYMES WHOSE ACTIVITIES ARE ALTERED BY INSULIN[1]

ENZYME	CHANGE IN ACTIVITY	POSSIBLE MECHANISM
cAMP METABOLISM		
PHOSPHODIESTERASE (LOW KM)	INCREASE	PHOSPHORYLATION
PROTEIN KINASE (cAMP-DEPENDENT)	DECREASE	ASSOCIATION OF R & C SUBUNITS
GLYCOGEN METABOLISM		
GLYCOGEN SYNTHASE	INCREASE	DEPHOSPHORYLATION
PHOSPHORYLASE KINASE	DECREASE	DEPHOSPHORYLATION
PHOSPHORYLASE	DECREASE	DEPHOSPHORYLATION
GLYCOLYSIS AND GLUCONEOGENESIS		
PYRUVATE DEHYDROGENASE	INCREASE	DEPHOSPHORYLATION
PYRUVATE KINASE	INCREASE	DEPHOSPHORYLATION
6-PHOSPHOFRUCTO-2-KINASE	INCREASE	DEPHOSPHORYLATION
FRUCTOSE-2, 6-BISPHOSPHATASE	DECREASE	DEPHOSPHORYLATION
LIPID METABOLISM		
ACETYL-CoA CARBOXYLASE	INCREASE	DEPHOSPHORYLATION
HMG-CoA REDUCTASE	INCREASE	DEPHOSPHORYLATION
TRIACYLGLYCEROL LIPASE	DECREASE	DEPHOSPHORYLATION
SIGNALING MOLECULES		
P42/44MAP KINASE	INCREASE	DEPHOSPHORYLATION
P90RSK	INCREASE	DEPHOSPHORYLATION
GSK3	DECREASE	DEPHOSPHORYLATION
P70 S6 KINASE	INCREASE	DEPHOSPHORYLATION
PHOSPHOPROTEIN PHOSPHATES 1G	INCREASE	DEPHOSPHORYLATION

Figure 11-2: Insulin stimulates the enzymes involved in anabolic (build up) processes and inhibits those involved in catabolism (break down).

[1] *Adapted from* **Diabetologia**, ©1981; 21:347. Denton, R.M., et al: *A partial view of the mechanism of insulin action.*

involved in anabolism and inhibits key enzymes involved in catabolism.

Similarly for protein, insulin stimulates the uptake of amino acids while simultaneously increasing the activity of some of the ribosomal enzymes that mediate the synthesis of protein from these amino acids and inhibits the enzymes that mediate protein catabolism.

Insulin is an anabolic hormone. It helps the body make and store energy from glucose. The higher the glucose levels in the blood, the more insulin secretion is stimulated (See **Figure 11-3**). Some of the effects of insulin binding onto the cell can occur within seconds or minutes, such as increased membrane transport, protein phosphorylation, enzyme activation and inhibition, and RNA synthesis, or after a few hours, such as protein and DNA synthesis and cell growth[1] (See **Figure 11-4**). When insulin is injected into the body, the actual insulin hormone is only in the serum for a few minutes, as insulin has a plasma

half-life of less than five minutes under normal circumstances. The major effects of insulin are indirect from the various products that are produced from insulin stimulation of cell receptors. Insulin receptors (IRs) are found on most mammalian cells, in concentrations of up to 20,000 per cell.[1] When insulin is missing (diabetes mellitus of childhood), or if the cell is insulin resistant (diabetes that occurs in overweight adults because the insulin receptor does not respond normally to the insulin that is present), the cell goes into the breakdown mode and becomes dehydrated and acidotic (See **Figure 11-5**). The similarities between this physiology and cancer should be obvious. When cancer goes unchecked, ultimately the person becomes acidotic, dehydrated, and extremely weak. Thus, being insulin deficient (or resistant) gives a similar body chemistry picture.

When the cells of the body do not respond normally to insulin, the condition is called **insulin resistance.** Its cause is excessive food intake, primarily in the form of carbohydrates (See **Figure 11-6**). The net effect of insulin resistance is an

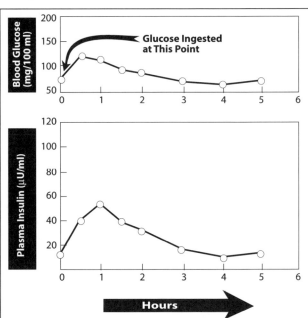

Figure 11-3: Blood Concentration of Glucose and Insulin in Normal Adults
Blood concentration of glucose and insulin following ingestion of 100 grams of glucose in normal human subjects. The higher the blood sugar, the more insulin is secreted.

Adapted from W. H. Daughaday, et al. The Regulation of Growth by Endocrines. Ann. Rev. Physiol., 37:211 (1977).

Figure 11-4: Relationship of the Insulin Receptor to Insulin Action

Insulin binds to its membrane receptor, and this interaction generates one or more transmembrane signals. This signal (or signals) modulates a wide variety of intracellular events, some of which occur in seconds; other events take hours.

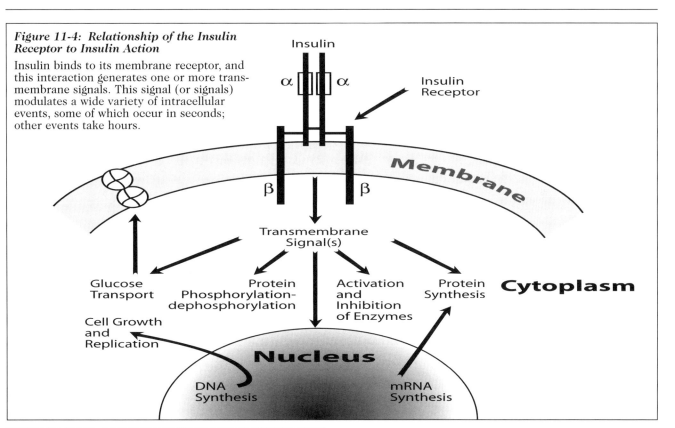

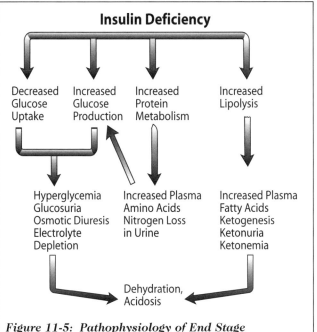

Insulin Deficiency

Figure 11-5: Pathophysiology of End Stage Insulin Deficiency

When insulin is deficient, the body becomes acidic and dehydrated, giving a similar physiologic picture as end stage cancer.

increase in blood glucose levels because insulin has lost the power to get into the cells. One could say this high blood glucose level actually poisons the body (See **Figure 11-7**). The glucose levels in the blood also cause more insulin to be secreted by the pancreas, and eventually (over many years) the number of insulin receptors declines (See **Figure 11-8**). The cells then become resistant to the effects of insulin.

The term *insulin resistance* requires explanation. Insulin is vitally important; therefore, pronounced resistance to its actions cannot be compatible with life; consequently, any resistance may be only partial and is usually defined as a decreased ability of insulin to stimulate glucose disposal and its storage as glycogen. Insulin resistance has been most studied in its association with atherosclerosis. Insulin resistance is known to be a causative factor in cases of hypertension, elevated cholesterol, and elevated triglycerides. The combination of all these conditions with insulin resistance is called *Syndrome X*.

Generally, a person does not become insulin resistant unless he or she has been eating poorly for years. This eventually causes the person to

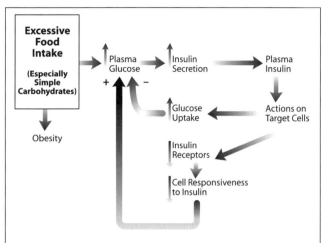

Figure 11-6: Insulin Resistance
Because of the excessive intake of simple carbohydrates, many overweight Americans have insulin resistance.

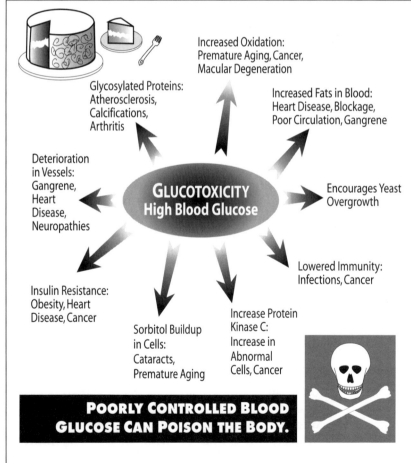

Figure 11-7: Poor blood glucose control can set the basis for cancer physiology.

Adapted from Advances in Care of Diabetes, *Vol. 15, No. 2, p.255, May 1999.*

become overweight. Interestingly, the more obese a person is, the greater his or her risk of cancer (See **Figure 11-9**). Specifically, obesity increases the risk of breast, prostate, colon, uterine, kidney, gallbladder, and pancreatic cancers. To stress the point even further, a person's blood sugar level most likely has an effect on his or her survival of cancer. **Figure 11-10** shows an animal study on breast cancer survival: the lower the blood sugar level is maintained, the higher the survival rate.[2] Researchers from the University of Toronto Mount Sinai Hospital followed 535 women with breast cancer for 10 years and studied the relation between breast cancer grade and stage and insulin concentration. Fasting insulin concentrations were measured to avoid postprandial (after meal) fluctuations. Patients enrolled in the study received standard accepted treatments of surgery with chemotherapy, hormonal therapy, and radiotherapy if indicated. *The researchers found that women with the highest insulin levels were eight times more likely to die during the study than women with the lowest insulin levels,* with 70% of such patients being alive after seven years compared with 95% of those with normal insulin levels.[3] The researchers found that those with high insulin levels were four times more likely to suffer metastatic disease and disease recurrence. In this study, fasting insulin levels alone were found to be an independent risk factor, as some women of normal weight also had high insulin levels, and the worse prognosis held for them as well. Other researchers have found that 50% of women with endometrial cancer and 22% with breast cancer had glucose intolerance, though the incidence of diabetic-type glucose tolerance curves could be over 50%.[4-7] It has been demonstrated that diabetes increases a woman's risk of breast cancer eightfold.[8] Diabetes has been shown to significantly increase the risk of other cancers, including liver and pancreatic cancer.[9]

FIGURE 11-8: INSULIN BINDING TO CIRCULATING MONOCYTES IN HYPERINSULINEMIC OBESE PATIENTS

CONDITION	PLASMA INSULIN CONCENTRATION	I^{125} INSULIN BINDING CONDITION		RECEPTOR CONCENTRATION	RECEPTOR AFFINITY
		WITH LOW INSULIN CONCENTRATION	WITH HIGH INSULIN CONCENTRATION		
HIGH-CALORIE, HIGH-CARBOHYDRATE DIET	ELEVATED	DEPRESSED	DEPRESSED	DEPRESSED	NORMAL
AFTER 72 HR TOTAL FAST	NORMAL	NORMAL	DEPRESSED	DEPRESSED	ELEVATED
72 HR FAST FOLLOWED BY 2 DAYS HIGH-CALORIE HIGH-CARBOHYDRATE DIET	ELEVATED	DEPRESSED	DEPRESSED	DEPRESSED	NORMAL
AFTER SEVERAL WEEKS OF 600-CALORIE DIET	NORMAL	NORMAL	NORMAL	NORMAL	NORMAL

Figure 11-8: The high-calorie, high-carbohydrate diet of many Americans leads to insulin resistance caused by a decline in insulin receptors.

Adapted from Robert Bar, Insulin Receptor Status in Disease States of Man. Archives of Internal Medicine, ©1977; 137:474-481.

ASSOCIATION BETWEEN OBESITY AND CANCER

Mortality Ratios for Cancer Site Relative to Percentage Over Average Weight

Cancer Type	10%-19%	20%-29%	30%-39%	≥40%
MEN				
Colon, Rectum	—	—	1.53	1.73
Prostate	—	1.37	1.33	1.29
WOMEN				
Endometrium	1.36	1.85	2.30	5.42
Uterus (unspecified)	—	1.81	1.40	4.65
Cervix	—	1.51	1.42	2.39
Ovary	—	—	—	1.63
Gallbladder	1.59	1.74	1.80	3.58
Breast	—	—	—	1.53

Data from the 12-year prospective American Cancer Society study of 750,000 men and women were analyzed to determine the relationship between obesity and cancer site. Overweight men had a higher mortality rate from colorectal and prostate cancer than men of average weight. Overweight women had a higher mortality rate from cancer of the gallbladder and biliary passages, breast, cervix, endometrium, uterus (unspecified), and ovary than women of average weight.

Figure 11-9: Association between Obesity and Cancer

Obesity is a risk factor for common forms of cancer, including breast, prostate, colon, uterine, kidney, gallbladder, and pancreatic. Ad libitum intake of excess calories in animal models has also been associated with enhanced tumorigenesis for breast, colon, and skin cancers. Because laboratory animals tend to develop obesity with age, the preventive effects of calorie reduction in animals are likely to be analogous to the prevention and treatment of obesity in humans by reduction in caloric intake or an increase in physical activity.

Adapted from L. Garfinkel: Overweight and cancer. Ann. Intern. Med. 1985. 103(6 [pt 2]): 1034-1036.

The above statistics confirm the fact that there is such a thing as cancer physiology. In regard to insulin and glucose tolerance, this can best be appreciated in a study done at New York State University, where parameters were checked after women (with and without breast cancer) were given a 100-gram glucose load.[10] This is the normal method to check for glucose intolerance. As can be seen in **Figure 11-11**, compared to healthy women, breast cancer patients had higher levels of glucose, insulin, and Growth Hormone. In regard to the latter point, other researchers have found that Growth Hormone levels are increased in women with endometrial and breast cancer.[11-13]

One of the main problems with high glucose levels in the blood is that it inhibits immune function. It has been found that just one 100-gram glucose load can suppress the *phagocytic index* (mean number of bacteria engulfed by neutrophils) for up to five hours.[14] For the person with glucose intolerance or insulin resistance, this means that immune functions are suppressed all day.

INSULIN STIMULATES CELL REPLICATION

Insulin stimulates the proliferation of a number of cells. Cultured fibroblasts, the cells that make collagen and connective tissues, are the most frequently used cells in studies of growth control. In such cells, insulin *potentiates* the ability of fibroblast growth factor, platelet-derived growth factor, epidermal growth factor, tumor-promoting phorbal esters, prostaglandin F2a, vasopressin, and cAMP (cyclic adenosine monophosphate) analogs to stimulate cell cycle progression of cells arrested in the G1 phase of the cycle.[2]

Insulin has other effects that stimulate cell growth. Insulin regulates more than 100 messenger RNAs (mRNA) in the cells (See **Figure 11-12**). Messenger RNA takes the message from the DNA in the nucleus of the cell and goes into the cytoplasm to direct the assembly of the proper sequence of amino acids to form proteins (enzymes). These mRNAs are the means by

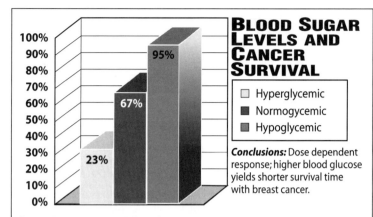

BLOOD SUGAR LEVELS AND CANCER SURVIVAL

- ☐ Hyperglycemic
- ■ Normogycemic
- ▨ Hypoglycemic

Conclusions: Dose dependent response; higher blood glucose yields shorter survival time with breast cancer.

STUDY DESIGN: Mice (BALB/C) injected with aggressive mammary tumor and then placed on three different diets to alter blood glucose. Survival after 70 days was eight of 24 (hyperglycemia), 16 of 24 (normoglycemia), and 19 of 20 (hypoglycemia).

Figure 11-10: This animal study shows that the higher the blood glucose level, the lower the survival rates are with breast cancer.

Adapted from Beating Cancer with Nutrition *by P. Quillin, Ph.D., R.D., CNS., with N. Quillin, Nutrition Times Press Tulsa, OK, 2001.*

which insulin (indirectly) modulates enzyme activity levels, embryogenesis, differentiation, and the growth and replication of cells.

These specific actions of insulin on growth and replication of cells can have some negative effects. The insulin receptor, along with receptors for many other growth-promoting peptides, including the ones stimulated by insulin, have tyrosine kinase activity. Many oncogene products, substances that are produced by genes that stimulate malignant cell replication, are tyrosine kinases. The cytoplasmic portion of the B subunit

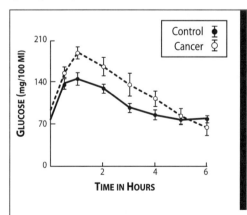
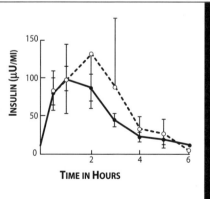
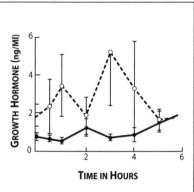

Figure 11-11: The Mean Plasma Glucose, Insulin, and Growth Hormone in 10 Patients with Metastatic Breast Cancer and 11 Healthy Women Given 100 Grams of Oral Glucose

The vertical lines represent ±1 standard error of the mean (SE). This is one of the many studies indicating that cancer patients often have higher glucose, insulin and Growth Hormone levels than people without cancer.

FIGURE 11-12: MESSENGER RNAs REGULATED BY INSULIN[1]

INTRACELLULAR ENZYMES
TYROSINE AMINOTRANSFERASE
PHOSPHOENOLPYRUVATE CARBOXYKINASE
FATTY ACID SYNTHASE
PYRUVATE KINASE
GLYCEROL-3-PHOSPHATE DEHYDROGENASE
GLYCERALDEHYDE-1-DEHYDROGENASE
GLUCOKINASE

SECRETED PROTEINS & ENZYMES
ALBUMIN
ADIPSIN
AMYLASE
α_{2u} GLOBULIN
GROWTH HORMONE

PROTEINS INVOLVED IN REPRODUCTION
OVALBUMIN
CASEIN

STRUCTURAL PROTEINS
δ-CRYSTALLIN

OTHER PROTEINS
LIVER (P33, ETC)
ADIPOSE TISSUE
CARDIAC MUSCLE
SKELETAL MUSCLE

Figure 11-12:
These mRNAs are the means by which insulin (indirectly) modulates enzyme activity levels, embryogenesis, differentiation, and growth and replication of cells.

[1] *This list is selective. Insulin has been shown to regulate at least 100 different mRNAs.*

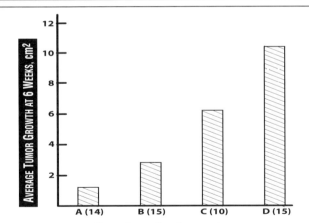

Figure 11-13: Effect of Insulin (2-5 Units per 100 grams Body Weight) and/or 10% Glucose Solution as Drinking Fluid on Growth of Rat Mammary Carcinoma

A: Control Group   **B:** 10% Glucose only
C: Insulin Only   **D:** Insulin plus 10% Glucose

Insulin and glucose both stimulated tumor growth in this study. Statistical significance (student's t test) of difference between matched groups: B—A, $p < 0.01$; C—A, $p < 0.02$; D—A, $p < 0.01$; D—B, $p < 0.01$; D—C, $p < 0.05$.

Adapted from Europ. K. Cancer, Vol. 6, pp. 349-351, by J.C. Heulson and N. Legros. 1970, Pergamon Press, Great Britain

of the insulin receptor has tyrosine kinase activity. This is probably one of the main reasons why people with insulin resistance have an increased cancer risk. The stimulatory effect of insulin on tumor growth can be seen in **Figure 11-13**. In this study, it is clear that glucose (simple carbohydrate) and insulin have a significant stimulatory effect on breast cancer growth.

The stimulatory growth effect on cancer cells by insulin is one of the mechanisms by which insulin potentiates the effects of chemotherapeutic medications. By giving a cancer patient insulin prior to the chemotherapy, the clinician is essentially turning on the cancer to proliferate. **This makes the cancer much more susceptible to the killing effects of the chemotherapy.** It would be like being on a desert island and finally being rescued by a ship. You are taken to the dining hall, and you see piles and piles of delicious, colorful food. You run to the food and just start gobbling. Within five minutes you drop dead because in your ravenous state, you drank some formaldehyde that someone had left accidentally by the food. In the ravenous state to nourish the body, the person is not selective in one's food choices. This is what insulin does to a cancer cell. It makes it hungry for food, and in this state, the cancer cell gobbles up everything, even the chemotherapy given, causing its own death (See **Figures 11-14A and B**).

This strange effect of the cancer cells to insulin may not be so strange as one considers the fact that it is probable that insulin is the sustaining force behind cancer survival. How else would you explain the fact that malignant breast tissue taken after a mastectomy or biopsy when grown in a media results in increased levels of insulin? Or the fact that breast cancer cells have seven times more insulin receptors on their cell membranes than on stromal cells within the tumors?[15-17] In one study, researchers checked the IR content in 27 normal breast samples and compared it to nine specimens of breast fibroadenoma and 159 breast cancer specimens.[16] The average content of insulin receptors in the breast carcinoma specimens was 6.1 ng IR/0.1 mg protein. This value was much higher than the mean value obtained in normal breast tissues (0.95 ng IR/0.1 mg protein) and in breast fibroadenoma tissue (1.09 ng IR/0.1 mg protein) (See **Figure 11-15**). Another fascinating fact of this study was that the IR receptor

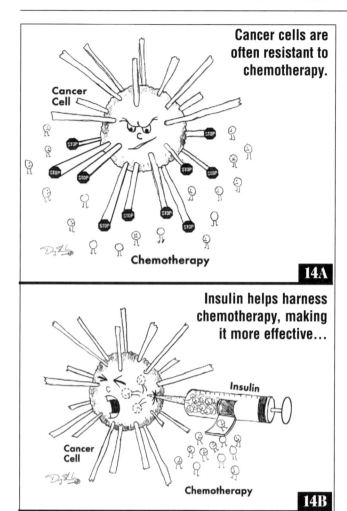

Cancer cells are often resistant to chemotherapy.

Insulin helps harness chemotherapy, making it more effective...

Figures 11-14A & B: Insulin Potentiation Therapy
Insulin stimulates cancer growth and membrane permeability—both of which enable chemotherapy's effectiveness in killing cancer cells.

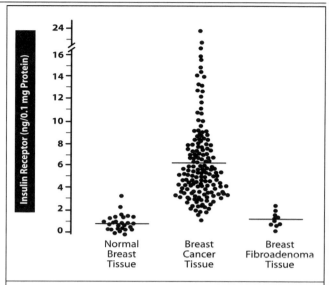

Figure 11-15: Insulin Receptor Content in Normal Breast Tissue, Breast Cancer, and Breast Fibroadenoma Specimens
Breast cancer tissue has significantly more insulin receptors than normal breast or breast fibroadenoma tissue.
Adapted from V. Papa, Status in human breast cancer, Journal of Clinical Investigation, 1990, 86, pp. 1503-1510.

count correlated with tumor size and histological grading (See **Figure 11-16**). The study also found that breast cancer tissue bound ninefold more insulin than normal breast tissue (4.60 of labeled insulin/0.1 mg of tissue protein vs. 0.51 of labeled insulin/0.1 mg of tissue protein). The researchers concluded:

> . . . that insulin receptors are markedly elevated in nearly all breast cancer specimens... Since insulin regulates breast cancer tissues, it is likely that insulin and its receptor plays a role in breast cancer biology.... These observations, although obtained in a limited number of patients, raise the possibility, therefore, that the insulin receptor may play

a role in the biology of breast cancers and that measurement of the IR content should be useful, in conjunction with other parameters, in the classification of breast tumors.[16]

It appears that certain cancer cells, besides producing more insulin and having more insulin receptors than normal cells, also have insulin receptors that have a great affinity for insulin. Researchers in the Department of Physiology at the University of Manitoba in Winnipeg, Canada, found that the binding capacity and affinity for 125I-labeled insulin was twice as great in breast cancer cells than in breast fat cells.[17]

To further promote the concept that insulin is vital to cancer survival, cancer cell insulin receptors do not down-regulate like normal cells. When insulin levels become too high, typically the number of insulin receptors on the cell surface declines. This process is called *down-regulation*. In a study done at Auckland Hospital through the University of Auckland School of Medicine in New Zealand, research found a significant difference in the down-regulation of insulin receptors in cancer cells than in normal cells. In tumor cell lines, grossly supraphysiological concentrations of insulin ($>10^{-6}$ M) were required to induce signifi-

INSULIN RECEPTOR LEVELS AND BREAST CANCER STAGING

Tumor Differentiation	Insulin Receptor Levels (ng IR/0.1 mg Protein)
Well	4.5
Moderate	4.8
Poorly	6.2
Node Status	
Node Negative	5.1
Node Positive	5.7
Tumor Size	
< 2 cm	4.6
2-5 cm	6.0
>5 cm	6.4

Figure 11-16: Insulin Receptor Levels and Breast Cancer Staging

Insulin receptor levels directly correlated with histological types, node involvement, and breast cancer size.

INSULIN, GROWTH HORMONE, AND INSULIN-LIKE GROWTH FACTORS

Insulin-like growth factors (IGFs, somatomedins) are structural homologues of insulin, with insulin-like biological activity. They are mainly synthesized and secreted by the liver but may also be produced by other tissues. When Growth Hormone is made by the pituitary gland, it interacts in the liver to cause the production of IGFs. IGFs are very close to the same structure as insulin, with IGF-1 sharing 43% of its main large sequence and IGF-2, 41%.[19] Since the structures of IGFs and insulin are so similar, they cross-react with each other's receptors.[20] (See **Figure 11-17**.) IGFs, therefore, have the same effects as insulin in their ability to stimulate cell differentiation, proliferation, and growth. IGFs and the IGF receptors have direct tyrosine kinase activity, along with the ability to increase cellular transformation and stimulate cell cycle progression.[21] It is not surprising, then, that elevated serum levels of free IGF-1 are considered a risk factor for major human cancers, including those of the prostate, colon, and breast.[22] Elevated levels of IGFs have been found in Hodgkin's and non-Hodgkin's lymphomas, renal adenocarcinoma, and carcinomas of the cervix and corpus uteri.

cant (>50%) receptor down-regulation. In contrast to results using tumor cells, a 50% reduction in IR levels was observed in human fibroblasts at levels of insulin 3.5 (10^{-9} M) only slightly above the physiological range.[18] This study showed that some tumor cells have a 1000-fold resistance to receptor down-regulation.

Treatment of the cancers caused the IGF levels to drop.[23,24] In these studies, it was also shown that high concentrations of IGFs were present in the homogenates of stroma-free tumor cells, strongly suggesting that the IGFs are secreted by the tumors themselves. Another interesting fact is that IGFs become normal when the person with cancer goes into remission.[25] Another study showed that IGFs in the serum in patients with uterine and cervical cancer was up to 20 times higher than in normal blood samples. The amount of IGFs found correlated with the stage of the disease. The more progressive the disease, the higher the blood level of IGFs. The author believed the IGFs were actually made by the tumors themselves because the levels decreased dramatically after surgery for the cancer.[24] This makes sense because just like with insulin, cancer cells apparently have more IGF receptors than normal cells. In one study, breast cancer cells were found to have ten times more IGF receptors than normal breast and other tissues within the host.[26] Since insulin cross-reacts with IGF receptors, the effects of insulin on tumor cells is compounded.[27] All of the above facts give credence to the notion that insulin will be able to and does stimulate cancer cells and thus will be able to potentiate the effectiveness of medications, especially chemotherapy.

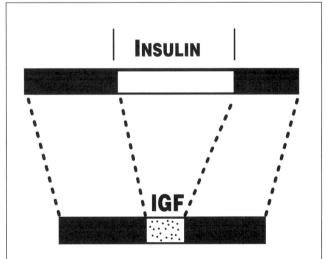

Figure 11-17: Diagrammatic Structures of Insulin and Insulin-Like Growth Factor (IGF-1)

IGFs are very close to the same structure as insulin, sharing over 40% of its main sequence.

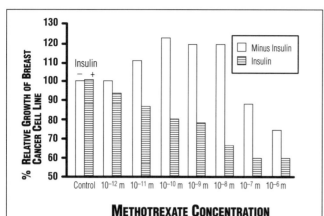

METHOTREXATE CONCENTRATION

Figure 11-18: Relative Growth Effect of MTX (Methotrexate) (10^{-12}M – 10^{-6}M ± Insulin on Breast Cancer Cell Line Cells)
DNA mass measurements were made on pooled cell samples from triplicate flasks on day 1 (24 hrs after cell planting) and day 7 (six days after the addition of MTX). The ratio of total DNA mass of the controls (-INS) on day 7 to the total DNA mass of the controls on day 1 (-INS) represents normal growth (100%). Similar ratios are presented between the total DNA mass on day 7 for each MTX concentration ± INS and the control total DNA mass (-INS) on day 1. Each ratio is then expressed as a percentage of the normal growth ratio. It is clear from this study that insulin potentiated the cancer-killing effects of methotrexate on this breast cancer cell line.

INSULIN THE POTENTIATOR

Knowing the various actions of insulin, the question is, "Can insulin potentiate the effects of various medications?" It is well established that rapidly growing, high-growth fraction tumors are more sensitive to chemotherapy than slow-growing, low-growth fraction tumors. It would therefore be desirable to modify the metabolic characteristics of slow-cycling and noncycling cancer cells in such a way that they develop drug sensitivity comparable to that of fast-cycling cells. The compounds most suited to increase the proliferation of slow or noncycling cancer cells in a controlled manner would be the various growth factors on which they depend. As has already been shown previously, insulin causes increased DNA, RNA, and protein synthesis and can increase the growth of various cancer cell lines.

To test the hypothesis that insulin can potentiate the effects of chemotherapy, researchers at George Washington University in Washington, DC, and the Laboratory of Pathophysiology at the National Cancer Institute in Bethesda, MD, studied the killing effects of methotrexate on breast cancer cells with and without insulin.[28] Methotrexate was chosen because it is more effective against fast cycling phase cells than against resting phase cells. The results of the study can be seen in **Figure 11-18**. The results showed that at concentrations of 10^{-10} M to 10^{-8} M, methotrexate had no cytotoxic effect in the absence of insulin. However, these concentrations were cytotoxic in the presence of insulin, so that 10^{-10} M with insulin was equivalent to 10^{-6} M without insulin. The authors found that insulin could increase the cytotoxic effect of methotrexate up to 10,000-fold. At every concentration of methotrexate used, insulin potentiated its killing effect. They concluded the research paper by saying:

> It is premature to extrapolate these in vitro observations to a clinical trial, but it is possible that the 10,000-fold increase in methotrexate cytotoxicity produced by insulin may establish not only a new way to increase the therapeutic effect of methotrexate but also the principle that metabolic modifiers should be examined as a means to increase the tumoricidal effects of chemotherapeutic agents.[28]

Further research found that insulin specifically enhances a high-affinity carrier system for methotrexate.[29]

The concept of enhancing the therapeutic index of chemotherapy was also the object of a study done at the University of Texas M. D. Anderson Hospital and Tumor Institute in Houston. The researchers noted:

> We have shown previously that a group of hormones stimulate the development and growth of the mammary gland also enhance the clonogenic growth of breast tumors. We have now explored if and to what extent these growth factors can modulate the sensitivity of cells to doxorubicin, an effective agent in the treatment of breast carcinoma.[30]

In this study, human breast cancer cells were incubated with four cell proliferating agents, including insulin. As can be seen in **Figure 11-19**, the percent cancer cell kill was significantly enhanced ($p > 0.001$) for both estrogen receptor-positive and -negative breast cancer cells. The study also showed that insulin and the other growth factors enhanced the doxorubicin cyto-

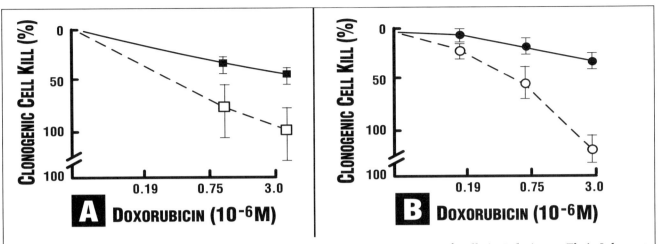

Figure 11-19: Hormone-Induced Modification of the Doxorubicin Sensitivity of Cells in Relation to Their Inherent Estrogen Dependence

Estrogen receptor-negative MDA 468 cells *(A)* and estrogen receptor-positive MCF-7 cells *(B)* were collected from monolayer cultures, and dose responses to doxorubicin in agar cultures were determined in the absence (——) and presence (– – – –) of 17 β-estradiol, epidermal growth factor, insulin, and hydrocortisone. The hormones increased doxorubicin sensitivity for both cell lines significantly (*P>0.001* for both cases). *Symbols,* mean values; *bars,* SD.

toxicity significantly more for the slowly growing (stationary) cell populations, and their effect resulted essentially in an approximation to the doxorubicin sensitivity of the rapidly (exponentially) growing cell populations. The growth factors increased the bone marrow progenitor cells to a much lesser degree to the doxorubicin, causing the author to conclude that "the in vitro therapeutic index of doxorubicin improved for most of the tumors tested."[30] In the discussion section, the author explained:

> The combination of these four growth-stimulatory hormones enhances the doxorubicin-mediated cell kill for most of the tumor cells. The effect was most striking on the subpopulations of the slowly growing cells, both of established and of fresh tumors. While the hormones increased the doxorubicin sensitivity of tumor cells, they did not increase the doxorubicin sensitivity of normal bone marrow cells, the target cells for the doxorubicin toxicity… . Hence, the results of our experiments indicate that tumor-specific growth stimulatory hormones can be utilized to overcome the cytokinetic drug resistance. They act by accelerating the traverse of cells through the cell cycle and by recruiting quiescent clonogenic cells into the cell cycle. They thereby render subpopulations of tumor cells vulnerable to the lethal effects of cell cycle-active drugs that other-

wise would have remained inert to their effects and might have constituted a potential source of late treatment failure.[30]

Remember, this is not Ross Hauser, or Donato Pérez García, Jr. (Donato 3), saying this; it is M. D. Anderson and Tumor Institute! What a promotion for IPT!

What the researchers are saying is that hormones, including insulin, recruit resting cancer cells to become active in protein and DNA synthesis. This is one of the main mechanisms by which insulin potentiates chemotherapy, as it has been found to increase the number of cells in the DNA synthesis part (S phase fraction) of the cell cycle (See **Figure 11-20**). In one study of an asynchronous population of breast cancer cells, the S phase fraction increased by 85% compared to controls.[31]

INSULIN THERAPY IN CANCER

For the fatigued, depressed, and anorexic cancer patient, nothing could be more helpful than insulin therapy. Patients with malignant neoplasms characteristically show progressive weight loss, yet the tumor tissue continues to grow even as the rest of the body becomes depleted. If one thinks about it, the terminal cancer patient resembles, clinically, a chronically starved person. Marion (Hauser) is a registered dietitian and is an expert in parenteral (intravenous) nutrition. She

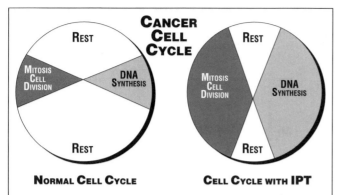

Figure 11-20: Insulin and the Cancer Cell Cycle
During rest periods, cancer cells are impenetrable by chemotherapy. *Note:* With IPT, the cell rest periods become shorter, and the times (during mitosis and DNA synthesis) that the cells can be penetrated by chemotherapy are greatly enhanced. Because the cancer cells are more easily penetrated, the amount of chemotherapy required to kill them is significantly reduced.

worked for many years on the nutrition support team at Hines VA Hospital in Hines, Illinois. At best, intravenous feeding or G-tube (stomach) feeding helps prolong life in the terminally ill, but by itself seldom turns a person around. It is a method to help give some time to allow other therapies to work. The terminal patient on this type of nutrition typically does not regain his or her strength or zest for life. **In contrast, cancer patients, even advanced cases, when given insulin therapy, quickly desire to eat and generally gain weight rapidly if malnourished.** In one study on seven terminally ill patients with cachexia and anorexia, "substantial increases in appetite and body weight, as well as voluntary increase in caloric intake, were observed during a course of daily insulin injections.... All seven patients felt better, and some even slightly euphoric."[32] Perhaps the most amazing part of this study is the insulin was given for only one month. These terminally ill cancer patients were turning their physiology around. What a great side effect of IPT—it gives patients their appetite back, increases their weight, and makes them euphoric!

One of the reasons insulin therapy may make patients feel better is that an insulin-induced coma was an old-time treatment for depression. It was commonplace for hospitals from the 1940s to 1960s to offer this treatment for many different types of mental illnesses, including depression, anxiety, and schizophrenia. According to one of the physicians we know, William Philpott,

M.D., who utilized the therapy, it was remarkably successful. Some psychiatrists utilizing insulin coma therapy for their patients noticed that their malignant tumors were also going into remission. One such physician reported on two cases, one involving metastatic adenocarcinoma of the cervix and the other metastatic melanoma. The only treatment these patients received for their inoperable cancers was hypoglycemic (insulin) comas. The author noted that "in both cases, there was remission of the mental, as well as of the cancer, symptoms."[33] The author felt that the hypoglycemic state causes unutilized oxygen to accumulate in the blood. This causes an alkalosis of the blood. These three cumulative effects then cause a destruction of tumor cells.

IPT AND THE BLOOD-BRAIN BARRIER

There are numerous conditions that affect the central nervous system, including strokes (also called cerebrovascular accidents), transient ischemic attacks, multiple sclerosis, Alzheimer's disease, dementia, amyotrophic lateral sclerosis (Lou Gehrig disease), and transverse myelitis, as well as infections from Borrelia (Lyme disease), syphilis, herpes, HIV (human immunodeficiency virus), and many other organisms. As seen from this list, the treatment options for these diseases are very scarce. The primary reason that treatments for these disorders are almost nonexistent is that **most medications do not adequately pass the blood-brain barrier.**

The blood-brain barrier retards the entry of many compounds into the brain, including chemotherapeutic agents.[34] Theoretically, if there were a way to increase the transport of substances into the central nervous system and through the barrier, the efficacy of treatment would be greatly enhanced.

A complex group of mechanisms closely controls both the kinds of substances that enter the brain and the rate at which they enter. The blood-brain barrier consists of both anatomical structures and physiological transport systems that handle different classes of substances. The anatomical basis of the barrier phenomena is the high resistance tight junction that joins more than 99% of the capillary endothelia of the brain.[35] Fenestrations that make the capillaries porous, as found in endocrine glands, intestines, or kidneys,

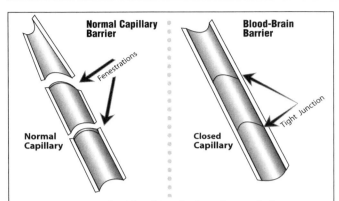

Figure 11-21: The Blood-Brain Barrier and the Normal Capillary

The tight junctions of the blood-brain barrier allow only very small molecules to pass into the brain tissues—thus keeping out most medications.

are absent in brain capillaries (See **Figure 11-21**). Thus, the free movement of circulating substances from the blood to the brain interstitial fluid is markedly retarded, and circulating molecules gain access to the brain only if the molecule has access to a specific transport system localized in the brain capillary epithelial cell. Specific transport systems in the blood-brain barrier have been identified for various different classes of nutrients, the most important of which is glucose (See **Figure 11-22**).

The most vital substance to the brain is glucose. Glucose is the only substrate that can usually be metabolized sufficiently rapidly by the brain to supply its energy requirements. Since the glycogen (storage form of glucose) stores of the brain are negligible, the brain is completely dependent on a continuous blood supply of glucose and oxygen. Although the adult brain is only 2% of body weight, it receives 15% of the total blood supply at rest to support its high oxygen utilization. If the oxygen supply is cut off for four to five minutes or if the glucose supply is cut off for 10 to 15 minutes, brain damage will occur.[36]

The blood-brain barrier, besides being a transport system for specific classes of nutrients, also possesses peptide receptors for insulin, IGF-1, transferrin, IGF-2, and albumin.[37] Various studies have confirmed that there is an insulin receptor localized on the luminal aspect of brain capillaries.[38,39] The receptor-mediated transport of insulin through the barrier explains the finding that **insulin is detectable in relatively high concentrations in the brain.** The insulin that is in the brain

has been found to come from the blood to the brain through this IR transport system.[40]

Although insulin mediates many cellular actions, it is traditionally associated with the enhancement of glucose transport. Insulin has been shown not to increase glucose uptake by the brain. Since insulin stimulates glucose transport and since glucose utilization by the brain is not limited by the transport step (unlike the case for muscle or fat), then it would not be expected that insulin should increase glucose uptake by brain. The exact action of insulin in the brain has not yet been elicited but may include regulation of appetite or other vital brain functions.[40] What is known is that insulin and its receptors are widely distributed throughout the central nervous system, which influences developing brain cells, including the regulation of neuronal maturation. Insulin is also known to stimulate the synthesis of nucleic acids and proteins in cultured brain cells. Of interest is the fact that fetal brain insulin-binding sites show a higher affinity and receptor number than reported for the adult human brain. These findings suggest that insulin plays a role in the growth and development of the nervous system.[41] This would explain some of the beneficial effects of IPT on central nervous system disorders such as multiple sclerosis, strokes, and Lou Gehrig disease. There are very few compounds that can stimulate neurological recovery, but research is showing that insulin is one of them.

In addition to the insulin receptor, there are separate receptors for IGF-1 and IGF-2 on isolated brain capillaries.[42] Although the affinity of the insulin receptor is about the same as the affinity of the IGF-1 or IGF-2 receptors for the respective ligans (compounds that bind to them), the capacity or maximal binding of the IGF receptors is approximately five-fold greater than that for the barrier receptor.[37]

Like insulin, IGF-1 and IGF-2 are internalized by isolated brain capillaries through the receptor transport system. The brain concentrations of IGF-2 exceed those of IGF-1. IGF-2, in particular, appears to be a potent growth factor in the developing central nervous system.[43] Since insulin can cross-react with IGF receptors, this would provide another mechanism through which insulin can stimulate the repair of central nervous system tissue and help curb the devastating effects of the diseases that affect it.

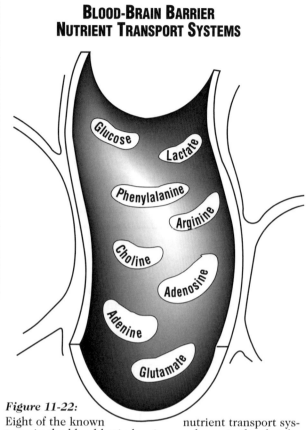

BLOOD-BRAIN BARRIER NUTRIENT TRANSPORT SYSTEMS

Glucose

Lactate

Phenylalanine

Arginine

Choline

Adenosine

Adenine

Glutamate

Figure 11-22:
Eight of the known nutrient transport systems in the blood-brain barrier are shown in the sketch of the brain capillary. The eight different carriers transport classes of nutrients, and the representative substrate is given for each system.

Adapted from Nutrition and the Brain, by W.M. Pardridge, edited by R.J. Wurtmann and J.J.Wurtman, Raven Press, New York, 1986, p. 106.

Just how good is the blood-brain barrier in keeping medications out of the brain? Very good. One of the best studied chemotherapeutic drugs, methotrexate, has been found to have a cerebrospinal fluid:plasma ratio of less than 0.05.[44] In other words, if a person has brain cancer and methotrexate is given, 20 times more of the drug will hit the tissues outside the brain, thus greatly increasing the risk of side effects. It is also doubtful that the little bit of methotrexate that gets to the brain cancer will be effective at eliminating the disease. Antibiotics, such as penicillin, are also normally excluded from the brain.[44]

To enhance drug uptake into the brain, various methods have been attempted, including injecting it directly into the brain or cerebrospinal fluid. Another method has been to make the drug more

lipid or fat soluble to help it cross the barrier. Both methods have had limited success and are often fraught with side effects.

Since the mid-1980s, another more physiologic approach has been studied. It uses the brain's own transport-directed mechanisms to enhance drug uptake into the brain. With the discovery of specific peptide receptor transport systems in the blood-brain barrier, a new strategy for peptide delivery to the brain was seen. The initial work involved the coupling of peptides or enzymes to insulin, which enhanced the uptake of the compound into the brain.[45-47] The main side effect was insulin-induced hypoglycemia, which could easily be eliminated by giving glucose along with the chimeric peptide (insulin-peptide complex).[48]

The initial work on using insulin to give compounds access to the central nervous system started some 50 years prior to the above research. The founder of IPT, Donato Pérez García, Sr., M.D. (Donato 1), showed that insulin given prior to the injection of mercury and arsenic salts could greatly enhance their uptake into the central nervous system.[49] Mercury and arsenic were the conventional antisyphilitic treatments before the advent of antibiotics (1937-1938). A study was then done at Austin State Hospital in Texas to evaluate this new treatment for neurosyphilis (syphilis infection of the central nervous system).[50] Of the nine patients who completed the course of treatment, six showed no more signs of the syphilis infection, as evidenced by clinical recovery and a reversal of their blood tests for syphilis. **A remarkable 66% of the patients tested were cured of their syphilis with IPT.** Syphilis infection of the central nervous system was thought to be incurable at the time.

As with syphilis, HIV infection can have just as devastating an effect on the central nervous system. Often, when HIV infection strikes the central nervous system, there is little that can be done from a pharmacological standpoint, and the disease often progresses to dementia (loss of memory). In November 1986, IPT was first utilized to treat a severely ill AIDS (acquired immunodeficiency syndrome) patient. Within three weeks of treatment in Mexico City by Donato Pérez García y Bellón, M.D. (Donato 2), the patient was in clinical remission, able to resume his normal activities of daily living.[50] He remained well during the next two years of follow-up. The primary treating agent in this case was ribavirin. Insulin was used to potentiate the effects of the drug and increase its transport into the central nervous system. Research by Dr. Ayre and associates confirmed that insulin could increase the concentration of the HIV drug, azidothymidine (AZT), now known as zidovudine, in the brain.[51]

In multiple correspondences between Ross and Donato 3, the efficacy of insulin in enhancing drug uptake into the central nervous system is inferred from the success of IPT in the treatment of such conditions as neurosyphilis, poliomyelitis, HIV, multiple sclerosis, and Lou Gehrig disease. Perhaps even more devastating than these diseases is brain cancer. Malignant gliomas constitute 35-45% of primary brain tumors. Glioblastoma multiforme tumors are gliomas of highest malignancy (grade IV) and are characterized by uncontrolled, aggressive cell proliferation and infiltrative growth with the brain and general resistance to conventional treatment.[52] **This is one of the deadliest cancers, being characterized by aggressive cell proliferation, thus making it an excellent candidate for IPT.** It is only a matter of time before IPT physicians start reporting successful treatment outcomes for brain cancers like glioblastoma multiforme. Insulin, by enhancing the chemotherapy drug's concentration into the brain, would be expected to significantly increase the person's chance of survival. Despite current efforts to improve therapies or to develop new ones, the outcome of treatment for malignant gliomas is very poor, as the median survival after therapy is about 10 months. And people call IPT experimental! IPT, in our opinion, based on what was discussed previously, would improve survival for conditions such as brain cancer because of its effect on the uptake of the chemotherapy drugs into the brain. Since glioblastoma multiforme is a rapidly dividing cell line, chemotherapy will kill it. The problem has been how to get the chemotherapy to the cancer cells. Normal brain cells for the most part would be spared, even with enhanced chemotherapy drug content in the brain, because of their slow cell turnover.

SUMMARY

Since its discovery in the early 1920s, insulin has been helping to save lives. Chris Duffield, the host of www.IPTQ.org, calls IPT "The second discovery of insulin."™ Shortly after the first discovery of insulin, the second occurred. A brave, young physician, Donato 1, decided to treat himself with this new hormone. When his own chronic malnutrition and gastrointestinal problem was cured, he then began using insulin to potentiate the effects of compounds and medications. Thus was born Insulin Potentiation Therapy.

Science has provided an explanation for the remarkable healing effects of insulin and the mechanisms by which IPT work. Though its main action is to lower blood glucose levels, its pharmacological effects are much more vast. Insulin stimulates glycogenolysis, proteogenesis, lipogenesis, and nucleic acid synthesis. It is an anabolic hormone that stimulates the growth or storage of muscle (protein), fat (lipid), and glycogen (glucose).

Insulin receptors are widely distributed over the cells of the body, including on the blood-brain barrier. It has been shown that some tumor lines (cancer cells) have more insulin receptors than normal cells. This mechanism, along with the fact that insulin can activate cancer cells into the S phase fraction of the cell cycle, explains the powerful selective cancer-killing effects of chemotherapy when combined with insulin. Insulin has also been shown to be secreted by various cancers. These cancers often have IGF and other growth factor receptors through which insulin can cross-react. These are other avenues through which insulin can potentiate the effects of compounds on tumor cells.

IPT is also a promising treatment for central nervous system infections, disorders, and cancers. Many diseases, such as multiple sclerosis, Lou Gehrig disease, and brain cancers, have poor treatment outcomes with conventional therapies. Donato 1 showed in the 1930s that insulin could be used to enhance the uptake of compounds in the central nervous system. He successfully treated such conditions as neurosyphilis and acute poliomyelitis. His son successfully treated HIV infection. Besides insulin's ability to enhance drug uptake into the central nervous system, it stimulates nerve cell growth. These are two of the mechanisms by which IPT offers hope to those with disorders that are causing central nervous system deterioration.

Because of the blood-brain barrier, many compounds, including beneficial medications, are kept outside the brain. Thus, the success rate of treatment for brain tumors, especially malignant gliomas, is poor. The most malignant of them is glioblastoma multiforme, which is characterized by uncontrolled, aggressive cell proliferation, making it an ideal candidate for the cancer-killing effects of chemotherapy. The problem is that the chemotherapy cannot pass through the barrier. Since normal brain cells have a very slow turnover, if chemotherapy can reach the brain, it is probable that the success rate for treating brain cancer would be enhanced. Insulin has the potential to do that.

Will IPT be the treatment of choice in the future for multiple sclerosis, Lou Gehrig disease, glioblastoma multiforme, HIV infection, and other central nervous system degenerative diseases? Only time will tell. Surely the scientific background is there to be using IPT in these diseases because the physiology of insulin is truly remarkable. ∎

Potentiation therapy involves Insulin and Chemotherapy.

Hopefully the last chapter convinced you that insulin does play a role in cancer development and, when used in IPT, a role in cancer cure. Most people have no problem with getting an insulin shot, but a shot of chemotherapy is another story. It is not the top thing on the average person's top 10 list…let's see, number five, get some chemotherapy.

It is for this reason that we have written six short chapters to explain why chemotherapy is needed in the majority of cancer patients. It is not the chemotherapy itself that is the problem; it is the way in which it is used. Traditional chemotherapy is given in massive doses, generally once per month. During IPT, low doses of chemotherapy are given typically once per week. Because the insulin helps target the chemotherapy, most patients go through the therapy with few or no side effects.

We can, of course, tell you all of the benefits of IPT, but if there is still that fear of chemotherapy, it will do no good. Just for the record, we shared your concerns about chemotherapy, and to be perfectly honest, Dr. Ayre told us about IPT a full three years before we started doing it in our office. The reason we did not do it when he first told us was the very fact that it involved chemotherapy. "A natural medicine doctor's office is not supposed to do chemotherapy. Chemotherapy is the enemy."

As you might well imagine, after some aggressive cancers went into remission with IPT, saving the patient from side effects and possibly death, our fears of chemotherapy soon evaporated. Chemotherapy, when used optimally, is a potent weapon against cancer. Perhaps it is best to consider IPT, a form of low-dose, high-frequency, targeted chemotherapy. The target is the cancer, and cure is our aim.

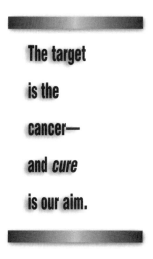

The target is the cancer— and *cure* is our aim.

CHAPTER 12

Chemotherapy—Don't Let the Word Scare You

Mention the word *chemotherapy* to someone, and he or she starts to sweat. Nothing can put fear into someone with cancer quicker than the word *chemotherapy.* What most people do not realize is that **for most cancers, a chemotherapeutic agent is necessary for healing.**

A chemotherapy drug is one that stops and then destroys cancer cells. So if one is to get well from cancer, then some agent that has cancer-destroying effects will have to be given to the patient. Thus, a chemotherapeutic agent is necessary for most cancer patients to heal.

Since the first dose of cytotoxic chemotherapy was given in 1942, hundreds of thousands of chemical agents have been tested for their activity in destroying cancer cells. Relatively few of these drugs reach the stage of clinical testing in animals, and fewer still are found to be safe and effective enough to be tested in humans.

For anticancer drug treatment to be effective, several features must be present. The drug must reach the cancer cells, sufficiently toxic amounts of the drug (or its active metabolite) must enter the cells and remain there for a long enough period of time, the cancer cells must be sensitive to the effects of the drug, and all this must occur before resistance emerges. In addition, the patient must be able to withstand the adverse effects of treatment.[1]

Traditional high-dose chemotherapy causes many side effects because very high doses of the medication are needed to get enough into the cancer cells to kill them. **IPT helps concentrate the chemotherapy into the cancer cells, thus toxicity to the cancer is enhanced, and toxicity to the patient is diminished.**

Anticancer drugs primarily work by stopping and destroying cancer cell division. Most cancer cells are not characterized by rapid growth. For example, breast, lung, and colon cancer cells may take up to 100 days to double their population.[1] The growth and division of normal and neoplastic cells occur in a sequence of events called the *cell cycle.* The various phases of the cell cycle can be seen in **Figure 12-1.** Chemotherapy works best when cells are making DNA in the synthesis (S)

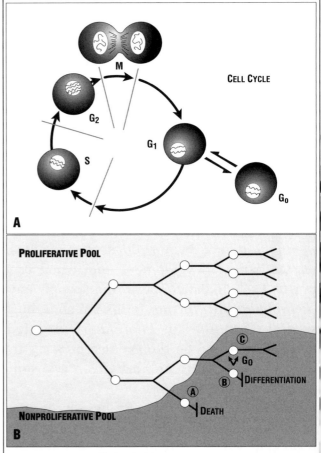

Figure 12-1: Cell Cycle Events

A is a diagrammatic representation of events during the cell cycle. "M" is the period of mitosis—approximately one hour from prophase to cell division. G_1 reflects the normal cell metabolism prior to DNA synthesis and usually constitutes more than half of the total cell generation time. Cells not actively undergoing replication are described as being G_0; they may remain here indefinitely or are recruited back into the cycle. The DNA synthetic (S) phase is generally six to 24 hours. **B** is a schematic representation of tumor growth. As the cell population expands, a progressively higher percentage of cells leave the proliferative pool by death (A), by differentiation (B), or by entering resting phase G_0 (C) from which they may be recruited back into the proliferative pool if the population size is reduced.

phase or are dividing (M phase). Cancer cells that are not actively replicating (G_0 phase) are resistant to chemotherapy medications. It is also possible for cancer cells to get out of the G_0 phase and back into the proliferative pool of cancer cells i[

the population of cancer cells is sufficiently reduced. In other words, the G_0 phase cancer cells represent the cells that chemo will not touch and also function as a reserve to ensure cancer survival. Because insulin helps cells go from the G_0 (resting) to the G_1 phase (proliferating), it increases the chances that the chemotherapy will be effective at destroying all of the cancer cells.

Chemotherapeutic agents that work at a certain point in the cell cycle are called cell cycle-specific agents and need the cancer cells to be actively dividing to work at maximum effectiveness. Since insulin increases cancer cell division, it potentiates the effects of these agents.

The cell cycle consists of various phases that allow cells, including cancer cells, to grow and divide. The cell itself is said to be nonproliferating or resting during the G_0 phase. When cells go into the G_1 phase, they are synthesizing RNA and protein. Once enough RNA and protein is made, the cells progress to the DNA synthesis phase or S phase. Once DNA synthesis halts, RNA and protein synthesis continues in the G_2 phase. During the final stage of the cell cycle, the mitotic or M phase, the cell undergoes cell division and produces two daughter cells.

As stated above, cell cycle-specific chemotherapy drugs work at a specific point in the cell cycle. For instance, Taxol, a common chemotherapeutic agent used in breast cancer, works between the G_0 and G_1 phases. Some of the more common generic chemotherapeutic drugs, such as cyclophosphamide, Cisplatin, and doxorubicin, are not cell cycle specific (See **Figure 12-2**).

What most people do not realize is that many of the chemotherapy drugs are actually extracts of plants. There are a whole host of natural chemotherapy medications, including bleomycin, vincristine, and Taxol (See **Figure 12-3**). Most of these natural chemotherapy agents act by disrupting DNA, which stops cancer cell division and ultimately causes cancer cell death.

During IPT, it is common for the person to receive three or four different agents during a treatment that each kill cancer cells by a different mechanism. This, at least theoretically, will decrease the likelihood of the cancer cells becoming resistant to the drugs used and also will increase the likelihood of cancer cell death.

Most regimes with IPT include an alkylating agent. These are the oldest class of chemotherapy drugs and include cyclophosphamide, chlorambucil, dacarbazine, and Cisplatin. They are not cell cycle specific. Alkylating agents are highly reactive compounds that easily attach to DNA and cellular proteins. The primary mode of action for most of these agents is via cross-linking of DNA strands, which stops the replication of the DNA (See **Figure 12-4**).

Another class of chemotherapy drugs used during IPT is the antimetabolites. This variety of chemotherapy medications works primarily during the S phase of the cell cycle by interfering with the synthesis of DNA. DNA is made up of nucleotides, and one that is specific to DNA is thymidine. Some of the more common antimetabolites work by interfering with the normal metabolism and incorporation of thymidine into

FIGURE 12-2: SOME CHEMOTHERAPY DRUGS AND THEIR RELATIONSHIP TO THE CELL CYCLE

PHASE OF THE CELL CYCLE	NAME OF DRUG PRODUCT	COMMON NAME	MOLECULAR TARGET
$G_0 \rightarrow G_1$	TAXOL	PACLITAXEL	MICROTUBULES
G_1	NONE	—	—
$G_1 \rightarrow$ S TRANSITION	HYCAMTIN, CAMPTOSAR	TOPOTECAN, CPT-11	TOPOISOMERASE I
S PHASE	CYTOSAR, CLADRIBINE	ARA-C, 2-CHLORODEOXYADENOSINE	DNA SYNTHESIS
S $\rightarrow G_2$ TRANSITION	ETOPOSIDE	VP-16	TOPOISOMERASE II
G_2	BLENOXANE	BLEOMYCIN	—
M	ONCOVIN, TAXOL	VINCRISTINE, PACLITAXEL	MICROTUBULES
NONSPECIFIC	PLATINOL	CISPLATIN	NUCLEOPHILES
NONSPECIFIC	ADRIAMYCIN	DOXORUBICIN	TOPOISOMERASE II, DNA
NONSPECIFIC	CYTOXAN	CYCLOPHOSPHAMIDE	NUCLEOPHILES

Adapted from The Biological Basis of Cancer *by Robert G. McKinnell, Ralph E. Parchment, Alan O. Perantonix, and G. Barry Pierce, ©1999, Cambridge University Press.*

FIGURE 12-3: NATURAL CHEMOTHERAPY AGENTS: MECHANISMS OF ACTION

DRUG	MECHANISMS
Aminocamptothecin	Inhibition of topoisomerase I
Asparaginase	Hydrolyzes the amino acid asparagine
Bleomycin	DNA strand scission by free radicals
Dactinomycin	DNA intercalation, inhibition of topoisomerase II
Daunorubicin	DNA intercalation, pre-ribosomal DNA and RNA inhibition, alteration of cell membranes, free radical formation
Docetaxel	Promotes microtubule assembly, stabilizes tubulin polymers resulting in formation of nonfunctional microtubules
Doxorubicin	Same as daunorubicin
Epirubicin	Same as daunorubicin
Etoposide	Inhibition of topoisomerase II
Mitomycin	DNA cross-linking and depolymerization, free radical formation
Mitoxantrone	DNA intercalation, inhibition of topoisomerase II
Paclitaxel	Same as docetaxel
Plicamycin	DNA intercalation and adlineation, osteoclast inhibition
Vinblastine	Tubulin binding (microtubule assembly inhibition and dissolution of mitotic spindle structure)
Vincristine	Same as vinblastine
Vinorelbine	Same as vinblastine

Adapted from The Cancer Chemotherapy Handbook, 5th Edition
©1997, Harcourt Heath Sciences Co.

The specific regime that is chosen for IPT depends on many variables, including the mechanisms of action of the various chemotherapy drugs. Another important factor is the possible side effects from the drugs. Because IPT uses such small doses of the various medications, this does not come into play as it does when traditional high-dose chemotherapy is used. The IPT clinician is primarily concerned with helping the patient do whatever it takes to get well. If it means praying, then pray. If it means taking a bunch of supplements, then bon appetite!

In regard to IPT, it may mean using multiple agents and changing the regime a few times. Whatever it takes is what the IPT clinician and the patient want. For most cancer patients, what it will take is chemotherapy. For this reason, chemotherapy is now a word that is no longer scary. "Chem-o-ther-a-py" is now a word that patients can say. ■

FIGURE 12-4: ALKYLATING AGENTS: MECHANISMS OF ACTION

DRUG	MECHANISMS
Busulfan	DNA cross-linking, alkylation of cellular thiols
Carboplatin	DNA cross-linking
Carmustine	DNA cross-linking; DNA polymerase repair, RNA synthesis inhibition
Chlorambucil	DNA cross-linking, alkylation of cellular thiols
Cisplatin	DNA cross-linking, DNA intercalation, DNA precursor inhibition, alternation of cellular membranes
Cyclophosphamide	DNA cross-linking
Dacarbazine	DNA methylation, alkylation
Ifosfamide	DNA cross-linking and chain scission
Lomustine	DNA cross-linking, DNA polymerase repair, RNA synthesis inhibition
Melphalan	DNA cross-linking, alkylation of cellular thiols
Procarbazine	DNA alkylation, inhibits methyl group incorporation into RNA
Streptozocin	DNA cross-linking, inhibits DNA repair enzyme guanine-0-methyl transferase
Temozlomide	DNA methylation, alkylation
Thiotepa	DNA cross-linking

DNA. Inhibition of DNA synthesis can be accomplished with 5-fluorouracil, which inhibits thymidylate synthase, and methotrexate, which inhibits dihydrofolate reductase. Often the combination of methotrexate and 5-fluorouracil is used to increase the effect.

There are many classes of chemotherapy drugs, including hormones, enzymes, mitotic inhibitors, topoisomerase inhibitors, and others. All have the net effect of killing cancer cells.

CHAPTER 13

Why I Believe Oncologists Are Good, but I Would Get a Second Opinion Before I Let One Treat Me

"A SOBER AND UNPREJUDICED ANALYSIS OF THE LITERATURE HAS RARELY REVEALED ANY THERAPEUTIC SUCCESS BY THE REGIMENS IN QUESTION."

–Ulrich Abel, M.D., in his 92-page review of the world's literature of survival of high-dose chemotherapy-treated cancer patients[1]

When confronted with the diagnosis of cancer, probably the best question to ask a doctor is, "If you were me, what would you do?" This one is easy for me to answer because I (Ross) believe oncologists are good, but I would most likely not let one treat me. They are good at giving chemotherapy. Oncologists in actuality are high-dose chemotherapy experts. They should be called chemotherapists, not oncologists. "Oncologist" comes from the Greek word *onkos*, which means mass or tumor. By definition, an oncologist is supposed to be an expert in cancer, and by inference, cancer physiology. It is my contention that because oncologists do not try to reverse cancer physiology while treating someone, they are not experts in cancer physiology and thus should not be called oncologists; if they know about cancer physiology and do not do anything to reverse it, then they at least are unethical. The later point about cancer physiology, of course, would be important to assist a person fighting cancer in beating the disease, and if oncologists do not tell a patient how to reverse cancer physiology, knowing themselves how to do it, then surely this is not someone I want treating me.

It is necessary to consult an oncologist when faced with the diagnosis of cancer because oncologists are the chemotherapy experts. According to Cecil's *Textbook of Medicine,* 18th edition (the internal medicine textbook used by many medical schools), the following cancers are curable with chemotherapy: choriocarcinoma, Burkitt's lymphoma, acute lymphocytic leukemia, Hodgkin's lymphoma, diffuse histiocytic lymphoma, nodular mixed lymphoma, testicular carcinoma (cyclist Lance Armstrong), childhood sarcomas, and childhood lymphomas. That is it. In the same textbook is a list of tumors responsive to chemotherapy (**Figure 13-1**). From these statistics, it is clear that for the majority of cancers, oncologists do not hold the key to long-term disease-free survival, and as such I would not let them treat me.

FIGURE 13-1: *TUMORS RESPONSIVE TO CHEMOTHERAPY*

CANCER TYPE:	PARTIAL RESPONSE (%)	LONG-TERM DISEASE-FREE SURVIVAL (%)
BREAST CARCINOMA (STAGE III-IV)	75	RARE
SMALL CELL CARCINOMA OF THE LUNG	90	10
GASTRIC CARCINOMA	50	RARE
OVARIAN CARCINOMA	75	10-20
MULTIPLE MYELOMA	75	RARE
ACUTE NONLYMPHOCYTIC LEUKEMIA	75	20
CHRONIC LYMPHOCYTIC LEUKEMIA	75	RARE
PROSTATE CANCER	75	RARE
HEAD AND NECK CANCER	75	RARE
MYCOSIS FUNGOIDES	75	RARE
BLADDER CANCER	60	RARE

"Doc, then why would you even consult an oncologist?" At Caring Medical, we treat many cancer patients. At any one time, we have between 100 and 200 patients who we are actively following. When someone is newly diagnosed with cancer, I recommend that he or she consult an oncologist to see what state-of-the-art modern medicine is doing for his or her disease. **The oncologist's recommendation can also be the starting point for that person's IPT regime.**

The problem with chemotherapy is not that it does not work. It does work. **Chemotherapy kills cancer cells.** The problem is that it kills the patient's immune system and eventually the patient. Since oncologists do not have a way to target the chemotherapy more toward the cancer cells and do not try to reverse cancer physiology, I would not let them treat me, unless after seeing an IPT physician, it was clear that I had a cancer that had a great chance of being cured with high-dose chemotherapy. So what would I do if I had cancer? I would definitely go to a physician who utilized IPT, along with a comprehensive natural approach to reversing cancer physiology. **One** such center is the **Caring Cancer and Interventional Natural Medicine Center (CCINMC) in Oak Park, Illinois.** I personally helped establish it as a place where comprehensive natural medicine services would be available to the cancer patient receiving IPT. There are other places to get IPT, and these can be found at www.IPTQ.org. In **Appendix E** is a list of physicians whom I personally know that perform IPT.

In one of the biggest reviews on the survival of chemotherapy-treated cancer patients, Ulrich Abel, Ph.D., of the Heidelberg Tumor Center in Germany found that chemotherapy alone can help only about 3% of the patients with epithelial cancer (such as breast, lung, colon, and prostate), which kills 80% of total cancer patients.[1] That is why a traditional oncologist for the majority of cancers does not have in his or her armamentarium the tools to cure a cancer patient.

A prominent scientist from the University of Wisconsin, Johan Bjorksten, Ph.D., has shown that high-dose chemotherapy alone destroys the immune system beyond the point of return, which increases the risk for early death from infections and other cancers in these immunodeficient patients.[2] Almost everyone involved in cancer therapeutics would also agree that high-dose chemotherapy substantially reduces a person's quality of life by the mouth sores, malaise, fatigue, hair loss, poor appetite, and numerous other side effects it causes. So if it doesn't increase survival, and decreases one's ability to enjoy life, then I am indeed justified in saying that I believe oncologists are good (at high-dose chemotherapy), but I would get a second opinion before I let one treat me. This conclusion is surely logical.

Donato 1 discovered that there is such a thing as cancerizable terrain. Surgery, radiation therapy, and high-dose chemotherapy do not change this terrain, and thus cancers do not shrink completely and have a high rate of return. He showed that insulin, combined with low dose chemotherapy, changed this terrain. Besides causing cancer cell death, the biochemical terrain of the patient was changed towards normal, thus, the high success rate with Donatian Therapy, later named Insulin Potentiation Therapy.

The only way cancer patients are going to survive longer is not with new chemotherapy drugs but by giving therapies that not only kill the cancer but help reverse cancer physiology. The biology of cancer is well known. Unfortunately, today's chemotherapists (oncologists) do not assist patients in reversing this biology, which is the only possibility of disease cure. IPT helps target chemotherapy and with nutrition and herbal supplementation can be part of a comprehensive program to reverse cancer and cancer physiology.

Where can you get a second opinion? I recommend that you find the best IPT doctor around. Only they have Insulin Potentiation Therapy as a treatment modality and understand that cancer physiology must be reversed through a comprehensive approach. I guess you could say I believe oncologists are good, high-dose chemotherapy is bad, but IPT physicians are excellent, and IPT as a therapeutic modality for cancer is great. ■

CHAPTER 14

Be Careful in Doing Only What Your Insurance Pays For

"WHAT IS THE DIFFERENCE BETWEEN A THREE-YEAR-OLD AND AN INSURANCE COMPANY? MOST THREE-YEAR-OLDS ARE TOILET TRAINED."
—*Anonymous*

Someday, we believe there will be justice. God says so in the Bible. We can only give you a glimpse of the horror stories our patients and we have had to endure at the hand of insurance companies. "Show me the double-blinded studies that it works." "We are not paying for it. Our 'medical expert' said the treatment wasn't warranted." "You should not have gone out of network." Insurance companies will use a million reasons why they will not pay for natural medicine services.

We have tried to talk to the medical experts who work for insurance companies. One such conversation went something like this:

Expert: "Dr. Hauser, why did you do the injections in the patient's neck?"

Hauser: "She had horrible neck pain radiating into her arm."

Expert: "I am sorry; that is not an indication for the injections."

Hauser: "You have to be kidding; the patient doesn't have any more pain. What criteria do you use to pay for the injections?"

Expert: "We aren't going to pay."

Hauser: "You are not answering my question. Tell me what criteria you use to pay for this type of injection."

The conversation quickly turned to me (Ross) yelling at the imbecile. This person is paid by the insurance company, and **if he has no criteria to pay for the procedure, then he is going to deny every claim on every one.** It is sad to say, but we have sometimes encouraged our patients to seek legal action against their own insurance companies (See **Figure 14-1**).

Sometimes this is the only way to get their attention. They do not want lawsuits because the pain and suffering to a cancer patient can be very costly. We sincerely believe that an insurance company that does not promptly pay a legitimate claim puts unnecessary strain on the patient, and for the cancer patient with limited resources, this can be deadly.

People underplay the role of stress. Stress can be the cause of many conditions. Stress puts a strain on the adrenal gland (stress gland), causing adrenal insufficiency, further decreasing a person's ability to handle stress. Stress can be caused by relationships, jobs, mind-set, and a host of other reasons. Stress can also come in the form of an uncaring physician. Often the cancer patient loses hope because of the poor care he or she receives at the hands of his or her oncologist. Too often, the traditional cancer specialist plan has drugs, surgery, and irradiation in his or her armamentarium, forgetting about kindness, the human touch, and caring.

Just like hopelessness can cause a person's health condition to deteriorate quickly, hope can restore one's health. The Bible says in Proverbs 17:22, "A cheerful heart is good medicine." A natural medicine specialist often has a myriad of treatment options available to the patient that the traditional physician knows nothing about. For the person with fatigue, the traditional physician will check thyroid levels, and, when these are normal, give the person an antidepressant even if the person is not depressed. The traditional physician does this because it is the only treatment option that he or she has. Compare this to the many treatment options that natural medicine specialists have at their fingertips to treat fatigue (See **Figure 14-2**).

The natural medicine specialist has many options to recommend (See **Figure 14-3**). In many respects, we believe the natural medicine specialist's remedies are more science-based than the traditional physician's counterpart. We practice good

---

FIGURE 14-2: **NATURAL MEDICINE TREATMENT OPTIONS TO CURB FATIGUE**

❖ CANDIDA PROGRAM
❖ DIETARY CHANGES
❖ DETOXIFICATION
❖ FOOD ALLERGY ROTATION
❖ DIET
❖ OZONE THERAPY
❖ SLEEP HYGIENE
❖ AMP SHOTS
❖ EXERCISE PROGRAM
❖ VITAMIN B SHOTS
❖ NATURAL HORMONE REPLACEMENT
❖ DIGESTIVE ENZYMES
❖ HERBAL SUPPLEMENTATION
❖ ADAPTOGENIC HERBS
❖ REST

DILLING & DILLING
ATTORNEYS AT LAW
ESTABLISHED 1917

1120 LEE ROAD
NORTHBROOK, ILLINOIS 60062
(312) 236-8417
TELEFAX NO. (312) 236-8418
EMAIL: dilling1@juno.com

CALIFORNIA LEGAL ASSOCIATE
R. CHANDLER MYERS
PASADENA, 91101

February 20, 2001

Blue Cross/Blue Shield of Illinois
300 East Randolph
Chicago, Illinois 60601-5099

RE: Your member's name: Paul Verest
Your Identification No.:
Your Claim Number:

Gentlemen:

We represent Paul Verest, Naperville, Illinois. Our client is a Cancer victim, with adenocarcinoma and lung and brain metastasis. In desperation last year he sought the services of Dr. Ross Hauser.   Dr. Hauser is an Internationally renowned specialist and medical author, with patients from all over the World seeking treatment from him. At the time Verest retained Dr. Hauser, his only prospect was that of early death with intensive suffering.

Dr. Hauser's treatment for Verest has resulted in a greater quality of life, a less severe cancer progress and undoubtedly extended Verest's survival time. Supporting Dr. Hauser's expert treatment of Paul Verest has been an amplitude of medical research and knowledge.

Dr. Hauser has treated Verest with chemotherapy modified so as to work favorably on cancer conditions but greatly lessen chemotherapy side effects while not impairing treatment effectiveness. Side effects minimized include nausea, vomiting, loss of appetite, diarrhea, anemia, hair loss, fatigue, mouth ulcers, yeast infections, depression, anxiety, insomnia, pain, and death under certain circumstances.

Needless to say, Verest is very satisfied with the treatment he has received.

Paul Verest has been covered by a health insurance policy issued by Blue Cross/Blue Shield of Illinois. However, the insurance has been rendered virtually valueless by your routine denial of any coverage, on the outrageous pretense that the treatments accorded to Verest are "medically unnecessary". Your arbitrary denials are wrong, unjustified and violate his insurance policy, well providing the basis for future awarding of compensatory and punitive damages. Understandably Dr. Hauser believes that it is the proper function of an insurance company to provide coverage for its policyholders, not to dabble in the practice of medicine.

A good illustration of your bad faith is shown by the statement dated January 29, 2001. $1,548.00 had been billed to Blue Cross/Blue Shield for laboratory services, radioisotope tests, injections, drugs, other treatment, and therapy.

The entire $1,548.00 amount was denied as "not covered", no exceptions even being made for any therapy, drugs or injections!

As a result of your bad faith and denial of coverage, Paul Verest has exhausted his meager resources and faces cessation of his vitally needed medical treatment.

Is it your aim to bring about Verest's premature and wrongful death?

It is hereby demanded that the sums you have heretofore wrongfully denied to Paul Verest, as due and owing under his policy of insurance with Blue Cross/Blue Shield of Illinois, shall be paid forthwith and without further delay. Unless we hear favorably that such payment is promptly to be made, we are authorized to institute a suitable lawsuit for damages, attorneys' fees and court costs.

Very truly yours,

DILLING AND DILLING, P.C.

Kirkpatrick W. Dilling

KWD:mem
bc: Paul and Carol Verest

ADELLE DAVIS FOUNDATION
AFFILIATE

NUTRADELLE LABORATORIES, LTD.
AFFILIATE

Figure 14-1

medicine. Natural medicine is science-based, good medicine. The problem is that much of the research performed on natural remedies or techniques is done in other countries or is anecdotal.

FIGURE 14-3: **NATURAL MEDICINE OPTIONS AVAILABLE TO THE CANCER PATIENT ***

- **Insulin Potentiation Therapy**
- **Adaptogenic Herbs**
- **Cancer Vaccines**
- **Chelation Therapy**
- **Detoxification**
- **Essiac Therapy**
- **Hydrogen Peroxide**
- **Hyperthermia**
- **Immunosupportive Herbs**
- **Intravenous Vitamin Therapy**
- **Laetrile Therapy**
- **Low-Dose Naltrexone**
- **Major Autochemotherapy**
- **Nutriceutical Support**
- **Photoluminescence**

What most people do not realize is that throughout most of history, "proof" of the safety and effectiveness of a new drug or therapy was provided by testimonials from satisfied patients or their doctors, which were then publicized. For many of the most famous treatments available, this is all that was used to get the treatment accepted. This includes penicillin for bacterial infections and insulin for diabetes.

Modern medicine demands that something be proven effective by a randomized controlled trial (RCT). The RCT is a human experiment in which the effects of one drug (or multidrug regime) are directly compared to those of another regimen (or placebo) given to patients with the same diagnosis. The patients are then randomized to either arm of the study and followed for a given length of time.

RCTs provide a lot of useful information, but there are many problems with them. They are still subject to researcher bias, especially if a drug company is paying for the study; researchers can manipulate the data and just report the response rate to show tumor shrinkage and not the survival data that may show that the drug hastened death. The nature of the study may be unethical for someone with a critical disease who needs comprehensive natural medicine care, not just some

drug or placebo. People can lie about whether they are taking the drug or not, and people often "sneak" other treatments while also participating in a drug trial. We have treated patients with natural medicine techniques while they were also in drug research trials. Problems can also occur because of poor design, loose criteria for patient selection, lack of ability to generalize results, journal bias for publishing "positive" results, and statistical inferences that are often of questionable clinical relevance. Some would say that tumor shrinkage is in the latter category if the treatment did not improve the quality of the person's life or extend longevity.

A major goal of the National Cancer Institute (NCI) is to increase patient entry into clinical trials. The NCI-designated high-priority trials program is aimed toward this end.[1] This is a noble goal, but 99.999% of these studies do not involve holistic care and see the cancer patient as a study participant, not as a human being who needs a flexible treatment program. There are many reasons for people not to enroll in clinical studies, the most significant of all is death from their disease. One should realize that even physicians often do not enroll patients in these studies for many reasons (See **Figure 14-4**). An important side note is that many of the experimental treatments done in these clinical trials are paid for by insurance companies. This is an important part of the NCI's agenda as told by their consensus statement back in the 1980s[2] (See **Figure 14-5**).

People with cancer who fail the usual and customary chemotherapy cocktail need to realize that whatever treatment they then do should be considered *experimental*. **Many times this fact wakes the patient out of his or her stupor that somehow modern allopathic medicine is scientific and natural medicine is quackery.** Just because a treatment is given by people in white coats in a sterile white building does not mean it is effective or scientific. Most of what is done to cancer patients is essentially experimental. So even in the worst-case scenario, if someone wants to say that IPT has not yet reached the gold standard of what modern medicine would consider the penultimate…the randomized double-blinded study, at least IPT is safe.

---

* *Having tried these and many other therapies on numerous cancer patients, it is our belief that by far the most successful therapy is Insulin Potentiation Therapy.*

FIGURE 14-4: REASONS FOR *NOT* ENROLLING PATIENTS ONTO A CLINICAL TRIAL

☆ It may harm the doctor-patient relationship

☆ Difficulty with informed consent

☆ Dislike of open discussions about uncertainty

☆ Conflict between roles of scientist and clinician

☆ Limited staff and financial support for research activities

☆ Practical difficulties with the protocol (e.g., procedures, data collection)

☆ Concern with the design of the study

☆ Not developed in collaboration with the other participants

☆ Significance of the scientific question not important

☆ Personal responsibilities if one of the treatments in the trial is found to be unequal

☆ Extra time involved to discuss protocol

☆ Lack of third-party reimbursement

Adapted from New England Journal of Medicine, *310:1363-1367, ©1984, Physicians' reasons for not entering eligible patients in a randomized clinical trial of surgery for breast cancer. K.M. Taylor, R.G. Morgdese, and C.L. Soskoline.*

FIGURE 14-5: IMPACT OF THIRD-PARTY REIMBURSEMENT ON CANCER CLINICAL INVESTIGATIONS: A CONSENSUS STATEMENT COORDINATED BY THE NATIONAL CANCER INSTITUTE

☆ [that] third party coverage should be allowed for patient care costs of all nationally approved (NCI or FDA) cancer treatment research protocols

☆ [that] third party coverage should be allowed for all cancer treatment research protocols, provided these protocols have been approved by established peer-review mechanisms, such as:

A. NCI and other designated cancer centers

B. Recognized national or regional cooperative groups

C. As a part of a peer-reviewed grant endeavor, or

D. Protocols entered into the Physician Data Query (PDQ) System

Adapted from Journal of National Cancer Institute *81:1585-1586, ©1989, Impact of third-party reimbursement on cancer clinical investigations: A consensus statement coordinated by the National Cancer Institute, M. McCabe, and M.A. Friedman.*

Many of the methods and madness used by traditional oncologists (and paid by people's insurance companies) that are touted as scientific have not been shown to extend a person's quality of life. "The reproach that clinical oncologists correctly raise against therapists favoring unconventional methods, that they are unable to give scientific support to their claims, reflects on themselves."[3] Or, to put it in biblical terms, orthodox medicine should first remove the beam from its own eye before criticizing the mote in another's.

We often get patients coming to the office who have been told by their oncologists that they have a "75% chance" of success with high-dose chemotherapy, which the patient interprets as a 75% chance of being cured. What it really means is that the patient has a 75% chance of getting shrinkage and about a 5% chance of being cured. This distinction has already been clearly seen in the previous chapter. Most tumors can be shrunk by high-dose chemotherapy, but few can be completely cleared. There is no arguing that traditional high-dose chemotherapy causes tumor shrinkage; it just destroys a lot of good stuff on the way, making cancer cure very difficult. This idea of response rates (percent chance or percent success) permeates oncology meetings and scientific studies. What a cancer patient is concerned with is survival and quality of life. Modern oncology seldom studies quality of life because **there is no quality while undergoing high-dose chemotherapy.**

Insulin Potentiation Therapy, a treatment that uses insulin and small doses of chemotherapy, will not be quickly picked up by the powerhouses of cancer therapy. There is too much at stake, and the insurance companies are flipping the bill. The world cancer therapeutics market reached $8.6 billion in 1995 and will top the $14 billion mark by 2000. The revenue growth rate in cancer therapeutics has gone up by at least 12% over the last decade.[4] The money in cancer therapy is not in the use of generic medications but in the latest cancer "breakthrough."

For some reason, however, the cost is tremendous for these latest FDA (Food and Drug Administration)-approved medications, and they are often covered by insurance. Blood tests, hospitalization caused by the "approved" medication, and CT scans and MRIs are all covered. The only thing that is not covered is the person's casket and funeral. Everything that kills the person is covered, but the remedies that could save the person, such as herbs, vitamins, YMCA membership, chelation therapy, ozone therapy, and other natural remedies, are not covered. It is sad to say but often IPT is not covered, even though it uses traditional "FDA-approved" medications. Insurance companies can deny coverage because it is not the "usual and customary" treatment; even if the usual and customary treatment hastens a person's death. The insurance companies make sure that this is the treatment he or she is to receive to obtain insurance coverage.

It is time for patients to take control of their health care and their health care coverage. If the insurance company will not cover a treatment that is as effective as the traditional therapy (and probably much more effective) but much safer, the patient should demand that it be covered. Any treatment that improves the person's quality of life should be covered. If the treatment is more effective than the "covered" treatment, again it is up to the patient to stand up for his or her rights. The system will not change unless patients change it.

Most chemotherapeutic agents are FDA approved for one or two cancerous conditions, but are used for many others. (See **Figure 14-6**). For example, Etoposide is FDA approved for use in refractory testicular tumors and small-cell lung cancer, but it is used in many protocols for almost all cancers, including cancers of the breast, brain, adrenal cortex, bladder, and stomach; Hodgkin's lymphoma; and many others. Many of these protocols have not undergone rigorous double-blinded studies. This is just another fact to show that even traditional chemotherapy drugs and protocols are primarily experimental.

FIGURE 14-6: **FDA APPROVED USES FOR ETOPOSIDE**

INDICATIONS AND USAGE:
Etoposide injection is indicated in the management of the following neoplasms:

REFRACTORY TESTICULAR TUMORS:
In combination therapy with other approved chemotherapeutic agents in patients with refractory testicular tumors who have already received appropriate surgical, chemotherapeutic, and radiotherapeutic therapy.

SMALL-CELL LUNG CANCER:
Etoposide injection and/or capsules in combination with other approved chemotherapeutic agents as first line treatment in patients with small-cell lung cancer.

Etoposide, like a lot of chemotherapeutic agents, have only been FDA approved for very limited indications. Yet oncologists use these medications to treat many other cancers. This fact alone proves that most of what is done in traditional oncology is truly experimental.

Adapted from Physicians' Desk Reference, *53rd Edition,* © 1999
Medical Economics Company, Publisher, Montvale, NJ

The fact is that most traditional treatments for metastatic cancer do not work. When high-dose chemotherapy is used for small tumor loads, the cancer goes into remission but then can come back five to seven years later because the cancer physiology has not been reversed. Even when it does not come back and high-dose chemotherapy "cured" the disease, most people vow, *never— and we mean never*—to get the treatment again. Ross' Aunt Karen is one of them. As we are writing this, Karen is fighting for her life. She received high-dose chemotherapy that got rid of the tumor for about six months, but now she has nodules in her lungs. She is a very upbeat person, and we believe her positive attitude is what helped her have such a dramatic response with high-dose chemotherapy. She is now very hopeless. She does not feel she has the strength to go through more high-dose chemotherapy. Many people describe the feeling during high-dose chemotherapy as a living death.

The majority of the people who go through traditional high-dose chemotherapy go through a period of hopelessness. In the words of Winston Churchill, "never, never, never, never give up!" **Where there is life, there is hope.**

One person who did not give up was Judith Meldahl. Despite already having gone through the horrors of traditional chemotherapy, only to have her breast cancer recur, she was determined to continue to fight.

Judy found out firsthand that IPT is not like other cancer treatments. One can go through it *without* side effects. She didn't lose her hair or her blood counts; she just lost her cancer. That was it.

It is exciting to think that now available to Judy and other cancer patients is a tremendously powerful and effective treatment. IPT can give others like Judy the cancer-killing effects they need without the side effects of the *living death*. Going through IPT is more aptly described as *living life*. The person has a choice to feel like *living death* or *living life*. The insurance company may just pay for the living death treatment, which is why people need to be cautious about doing just the treatments that insurance companies pay for. You cannot put a price on life, but apparently the insurance companies have. Choose life. Choose IPT. ■

CHAPTER 15

Understanding the Pharmacokinetics of Cancer Therapy— It Could Save Your Life

Everyone has their top three boring classes in school. Mine would have been geometry, statistics in biology, and pharmacokinetics. The word *pharmacokinetics* comes from the Greek word *pharmakon*, which means "drugs" or "medicines," and the Greek word *kinesis,* which means "movement." Thus pharmacokinetics is the movement of drugs within the human body as affected by uptake, distribution, binding, elimination, and biotransformation. The importance of this field is best stated by the fact that understanding the pharmacokinetics of cancer therapy could save your life!

According to *Cecil's Textbook of Medicine,* 18th edition, approximately 40% of patients with cancer are cured by local or regional forms of treatment. For the remainder, systemic therapy is used at some point during their illness, and in selected diseases and clinical situations, this therapy may be curative. Unfortunately, for the other 60%, death is the usual outcome. As depicted in *The Biological Basis of Cancer,* about 1,228,600 new cases and approximately 560,000 deaths from cancer in the United States occurred in the year 1998.[1] In blunt terms, **modern medicine has little to offer people with cancer metastases. Their only hope is a different approach.**

It is for this reason we founded CCINMC. The only hope for the cancer patient with metastases is to receive therapy at a comprehensive natural medicine center that utilizes the best treatment modalities from around the world. The best treatment for cancer that we have found is IPT, as taught by Donato Pérez García, Jr., M.D., of Tijuana, Mexico, and Steven G. Ayre, M.D., of Burr Ridge, Illinois. The therapy must also be able to reverse the cancer physiology that led to the cancer in the first place. In addition, the natural medicine specialist must understand not only cancer physiology but also the kinetics of cancer and, as importantly, the pharmacokinetics of the agents used to kill the cancer cells.

As I (Ross) am a very visual person, much of what needs to be explained will be in graph form. **Figure 15-1** describes the kinetic phases of tumor growth. Cancer usually cannot be diagnosed until the tumor burden in the patient

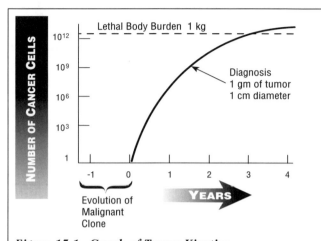

Figure 15-1: *Graph of Tumor Kinetics*
Once a tumor is diagnosed, only ten further doublings are required for the tumor (cancer) to be lethal.

reaches at least 10^9 malignant cells; a tumor burden of 10^{13} cells is lethal.

The kinetics of tumor growth are crucial in determining the prognosis and are also factors in determining response to chemotherapy. The "doubling time" is the time that it takes for the amount of tumor cells to double. The faster the doubling time, the more likely the cancer will respond to chemotherapy but also the quicker (if no therapy is given) the cancer will kill the person. It is felt that a tumor that has reached the size of clinical detectability (1-cm size) has already undergone approximately 30 doublings to reach 10^9 cells.[2] Only 10 further doubling cycles are required to produce a tumor burden of approximately 1 kg (2.2 pounds), which is usually lethal.

During the subclinical phase of the disease (the person does not know he or she has cancer), there are few nondividing cells that have a uniform cell population. In other words, the cancer is made up of rapidly dividing cells that are all about the same type. These are the types of cells that are killed very easily with chemotherapy, since chemotherapy kills rapidly reproducing cells (as evidenced by a person's hair falling out with high-dose chemotherapy). Chemotherapy often does not work with metastatic disease because as a tumor burden increases, the cell population becomes heterogeneous, with some cells resting or nondividing at any given time. These cancer cells have a longer cell cycle, and their growth phase decreases. Thus the percent of cancer cells killed with a given dose of chemotherapy diminishes. Thus, for a given therapy to be effective at curing the person of cancer, it must kill more cells than are regenerated before the next therapy is given. In addition, it must eventually kill enough cancer cells to allow the immune system to finally kill every last one of the cancer cells. The therapy must also do so without killing the patient. The study of the above factors is called *pharmacokinetics*. Do you now understand why understanding pharmacokinetics may one day save your life?

Let's now look at some visual examples. For example, a common cancer that is treated with surgery is breast cancer. Some women receive no other treatment after a mastectomy, whereas some receive radiation and/or chemotherapy. **Figure 15-2** shows three different patients who

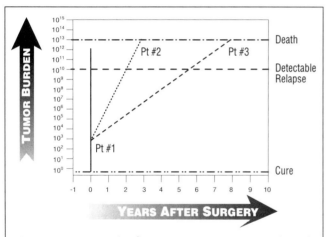

Figure 15-2: Graph of Post Surgery Treatment (Only)
This shows the results of cancer treatment with surgery alone. Three patients each with tumor burdens of 1×10^{12} were treated with surgery alone. In patient one, all of the tumor burden was localized within the resected tissue, and the tumor burden remaining after surgery was an average of <1 cell, so cure resulted. In both patient two and three, 1,000 malignant cells had spread outside the resected area by the time of surgery. Consequently, patient two suffered a relapse from disseminated disease two years after surgery and death at three years from a lethal tumor burden. Patient three did not reach these end points until six and eight and a half years, respectively, even though surgery was equally effective in the two patients, because the residual tumor multiplied more slowly in patient three than in patient two.

Adapted from The Biological Basis of Cancer *by Robert G. McKinnell, Ralph E. Parchment, Alan O. Perantonix, and G. Barry Pierce, ©1999, Cambridge University Press.*

each elected to do nothing after the surgery because it was felt that the disease was localized. In patient one, the surgery cured the disease because there were essentially no cancer cells left in that person's body after the surgery. Unfortunately, patients two and three had 1,000 malignant cells left after surgery that continued to multiply. They each had a recurrent nodule form and eventually died of the disease some three years (patient two) and eight and a half years (patient three) after the surgery. They had recurrences and died at different times because their tumors grew at different rates. Thus, **tumor growth rates will determine the aggressiveness of the cancer and should help determine the aggressiveness of the treatment needed.**

Knowing the doubling time or growth rate of your particular cancer is important and can easily be determined by giving the pathologist a specimen of the live tumor. Anyone undergoing cancer surgery or a biopsy needs to make sure that the doubling times of the cancer cells will be determined from the tumor tissue itself. A person who has a tumor with a doubling time of less than 60 days needs to start treatment today! In such an instance, an aggressive treatment program with IPT would be recommended. The person in such an instance does not have the time to wait to see if herbs and vitamins will work.

VANESSA DOWNEY, LEFT BREAST CANCER HISTOLOGY

Vanessa came to CCINMC because of breast cancer. She did not want to get high-dose chemotherapy. One of the first items that was reviewed was the pathology report on her particular cancer. From **Figure 15-3**, one can see that 7.8% of her cancer cells were in the S phase, which meant that it was fairly rapidly dividing; but what was especially disturbing was that her cancer had a potential doubling time of 19 days. She needed aggressive treatment, so IPT was recommended. She insisted on just doing aggressive natural medicine care. Her case is further explained in **Chapter 23** and shows how in some instances all a person needs is diet and herbal remedies; this is not the prudent course of action, however, when a person's tumor load is great. Vanessa was able to just do natural medicine because the majority of her cancer was removed with the mastectomy and she was diligent in her natural medicine program.

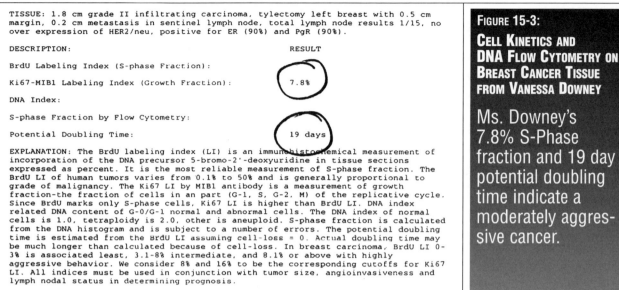

```
TISSUE: 1.8 cm grade II infiltrating carcinoma, tylectomy left breast with 0.5 cm
margin, 0.2 cm metastasis in sentinel lymph node, total lymph node results 1/15, no
over expression of HER2/neu, positive for ER (90%) and PgR (90%).

DESCRIPTION:                                         RESULT

BrdU Labeling Index (S-phase Fraction):

Ki67-MIB1 Labeling Index (Growth Fraction):          7.8%

DNA Index:

S-phase Fraction by Flow Cytometry:

Potential Doubling Time:                             19 days

EXPLANATION: The BrdU labeling index (LI) is an immunohistochemical measurement of
incorporation of the DNA precursor 5-bromo-2'-deoxyuridine in tissue sections
expressed as percent. It is the most reliable measurement of S-phase fraction. The
BrdU LI of human tumors varies from 0.1% to 50% and is generally proportional to
grade of malignancy. The Ki67 LI by MIB1 antibody is a measurement of growth
fraction-the fraction of cells in an part (G-1, S, G-2, M) of the replicative cycle.
Since BrdU marks only S-phase cells, Ki67 LI is higher than BrdU LI. DNA index
related DNA content of G-0/G-1 normal and abnormal cells. The DNA index of normal
cells is 1.0, tetraploidy is 2.0, other is aneuploid. S-phase fraction is calculated
from the DNA histogram and is subject to a number of errors. The potential doubling
time is estimated from the BrdU LI assuming cell-loss = 0. Actual doubling time may
be much longer than calculated because of cell-loss. In breast carcinoma, BrdU LI 0-
3% is associated least, 3.1-8% intermediate, and 8.1% or above with highly
aggressive behavior. We consider 8% and 16% to be the corresponding cutoffs for Ki67
LI. All indices must be used in conjunction with tumor size, angioinvasiveness and
lymph nodal status in determining prognosis.

ELECTRONIC SIGNATURE FOR JOHN S. MEYER, M.D. - 06/04/99 16:45
```

FIGURE 15-3:

CELL KINETICS AND DNA FLOW CYTOMETRY ON BREAST CANCER TISSUE FROM VANESSA DOWNEY

Ms. Downey's 7.8% S-Phase fraction and 19 day potential doubling time indicate a moderately aggressive cancer.

A further explanation of Vanessa's cell kinetic and DNA flow cytometry is needed to really understand why IPT is needed in the majority of cancers for treatment. Remember that chemotherapy works best when cells are in the S phase of the growth cycle. In Vanessa's case, according to the pathology report from her surgery, only 7.8% of her cells are in the S phase, which means that if the chemotherapy drugs just work in that phase, 92.2% of them will not be killed by the therapy. Remember that IPT recruits cancer cells out of the rest phase and into the growth phase, so in Vanessa's case, it would be a great advantage to her to increase the ability of the chemotherapy to target the cancer.

Some practical examples of this need to be explained further. Let's say that a person has metastatic disease, and the pathology report shows a doubling time of two months. By definition, a 1-cm nodule has 10^{10} cells. If the tumor doubles in two months, it will take that person only about seven months to have 10^{11} cells. (This is 10 times the number of cells that occur because with a doubling time of two months, this means that in two months the number of cancer cells doubles; in just four months, it quadruples; in six months, it is eight times the number; and around one year, it will be 48 times the number of cells.) Thus, to meet the lethal tumor burden of 10^{13} will take only two years. Realize, however, that 10^{10} cells represents a 1-cm lesion; if a person has a 2-cm lesion, it is likely that the tumor burden is 10^{11} cells. If metastases are present (in the lymph nodes and beyond), it could well be that the tumor load is 10^{12} cells, and the lethal burden of cancer will be met within a year. *The bottom line with all of this is that by the time a cancer is detected, the disease process is well on its way to killing the person. Treatment needs to start today. There is no time for "thinking."*

A common question that is asked of IPT physicians is, "If the surgery removed all of the tumor, why is chemotherapy recommended?" Well, a physician doing IPT would not say that high-dose chemotherapy is recommended, but IPT and low-dose chemotherapy are recommended. The reason that these are recommended is because cancer is a systemic disease. It is doubtful that any cancer is truly completely localized. Let's say a woman has a mastectomy that reduces the tumor burden from 10^{11} to 10^{6}. In other words, the surgery removed a 2-3-cm nodule in her breast and now there are only 10^{6} or 1 million cancer cells in her body. Using this example, it would mean that the surgery was effective at removing 99.9999% of the cancer cells. This is great, correct? Yes, it is great, but there are still 1 million cancer cells in her body. If she had the same cell kinetic study as Vanessa above, how long would it take for a mammogram to pick up a cancerous nodule? These one million cancer cells will then double every 19 days. So 19 days after the surgery, there will be two million cancer cells; in 38 days, four million cells; within a year, you guessed it…a positive mammogram. Even though surgery helped remove 99.9999% of the cancer cells, if they have a high doubling time, the woman has a chance that the nodule will be back within a year. Once a cancer is diagnosed, it is imperative that some type of systemic therapy be done, and the one we recommend is IPT.

A person with cancer who does no type of treatment to reverse cancer physiology must remember that in between cancer-killing therapies *the cancer is growing*. Even if a person is on a high-dose chemotherapy regime that kills 99.9% of his or her cancer each visit, it probably will

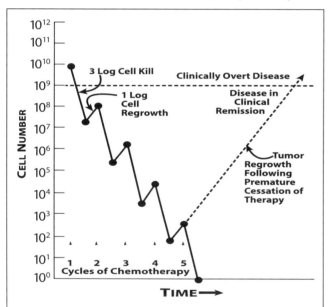

Figure 15-4: Relationship between Tumor Cell Survival and Chemotherapy Administration
The exponential relationship between drug dose and tumor cell survival dictates that a constant proportion—not number—of tumor cells be killed with each treatment cycle. In this example, each cycle of drug administration results in 99.9% (3 log) of cell kill, and 1 log of cell regrowth occurs between cycles. The broken line indicates what would occur if the last cycle of therapy were omitted. Despite complete clinical remission of the disease, the tumor would ultimately recur.

take at least six visits to be cancer free because of the tumor growth that occurs in the four weeks between treatments. Stopping the chemotherapy before complete tumor kill is a sure way to allow tumor regrowth. (See **Figure 15-4**). This is often

what happens with traditional high-dose chemotherapy because cancer terrain is not addressed. IPT, by reversing this terrain and giving the treatments more frequently, typically once per week, reduces the ability of cancers to gain strength between treatments.

Fortunately, most cancers do not grow so quickly, but one should now easily see why oncologists are so quick to rush to chemotherapy. Even in Stage One breast carcinoma, the 10-year survival rate with surgery alone is only 38% in some studies. It is for this reason that even apparent localized disease should be assumed to be systemic metastatic disease and treated as such.

The above principles show that **cancer cure occurs only when the total kill from all therapies used has eliminated the last malignant cell because a single malignant cell has the capacity to regrow into a symptomatic tumor and kill the host.** This is one of the reasons that cancer patients at CCINMC have their cancer markers checked so frequently. One of the specialty tests used is the AMAS test. The AMAS test is an anti-malignin antibody screen and can tell when there are just a few cancer cells in the body or a person's physiology is abnormal (has a cancer milieu).

Theoretically, all of the above examples can occur. We all know people who apparently were "cured" of their cancer only to die two, three, or six years later. Why? Because they formed a new cancer? Not likely. A more plausible explanation is that they were never cured of their cancer in the first place. They still had some cancer cells in their system that probably could have been seen by doing natural medicine cancer marker and physiology testing. The goal of cytoreductive therapy is to reduce the surviving number of malignant cells to less than one cell. It is the belief of most practitioners in natural medicine that if a person's tumor load can be substantially reduced (by traditional therapies or IPT), any residual cancer cells can be killed by a person's immune system, even if some cells remain after treatment. This most likely is the case, but it is false to believe that cancer, by definition, is an immunodeficiency disease. It is possible to have a very strong immune system and not only get cancer but have it thrive. This is why laboratory testing is needed to determine immunoincompetence. If a person has a strong immune system but still has cancer surviving and thriving in his or her body,

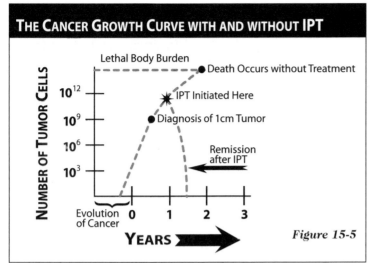

THE CANCER GROWTH CURVE WITH AND WITHOUT IPT

Figure 15-5

then a treatment such as IPT, which has shown remarkable and demonstrable results, is needed. This minimizes the chances of the cancer becoming resistant to the chemotherapy drugs.

By understanding pharmacokinetics, it is clear why traditional chemotherapy for solid tumors (adenocarcinomas) does not work. The following are some of the reasons:

- Solid tumors are composed of slow-growing, heterogeneous cells.

- Some of the cells are in the rest phase of the cell cycle.

- Chemotherapy does not correct cancer physiology.

- Because cancer physiology is not addressed, the cancer cells grow between treatments.

- Cancer cells become resistant to the chemotherapy agent.

IPT helps overcome these concerns. By giving IPT weekly or biweekly, the cancer cells that are not destroyed are not given a chance to repopulate (unlike high-dose chemotherapy, which is given once every three or four weeks, giving cancer cell populations ample time to regrow and regain strength). In addition, IPT is given with multiple agents, with the regime being changed as needed. This minimizes the chances of the cancer becoming resistant to the chemotherapy drugs.

By understanding cancer physiology, it is evident why high-dose chemotherapy with one or two agents, by definition, has to fail. First of all,

nothing is being done to reverse the cancer physiology. Even more important is the fact that because tumors in humans are large (adenocarcinomas are not discovered until a nodule is present with a large tumor load) and are composed of heterogeneous cell populations, treatment will eliminate the most sensitive cells, leaving behind the more drug-resistant population. In addition to the problem of drug resistance, most human neoplasms contain a large fraction of slowly dividing or nondividing cells (up to 90%). Thus for total cancer cell kill to be achieved, the problem of drug resistance and slowly dividing and nondividing cells must be addressed. By giving insulin prior to the chemotherapy, the slowly dividing and nondividing cells are recruited into the growth phase prior to administration of the chemotherapy. By using multiple agents at once (not relying on the cancer being sensitive to a single agent), the problem of drug resistance is minimized. In the course of IPT, it is possible to use multiple agents and to receive multiple and different protocols during a course of therapy to minimize the chances of a cancer becoming resistant to a particular regime or agent. The result for many cancer patients treated with IPT is remission (See **Figure 15-5**). If a person's cancer physiology has been corrected, then the odds of a complete cure are enhanced.

While traditional oncology waits three or four weeks between chemotherapy treatments, the patient's cancer often becomes repopulated, and the person becomes immunosuppressed. This is a formula for continued cancer growth and ultimate spread—metastases and death. A better approach would be to give immunostimulant treatments in between the IPT treatments. Some of these include nutriceutical agents like herbs, a healthy diet, ozone therapy, and other intravenous therapies that help encourage normal organ repair and regeneration. There is now a wide array of intravenous nutriceutical agents available to the natural medicine specialist. Many of these are used with great success at CCINMC or other natural medicine practices, including astragalus, germanium, quercetin, DMSO, licorice root, chelating substances, minerals, vitamins, and other herbal remedies.

The ultimate goal of all of the above is tumor regression and hopefully cure. An objective assessment of the response of a tumor to treatment is of vital importance. Too often subjective impressions of improvement based on a patient's sense of well-being or performance status are not borne out of objective criteria. This is why it is vital for a person to be treated until the blood cancer markers and x-rays/CT scans show that a person is clear of cancer. Then during the first year after treatment, the tests are repeated at least every three to four months. Generally, tests are taken every six months for the next year after that. If after two years the person is still apparently cancer free, then the first piece of chocolate can be eaten! Just joking—a little humor. All this talk about cancer is depressing. After the second year, yearly blood, urine, saliva tests, and CT scans/MRIs are done. Failure to do so puts the person at risk of recurrence. During this time period, markers of cancer physiology are also tested and treated.

Cancers recur even if people start feeling good! Feeling good is a poor indicator of the presence or absence of cancer. Please get regular checkups; and for those fighting cancer, please understand the pharmacokinetics of cancer therapy because it could save your life! ■

CHAPTER 16

Chemotherapy: The Good, the Bad, and the Ugly

"THERE IS A GREAT NEED FOR AGENTS THAT DO NOT INTERFERE WITH HOST IMMUNE REACTION CAPABILITIES, AND FOR AGENTS THAT STIMULATE HOST RECOGNITION OF AND REACTION TO WEAK TUMOR ANTIGENS."
—American Cancer Society

"THE GREATEST FEELING IS BEATING CANCER WITHOUT HAVING TO GO THROUGH ALL THE TERROR OF CHEMOTHERAPY. I WOULD 'ABSOLUTELY' RECOMMEND IPT TO ANY CANCER PATIENT."
—Milenka Glasscock

"ALL I CAN SAY IS 'IT WORKED.' I HAD NO SIDE EFFECTS WITH IPT PHYSICALLY, WHICH DEFINITELY MADE THINGS BETTER FOR ME EMOTIONALLY. I WAS VERY COMFORTABLE DURING THE PROCEDURE AND CAME OUT OF THE HYPOGLYCEMIC STATE RAPIDLY. IPT IS SO MUCH SIMPLER ON A PATIENT THAN CHEMOTHERAPY. THANK YOU FOR HELPING SAVE MY BREAST BUT MORE IMPORTANTLY—MY LIFE."
—Judith Meldahl

The word *cancer* in many people's minds is synonymous with death. All one has to do is consider the statistics to see why this is true. In 1968, the American Cancer Society predicted that one in four people would die of cancer by 1980 and that in the year 2000 it would be one in three (See **Figure 16-1**).[1] By the year 2000, they felt 400,000 Americans would die of cancer each year. It is sad to say that they underestimated it by a large margin, as 552,200 Americans died of cancer that year.[2] Cancer is the second leading cause of death in the United States, exceeded only by heart disease. According to a Reuters Wire Service e-newsletter (March 26, 2001), the World Health Organization (WHO) estimated that the number of new cases of cancer would increase from 10 million to 20 million per year and the number of deaths from six million to 12 million per year.

In 1971, then-president Richard Nixon declared a "war on cancer" to eradicate the disease by the year 2000; needless to say, the National Cancer Institute is losing the war badly. Cancer is the number one health concern of most Americans and for good reason. Each year, about 1.3 million people in the United States are diagnosed with cancer and more than half this number will probably die from the disease or its treatment (See **Figure 16-2**). That is about one

American life lost to cancer every 45 seconds.[3] These statistics do not include the one million cases of basal and squamous cell skin cancers that will occur.

For the past half century, the theory behind cancer chemotherapy has been this: Hit hard, with as much drug as the patient can stand. Kill every tumor cell possible. Give the patient a few weeks to recover. Then do it again. It makes sense because the goal essentially is to poison cancer cells. This works in some cases, but in most cases it fails. The resistant cancer cells seem to gain strength, and once this happens, there is little hope of cure.

It is routine in medical practice for a person diagnosed with cancer to be advised to undergo chemotherapy. What most people do not know is that for most cancers, chemotherapy is ineffective. Although 30% of patients with solid tumors respond to aggressive combination chemotherapy, **Figure 16-3** shows that the vast majority are

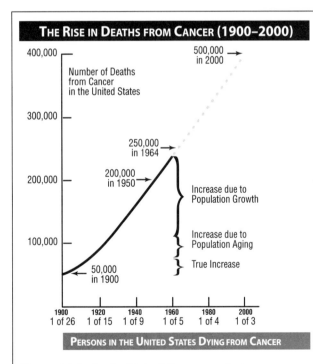

THE RISE IN DEATHS FROM CANCER (1900–2000)

400,000 —
Number of Deaths from Cancer in the United States
500,000 → in 2000
300,000 —
250,000 → in 1964
200,000 — 200,000 in 1950 →
Increase due to Population Growth
100,000 —
Increase due to Population Aging
True Increase
← 50,000 in 1900

1900 1920 1940 1960 1980 2000
1 of 26 | 1 of 15 | 1 of 9 | 1 of 5 | 1 of 4 | 1 of 3

PERSONS IN THE UNITED STATES DYING FROM CANCER

Figure 16-1: In the United States, one in two women, and one in three men will die from cancer.
Adapted from Cancer Statistics, *The American Cancer Society,* ©1968

FIGURE 16-2: **ESTIMATED NEW CANCER CASES AND DEATHS BY SEX FOR ALL SITES, UNITED STATES, 2000***

	ESTIMATED NEW CASES			ESTIMATED DEATHS		
	BOTH SEXES	**MALE**	**FEMALE**	**BOTH SEXES**	**MALE**	**FEMALE**
All Sites	1,220,100	619,700	600,400	552,200	284,100	268,100
Oral cavity & pharynx	30,200	20,200	10,000	7,800	5,100	2,700
Digestive system	226,600	117,600	109,000	129,800	69,300	60,500
Respiratory system	179,4000	101,500	77,900	161,900	93,100	68,800
Bones & joints	2,500	1,500	1,000	1,400	800	600
Soft tissue (including heart)	8,100	4,300	3,800	4,600	2,200	2,400
Skin (excluding basal & squamous)	56,900	34,100	22,800	9,600	6,000	3,600
Breast	184,200	1,400	182,800	41,200	400	40,800
Genital system	265,900	188,400	77,500	59,000	32,500	26,500
Urinary system	86,700	58,600	28,100	24,600	15,700	8,900
Eye & orbit	2,200	1,200	1,000	200	100	100
Brain & other nervous system	16,500	9,500	7,000	13,000	7,100	5,900
Endocrine system	20,200	5,600	14,600	2,100	1,000	1,100
Lymphoma	62,300	35,900	26,400	27,500	14,400	13,100
Multiple myeloma	13,600	7,300	6,300	11,200	5,800	5,400
Leukemia	30,800	16,900	13,900	21,700	12,100	9,600
Other & unspecified primary sites	34,000	15,700	18,300	36,600	18,500	18,100

* Excludes basal and squamous cell skin cancers and in situ carcinomas except urinary bladder. Carcinoma in situ of the breast accounts for about 42,600 new cases annually, and melanoma in situ accounts for about 28,600 new cases annually. Estimates of new cases are based on incidence rates from the NCI SEER program (1979-1996).

Adapted from Facts, The American Cancer Society. ©2000.

resistant. Thus, although combination chemotherapy sometimes cures acute cases of leukemia, Hodgkin's lymphoma, high-grade lymphomas, and testicular cancer, therapy for most solid tumors is administered with a palliative intent. The problem with this approach is that the person lives two months longer but is in misery because of the side effects from the chemotherapy, including hair loss, mouth sores, weakness, depression, poor appetite, and apathy. *The cure rate of traditional chemotherapy for most cancers is almost zero* (See **Figure 16-4**).

The primary factors that determine the response to treatment are the extent of the disease and the type of treatment given. Most tumors are staged by the TNM categories:

T—primary lesion size: T0, T1, T2, T3, T4
N—nodal involvement: N0, N1, N2, N3
M—metastasis: M0, M1

This system allows consideration for the type of malignant spread: T or *primary* for local extent, N or *secondary* for lymphatic involvement, and M for *vascular* dissemination. It is important to appreciate that staging does not imply a regular and inevitable progression. Although some cancers proceed in a typical course by advancing from a primary tumor into secondary nodal disease and eventual remote metastases, many variations exist.

Cancer staging allows the patient and the physician to understand the exact known extent of the disease (See **Figures 16-5A** to **16-5E**). Staging of cancer is an evolving science but generally is as follows:

- **STAGE ONE:** T1, N0, M0—Clinical examination reveals a mass limited to the organ of origin; an operable, resectable, favorable lesion with only local involvement and absence of nodal and vascular spread. Best chance for survival—ranges from 70 to 90%.*

---

* *Survival rates are quoted for patients just using traditional methods of care (surgery, radiation, high-dose chemotherapy).*

Figure 16-3: **IMPACT OF CHEMOTHERAPY ON MALIGNANT DISEASE**
Just a few cancers can be cured with traditional high-dose chemotherapy.

Curable by Chemotherapy:
- Embryonal testicular carcinoma
- Choriocarcinoma
- Acute lymphocytic leukemia of childhood
- Acute promyelocytic leukemia
- Burkitt's tumor
- Hodgkin's disease
- Diffuse mixed and large cell lymphoma

Chemotherapy Improves Survival:
- Wilm's tumor
- Ewing's sarcoma
- Osteosarcoma
- Breast adenocarcinoma
- Ovarian adenocarcinoma
- Acute lymphocytic leukemia of adults
- Acute myeloid leukemia
- Hairy cell leukemia
- Small-cell lung carcinoma
- Colorectal Cancer

Palliation (Comfort) Only:
- Colorectal cancer
- Lymphocytic lymphoma
- Multiple myeloma
- Chronic leukemias
- Prostate cancer
- Metastatic unknown primary cancer
- Kaposi's sarcoma
- Endometrial carcinoma
- Adrenal carcinoma
- Islet cell carcinoma
- Bladder carcinoma
- Neuroblastoma
- Extragonadal germ cell carcinoma
- Soft tissue sarcoma
- Mycosis fungiodes
- Carcinoid
- Malignant melanoma
- Brain tumors
- Esophageal carcinoma
- Head and neck cancer

Adapted from James B. Wyngaarden, Lloyd H. Smith Jr., Cecil Textbook of Medicine, *18th Edition ©1988, J.B. Saunders, Philadelphia.*

FIGURE 16-4: **TUMORS RESPONSIVE TO CHEMOTHERAPY**

	AGENTS*	PARTIAL OR COMPLETE RESPONSE (%)	LONG-TERM DISEASE FREE SURVIVAL (%)
Breast Carcinoma (Stage III-IV)	MTX, FU, Alk, Anth	75	rare
Small Cell Carcinoma of the Lung	Alk, MTX, Pro, Anth, VP-16	90	10
Gastric Carcinoma	FU, Anth, Mit	50	rare
Ovarian Carcinoma	MTX, FU, Alk, Plat, Hex	75	10-20
Multiple Myeloma	Alk, Pred, Vin, Anth	75	rare
Acute Nonlymphocytic Leukemia	Ara-C, Anth, Alk	75	20
Chronic Lymphocytic Leukemia	Alk, Pred	75	rare
Prostate Cancer	HT	75	rare
Head and Neck Cancer	Bl, MTX, Plat	75	rare
Mycosis Fungiodes	Alk, MTX	75	rare
Bladder Cancer	Alk, MTX, Plat, Vel	60	rare

* Combination therapy yields responses in the majority of patients but less than 25% have long-term disease-free survival. Median survival of treated patients is prolonged.

Alk = alkylating agents; Anth = anthracycline (Adriamycin or daunomycin); Ara-C = cytosine arabinoside; Bl = bleomycin; FU = 5-fluorouracil; Hex = hexamethylmelamine (investigational drug available from National Cancer Institute); HT = hormonal therapy; Mit = mitomycin C; MTX = methotrexate, Plat = cisplatin; Pred = prednisone; Pro = procarbazine; Vel = vinblastine (Velban); Vin = vincristine.

Most cancers kill their hosts despite high-dose chemotherapy. IPT, by targeting the chemotherapy, is reversing this trend (cancer death, host alive).

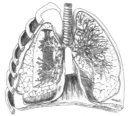

A *Figure 16-5A-E: New International Staging Systems for Lung Cancer*
Cancer generally progresses from Stage 1 (localized) to stage 2 (extended) to Stage 3 (lymph node involvement) to Stage 4 (metastases)—that is if aggressive treatment isn't started.

Normal Lung

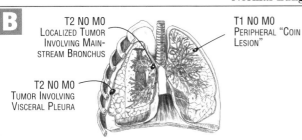

B
T2 N0 M0
LOCALIZED TUMOR INVOLVING MAIN-STREAM BRONCHUS

T1 N0 M0
PERIPHERAL "COIN LESION"

T2 N0 M0
TUMOR INVOLVING VISCERAL PLEURA

Stage 1: No Lymph Node Involvement

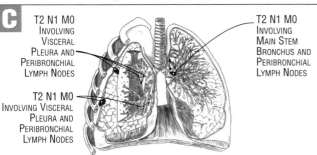

C
T2 N1 M0
INVOLVING VISCERAL PLEURA AND PERIBRONCHIAL LYMPH NODES

T2 N1 M0
INVOLVING MAIN STEM BRONCHUS AND PERIBRONCHIAL LYMPH NODES

T2 N1 M0
INVOLVING VISCERAL PLEURA AND PERIBRONCHIAL LYMPH NODES

Stage 2: Intrapulmonary and/or Hilar Lymph Nodes

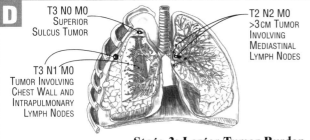

D
T3 N0 M0
SUPERIOR SULCUS TUMOR

T2 N2 M0
>3CM TUMOR INVOLVING MEDIASTINAL LYMPH NODES

T3 N1 M0
TUMOR INVOLVING CHEST WALL AND INTRAPULMONARY LYMPH NODES

Stage 3: Larger Tumor Burden

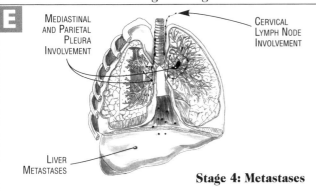

E
MEDIASTINAL AND PARIETAL PLEURA INVOLVEMENT

CERVICAL LYMPH NODE INVOLVEMENT

LIVER METASTASES

Stage 4: Metastases

- **STAGE TWO:** T2, N1, M0—Clinical examination shows evidence of local spread into surrounding tissue and first station of lymph nodes. It is operable and resectable, but because the local extent is greater, there is uncertainty as to completeness of removal. The specimen shows evidence of microinvasion into capsules and lymphatics. Good chance for survival (about 50% ± 5%).

- **STAGE THREE:** T3, N2, M0—Clinical examination reveals an extensive primary with fixation to deeper structures, bone invasion, and lymph nodes of a similar nature. It is operable but not resectable, and gross disease is left behind. Some chance for survival (20% ± 5%).

- **STAGE FOUR:** T4, N3, M1—Evidence of distant metastases beyond local site of origin. Inoperable. Little to no chance for survival (less than 5%).

This staging notation is from the American Cancer Society in 1970.[1] The second edition of *Clinical Oncology,* though, confirms that once distant metastases are found, the outlook for cure is dismal[4] (See **Figure 16-6**).

It is important for patients with cancer to realize that the so-called science-based oncological treatments for metastatic cancer for the over-

FIGURE 16-6: FIVE-YEAR SURVIVAL RATES* FOR SELECTED SITES BY STAGE			
	ALL STAGES %	**LOCAL %**	**REGIONAL %**	**DISTANT %**
ORAL	53	78	42	19
COLON-RECTUM	58	89	58	6
PANCREAS	3	8	4	2
LUNG	13	46	13	1
MELANOMA	84	92	55	14
FEMALE BREAST	79	93	72	18
CERVIX UTERI	67	90	52	13
CORPUS UTERI	83	94	69	27
OVARY	39	88	36	17
PROSTATE	77	92	82	28
BLADDER	79	91	46	9
KIDNEY	55	86	57	10

* *Adjusted for normal life expectancy. This chart based on cases diagnosed in 1983-87, followed through 1990.*

Adapted from Cancer Statistics Branch, The National Cancer Institute.

whelming majority do not work. For a person with cancer or an oncologist to claim that IPT or other alternative medicine is experimental is somewhat hypocritical when one looks at the results with traditional chemotherapy. Giving traditional chemotherapy to a person with a metastatic cancer of a solid tumor is not only experimental but also should be considered unethical considering the dismal results.

Besides dismal results, the high-dose chemotherapy given to people with cancer has horrendous side effects. A good friend of ours, Steve Meyer, recently survived a bone marrow transplant and is now a member of some cancer chat groups. He let us look at some of his e-mails, and here is what we came up with in just a few minutes:

> My experience with Cisplatin, part of ESHAP, was most unpleasant. It is the only thing I have taken that really did bad things to my head. It gave me trouble with vision, concentration, and reading and resulted in an uncharacteristic depression...I also believe that vincristine is responsible for the numbness and tingling in my hands and feet since 1996. (B.H.)

> My husband's treatment with fludarabine caused an acute reaction that caused his body to destroy his own red blood cells (hemolysis). Therefore the doctor does not want to use it again. (J.R.)

> Randy has had neutropenic fever for four days with fevers of 103.8, and his WBC dropped to 0.27. He has no platelets to speak of. He is not eating well and is as white as a sheet. (E.W.)

> I gained a lot of weight during chemo. I went from 178 to 218 and was a bloated looking man with no hair. Needless to say, I had to

Chemo and Me
LESLIE PENNA, BREAST CANCER SURVIVOR

Figure 16-7

When I found out the small percentage that chemotherapy actually improves the odds of no reoccurrence of breast cancer in my case, I decided not to do it. I looked for alternatives and was eager to get Insulin Potentiation Therapy instead of high-dose chemo. Ultimately, however, our conventional doctor friends convinced my husband otherwise, that not doing high-dose chemo was not an option.

The drugs that they used on me were Cytoxan and Adriamycin. My treatments always started with intravenous Compazine to help with the nausea. It didn't help much, and I always felt horrible afterward. All I could eat was rice, mashed potatoes, and yogurt.

My first treatment felt like it lasted six hours instead of two. I had a very hard time staying awake. My head got very stuffed up and foggy. When I got home at about 4 p.m., I went right to bed and didn't wake up again until 1:00 p.m. the next day.

Every time I watched the I.V. being inserted into my arm, I felt like I was getting poison pumped into my body for no good reason. This feeling became worse as I started experiencing side effects. I first was nauseated and then sores started appearing in the back of my mouth and down my throat. The sores stung and made eating a misery instead of a joy. My long hair all fell out, as did the rest of the hair on my body. I felt ugly. I had to buy a wig that the insurance company wouldn't pay for. My fingers turned a dark color and my skin, especially on my face, dried out so much that it felt like sandpaper. Not only did I feel like death, I looked like it. My face gained years of age over the three months of chemo. I got a lot of wrinkles. I had to stop wearing my contact lenses because when I put them in it felt like they were scratching my eyes. At one point my feet hurt so bad that I could hardly walk for three days. I have not recovered from the tenderness to my feet and still can't wear most of my shoes—only gym shoes and shoes with thick, soft soles. My blood cell count dropped and I got a bad sinus infection as well as anemia. Lastly, but not least, the chemo induced me into going into menopause and I am now dealing with irritability, depression, hot flashes, and an overall sense of fatigue and malaise.

I have vowed to never go through that experience again. Through Dr. Hauser's help I am on a natural medicine program and if needed, I plan to do IPT.

I am grateful for the support of friends, family and of course my husband. Our congregation fed us for four months, although it was hard to cook again when they stopped. My husband and I were shown so much love and concern. The one benefit through the whole experience was watching God's hand at work and his magnificent love.

Yes, I am a breast cancer survivor—but perhaps more appropriately—I am a chemo survivor. ◆

get some fat clothes. I bought an inexpensive suit, size 46, to attend a wedding. While the chemo fueled my hunger, I believe that depression was my main problem. (H.H.)

A good friend of ours, Leslie Penna, calls herself not only a breast cancer survivor but a chemotherapy survivor (See **Figure 16-7**). People do not fear chemotherapy; they fear the chemotherapy-induced side effects, which can be

FIGURE 16-8: **POTENTIAL SIDE EFFECTS OF CANCER CHEMOTHERAPY**

ORGAN AFFECTED	SIDE EFFECTS
Bone Marrow	Immune suppression; Low RBCs (red blood cells), WBCs (white blood cells), and Platelets; Increased Risk of Infection; Cancer
Gastrointestinal Tract	Nausea, Vomiting, Anorexia, Weight Loss
Reproductive System	Irregular or Loss of Menses, Infertility, Poor Sex Drive, Early Menopause, Birth Defects
Skin/hair Follicles	Mouth Sores, Hair Loss, Dry Skin
Nervous System	Numbness and Tingling in Feet and Hands, Anxiety, Depression, Inability to Handle Stress
Heart	Cardiomyopathy, Heart Damage, Fluid Retention
Kidneys	Kidney Failure, Kidney Damage, Fluid Retention
Liver	Liver Failure, Liver Damage, Fluid Retention
Muscles	Malaise, Achiness, Weakness, Headache

numerous, including causing cancer itself (See **Figure 16-8**)! Burton Goldberg, publisher of *Alternative Medicine Digest and Cancer Diagnosis: What to Do Next,* put it this way:

> There is a famous saying I love to quote: "Science and medicine advance funeral by funeral." This means old beliefs and practices die out and give way to new approaches only when the older generation of scientists holding them literally die off and leave the fold. We no longer have time to wait for those who swear by conventional medicine to leave the field. The escalation of the rate of cancer demands this urgency. Doctors of all ages must open their minds to new possibilities, to alternative approaches that have been clinically proven to work. Otherwise, the toll of cancer deaths will continue to mount as thousands of cancer patients fail to hear about alternatives that could save their lives.

> Let me adapt that previous famous quote to say: "Cancer care will advance patient by patient." As each cancer patient recovers (his or her) health, thanks to alternative medicine, and tells a friend and the family doctor, this will transform Western medicine.[3]

In September 2000, Dr. Donato Pérez García, Jr. (Donato 3), Dr. Steven G. Ayre, and I went to Bethesda, Maryland, to discuss IPT with the Cancer Advisory Panel (some of the most influential people in cancer care) as part of the National Cancer Institute's Office for Cancer Complementary and Alternative Medicine best case series. The panel of 15 people was somewhat open-minded to the idea of IPT but not as much as Dr. Ayre, the person who arranged the meeting, would have liked. Dr. Ayre spoke for three hours on the science behind IPT, and then we each presented a case of a person who benefited from IPT. The main point I (Ross) discussed and wanted to get across was that **IPT makes it possible for non-cancer specialists, the family physicians of the world, to give chemotherapy in their office.** I am convinced of the increased effectiveness of IPT over traditional chemotherapy, but some on the panel were so ingrained in traditional chemotherapy that it was difficult for them to see this fact. In the middle of the discussion, Dr. Ralph Moss, author of *Questioning Chemotherapy* and *The Moss Reports,* noted that "If Insulin Potentiation Therapy is found to be as efficacious as traditional chemotherapy but minimizes its side effects, then it would mark a great advance in cancer therapy." Dr. Moss went on to explain the issue is not the fact that chemotherapy kills cancer cells but whether IPT is a safer way to do it.

In regard to the cancer grading system, Dr. Ayre came up with an additional layer of disease classification beyond the classical clinical staging. He calls it the SCR score, which stands for

S—Surgeries
C—Courses of chemotherapy
R—Radiation therapy rounds

A breast cancer patient, for instance, may be labeled Stage Four (S1, C6, R8). This would mean the person had one surgery for the cancer, six courses of chemotherapy, and eight rounds of radiation therapy. The SCR score would have a significant impact on the efficacy of treatments, including IPT. **It is best to get IPT as the first-line treatment.** When a person gets IPT as a first-line therapy, there is an excellent chance that his or her immune system is still in good shape, which provides another weapon against the cancer. This is why we have hammered home this point so often. **It is in the cancer patient's best interest to**

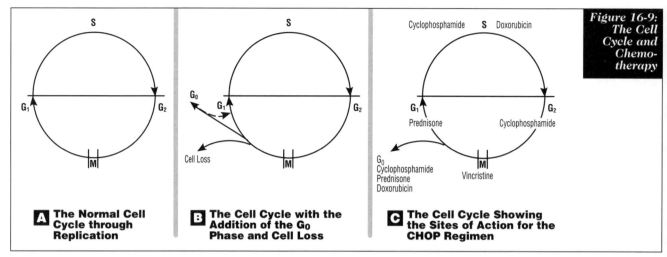

Figure 16-9: The Cell Cycle and Chemotherapy

A The Normal Cell Cycle through Replication

B The Cell Cycle with the Addition of the G_0 Phase and Cell Loss

C The Cell Cycle Showing the Sites of Action for the CHOP Regimen

seek out a consultation with a doctor who performs IPT before he or she is immunosuppressed and malnourished from the ravages of high-dose chemotherapy. The notion that results are excellent with IPT if it is given as a first-line therapy is something that is taught by Donato 3, the world expert in IPT. In the patients whom we have treated with IPT, we have also noted that there is a greater chance of complete tumor regression with IPT if IPT is given as a first-line therapy.

CHEMOTHERAPY KILLS CANCER

Chemotherapy is the treatment of cancer with anticancer drugs. Chemotherapy is typically given by mouth or injection into the veins. The drugs reach and destroy cancer cells in nearly every part of the body. Because anticancer drugs can reach sites that are far away from the original cancer site and can destroy cancer cells circulating in the body, chemotherapy is the primary treatment for many kinds of recurrent cancers and for those that involve metastases in the lung and liver.

Chemotherapy drugs typically kill cancer cells by interrupting DNA synthesis in all cells but will most significantly inhibit the cells that are multiplying the fastest. An aggressive cancer has a doubling time of 60 days or less (meaning how long it takes for the cancer mass to double its size); a moderate cancer doubles in 61-150 days; an indolent cancer doubles in 151-300 days. For a sense of perspective, the average size of a breast cancer when first detected by mammography is about 600 million cells, or about ¼-inch across; the average size detectable by manual palpation has about

45 billion cells and may have a diameter of 1¾ inches.[3] A lump appears after about 30 doublings and only 10 more doublings are needed for death.

Most people with metastases have cancers that have doubling times less than 60 days. These results should be pretty frightening, but not as much as when one considers the potential doubling time of most cancers is actually around 16 days.[5]

Most antineoplastic drugs are therapeutic because they interfere with cell replication, causing death. As has been discussed elsewhere, the typical cell undergoes a cycle that involves four phases: G_1, S, G_2, and M. The phase in which enzymes, structural proteins, and cell organelles are synthesized is G_1 and is sometimes called the first gap or the first growth period. The S phase is the period of DNA synthesis. The second growth period is G_2 or the second gap. The M phase, or mitosis, is the phase when cell division takes place. The rapidity with which cells complete this cycle depends on the generation time for the particular cell population. Cells with a short generation time may reproduce within hours; others may require days, weeks, months, or years.

Beyond a certain point during the G_1 phase, cells will continue through the cycle, but some cells go into a resting phase and for a time do not reproduce. It is these cells that can leave the cell cycle and rest in G_0 that escape the drug-killing effects of chemotherapy and reenter the cycle later (See **Figures 16-9A, B, and C**). After a certain percentage of proliferating cells have been killed, G_0 cells are recruited into the cycle. Cellular function continues without interruption because the surviving cells from the G_0 phase replace the killed cells.[6]

Chemotherapy drugs are classified according to their mechanism of actions and source.

- **ALKYLATING AGENTS:** These act by directly attacking body compounds of importance, such as DNA and enzymes, and usually attack a critical portion of a physiologically important molecule by a covalent bond, thus rendering the molecule unavailable for normal metabolic reactions. Some examples are mechlorethamine, melphalan, chlorambucil, busulfan, cyclophosphamide, ifosfamide, and carmustine.

- **ANTIMETABOLITES:** These drugs cause cancer cells to die by preventing the production of proteins and nucleic acids that cancer cells require in order to form DNA. An antimetabolite is a molecule designed to closely resemble a necessary, well-tolerated substance, such as a vitamin or an amino acid. Once the look-alike is taken up by the cell, its slight difference puts a monkey wrench into normal cellular functioning, interfering with the metabolic pathways of dividing cells and usually interrupting DNA synthesis. Some examples are Methotrexate, 5-Fluorouracil, Cytarabine, Mercaptopurine, and Thioguanine.

- **ANTI-TUMOR ANTIBIOTICS:** These are natural products derived from microbial culture broths of various kinds of Streptomyces bacteria or fungi. These antibiotics interfere with cancer-cell functioning and can inhibit DNA, RNA, or protein synthesis. Some examples are Bleomycin, Daunorubicin, Adriamycin, Mitoxantrone, Mitomycin, and Dactinomycin.

- **PLANT-DERIVED AGENTS:** A number of cytotoxic drugs are derived from plants. These act by disrupting microtubules, which inhibit the cancer cells from replicating. Some examples are Vincristine, Vinblastine, Etoposide, and Taxol.

- **PLATINUM ANALOGUES:** These are substances that contain platinum. They bind to DNA and produce lesions (cross-links) within the genetic material. Cytotoxic effects are derived from these effects on the genetic material. Some examples are Cisplatin and Carboplatin.

The success of any antineoplastic agent is not based solely on the patient's biochemical, cytokinetic, pharmacologic, toxicologic, and therapeutic response. There is a good possibility that malignant cells vary in their sensitivity to cytotoxic agents for reasons other than cell cycle kinetics.

The target of most chemotherapy is DNA synthesis, so cells in the S phase are affected. Antineoplastic drugs damage DNA by:

1. Replacing a hydrogen ion in a substance with an alkyl group (alkylation)
2. Replacing the correct building materials, the purine and pyrimidine bases, with their incorrect analogs
3. Blocking the needed nutrient with antimetabolites
4. Interfering with cell division through a reaction of anti-tumor antibiotics with DNA

Since tumor cells are more rapidly dividing than most normal cells and chemotherapy kills growing cells, why does chemotherapy work so poorly? The answer can be easily answered when one considers that at any one time less than 10% of the cancer cells from solid tumors are in the S phase. In a study done at Washington University Medical Center in St. Louis, Missouri, the percentage of S phase cancer cells varied from 1.1% to 24.4% with a mean of 8.0%.[7]

What is one to do if presented with a recurrence of cancer or metastases? The outlook is bleak if one considers traditional high-dose chemotherapy. To give an example, consider a study on 758 patients who were treated for recurrent or metastatic breast cancer at the Clinical Oncology Unit at Guy's Hospital in London. The response rate following first-line chemotherapy was 34%. The median duration of response was 7.8 months, median time to progression was 3.7 months, and median survival was 7.9 months.[8] From **Figure 16-10**, it can easily be seen that the result for over 99% of the women was death.

There are many reasons why traditional chemotherapy does not cure the majority of cancers:

- Constant fractional survival of cancer cells despite maximum therapy

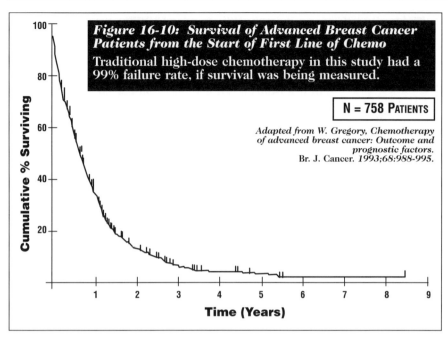

Figure 16-10: Survival of Advanced Breast Cancer Patients from the Start of First Line of Chemo
Traditional high-dose chemotherapy in this study had a 99% failure rate, if survival was being measured.

N = 758 PATIENTS

Adapted from W. Gregory, Chemotherapy of advanced breast cancer: Outcome and prognostic factors. Br. J. Cancer. 1993;68:988-995.

- Small fraction of cancer cells with sensitivity to chemotherapy
- Insufficient chemotherapy kill with each round
- Lack of drugs with sufficient cytotoxic specificity for neoplastic cells
- Lack of drugs with sufficient therapeutic index
- Limitation of host toxicity
- Failure of the drug to get to the cancer site
- Failure of the drug to cross the blood-brain barrier
- Cancer cells resistant to chemotherapy

In cancer chemotherapy, the situation is discouraging because accurate predictions cannot be made concerning the initial effectiveness of a given drug in any individual or concerning the duration of a remission if one is obtained. One might ask, "How can this be?" In human cancer, one is dealing with neoplastic cells that arise from normal cells of the host and whose biochemical mechanisms appear to differ little, but often quantitatively, from those of rapidly reproducing normal cells in the same person. As a consequence, the most potent weapons that chemistry has so far provided, though possessing the potential of preventing the reproduction of all malignant cells in a human individual, cannot accomplish this in the environment of the host. This is because of several factors; probably of greatest importance, however, is the fact that the selective toxicity of the agent for the cancer cells may not be very great.

Modern medicine is finally realizing that the best way to give chemotherapy is not by killing the host along with the cancer by high-dose, low-frequency chemotherapy. Recent research by Canadian and US researchers have shown that in animal studies, small but continuous (high-frequency) doses of cancer drugs can permanently eradicate tumors. The University of Toronto's Robert Kerbel and Harvard University's Judah Folkman, two of the principal investigators into this method of giving chemotherapy, believe that low-dose treatments do not target tumor cells directly but the blood vessels that nourish them.[9] Researchers are now using this method in clinical trials on humans and are noting "the patients also report few or no side effects."[9] As reported by the *National Post,* "Oncologists are being absolutely bombarded."[10] They also stated, "The use of low-dose drugs means the hair loss, pain, nausea, and loss of bone marrow suffered by millions of chemotherapy patients may become a thing of the past."[10] Apparently the three-week break given to cancer patients between their "rounds" of chemotherapy gives the blood vessels supplying the tumor an opportunity to regrow. Chemotherapy given at more frequent intervals does not allow this to happen. Of interest is that other researchers have noted that low doses of the anti-tumor agents cytosine, arabinoside, Adriamycin, and Methotrexate may produce immune stimulation. The theory is that low-dose therapy with an appropriate agent induces the synthesis of one or more of the lymphokines, including interferons, interleukins, and tumor necrosis factor, to increase.[11]

TARGETED CHEMOTHERAPY IS NOW HERE

IPT is able to target chemotherapy because of the many insulin receptors on cancer cell surfaces. Pharmaceutical companies are very aware of the various components of the cancer cell surface. One of the most innovative of these companies is NeoPharm, which has developed liposome-encapsulated drugs to target tumor cells. Liposomes are microscopic membrane-like structures created from lipids (fats). They:

1. Protect the active drug from degradation from the body's natural defenses against foreign objects and

2. Deceive the tumor cells into recognizing the liposome-encased drug as a potential source of nutrition.

So, this company has liposome-encapsulated many chemotherapy drugs including Paclitaxel, Doxorubicin, Mitoxanthrone, and Epirubicin. They also developed pharmaceuticals that contain specifically designed toxins (chemotherapy drugs) that are linked with agents that bind selectively with components on the surface of cancer cells. For example, their tumor-cell identifier, called "Illinois13-PE38," combines with the target receptor "Illinois 13" found in kidney cancer, brain cancer, Kaposi's sarcoma, breast cancer, and head and neck cancer.* These products are currently going through the FDA-mandated drug approval process. Once approved they will be a potent weapon to combine with IPT.

IPT—THE CHEMOTHERAPY OF THE FUTURE

For over 50 years, the Pérez family of doctors have been doing low-dose, high-frequency chemotherapy in the form of IPT. Modern medicine is finally realizing that there are ways to give chemotherapy to get a cancer-killing effect without a patient-killing effect. Do I believe this "new" research will change modern oncology? It is doubtful. Cancer-drug sales are big business in the United States, topping the $5 billion mark (See **Figure 16-11**).

IPT negates many of the reasons that traditional chemotherapy fails. Although giving the same medications, the two therapies are quite different. Consider **Figure 16-12**.

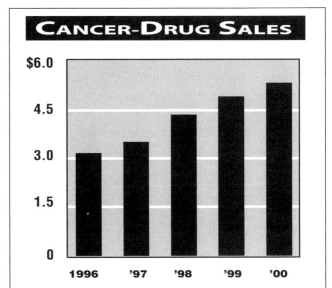

CANCER-DRUG SALES

Total Cancer Drug Sales in the US, including Leukemia Drugs, in Billions

Figure 16-11

FIGURE 16-12: **A COMPARISON OF TRADITIONAL CHEMOTHERAPY AND IPT**

	TRADITIONAL CHEMOTHERAPY	IPT
ENERGY LEVEL	TERRIBLE	GREAT
EXPERIENCE	LIKE HELL	LIKE HEAVEN
FREQUENCY	LOW (GIVEN EVERY 3 TO 4 WEEKS)	HIGH (GIVEN ONCE TO TWICE/WEEK)
HAIR	LOST	KEPT
HOW THEY FEEL DURING	WORSE	BETTER
IMMUNE SYSTEM	SUPPRESSED	STIMULATED
MENTAL STATUS	DEPRESSED/FATIGUED	ENCOURAGED
SIDE EFFECTS	HIGH	LOW
SUCCESS	POOR	HIGH

Traditional chemotherapy involves giving massive doses of medications once every three to four weeks, compared to IPT where low doses (about 10-15% of normal doses) are given once or twice per week. Most patients receiving IPT are seen once a week. Though the same medications are used, IPT is remarkably safe and free of side effects.

In May 2001, Barry Weiner, publicity director for Caring Medical, observed IPT in the office for the first time. The first patient was Harold who

---

* *Information is from* NeoPharm Annual Report 2000. *For more information go to www.neophrm.com*

Dr. Frank C. Noonan

The Lincoln Building
1248 West Main Street • Ephrata, PA 17522
(717) 733-1736

FAMILY PRACTICE

Ross Hauser, MD – Sent Via Fax   May 14, 2001

Dear Ross,

As you are aware, we are utilizing a new approach to cancer therapy called Insulin Potentiation Therapy (IPT). This therapy is relatively new to the United States, but was pioneered and employed in Mexico for many years.

This therapy involves pre-treating the patient with an intravenous dose of insulin, thereby setting up a condition whereby the cancer cells are more sensitive to the chemotherapy agents. This provides a setting where we can administer only 10-15% of the normal chemotherapy dose and yet achieve equal or superior cancer killing rates when compared to the normal high-dose chemotherapy which is generally used by traditional medicine.

The exciting news about IPT cancer treatment is that we achieve excellent results and side effects are practically non-existent. We feel that IPT represents an excellent choice for patients in need of chemotherapy but reluctant to take treatment because of the well-documented side effects of traditional chemotherapy.

The following cases represent some of the patients that we have treated with IPT:

Case #1

A 28-year-old white male with desmoplastic round small cell tumor; this was an extra-testicular tumor with metastasis to the pelvis, abdomen and lymph nodes in the neck. This patient had a large mass in the pelvis and the pancreas, and small bowel were surrounded by tumor. After approximately fifteen treatments, the pelvic tumor had decreased 50% in size and the tumor surrounding the pancreas and small bowel is no longer detectable on CT scan.

Case #2

A 72-year-old white male with non-Hodgkin's lymphoma (Stage IV); large lymph nodes which were malignant in the groin and neck. The patient was given eight IPT treatments and has been in complete remission for the past nine months.

Case #3

A 57 year old white male with a malignant mass in the neck; when we initially saw him the mass was the size of a grapefruit and he could not turn his head to the left. We administered ten IPT treatments to this patient and the mass is completely gone and he moves his head freely in all directions.

Approximately one week ago I received a telephone call from a doctor at the National Cancer Institute in Bethesda, Maryland. They are interested in doing a prospective study to officially investigate IPT as a recognized cancer therapy program.

Thank you, Ross, for your wisdom and encouragement.

Yours truly,

FRANK C. NOONAN, DO

Figure 16-13: As this letter from Dr. Frank Noonan testifies, IPT can be safely done in the office of a family practitioner.

has Stage Four lung cancer. Barry asked him about his experience:

> I feel a little tired, but otherwise I feel great. I know it is working, because the neck mass that I had is completely gone. As I said, I feel great. I do everything I normally do. I knew I didn't want to do regular chemotherapy. Whatever Dr. Hauser says, I do. IPT has worked for me.

The next patient was Ernie who has Stage Four non-Hodgkin's lymphoma. Ernie was explicit:

> I have never felt better. I have had no side effects. I was getting yellow, was jaundiced, and had abdominal pain from my tumor. After the third IPT treatment, my jaundice was gone as well as my pain. I have a great appetite. My energy level is terrific. I would highly recommend IPT to anyone with cancer. There is no comparison to the type of chemotherapy given at hospitals.

We think Barry was in shock. These people had no side effects, yet their cancers were shrinking. Imagine a potent, remarkable cancer therapy that has demonstrable results and the person **feels better** as he or she goes through it. This is IPT.

Besides the low-dose chemotherapy, there are other factors involved in IPT that make it more appealing than traditional chemotherapy. Insulin allows lower doses of chemotherapy to be given and yet maintains a potent cancer-killing effect. Frank Noonan, M.D., a family physician in Ephrata, PA, who works with Gail Gelsinger, R.N. (a long-time friend), wrote me recently of some of his results with IPT (See **Figure 16-13**). This is very exciting for cancer patients because this means they can receive safe treatments by generalists instead of receiving toxic therapies by oncology specialists.

There are many reasons to explain IPT's success. The primary one is the fact that it helps correct almost all of the reasons for chemotherapy failure. IPT potentiates the effects of chemotherapy because of the response of insulin on cancer cells. Insulin, by stimulating cells into the proliferative phases of the growth cycle, allows a greater percent kill with each treatment. Because cancer cells have more insulin receptors than normal cells, the chemotherapy gets into the cancer cells in greater quantities. Insulin allows lower doses of chemotherapy to be used, thus eliminating much of the toxicity of the treatment. To overcome the drug resistance factor in chemotherapy failures, several chemotherapy medications are given with each IPT treatment in order to attack the cancer cells by many different mechanisms. Many physicians who utilize IPT also give immune-stimulating agents during IPT, including interferon, ozone, and vitamins, to maximize immune function.

SUMMARY

Chemotherapy can kill cancer cells but has a low efficacy in curing many cancers. Cancer cells become resistant to chemotherapy for various reasons, including a low percentage of cancer cells in the S phase of the cell cycle during which chemotherapy is most effective, the toxicity of the treatment, the inability of the chemotherapy to get to the cancer site, cancer cells in the G_0 (resting) phase that repopulate the cancer between chemotherapy treatments, and a lack of drug specificity to cancer cells.

Traditional chemotherapy is given in high doses every three to four weeks (low frequency). This is in contrast to IPT where lower doses of chemotherapy are given once or twice a week (high frequency). IPT corrects the reasons for traditional chemotherapy failure because of the physiological reactions of cancer cells to insulin. Insulin stimulates cancer cells to go into the proliferative phases of the cell cycle, thus making chemotherapy more effective. Because cancer cells have more insulin receptors than normal cells, the chemotherapy is preferentially taken up by cancer cells during IPT. To overcome drug resistance, multiple antineoplastic agents are used during the IPT treatments. For all of these reasons, IPT helps chemotherapy hit the target, and when it does, cancer cells are in trouble. ∎

CHAPTER 17

Insulin Potentiation Therapy: The Method

Betty Jo Davis gladly volunteered to show people IPT. Her two-inch by three-inch breast mass completely dissappeared according to her MRI report. IPT helped save her breast—and her life.

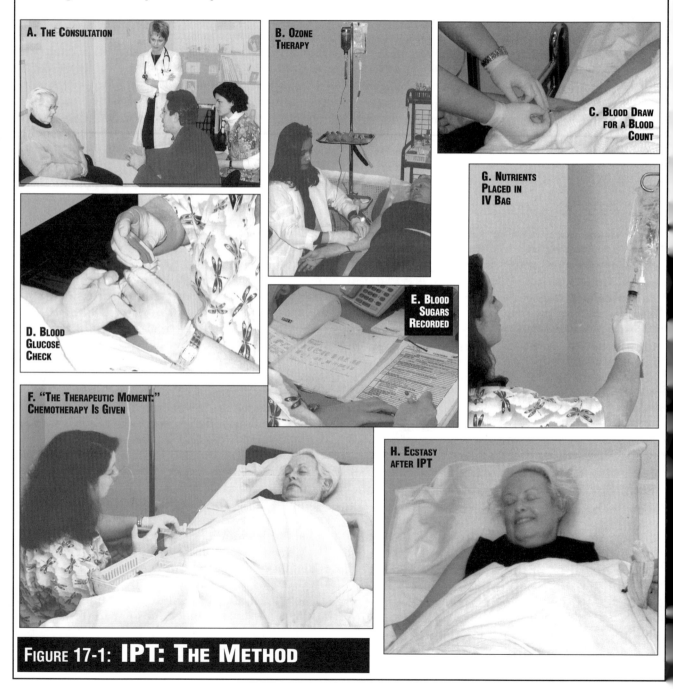

A. THE CONSULTATION

B. OZONE THERAPY

C. BLOOD DRAW FOR A BLOOD COUNT

D. BLOOD GLUCOSE CHECK

E. BLOOD SUGARS RECORDED

G. NUTRIENTS PLACED IN IV BAG

F. "THE THERAPEUTIC MOMENT:" CHEMOTHERAPY IS GIVEN

H. ECSTASY AFTER IPT

FIGURE 17-1: **IPT: THE METHOD**

Insulin Potentiation Therapy is a treatment performed in a doctor's office under his or her supervision. Typically, the treatment is administered by a nurse who has been trained in the technique and is familiar with chemotherapy medications. Throughout the whole procedure, the patient is monitored by the nurse.

On the day of the IPT procedure, the patient is first seen by one of the natural medicine specialists, which in our office is a physician or physician assistant. At this time, the person's questions and concerns are answered. It is also important that the person's progress with IPT be ascertained. For example, "Does the breast mass feel softer?" "Does the breast feel less heavy?" "Has appetite come back?" "Is the bone pain less?" It is very common that the person improves and can "sense" the improvement with each treatment. Small increases in energy, slightly better skin color, improvements in weight, and a happier outlook are all signs that the person's cancer physiology is improving—that the disease process is starting to reverse.

What each IPT treatment involves after this will vary somewhat. Depending on the cancer, the experience of the individual practitioner, and the health of the patient, the protocol can vary. The actual insulin shot and the chemotherapy doses are similar in various offices. The most important aspect of the IPT method is the insulin shot and the chemotherapy; everything else is just gravy.

At CCINMC, the next step that occurs is that a person gets a complete blood count (CBC) done. We have a CBC machine in the office. This measure gives us an idea as to how the person's immune system is handling the treatment. It is typical with traditional high-dose chemotherapy for a person's blood counts to plummet with the first treatment. When receiving IPT, the blood counts may drop, but they drop slowly and can be easily corrected with supplements, medications, or decreasing the frequency of treatments.

The IPT protocol is started after the CBC is verified. At our center, this begins with the patient receiving major autochemotherapy. This involves withdrawing 100-150 cc of blood into a glass bottle and injecting a similar amount of ozone. The blood-ozone mixture is then transfused back into the patient (See **Figures 17-1A** to **17-1F**). The healing effects of major autochemotherapy can be seen immediately as the blood turns a bright red color after the ozone is added.

The patient is next taken to a private room to receive the IPT treatment. He or she is dressed in a hospital gown because there will be some sweating with the treatment. The patient then lies down on the hospital bed, where the nurse takes the patient's vital signs and further explains the technique. A saline bag is added to the intravenous line (which is where the ozone therapy was given). The intravenous bag will eventually contain some nutriceutical agents, which could include selenium, zinc, molybdenum, germanium, B vitamins, vitamin C, glutathione, and DSMO (another potentiating agent).

The patient's blood sugar is then taken. An acid-blocking medication is taken by mouth, which is used to decrease the chance of any gastrointestinal upset occurring. The IPT procedure is then started as the insulin shot is given (See **Figure 17-2**). The time of the insulin shot is recorded (as are all the injections or blood sugar measurements). Approximately 10 minutes after this, the patient receives some intramuscular (buttock area) and subcutaneous (under the skin)

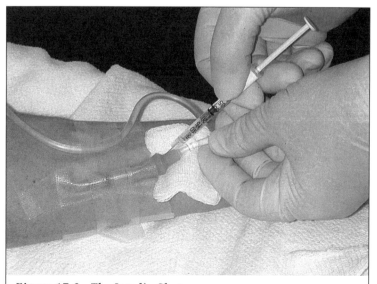

Figure 17-2: The Insulin Shot
Insulin is the main substance that potentiates the cancer-killing effects of chemotherapy during IPT.

shots. These can include a variety of medications and nutriceutical agents, including Toradol (anti-inflammatory), Kutapressin (liver extract, anti-inflammatory), interferon-alfa (immune stimulant), testosterone/progesterone (hormones), and a host of others.

About 15 to 20 minutes after the insulin shot, the patient begins feeling fatigued/sleepy as his or her blood sugar starts to drop. While going through the hypoglycemic symptoms, including a fast heart rate and sweating, the blood sugars are checked. It is generally at the 25- to 35-minute mark after the insulin is given that the person becomes "real hot" and starts profusely sweating. This is the "therapeutic moment," where the person's blood sugar reaches its lowest point (See **Figure 17-3**). The blood sugar is then checked again. The various chemotherapy medications are then injected intravenously. The usual IPT patient receives three or four chemotherapy agents at this time.

The patient is then held in the low blood sugar state for various lengths of time depending on his or her tolerance. Some patients are given a fruit drink to drink immediately after the chemotherapy is given, though some believe that there is a benefit to keeping the blood sugar low for another 20 to 60 minutes. After the chemotherapy is given, the various nutrients are added to I.V. bag.

The patient then generally rests for another 30 to 45 minutes while the blood sugar comes back to normal and the symptoms of hypoglycemia resolve. The patient then puts on his or her clothes and walks out of the office. Most people then go out for a light lunch after the treatment. The average person feels a heightened awareness during and after IPT. Because of the sweating (detoxification) during the procedure, most people feel refreshed after IPT.

Believe it or not, that is it. A person receiving IPT is often nervous on the first visit, but thereafter does not mind the treatment because he or she starts feeling better. This is because the IPT is reversing cancer physiology. Once the tumor load

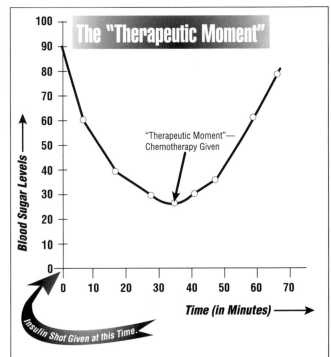

Figure 17-3: The "Therapeutic Moment"

When the blood sugar is at its lowest point, this is called The "Therapeutic Moment." It was given this name by Dr. Donato Pérez García to signify that moment when drugs should be given by an intravenous push. It is at this time that the physiological aspects of insulin maximally target the chemotherapy to the cancer site.

starts decreasing, the person really starts feeling better. In our experience, this occurs between the fourth and the sixth treatment.

Most doctors do some routine blood tests at every other IPT treatment to check liver, kidney, and immune function. About every six IPT treatments, cancer markers are checked. A CT scan, mammogram, or other radiographic study is generally done after eight to twelve IPT sessions. The average number of treatments a person needs is highly variable, from ten sessions for a woman after a mastectomy and very little tumor load to 25 sessions for a large tumor load. Dr. Donato Pérez García, Jr., says the most number of treatments that he has ever given to a patient was 28. ■

CHAPTER 18

Insulin Potentiation Therapy: The Results—
An Interview with Donato Pérez García, M.D.

Dear Donato,

Per our conversation on the phone, I am sending you the interview questions via e-mail. Please answer them as completely and accurately as you can. This information will be used in various publications, but primarily in the IPT book that is soon to be released. This information will be very valuable to patients, and your inclusion in the book will be very helpful for your practice.

For the IPT book, it would also be helpful to have a picture of your grandfather, father, and you together, as well as separate pictures for various parts of the book. Also, a copy of anything about the history of IPT that you feel would be helpful would be welcome. Also, please try to find a picture(s) of you, your father, and your grandfather treating a patient (separately). Each picture you send, if it is used in the book, will have a caption that it is used with permission from you.

The pictures need to be very clear. You cannot send them by e-mail. e-mail pictures do not show up well in print. I need copies of actual photographs. Go to a camera shop and get copies of the photographs and send them to me.

I need these interview questions answered, any other printed material from you that you want in the book, and the photographs in one month. Please do not take longer because the book is almost completed. It goes to the person who is putting it together in early July, and it is planned to be in printed in early 2002.

Ross Hauser

The above e-mail with the questions below was sent to Dr. Pérez in May 2001. He answered them promptly. Dr. Pérez is a very humble, gracious man. He is the world's expert on IPT and has by far the most experience in the treatment. It was his grandfather who discovered Insulin Potentiation Therapy, and he was taught the technique by his father. His opinion is authoritative on the subject of IPT, and, as such, it makes sense to have him answer any questions in regard to the results with IPT. He has been extremely kind and generous to Marion and me.

We have met him on several occasions, most notably at his office in Tijuana, Mexico, where we were trained by him to do IPT (see **Figures 18-1, 18-2, 18-3,** and **18-4**).

THE INTERVIEW
R = Ross

D = Donato

R: Dr. Pérez, thank you for your willingness to participate in this important project.

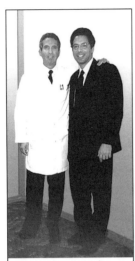

Figure 18-1: After IPT Training

Dr. Donato Pérez García at his office in Tijuana, Mexico with Dr. Ross Hauser.

D: Thank you for inviting me to participate in your project.

R: Can you briefly explain how you and I met?

D: Our first contact was by e-mail. You requested information about the medical technique that I use to treat my patients and asked me if I could teach you and when.

R: Could you please tell us what you recall from your father and grandfather in regard to Insulin Potentiation Therapy?

D: The memories that I have of my grandfather, because I was in seventh grade when he died, are mainly of his relationship as a granddad. He was very kind and always laughed. He enjoyed what my sister and I did as kids.

I learned Insulin Potentiation Therapy from my father. I heard almost daily at home the results he had with patients. And I very often opened the door at home or answered a phone call from distinguished people in politics or the arts who had been successfully treated by my father and who were grateful to him for curing them. During the late 1970s, my father took our family (mother, sister, him, and myself) to Europe during the summertime. It was part holiday and sometimes to visit a pharmaceutical drug company where he presented his papers or a movie about the treatment of cancer. We visited institutions/drug companies in Finland, Germany, Denmark, Holland, and Switzerland.

R: Should your grandfather have received a Nobel Prize in Medicine?

D: I remember that I heard at home the words *Nobel Prize*, not knowing exactly what it was the first time I heard it until years later. Some of my father's friends or patients from the United States or Europe told him that his father

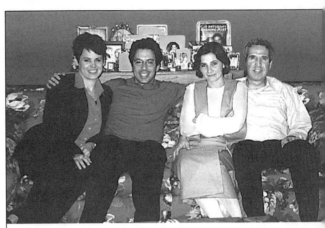

Figure 18-2: The Hauser and the Pérez couples enjoy some time together at Dr. Donato's home in Tijuana.

should have received that prize. Today, April 30, 2001, and after 18 years of experience with the procedure, I am still surprised by all that my grandfather proposed as explanations of his technique with the limited knowledge that he and the scientific world had.

As I once told you, he treated peptic ulcers in the early 1950s with IPT, using penicillin and bismuth salts at a time when surgery was the standard form of treatment, and, of course, *H. pylori* was a mystery. He also treated polio with IPT with complete success at a time when science stated that regeneration of nervous cells did not take place. He treated tertiary syphilis and cured patients at a time when there were no antibiotics. As evidence, a *Time* magazine reporter in 1944 wrote an amazing note about my grandfather's treatment when he was invited to the Naval Hospital in San Diego, Calif.

I now believe that my grandfather was ahead of his time by at least 70 years. And I now believe that he really did deserve that prize. As a medical doctor, he had vision, but he was not understood by medical science of his time. What he discovered and repeated several times in almost all his patients in Mexico and the United States was way ahead of the technological developments of his time. And thanks to my father, who was the only doctor who learned the technique and who endured humiliation by his peers, we are here writing/talking about it.

R: Tell us about his and your patents for IPT.

D: Official U.S. Patent Office high-resolution image files (TIF format) of the original IPT patents are now available free on www.IPTQ.org.

Back in 1934 when my grandfather went to Washington, D.C., he prepared a U.S. patent application for his procedure, which was filed in 1935 and granted in 1939. Then in the early 1990s, two more patents, more detailed and with a wider spectrum, were obtained.

R: Did you know early on when you were in medical training that you would be practicing Insulin Potentiation Therapy?

D: Yes. Why? Well because it was there; I have heard about it since I was, well since the beginning of my beginning.

R: How long have you been practicing IPT?

D: For 18 years. I started in June 1983.

R: Some people have concerns about the safety of IPT. What is its track record?

D: There are two types of people who have concerns about IPT: **1.** doctors who fear what they do not know and who do not read the manuals as they learn a new technique and **2.** ignorant people who enjoy talking about something without getting information from the source. In my experience, my father's 44 years of practice, and my grandfather's 41 years of experience with IPT, no patient has died as a result of the procedure, during the procedure, or after the procedure.

R: How does a person feel during and after IPT?

D: During the mild induced hypoglycemia, you feel relaxed and hungry; sleepy and comfortable. After the IPT treatment is finished, you feel that your energy is increased, and, depending on the disease, some improvement. I had three IPT treatments back in 1983 to experience what my patients would feel.

R: Do people throw up and lose their hair?

D: I can give you two answers to this question. The medical answer is *no*. And the answer I give my patients is: If you lose your hair, please let me know as soon as possible because you would be my first bald patient. Oh! I forgot: no need to worry about embarrassing and disgusting moments with vomit.

R: Whenever a therapy has been around a long time and is not well known, people are skeptical of it. How come IPT is not better known?

D: I can think of several answers or excuses, but the real truth is that doctors in power have made all efforts to ignore it. When something is ignored, it is not in the news. Why do I think they have done that? Mainly ignorance from their part. Also, the name my grandfather used to refer to his work was inappropriate because scientists and doctors misunderstood the concept. And when you are 70 years ahead of your time…well, try talking about software and personal computers to people in the 1930s and try to sell them one, telling them, of course, that for their convenience you accept VISA or MasterCard. [laughing]

R: It is common to use chemotherapeutic drugs with IPT in the treatment of cancer. The word *chemotherapy* scares a lot of people. Does the chemotherapy in IPT cause side effects?

D: I cannot change the common sense about the word *chemotherapy*, but the word only means that we are using a chemical substance to do some therapeutic effect. Treating cancer with IPT means that a doctor will be targeting only the malignant cells, using small doses, thus leaving the normal cells unaffected. So side effects are rare.

R: What conditions is IPT most helpful for?

D: For all diseases for which there is a prescription drug or chemical substance with a known and scientifically proven effect on that condition. Examples are asthma, bronchitis, gastritis, peptic ulcers, prostate enlargement, viral infections, solid tumors (benign and cancerous), and arthritis.

R: Could you tell us about some of the cases you have treated?

D: I will describe four cases, and I am sure you will understand the importance of these.

My first patient, I mean, the very first time I was in charge of a patient, was in early December 1983. He was an 85-year-old male with a 40-year history of emphysema. He was referred by a patient who had been successfully treated by my father. He had a consultation with both of us, and then my father told me to write my treatment in the chart and give it to the nurse. At this point, I was really doing an excellent job.

But first let me tell you an anecdote about the nurses at our clinic in Mexico City. One morning, the three nurses my father had, including the most experienced who was trained by my grandfather and working there for at least 16 years, did not show up to work. Why? I had caught them in a business of reselling prescription drugs to patients, saving patients a trip to the drugstore. So they quit. Well, I solved the emergency by calling a service, and they sent two nurses to help out with patient cleaning and nursing duties other than drug administration.

The youngest nurse, Petra Calixto Morales, saw no problem, and she was determined to do IPT with me and my father. She received my chart, began to fill syringes and prepare the medications, and took them to my patient. He had gone to the second floor in his wheelchair with an oxygen tank, into room number 3. Our clinic in Mexico City had ten rooms, eight private with full bathrooms, and two double-bed rooms, also with full bathrooms.

The nurse administered the insulin and left the patient. When she returned to his room, she found him lying in bed, sweating, sleepy, and with blue lips. She rushed out of the room to get me because the patient was not looking good. I ran upstairs, also scared, entered room 3, and saw the patient, not with blue lips, but purple-black lips, and only able to answer questions yes or no. I began to administer the intravenous drugs, then the glucose. When the patient was more alert in a matter of four minutes, I told Petra to give him the intramuscular and oral drugs. Cool, hey. Well, I sweated, but that was my first contact with hypoglycemia and IPT in full.

The patient went out of the clinic feeling much better and returned for a follow-up the next morning. And I was surprised to see him, as were my father and the nurses. He came back and entered the clinic with no wheelchair and

no oxygen. And, yes, his condition had improved about 45%.

My second example goes back to September 1990. A female living in Texas, Teresa Miller, with a diagnosis of lung cancer, came to see me at my Tijuana office. She had not been treated and only had a biopsy. She was treated with IPT, and the tumor disappeared. It is still gone as of today, April 30, 2001. The amazing story here is that I learned that IPT from the radiologist's point of view can make tumors "barely visible to x-rays." And, well, I am excited to know that after completing treatment with IPT, my patients will read in their reports the nice words *barely visible.*

A third case is that of a young female patient with kidney failure, Susan A. She was taking prednisone prescribed by her doctor in Los Angeles. Her father brought her to my office and asked me to treat her, to please do something, knowing that she was very ill and giving me his permission. Susan was perspiring serum. Her grandmother told me that she changed the girl's bed daily because she was sweating blood. She had the first IPT treatment and left my office with less edema. She returned the next Saturday. Wow. No more "blood sweating," and edema had almost disappeared from her legs and eyelids. She did very well for four years. Then one day she caught a flu, developed a cough, and began to take a cough syrup that increased her blood pressure and damaged her kidney irreversibly.

A fourth case is that of my first American female with a diagnosis of breast cancer, Donna McDermott. The relevant fact with her is that she had no previous treatment, and she decided to do IPT as her first form of treatment. I saw her first in December 1996. She is a survivor, too. No tumor is seen on x-rays, and she is doing great as of April 2001.

R: How does IPT help autoimmune diseases such as rheumatoid arthritis?

D: Unfortunately, little can be done to cure rheumatoid diseases. In my experience with arthritis in the last 12 years at my Tijuana office, I help patients feel pain free for a period of two months up to 6.5 years. Some have been able to walk again. And all, yes all, do things without using orthopedic devices such as walkers. The most rewarding fact is that they all report that the effect of IPT is superior to home remedies, prescription and nonprescription drugs, food supplements, and herbs or shark capsules.

R: Can IPT help other autoimmune diseases such as systemic lupus and scleroderma?

D: Yes, it can help to improve the quality of life.

R: What is the chance that IPT could help those conditions?

D: It depends on the prescription drugs you have available to administer plus the natural supplements you can give to improve the body's immune response.

R: What types of agents (medications/compounds) would be used?

D: Preferably agents that will increase the immune response, control the immune reaction, and agents to help liver function.

R: How often would someone receive IPT for those conditions and for how long?

D: Once a week, until the patient's condition in general is improved compared to his or her initial state. That could take four to six weeks.

R: Can IPT be used to treat infections?

D: Yes.

R: What types of infections can be treated successfully with IPT?

D: Lung, renal, bone, and others.

R: Can IPT be used to treat the following infections and what is the success rate?

R: Herpes?

D: Yes, 100%.

R: Hepatitis A and B?

D: Yes. 90%.

R: Hepatitis C?

D: Yes, 80%.

R: Cytomegalovirus?

D: Yes.

R: Epstein-Barr virus?

D: Yes.

R: Mycoplasma?

D: Yes.

R: IIIV?

D: Yes. I treated three cases with a survival of three years. I lost them to follow-up.

R: Candidiasis?

D: Yes, 95%.

R: Other fungal infections?

D: Yes, 90%.

R: Lyme disease?

D: Yes, 70%.

R: Can IPT help a person become HIV negative?

D: Since I only treated three cases back in 1985, I am not sure what the results would be.

R: There have been successes in treating poliomyelitis with IPT, and this same protocol can be used for amyotrophic lateral sclerosis (Lou Gehrig disease). Could you tell us about that?

D: My grandfather treated polio in the early 1950s with excellent results. He and my father filmed several child patients who recovered from polio with no damage to their limbs.

R: What types of medications (compounds) would be used?

D: Intravenous drugs: ascorbic acid, 250 mg; calcium gluconate, 0.116 mEq/mL; and ceftazidime, 250 mg. Intramuscular drugs: ergocalciferol, 125,000 units; liver extract, 1 cc; B complex (B_1, B_2, B_3, and B_6), 1 cc. Oral drugs: nylidrin HCl, 3 mg; artichoke, 1 capsule; nicotinic acid, 250 mg; and doxycycline hyclate, 50 mg.

R: What is the chance that IPT could help these infections?

D: Very good.

R: How often would someone receive IPT for those conditions and for how long?

D: Every week in the acute phase, until signs and symptoms disappear.

R: Some of the more disabling conditions are those that affect the central nervous system. What is unique about IPT and the central nervous system?

D: IPT can breach the blood-brain barrier, allowing specific prescription drugs to enter the central nervous system.

R: Some of the more common central nervous system diseases are multiple sclerosis and stroke. Can IPT help these conditions?

D: Yes.

R: What types of agents would be used in these conditions (along with the insulin)?

D: Substances that increase some of the low neurotransmitters as well as anti-inflammatory agents.

R: What is the likelihood of IPT helping such conditions?

D: Good.

R: Could you tell us of a case or two that you recall IPT helping with this (these) condition(s)?

D: My father was treating one when I began to learn at the clinic in 1983. Although not cured, the patient improved about 85%.

R: Are there any other conditions that you feel IPT would be especially helpful for? Please explain.

D: Again, if there are chemical substances for a particular disease, IPT can work.

R: Your particular interest in using IPT is in cancer. How did you become a cancer specialist?

D: It is a peculiar story how I became involved in treating cancer patients. After learning IPT with my father back in 1983, the majority of patients seen in a week were cancer patients. I was administering 12 IPT treatments daily at our clinic in Mexico City. One day in 1988, on which I could blame my Celtic genes, I shook my bones and took my family to Tijuana, where I opened an office. Initially, I advertised to treat arthritis. But one day, a patient named

Catalina Escobar living in Los Angeles saw my ad in *La Opinion*, a local newspaper for Hispanics, called to find out who I was, made an appointment, and later spread the word to her relatives and friends because she is a living example of a successfully treated patient with IPT back in the late 1960s.

R: What are the most common cancers that you see in your practice?

D: Breast, lung, colon, prostate, ovarian, uterine, and bone.

R: Are these the cancers that are best treated with IPT?

D: Yes.

R: Who would be the ideal IPT patient candidate?

D: For cancer treatment, the one who has had only a biopsy to confirm the diagnosis.

R: What if a person already had radiation therapy and chemotherapy?

D: Improvement in quality of life can be achieved.

R: Are there some cancers that in your experience do not respond well to IPT?

D: Yes, liver and brain.*

R: Why does traditional chemotherapy not work, whereas IPT does work?

D: Using IPT means targeting the cell membrane of cancerous cells only and leaving the nonaffected cells intact, thus avoiding side effects.

R: If a woman came to you with a lump in her breast that was cancerous, would you recommend surgery or IPT?

D: After evaluating her case, I would recommend IPT first.

R: Can IPT save a woman from having a mastectomy?

D: Yes, if IPT is instituted as the first form of treatment right after the initial diagnosis is given.

R: For the woman considering chemotherapy after a mastectomy, would IPT be a better option?

---

* For such cases as these, we added DMSO as a potentiating agent which gives increased access for the chemotherapy drug to the brain. We have found IPT to be effective for these cancers.

D: Yes.

R: How often are treatments typically given, and how many treatments are generally needed to successfully treat cancer, assuming the person is a good IPT candidate?

D: Each person must be evaluated, and a personal program instituted. There is no recipe to follow. Why? Because our body is a dynamic entity that changes constantly, and IPT is a dynamic treatment that interacts with the patient's body and disease. In general, we suggest weekly applications until 50% remission is achieved. Thereafter, we suggest applications every 14 or 21 days, until full remission, or when the radiologist sends a report that the tumor is barely visible and wants to know what treatment the patient had.

R: What is the likelihood of success in using IPT to treat breast cancer?

D: There is 100% success for good candidates, when the patient receives IPT right after the diagnosis is made with biopsy. And there is no fear of recurrence, even after five or 10 or more years.

R: What is the likelihood of success in using IPT to treat cancer in general, assuming someone is a good candidate?

D: As with breast cancer, 100%.

R: Are you saying that for the cancers mentioned above, many people could use IPT as their first-line therapy?

D: Yes.

R: Treating cancer can sometimes be frightening for doctors who are not oncologists. Do you feel it is safe for regular family doctors to be using IPT in their practices to treat cancer?

D: To do any new procedure or technique, you need training. Time and practice (repeating the procedure several times per day over the years) will give you experience and knowledge.

R: How can a person get trained in IPT?

D: Attending a workshop. Updated information is given at http://www.IPTQ.org.

R: Back to IPT cancer therapy. Lung cancer is very prominent. Can IPT successfully treat this condition?

D: Yes.

R: Does it work better for certain types of lung cancers?

D: It is better for the small cell type.

R: How often and how many treatments are typically needed?

D: Weekly applications until 50% reduction in tumor size, then less frequently until finished.

R: What is the chance of success that IPT will work for lung cancer?

D: If treated right after the diagnosis is made in a good candidate for IPT, 100%.

R: Please describe the chance of success for the following cancers with IPT.

R: Hodgkin's lymphoma?

D: 100%.

R: Non-Hodgkin's lymphoma?

D: 80%.

R: Chronic leukemia?

D: 80%.

R: Acute leukemia?

D: 80%.

R: Pancreatic?

D: 50%.

R: Stomach?

D: 80%.

R: Colon?

D: 80%.

R: Kidney?

D: 50%.

R: Bladder?

D: 60%.

R: Unknown primary?

D: Unknown %.

R: Uterine?

D: 90%.

R: Cervical?

D: 100%.

R: Ovarian?

D: 90%.

R: Sarcoma?

D: 90%.

R: Glioblastoma multiforme?

D: 10%.

R: Astrocytoma?

D: 10%.

R: Any others?

D: ?%.

R: What if a person finds out the cancer already has metastasized. Can IPT still help?

D: IPT can help, but metastasis means the cancer has breached the immune system, and organs such as the liver may have an impaired function.

R: What is the likelihood of success?

D: Just improvement of quality life for most cases. A few patients can expect 50% remission.

R: What if the cancer has spread to the brain. Can IPT still help?

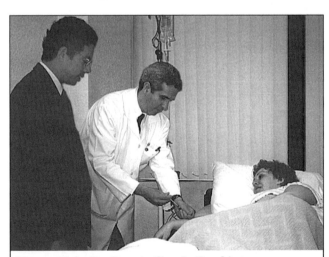

Figure 18-3: Dr. Donato García Teaching Dr. Ross Hauser the Technique of IPT at His Tijuana, Mexico Office.

D: No.

R: What is the likelihood of success?

D: Little.

R: When IPT fails to cure a cancer, does it still help a person's quality of life?

D: In all cases, IPT will improve quality of life.

R: How does it help the quality of life? If a person is on morphine because of pain, can IPT help the person get off it?

D: Yes, by reducing the dose, and in some cases by using other painkiller agents with fewer side effects.

R: Anorexia and malnutrition are often found in cancer patients. Can IPT help this? How?

D: Almost all patients will experience increased appetite by the second or third IPT treatment.

R: What would be your take-home message about IPT to people who are reading this?

D: IPT is a safe, highly effective medical treatment for cancer, with minimal side effects (such as pain at the site of needle puncture). For cancer, it can typically achieve 50% remission, with the possibility of a 100% remission when used as the first choice of treatment, with no fear of recurrence. For many infections, a one-day half-morning cure to get back to enjoying your life, with no fear of developing a serious complication, unless you do all possible things to get ill again. For rheumatic pain, think of life with little or no pain and being able to comb and dress by yourself.

R: What would you like to see in the future in regard to IPT?

D: New prescription drugs for diseases that are considered rare and better ones for the diseases that affect the majority of us.

R: What is the future of IPT?

D: My grandfather developed the idea. My father preserved it for us and began to spread it among two doctors. They always dreamed of seeing this method used by doctors around the world to treat many diseases. I am sharing what I know with you so that other doctors with different interests can start to treat diseases that are considered incurable today.

R: Dr. Pérez, it has been a pleasure talking with you today. Marion and I think highly of you and your family. You are a true gentleman and a scholar. You are a credit to your family. Your work in the cancer field is remarkable, incredible. I wish you much continued success in your IPT practice and research.

D: Thank you for your comments. Thank you for your interest in this medical procedure that now is part of your professional life. I ask you to always give credit to the original developer of IPT, the late Dr. Donato Pérez García, Sr. (1896-1971), because without him, his perseverance and great wisdom, this interview would never have taken place. ■

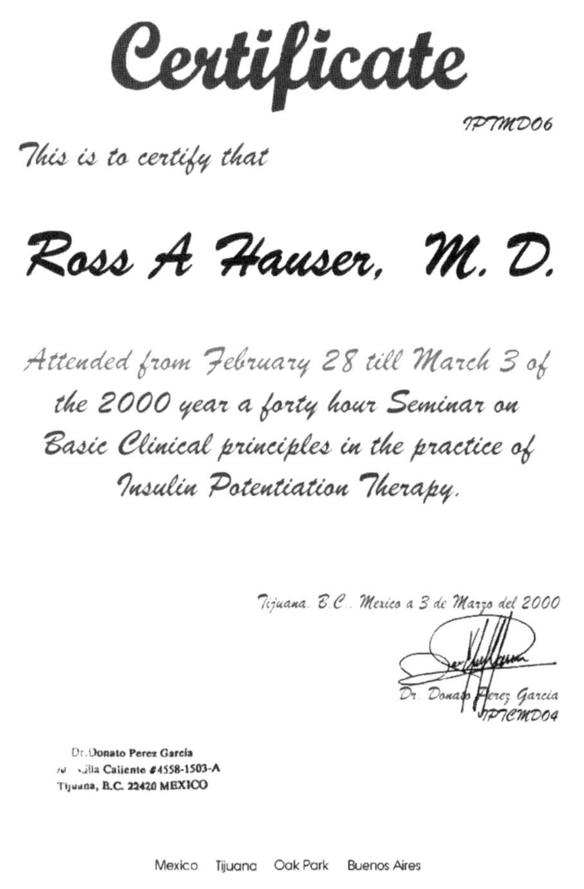

Certificate

IPTMD06

This is to certify that

Ross A Hauser, M. D.

Attended from February 28 till March 3 of the 2000 year a forty hour Seminar on Basic Clinical principles in the practice of Insulin Potentiation Therapy.

Tijuana. B.C., Mexico a 3 de Marzo del 2000

Dr. Donato Perez Garcia
IPTCMD04

Dr. Donato Perez Garcia
.. .lia Caliente #4558-1503-A
Tijuana, B.C. 22420 MEXICO

Mexico   Tijuana   Oak Park   Buenos Aires

Figure 18-4: Dr. Ross Hauser's Certificate of IPT Training Presented to Him by Dr. Donato Pérez García.

Chapter 19

Insulin Potentiation Therapy—Common Questions and Answers

Insulin Potentiation Therapy is very good medicine. By using the scientific method, regular allopathic medications are given but used in a manner consistent with molecular biology and natural medicine principles.

People with cancer and those who love them have many valid concerns and questions. It is often comforting for them to receive care in a comprehensive natural medicine cancer center such as CCINMC. In such a setting, there is time to ask questions and have them answered. Below is a sampling of the types of questions that are often asked.

Will IPT Help Me?

This is, of course, the end-all question. "Am I an appropriate IPT candidate?" To fully assess a cancer patient and which treatment would be most helpful for the patient, it is important for the physician or natural medicine specialist to review the following information:

- Biopsy results of cancer
- CT/MRI reports
- History of previous treatments used for cancer
- Surgical report
- Blood cancer marker results
- Blood tests for kidney, liver, and immune function
- Initial PET scan

We believe it is always best to see the patient and talk to the family in person. There is the old saying, "People are never the same when they have shared a meal together." Well, the same goes for office consultations. We have had many cancer patients simply not like their oncologists, a major reason for not doing conventional therapy. **It is imperative for the cancer patient and his or her family to feel comfortable and to trust their health care providers and the therapies provided.**

For patients who live far away or are still in the hospital, we do phone consultations with patients and their families to assess as best we can if someone is an appropriate IPT candidate. The phone consultation is usually done after the above information has been sent to the office. The main information that is assessed is the type of cancer to be treated and what will be required to get a good response. In regard to IPT, a person with the following would make an ideal candidate:

- Cancer newly diagnosed
- Small tumor load
- No metastases
- No previous treatment
- No concomitant medical conditions

For the person with these criteria, the likelihood of success with IPT is tremendous. This does not mean that someone who has had previous chemotherapy, has multiple medical conditions, or has a high tumor load cannot get IPT, but it does signify that the prognosis is not as good. For less than ideal candidates, the number of sessions of IPT and the amount of medications used may need to be increased.

How Many IPT Treatments Will Be Needed?

Most cancers are evaluated after six to twelve IPT treatments. Generally, IPT is utilized to treat a cancer until one of the following responses occurs:

- Cancer goes into remission.
- Cancer is arrested.
- IPT is clearly not working.

If after six to twelve IPT treatments there has been no tumor regression, the treatment regime is either stopped or changed. IPT is a pliable treatment. The regime can be changed and sometimes change is needed to decrease the chance of drug resistance or because of drug resistance. IPT helps potentiate the effects of chemotherapy medications but still depends on the particular cancer being sensitive to the chemotherapeutic agents that are used.

In regard to the total number of treatments needed, it often depends on how aggressive and rapidly the cancer is growing. For the person with a newly diagnosed, rapidly growing cancer (cancer diagnosed within a month or two), the response with IPT is often quite rapid within the first round of IPT treatments. For someone with a more indolent type of cancer that is very slow growing, the number of treatments typically will be higher.

For the person who has been recommended to get "preventive chemotherapy" by his or her oncologist, such as a woman after a mastectomy, we give one IPT treatment weekly for 10 weeks, in lieu of the patient receiving high-dose chemotherapy. For other cancer patients, it is truly impossible to tell how many IPT treatments will be needed; it obviously depends on the response. One thing can be said for sure. **If the person has a tumor that is shrinking with IPT, do not take a break from IPT! While a tumor is being destroyed, it needs to be *even further attacked!***

Tumors have tremendous resiliency. Just because IPT is causing tumor regression today does not mean it will still work after a two-month break from treatment. The tumor could build up drug resistance during that time.

How Often Do I Need to Get IPT?

The success of IPT depends on its ability to kill more cancer cells than will be replicated between each treatment. Between IPT treatments, there is always a risk of cancers being replicated and getting bigger, so IPT is generally given at least weekly. Some people require more frequent treatments, such as two or three times per week.

For the person who for whatever reason can only get IPT once per week but needs more cancer-killing effects between treatments, low-dose oral chemotherapy is sometimes given. In our office, natural chemotherapeutic agents such as high-dose vitamins A and D are also given.

How Long Do I Have to Fast before IPT?

It is best to fast overnight before getting IPT. It is okay to drink water in the morning of the treatment, but nothing else. Any medications or herbs should not be taken on the day of treatment unless they have been reviewed. For people receiving IPT in the afternoon, a person should fast at least four hours. After saying this, we would still reiterate that it is best not to eat from the evening before a treatment is to be given.

How Will I Feel during IPT?

IPT is predicated on the fact that insulin opens up the membranes surrounding cells to help them "feed" by increasing their intracellular glucose concentration. This has the effect of decreasing blood sugar levels and inducing a hypoglycemic reaction. Because of these hypoglycemic symptoms, at CCINMC, the IPT is administered in rooms with hospital beds. The person puts on a hospital gown and lies on a very comfortable hospital bed (as comfortable as hospital beds can be).

Generally beginning 15 minutes after the insulin is given, the person will begin to feel fatigued or sleepy. This will then progress to sweating, rapid heart rate, and eventually a very hot feeling. The maximum hypoglycemic effect is typically around 30 minutes after the insulin is given. Once this tremendous "hot" feeling occurs, the person is at the "therapeutic moment." The "therapeutic moment" of IPT is that point when the person has the maximum symptoms of hypoglycemia. It is important because this is when the chemotherapy drugs are given to maximize their potentiation effects.

Once the chemotherapeutic agents are given, the person is then given a fruit drink to reverse the hypoglycemic symptoms. Often after just a few ounces of fluid, the person feels better and then is just tired. After a 45-minute rest, the person gets dressed in his or her own clothes and simply walks out of the office.

Can I Eat after IPT?

Food never tasted so good as it does after IPT. Immediately after IPT, a very small, easily digested meal can be eaten, such as soup, fruit, or a salad. For the evening meal, the same types of foods can be eaten. IPT is generally very well tolerated, but eating too much food after IPT can make a person feel nauseated.

How Low Does the Blood Sugar Go with IPT?

Insulin causes a person's blood sugar to drop. Typically during IPT, the blood sugar drops to around 30 but can vary from about 20 to 40. A normal blood sugar level is between 75 and 110. Because individual responses to insulin vary, it may take a few visits to get the blood sugar to drop that low.

FIGURE 19-1: **MORTALITY RATES WITH IPT**		
WHO	**YEARS DOING IPT**	**MORTALITY**
Donato Pérez García, Sr., M.D. (originator of IPT; 1896-1971)	1930-1971: 41 Years	0%
Donato Pérez García y Bellón, M.D. (1930-2000)	1956-2000: 44 Years	0%
Donato Pérez García, Jr., M.D. (Still living)	1983-2002: 19Years (Still practicing)	0%

ARE THERE ANY SIDE EFFECTS TO IPT?

At the IPT course in Las Vegas, Nevada, in February 2001, Dr. Donato Pérez García, Jr., showed a slide of the morbidity that his family (three generations of physicians) have had using IPT (**Figure 19-1**). The group of physicians who founded IPT have over 100 years of experience with it and have never seen a person die because of IPT. (This is a mortality rate of 0%.) Because the doses of chemotherapy medications used during IPT are 10-15% of the amounts given during traditional cancer care, the side effect risk is greatly diminished. The most common side effect from IPT is fatigue during the day of treatment. Some nausea occurs only rarely.

One of the main reasons that people get IPT is because it is a great alternative to high-dose chemotherapy with all of its side effects that can include immunosuppression; hair loss; and nerve, heart, kidney, and liver damage. IPT can cause these side effects also, but it is much less likely because of the low dose of medications used.

ARE THERE ANY ABSOLUTE CONTRAINDICATIONS TO IPT?

There are no absolute contraindications to getting IPT.* There are factors that can decrease a person's response to IPT, such as previous chemotherapy, radiation therapy, poor immune function, and hopelessness, but these do not preclude someone from having IPT. One should always remember that **where there is life, there is hope.** (This is a saying we picked up from Dr. Ayre.)

CAN I TAKE SUPPLEMENTS WHILE UNDERGOING IPT?

True comprehensive natural medicine care for cancer involves potent nutriceutical supplementa-tion. Appropriate nutritional supplementation during IPT can have multiple beneficial effects, including immune stimulation, liver detoxification, protection of normal cells against chemotherapy, potentiation of the chemotherapy effect on the cancer cells, as well as many others. Nutritional supplementation is a vital part of any cancer treatment protocol. (**This topic is covered in detail in Chapter 30, Appendix A, and B.**)

CAN I GET OZONE THERAPY OR NUTRITIONAL THERAPIES WHILE UNDERGOING IPT?

At CCINMC, ozone therapy and/or other oxidative therapies are generally part of the IPT protocol. To optimize treatment goals, other nutritional therapies such as high-dose vitamin C drips are often given on days when a person is not getting IPT. For the person with cancer, aggressive interventional natural medicine treatments including ozone therapy, intravenous vitamin drips, and potent nutriceutical supplements all appear to increase the effectiveness of concomitant therapies, whether they be conventional chemotherapy or IPT.

CAN MY ONCOLOGIST DO IPT?

IPT can be done by any licensed physician. Because most oncologists are not trained in IPT, it is best to have the treatment done by someone experienced in the technique.

WHY HAS MY ONCOLOGIST NOT HEARD OF IPT?

IPT throughout most of its history was done exclusively in Mexico. There are many successful treatments that are done throughout the world, yet these are not done in the United States.

---

* *The benefit/risk ratio of doing IPT during pregnancy would have to be decided on a case-by-case basis between the patient and their private physician.*

There are also successful treatments for chronic diseases that have been done in the United States for many decades, yet the majority of physicians have not heard of them. A good example of the latter is Prolotherapy. Prolotherapy has been done in the United States since the 1930s, yet most physicians do not know that it can cure most chronic pain. Prolotherapy is a treatment that stimulates the body to heal painful areas. It must be done by a licensed physician or physician assistant and involves the injection of substances to stimulate the healing of such structures as ligaments, tendons, menisci, and cartilage. The sad fact is that most people in chronic pain do not know about it.*

Just because a traditional oncologist or physician has not heard of a specific treatment or knows nothing about it does not mean the treatment is not valuable. IPT, like Prolotherapy, has been helping people for decades. The fact is that a traditional physician is trained to use conventional methods. IPT, Prolotherapy, and other techniques like them fall into the realm of natural medicine. Traditionally trained physicians do not know much about natural medicine. For natural medicine treatments, it is best to seek the expert opinion of a natural medicine specialist, not a traditional physician.

Is IPT Approved by the FDA?

The medications used in IPT are FDA approved, but they are given in an off-label use.

The following is from the *FDA Drug Bulletin,* April 1982, under the section of "Use of Approved Drugs for Unlabeled Indications:"

> The FD&C Act does not, however, limit the manner in which a physician may use an approved drug. Once a patent has been approved for marketing, a physician may prescribe it for uses or in treatment regimens or patient populations that are not included in approved labeling. Such "unapproved" or, more precisely, "unlabeled" uses may, in fact, reflect approaches to drug therapy that have been extensively reported in the medical literature.

The *FDA Drug Bulletin* goes on to say, "Valid new uses for drugs already on the market are often first discovered through serendipitous observations and therapeutic innovations, subsequently confirmed by well-planned and executed clinical investigations."

Can IPT be Used for Other Conditions?

IPT was first used to treat tertiary syphilis, a condition caused by an infection. IPT in its history has been used for many conditions, including infections and autoimmune and various neurological conditions. (These are covered in great detail in the next two chapters.)

Insulin has been shown to potentiate the effects of antibiotics and antiviral medications. Thus, at least theoretically, any condition that has an infectious etiology would be helped by IPT using antimicrobial agents. Modern medicine is realizing that many conditions, including autoimmune diseases, rheumatological conditions, some cancers, chronic fatigue syndrome, and even heart disease, may have an infectious etiological basis.

Where Can I Find Out More Information on IPT?

There are many good places on the Internet to learn about IPT, including www.iptcancer.com. Donato 3 and Chris Duffield, Ph.D., have done a great job with www.IPTQ.org. For anyone desiring to ask Dr. Donato Pérez García specific questions, his e-mail address is donatopg3@yahoo.com. Chris Duffield, is owed a great debt for the time and effort that he personally donates to www.IPTQ.org. This web site has a list of the doctors who have been trained in IPT. They also have information on how a physician can get information on IPT training.

Another great resource for information on IPT are two books that have been translated into English by Aimé Ricci. *Donatian Cellular Therapy* was written by Donato 1, the originator of Insulin Potentiation Therapy, and *Medicine of Hope* was written by Dr. Paquette, a Canadian doctor who had been taught the technique by Donato 2. The first book is available at www.IPTQ.org. The latter book can be purchased at www.benuts.com. ■

---

* For people who desire to learn more about Prolotherapy, call 1-877-RX-BEULAH, or go to www.prolonews.com, www.sportsprolo.com, or www.beulahlandpress.com. There, one can order any of the books we have written on Prolotherapy, including Prolo Your Pain Away! and Prolo Your Sports Injuries Away!

CHAPTER 20

IPT as a General Medical Technique

If one closely examines what was written about Donato 1's cellular therapy, such as from the *Time* magazine article and certifying letter from the Secretary of Defense of Mexico, J. Agustin Castro, it is clear that IPT is a very safe procedure. Donato's 1, 2, and 3 all practiced it as an outpatient procedure in a private practice physician's office. This is one of the primary benefits of the procedure because it puts a very potent weapon for cancer and other chronic diseases in the hands of the family physician.

In this age of HMOs (health maintenance organizations) and managed care, many people are turning to more holistically-minded practitioners for their health care. We personally like the term *natural medicine*. I (Ross) am a natural medicine specialist who practices family medicine (though my AMA-approved board certification is in physical medicine and rehabilitation). For many people, they would prefer to have such a physician take care of their cancer and other health conditions rather than a medical specialist such as an oncologist, whose cancer treatment is primarily high-dose chemotherapy. Most cancer physicians know very little about natural medicine, generally discourage it, and leave the patient feeling like a disease rather than a human being. The natural medicine specialist looks at the whole person and believes that the spirit, mind, and body of a person should be treated for optimum results. The natural medicine specialist also has

many different ways to attack conditions such as cancer and often utilizes several or all in treating a patient (See **Figure 20-1**).

We believe it is prudent for a person with cancer to be followed by a medical doctor or osteopathic physician. It may be surprising to some, but many people, even with advanced cancers, treat themselves or take advice from the Internet, a friend, or the latest natural health journal. We get letters all the time from prospective patients telling us the treatment regimes they are using on themselves (See **Figure 20-2**). **A cancer patient not being followed by a physician competent in the treatment of cancer is a quick way to the grave.** Highly talented people have been referred to our office, including television stars and beauty queens, with advanced cancers who completely denied the severity of the illness and monkeyed with herbs until it was too late. (Some of their actual case histories are included in this book.) The time to get under the care of a physician whom a cancer patient trusts is not when, for example, the cancer-infested breast is twice its normal size but when the person first knows that something is wrong (See **Figure 20-3**). As soon as a change is noticed in the breast, such as a heaviness, swelling, nipple retraction, or a nodule, an appointment with a competent, natural medicine specialist should be made.

The person with early-stage cancer often feels fine and has a difficult time believing that there is a life-threatening mass growing in his or her body. **How a person feels is a poor indicator of prognosis or the seriousness of the cancer condition.** A person with cancer needs to be followed by a

> Most cancer physicians know very little about natural medicine, generally discourage it, and leave the patient feeling like a disease rather than a human being.

FIGURE 20-1: NATURAL MEDICINE APPROACHES TO CANCER

Herbal Medicine	Intravenous Nutriceuticals
Hyperthermia	Natural Chemotherapy
Immune Stimulation	Positive Attitude
Insulin Potentiation Therapy	Prayer
Interventional Natural Medicine Techniques	Proper Nutrition
	Reversing Cancer Physiology

Natural medicine seeks to treat the whole person because all aspects of a person's being are affected by disease.

3.15.01

Hello,

I was given your address by Second Opinion Pub. Co.. I am interested after reading "Into the Light" by W.C. Douglas M.D. in the photoluminescent therapy. I read and saw a video on the practices of oxygenation therapies in Russia. They have had wonderful results for years now.

I had a mastectomy of the right breast two years ago. I did this after my soul search and deep-long studies of all my alternatives. I let them take only 2 lymphnodes, because I felt one was involved in my right armpit, and it was. Now I have a swollen armpit lymphnode in the left side. (approx 2 mos.) I am on a herbal regime - Essiac that I make myself, CELLFORTE, and other herbs, foods and teas, too many to mention here, that help my immunity and are especially good for healing cancer and strengthening the liver etc. If I feel I need to "step-it-up" I would like to do the photoluminescence / oxygenation route. Could you help me? What exactly do you do? Are your charges for this reasonable?

I do appreciate your time and attention to this matter.

Sincerely,
K.B.

Nisconsin

Figure 20-2: *Actual Patient Letter Sent to Caring Medical*
This person is playing Russian Roulette with her health and even her life by *not* having a physician follow-up for her breast cancer.

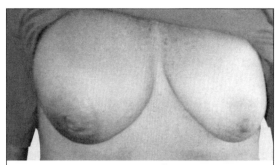

Figure 20-3: *Appearance of a Massive Right Breast Mass*
This cancer had been growing for a year prior to the person going to a doctor for evaluation. As has been repeated several times in this book: The day that a person notices something wrong—that is the day to seek out the counsel of a natural medicine doctor, a physician who practices IPT and other natural medicine techniques.

encourage our cancer patients to get an oncology consultation so they can find out what the best modern medicine has to offer. Subsequently, most cancer patients realize that the risks of high-dose chemotherapy are significant in relation to the benefits. It also becomes quite obvious to them that the traditional oncologist knows very little about herbs, vitamins, natural ways of immune stimulation, and natural medicine principles except that they play no role in cancer therapy. To any intelligent individual, this does not sit right because both **the immune system and nutrition have to play a role in overcoming cancer.** To ignore this avenue of care makes no sense for the person fighting for life. Natural medicine methods to improve immune function and nutrition have virtually no side effects and clearly would help a person's quality of life and at best help one's body destroy the cancer.

Because IPT is so safe, it gives the family physician a modality to aggressively treat cancer. This has many benefits. Perhaps the greatest of these is that the cancer patient does not have to be shipped off to some impersonal cancer ward to be treated. Nothing is more depressing and discouraging than seeing a bunch of balding, dusky people after high-dose chemotherapy. High-dose chemotherapy makes people feel terrible, whereas IPT generally makes people feel great. Consider this letter sent to us by one of our

physician who can monitor the cancer via radiographs (CT scans, PET scans, MRIs, and x-rays) as well as blood tests including cancer markers. The person whose cancer is not closely monitored via these methods is playing Russian roulette; unfortunately, in such cases, the cancer generally wins.

Most people want to be monitored by their family physician or a natural medicine specialist. This is the person who knows them the best. We

March 29, 2001

Dear Dr. Hauser,

I want to let you know how wonderful I have been feeling since I finished with IPT. As you know, I was diagnosed with breast cancer in March 2000. I had a mastectomy that April and the oncologist wanted me to undergo 6 months of chemotherapy and radiation because the cancer had spread to my lymph nodes. I was <u>petrified</u>. I did not think I had any other option for treatment so I went in for 1 chemotherapy treatment. It was a terrible experience. I didn't feel recouped from chemo until 4 or 5 days later, I lost all my hair, and did not want to go back again. I never felt good about getting it. That same week I heard about IPT and I decided to make an appointment to see you.

I had 10 sessions of IPT and couldn't be more pleased. I had no side effects! I was able to do things after my IPT treatments unlike with chemotherapy. I also regrew all of my hair, much of it <u>during</u> the treatment. That's a switch isn't it? Get a cancer treatment and grow your hair instead of lose it! My body is cancer free and so am I! I can now go on with my life.

I have even joined an online support group of alternative medicine. I would "absolutely" recommend IPT to any cancer patient. The greatest feeling is beating cancer without having to go through all the terror of chemotherapy.

Thank you Dr. Hauser for your ongoing work and research in alternative cancer treatments.

Best wishes,

Milenka Glasscock

Milenka Glasscock

Figure 20-4: This letter says a lot about the differences between traditional chemotherapy and IPT. Using one method of treatment, you lose hair, and with the other—it grows back. We wonder which treatment you'd rather have?

patients, who was given a single treatment of high-dose chemotherapy with all of its side effects and then ran to get IPT. Milenka lost all of her hair with one high-dose chemotherapy treatment, and during the ten sessions of IPT, her hair grew back. What a contrast! (See **Figure 20-4**.)

The family practitioner sees every human disease. It becomes quite evident that even with the best natural medicine approach, there are going to be conditions that just do not respond. For conditions such as cancer, viral infections, Lyme disease, mycoplasma infection, multiple sclerosis, systemic lupus erythematosis, rheumatoid arthritis, chronic body pain, and other neurological conditions, a more aggressive approach than the usual diet and herbal remedies is needed (**See Figure 20-5**).

Because Caring Medical is a comprehensive *interventional natural medicine clinic*, some of

the modalities available for patients include photoluminescence; ozone therapy; chelation therapy; intravenous vitamins, minerals, and herbs; mesotherapy; neural therapy; Prolotherapy; and Insulin Potentiation Therapy. For a complete explanation of these various therapies, please see www.caringmedical.com. These are all done as an outpatient, in the clinic with the patient going home on his or her own accord after the procedure. For the person with a serious disabling condition that significantly alters his or her quality of life, some type of interventional natural medicine procedure most likely will be needed.

In the past, serious medical conditions such as heart disease and cancer were quickly referred to the local "specialist." For many family medicine doctors such as myself who utilize interventional natural medicine procedures, it becomes evident that **most serious, general medical conditions can be reversed with interventional natural medicine.** (Ross is actually a physical medicine and rehabilitation specialist who practices family or general medicine.) We feel so strongly about this that our next book, *Interventional Natural Medicine Techniques: Reversing Chronic Degenerative Diseases*, discusses many of the allopathic and surgical proce-

FIGURE 20-5: SOME GENERAL MEDICAL CONDITIONS MAY REQUIRE AN AGGRESSIVE INTERVENTIONAL NATURAL MEDICINE PROGRAM.	
AUTOIMMUNE DISEASES	EPSTEIN-BARR VIRUS
CANCER	HEPATITIS
CENTRAL NERVOUS SYSTEM DISEASES	HERPES
CHRONIC BODY PAIN	LYME DISEASE
CHRONIC FATIGUE SYNDROME	MENTAL DEFICIENCIES
CYTOMEGALOVIRUS	MULTIPLE SCLEROSIS
DEBILITATING FATIGUE	MYCOPLASMA
DIZZINESS	RHEUMATOID ARTHRITIS

CONDITION	INTERVENTIONAL NATURAL TECHNIQUE	ALLOPATHIC PROCEDURE
Coronary Artery Disease	Chelation Therapy	Heart Bypass Surgery
Peripheral Vascular Disease	Chelation Therapy	Extremity Bypass Surgery
Severe Joint Arthritis	Prolotherapy	Joint Replacement
Degenerative Disc Disease	Prolotherapy	Neck/Back Surgery
Cancer	IPT	High-Dose Chemotherapy
Hepatitis	Ozone Therapy/IPT	Interferon
Herpes	Ozone Therapy/IPT	Antiviral Medications
Neuritis/Nerve Entrapment	Neural Therapy	Radiofrequency Ablation
Lyme Disease	Ozone/Photoluminescence/IPT	Intravenous Antibiotics
Allergies	Serial Dilution Therapy	Long-Term Allergy Shots
Chronic Sinus Infections	Neurocranial Restructuring	Sinus Surgery
Facial/Hip Obesity	Mesotherapy	Plastic Surgery
Rheumatoid Arthritis	Ozone Therapy/IPT/Prolotherapy	Joint Replacements
Multiple Sclerosis	IPT	Interferon/Medications

Figure 20-6: Interventional Natural Medicine Techniques Versus Allopathic Treatments
Interventional natural medicine procedures help reverse many chronic degenerative diseases, thereby abating the need for the patient to get more invasive and dangerous allopathic treatments.

dures that are eliminated by people receiving interventional natural medicine procedures (See **Figure 20-6**).

STATE OF THE UNION: WE ARE AN UNHEALTHY BUNCH

There is a chronic disease epidemic in the United States. Consider these facts:[1]

- 1.2 million people diagnosed with cancer every year
- 43 million people have asthma or allergic disease
- 73 million have chronic respiratory problems
- 38 million suffer with arthritis
- 500,000 have systemic lupus erythematosus
- 11 million people have diabetes
- 1 million are infected with the AIDS virus
- 2 million have ileitis and colitis

We are getting to the point in America that it is typical for people over the age of 60 to suffer from a chronic medical condition that affects their life on a regular basis. It is for this reason that many patients are turning to more natural remedies for their care because the traditional allopathic care for most of these conditions is suboptimal, producing very few long-term cures and, at best, typically only temporary help. IPT and other natural remedies and interventional techniques help correct the underlying altered biochemistry, helping many of the symptoms of these chronic diseases at the same time. These types of treatments do this safely without the risk (or a substantial decrease in risk compared to typical allopathic treatments) of side effects.

INSULIN POTENTIATION THERAPY IN GENERAL MEDICAL PRACTICE

"Nothing new, but in a new way." Jean-Claude Paquette, M.D., stated this in *Medicine of Hope*. He said the motto applies curiously to Insulin Cellular Therapy. He explained:

> We use the same medications as in conventional medicine, the best we can find and whatever is the country of origin. The administration of these medicines is done in the same ways: orally, subcutaneously, intramuscularly, intravenously, locally, vaginally, or rectally.[2]

In other words, IPT can potentiate the effects of all or at least most of these medications.

Insulin Potentiation Therapy is the cancer therapy for the new millennium, but it may be the general medicine treatment for the new millennium as well. It is clear in reviewing the writings of Donato 1 and 2, as well as Jean-Claude Paquette, that IPT can help reverse many chronic diseases.[2,3]

The list of medical conditions for which IPT has been successfully utilized is quite vast. It includes various infections, autoimmune diseases, allergies, cancer, and neurologic conditions (See **Figure 20-7**). The conditions that can be helped with IPT are significant. Since most doctors who do IPT are specialists in natural medicine, IPT is often utilized only after other treatment regimes have failed. Dr. Paquette put it best in *Medicine of Hope* when he wrote in the section entitled "My Code of Treatment with ICT:"

> In fact, I have applied it only in a very small percentage of my practice, and still with much understanding, prudence, attention, and circumspection. It is only in exceptional cases where I consider it my duty to intervene, for example, in chronic cases where conventional medicine has reached a ceiling between relief and symptomatic treatment

and was acknowledged powerless; among patients having made the round of specialists, of orthodox medicine or not, conventional or alternative; in irremediable cases who were abandoned or who had capitulated to failure; in complex cases where one would be lost facing a multitude of diagnoses. These were the most enthralling cases that I adored to solve.

There are times when the patient wonders if he or she is ever going to get better. The patient feels exhausted, exacerbated, and downright depressed. In such a situation, the patient and the clinicians should consider IPT. IPT helps reverse toxicity and alters physiology for a multitude of conditions and is especially helpful for the chronically ill patient.

It is important to understand some of the mechanisms as to how IPT assists the healing of some of the general medical conditions described above. Since the definitive cause of many chronic diseases is not known, IPT may be helping the condition by any number of mechanisms. (See **Figure 20-8**.)

FIGURE 20-7: **GENERAL MEDICAL CONDITIONS THAT HAVE BEEN SUCCESSFULLY TREATED WITH IPT***

RESPIRATORY:	asthma, allergic bronchitis, respiratory allergies, vasomotor rhinitis, emphysema, and chronic sinusitis
CIRCULATORY:	migraine, cephalgias (headaches), obliterating endarteritis, hypertension, acrocyanosis, angina, and hemorrhoids
DIGESTIVE:	viral hepatitis, ulcerous colitis, hypoglycemia, and bilary dyskinesia
NERVOUS OR NEUROLOGICAL:	multiple sclerosis, migraine, facial paralysis, hemiplegia, slipped disk (herniated disk), sciatica, and thoracic shingles
GENITO-URINARY:	cystitis, pyelonephritis, prostatitis, neoplasia of the prostate, and of the cervix
RHEUMATIC:	rheumatoid arthritis, arthrosis, gout polyarthitis, osteo-arthritis, and chronic osteomyelitis
DERMATOLOGICAL:	psoriasis, eczema, contact dermatitis, acne, urticaria, dermographism, thoracic shingles, and erythematous lupus
ALLERGIES:	food, medicinal, respiratory, or contact with metals, the sun, chemicals
INFECTIONS:	chronic, viral hepatitis, bronchitis, cervicitis, osteomyelitis, etc.
INTOXICATIONS:	a) General: (present in all the chronic cases) b) Specific: to drugs, alcohol, and tobacco
CANCERS:	breast, prostate, lung, liver, intestine, cervix, skin (melanoma), bone (osteosarcoma), and thyroid

* *This list is from the experience of Dr. Jean-Claude Paquette in Medicine of Hope.*

FIGURE 20-8: **PROPOSED MECHANISMS OF ACTION OF IPT**

- ENHANCED CELL MEMBRANE PERMEABILITY
- INCREASED PERMEABILITY OF THE BLOOD-BRAIN BARRIER
- RECRUITMENT OF CANCER CELLS INTO THE S PHASE
- DETOXIFICATION
- ENHANCED CELLULAR OXYGENATION
- IMPROVEMENT IN CELL NUTRITION
- INCREASED CELL ENERGY PRODUCTION
- INCREASED UPTAKE OF MEDICATIONS INTO THE CELL
- ENHANCED TRANSPORT OF MEDICATIONS INTO THE CENTRAL NERVOUS SYSTEM
- STIMULATION OF STEM CELL AND FIBROBLAST DIFFERENTIATION*

In a more practical sense, it becomes evident how IPT could help chronic, degenerative disease because it helps reverse the "sick" physiology that is found with these conditions. In our office, we perform extensive biochemical tests that show the altered physiology. Dr. Donato Pérez García, Sr.

* *From http://www.IPTQ.com/howipt.htm, posted March 4, 2000 by web site host Chris Duffield, Ph.D.*

(Donato 1), was the first to show that IPT reverses altered physiology. The most obvious example is cancer, where the body becomes toxic and anaerobic. All these conditions can be reversed with IPT. In regard to multiple sclerosis, the condition by definition involves the central nervous system. By enhancing drug uptake into the brain and the central nervous system, IPT increases the likelihood of improvement with such medications as interferon and various antimicrobials if an infection is found in the patient.

Many of the conditions helped by IPT are ones where no good allopathic treatment exists, or if they do exist, they are horribly expensive, fraught with side effects, and not curative. There are many chronic conditions, such as autoimmune diseases, viral infections, cancer, and various neurological diseases, that are not substantially helped by allopathic medications and treatments. For people suffering from a chronic condition that has viable allopathic treatment options, these are often fraught with significant side effects and morbidity. For this reason, patients are turning to more natural treatments such as diet, vitamins, and herbs. For the person who is not helped by this type of treatment, care from a physician who utilizes interventional natural medicine should be done.

Such a physician has a wide array of interventional natural medical techniques, including Prolotherapy, Neural Therapy, chelation therapy, ozone therapy, IPT, and many others to help severe medical conditions. Generally, chronic medical conditions cause a significant alteration in the biochemistry of the body that is not addressed with modern therapeutics. By giving insulin prior to traditional, injectable medications, the concentrations of medications transported into the cell and central nervous system (brain) are enhanced, which helps to reverse the altered physiology, thereby significantly aiding recovery.

IPT has been used successfully to treat many general medical conditions, including asthma, allergies, infections, colitis, rheumatoid arthritis, toxicity, cancer, and many others. It does so by many proposed mechanisms, including enhanced immunity, increased cellular oxygenation and energy production, detoxification, and the potentiating effects of other medications.

Because of enhanced diagnostic testing procedures such as polymerase chain reaction (PCR), blood infections can now be documented with enhanced sensitivity and accuracy. Researchers are finding that conditions such as rheumatoid arthritis (autoimmune diseases), multiple sclerosis (neurological diseases), and coronary artery disease sometimes have an infection as their etiological basis. By giving appropriate antifungal, antibiotic, or antiviral medications, the condition can often be eradicated or slowed. Because some organisms are intracellular, such as viruses, mycoplasma, chlamydia, or Borrelia (Lyme disease), insulin is sometimes needed to increase drug levels inside the cell. If the infection is the primary cause of the person's chronic medical conditions or symptoms, the results can be dramatic.

Here are a few case studies that can give good credence to the notion that IPT may be the general medical technique of the new millennium.[2,3] The following two cases were treated by Dr. Paquette and are from *Medicine of Hope*.*

- **ASTHMA:** T.J. suffered from asthma for 12 years and became symptom-free for four years after nine IPT treatments.

- **RHEUMATOID ARTHRITIS:** C.W. had rheumatoid arthritis for 24 years and became symptom-free for six years after four IPT treatments. Mild symptoms returned, and after one IPT treatment, she became symptom free again for at least four more years.

The following pneumonia case was treated by Frank W. George, D.O., M.D. of Sun City, Arizona (See **Figure 20-9**):

G.E. is an 84-year-old male who presented at the end of April 2001 after an extended vacation out of the country with his wife with symptoms of a chest cold with cough worse at night, sinus congestion, and rhinitis for the past three days. He was treated for sinusitis and viral upper respiratory infection with Neural Therapy, osteopathic manipulation, combination homeopathy, and intravenous hydrogen peroxide.

Over the course of the week, the patient's condition did not improve. He developed a

---

* *This book can be ordered at www.benuts.com. For many additional general medical cases, please see www.IPTQ.org.*

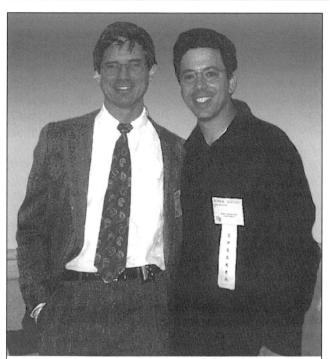

Figure 20-9: Drs. Frank George and Ross Hauser at an IPT Conference

rattling, hacking productive cough and some night sweats, without chills or fever. His appetite diminished, and this previously asthenic man had lost approximately 10 pounds since prior to leaving on vacation. Findings upon reexamination were a gaunt and weary appearance, afebrile state, increase respiratory rate of 36, and coarse rhonchi localized to the left lung base. Neural autologous hemotherapy was administered to the lung fields. An unsuccessful attempt at ultraviolet blood irradiation led to hydration with normal saline and the start of oral Zithromax. He was diagnosed with left lower lobe bronchopneumonia, which was later confirmed by chest x-ray. Sputum cultures revealed *Haemophilus influenza*, which was sensitive to the above prescription.

Over the course of the next three weeks of treatment with antibiotics and intravenous vitamins with minerals, the patient improved a little, with partial improvement in appetite and lessening of cough. He developed bilateral pedal edema, was still very weak, but had no further night sweats. Follow-up exam and x-ray indicated that there was minimal clearance of the left lobar pneumonia with expansion to the right lower lobe.

At this juncture, I decided to treat him using insulin as a potentiating and biological membrane modifier. He received three treatments over the course of three weeks. After the first day of the first treatment, he noted how much improved his appetite and energy level had become. The treatments consisted of oral vitamin A, magnesium and potassium, clostrum (transfer factor), and artichoke extract. Intramuscular injections included thymus, utilin 6X, gomenol, and 500 mg of Rocephin. Before the nadir of hypoglycemia, the patient had 140 mL of autologous blood irradiation, followed by intravenous vitamin C, minerals (magnesium, zinc, chromium, and selenium), homeopathic heel remedies (mucosa compositum, Gripp heel, Echinacea compositum forte S, and coenzyme compositum). Notakehl and Flagyl were also given. Many of these medicaments had been given during the course of the first three weeks of his illness with the exception of utilin, Flagyl, artichoke extract, and Rocephin. By his third treatment, this 84-year-old man felt back to normal, and two days later he flew cross-country for his 65th year college reunion.

There are many medical conditions where traditional allopathic medicine offers little hope of curing the condition including autoimmune diseases, chronic body pain, chronic fatigue syndrome, hepatitis, multiple sclerosis, many forms of cancer, central nervous system diseases, and viral infections. The primary reason for the failure of traditional medicine in many of these conditions is that the pharmaceutical drugs can not get into the cell, central nervous system, or other places it needs to go to get a healing effect.

Insulin Potentiation Therapy can be used as a general medical technique for many chronic medical conditions because it can potentiate the effects of medications for these conditions. Insulin Potentiation Therapy has many proposed actions which would help reverse the physiology of chronic diseases including enhanced cell membrane permeability, increased permeability of the blood-brain barrier, recruitment of cancer cells into the S phase, detoxification, enhanced cellular oxygenation, improvement in cell nutrition, increased cell energy production, increased uptake of medications into the cell, enhanced transport of medications into the central nervous system, and stimulation of stem cell and fibroblast differentiation.

FIGURE 20-10

POLIO CASE STUDY OF JUAN CARLOS SANCHEZ CORTINA

Dear Dr. Donato Péres García:

We thank you very much for the letter that you sent us. It is possible that you do not remember us, because I imagine that you have a lot of patients. My son, Juan Carlos Sanchez Cortina, was a patient of yours in 1988 when he was three years old and was suffering of polio problems when we were with you and your father. My son had already serious polio problems. He had completely lost the use of his right hip and foot. Thanks to you and your father—and with the intramuscular medical technique that you applied to my son in seven treatments—my son remained very well. Thanks to your medicine and treatment, my son has been playing soccer since the first grade. He is now 15 years old and continues playing his favorite sport as already I have previously mentioned.

For my husband and your humble servant, this has been a wonderful miracle as (thanks to the grace of God and you) my son has been able to walk again and he is now a healthy and strong adolescent. I do not know what we would have done without your help and whether our son would now be walking.

Again, my family and your humble servant, we thank you infinitely for your help, may God give you all the blessings so that you can continue to help the whole humanity with your treatments.

Warm Greetings from the Sanchez Cortina Family,
Mrs. Norma Cortina

(Translated from the original Spanish)

It is probable that in the future, the treatment of many chronic conditions will include Insulin Potentiation Therapy. As IPT was shown to reverse tertiary syphilis and polio by Dr. Donato Pérez García (Donato 1) prior to the modern antibiotic era, physicians of today are continuing to utilize IPT to reverse many so-called "irreversible" conditions (See **Figure 20-10**). Because IPT can help target medicines and reverse the physiology of various conditions, its role in the treatment of chronic medical conditions will undoubtedly expand as more patients discover its life-changing abilities.■

Insulin Potentiation Therapy: The Treatment of the Future for Infections and Autoimmune Diseases

Modern medicine has yet to cure the common cold virus. We vaccinate millions of people against the flu every year because the modern allopathic treatments for the flu are ineffective. People would be astonished to know how many conditions are caused by low-grade indolent infections. Modern medicine is still in the dark ages, believing that all infections cause fever, chills, and overt illness. Nothing could be further from the truth. Most infections cause covert symptoms such as malaise, fatigue, and mental fog.

OUR IMMUNE SYSTEMS ARE BREAKING DOWN

Disorders and diseases of the immune system affect the health and quality of life of every American. It has been estimated that approximately one in four Americans, or in excess of 65 million people, has a dysfunction of the immune system.[1] This does not take into account the number of work and school days lost, the cost of medications, hospitalizations, diminished quality of life, and involvement of family and friends during immune deficiency illnesses.

THE IMMUNE DEFENSES OF OUR BODY

The immune system is a complex network of specialized organs, cells, and cell products that protects the body from bacteria, viruses, infectious agents, and other substances that the body recognizes as foreign or abnormal. Its job is to neutralize or eliminate them. The immune system, however, has more diverse functions than this. It is involved both in the elimination of "worn-out" or damaged body cells (such as old red blood cells) and in the destruction of abnormal or mutant cell types that arise within the body. The latter can cause tumors or cancer. This last function, known as immune surveillance, constitutes one of the body's major defenses against cancer.

Specifically, the immune system consists of the organs that make immune cells, such as the thymus gland and bone marrow. Another major part is the lymph nodes where the immune system resides, and the gut-associated lymphoid tissue, which lines the intestinal tract (See **Figure 21-1**). The immune system also depends on the liver, spleen, and endocrine glands working in the proper coordination with other body systems for optimal function.

AUTOIMMUNITY: WHEN THE BODY TURNS ON ITSELF

One of the primary jobs of the immune system is to distinguish between what is "self" and what is "not self." Once this has been made, "self" is preserved, and "not self" is destroyed. In autoimmunity, the immune system recognizes and attacks the self's own tissue. The reason for this is still speculative, but some research indicates that the basis of autoimmunity may be a resemblance between a specific foreign molecule and a molecule of self.[1]

The list of autoimmune diseases is both long and disturbing. It includes multiple sclerosis, in which the tissue attacked is myelin (the coating of the nerve cells); myasthenia gravis, in which the target is a receptor molecule for the important neurotransmitter

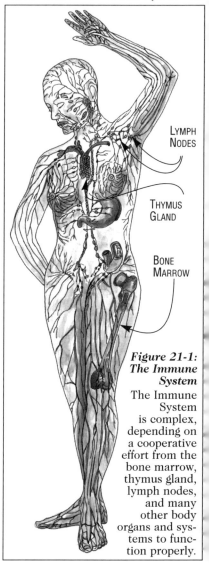

LYMPH NODES

THYMUS GLAND

BONE MARROW

Figure 21-1: The Immune System

The Immune System is complex, depending on a cooperative effort from the bone marrow, thymus gland, lymph nodes, and many other body organs and systems to function properly.

Figure 21-2: WHERE AUTOIMMUNITY MAY STRIKE

DISEASE	TARGET
Addison's Disease	Adrenal gland
Autoimmune Hemolytic Anemia	Red blood cell membrane proteins
Crohn's Disease	Gut
Goodpasture's Syndrome	Kidney and lungs
Graves' Disease	Thyroid
Hashimoto's Thyroiditis	Thyroid
Idiopathic Thrombocytopenic Purpura	Platelets
Insulin-Dependent Diabetes Mellitus	Pancreatic beta cells
Multiple-Sclerosis	Brain and spinal cord
Myasthenia Gravis	Nerve/muscle synapses
Pemphigus Vulgaris	Skin
Pernicious Anemia	Gastric parietal cells
Poststreptococcal Glomerulonephritis	Kidney
Psoriasis	Skin
Rheumatoid Arthritis	Connective tissue
Scleroderma	Heart, lungs, gut, and kidney
Sjogren's Syndrome	Liver, kidney, brain, thyroid, and salivary gland
Spontaneous Infertility	Sperm
Systemic Lupus Erythematosus	DNA, platelets, and other tissues

acetylcholine; rheumatoid arthritis, whose target is the peripheral joints; type 1 (juvenile) diabetes mellitus, in which the cells producing insulin are destroyed; systemic lupus erythematosus, in which DNA, blood vessels, skin, and kidneys are attacked; as well as many other conditions (See **Figure 21-2**).

AUTOIMMUNITY DETECTION IS ONLY A BLOOD TEST AWAY

Many people are afflicted with an autoimmune disease and do not even know it. Sensitive blood tests are now available that show the autoantibodies that are produced in various diseases. Antibodies are specialized proteins capable of combining with a specific antigen or foreign substance that stimulated its production. Once the antibody-foreigner connection is made, immune cells called phagocytes destroy (eat up) the complex. This is great if the foreigner is a bacteria that needs to be eaten but bad if it is the person's own joints (rheumatoid arthritis). The way to diagnose autoimmune diseases is by detecting the various autoantibodies in the blood (**See Figure 21-3**). Unfortunately, many traditional medical doctors do not know about the vast array of autoantibodies, so they are not tested, and people go undiagnosed with these conditions. Caring Laboratory Services, conveniently located in the Caring Medical complex, has the capability to do blood tests for just about every autoantibody, as well as the other tests that are needed to fully evaluate someone with an autoimmune disease.

FIGURE 21-3: AUTO-ANTIBODIES AND DISEASE

Auto-antibodies can attack cells and organs of the body, causing a myriad of symptoms and medical conditions.

AUTOANTIBODY	CONDITION
Anti-DNA	Sjogren's Syndrome
Anti-Nuclear Antibody	Systemic Lupus Erythematosus
Anti-Parietal Cell	Hypochlorhydria
Anti-Thyroglobulin	Hypothyroidism
Rheumatoid Factor	Rheumatoid Arthritis
Anti-Adrenal Gland	Adrenal Insufficiency
Anti-Collagen	Dermatitis
Anti-Insulin	Diabetes Mellitus
Anti-Sperm	Infertility
Anti-Estrogen	Menstrual Irregularities
Anti-Testosterone	Low Libido
Anti-Serotonin	Depression
Anti-Myelin Basic Protein	Multiple Sclerosis

AUTOIMMUNE DISEASES CAUSE A CONSTELLATION OF SYMPTOMS

Autoimmune diseases cause a destruction of normal body tissues or block regular bodily processes. For instance, in Sjogren's syndrome, the salivary glands, liver, and kidney can be damaged, whereas if a person is producing antiestrogen antibody, the body will act as if estrogen is missing, causing such symptoms as hot flashes, hair growth, and infertility. As a matter of fact, autoimmunity can cause very common symptoms (**See Figure 21-4**). This is another reason the condition goes undiagnosed.

143

FIGURE 21-4: COMMON SYMPTOMS FROM AUTOIMMUNITY

DEPRESSION	JOINT PAINS	STIFFNESS
DRY SKIN	MALAISE	STOMACH UPSET
FATIGUE	SKIN RASHES	WEAKNESS

THE NATURAL MEDICINE APPROACH MAKES MORE SENSE THAN THE ALLOPATHIC ONE

If one looks at the list of autoimmune diseases in **Figure 21-2,** it is clear that the main allopathic treatment used for many of these conditions is prednisone or some other corticosteroid. At best, this approach only slows down the progression of the disease; however, long-term prednisone can cause a host of its own problems, including osteoporosis, immune suppression, weight gain, bloating, thin skin, easy bruisability, many other bad side effects and even death. Prednisone is used because it is good at symptom control, but it does not address the etiology of the problem. The natural medicine approach is to look for the cause of the problem. In other words, since autoimmune diseases are caused by autoantibodies, the question is, "Why is the person making these antibodies in the first place?" This is why the natural medicine approach to autoimmune diseases makes more sense than the allopathic one.

AUTOANTIBODIES: THINK OF THEM AS FRIENDLY FIRE

The immune system is continually making antibodies to help rid the body of substances it sees as "nonself." Antibodies can then be compared to torpedoes, which are launched to get rid of one's enemies. Two enemies the body normally produces antibodies against are infections and food allergens. When the immune system is exposed to an infection or an allergen, it will produce antibodies against the offending organism or substance, so it can be eliminated by the immune surveillance system. Some experts in the natural medicine field believe that some autoantibodies are produced in response to the body fighting an infection or an allergen. When the offending infection(s) or allergen(s) are removed, the autoantibodies stop being produced (**See Figure 21-5**). Thus one can think of autoantibodies as "friendly fire" that occurs in battles when one is shot down or hit by a torpedo from one's own troops.

CASE STUDIES ILLUSTRATE THE POINT
JAN WITH SCLERODERMA

Jan and her husband were frantic; you could see it on their faces. She had a diagnosis of scleroderma and an ANA (antinuclear antibody) titer of 1280 (normal is 0). As if this was not bad enough, she was two months pregnant. Abortion was out of the question, as they were devout Christians. Her allopathic physicians did not leave them many options, so they came to Caring Medical. After hearing their story, Dr. Hauser informed them that he would like to try and make Jan ANA negative. The husband spoke in disbelief asking, "Is that possible?"

Like many others, this family did not understand the power of natural medicine. After some testing, Jan was placed on a hypoallergenic diet, and in six weeks she was ANA negative. She subsequently

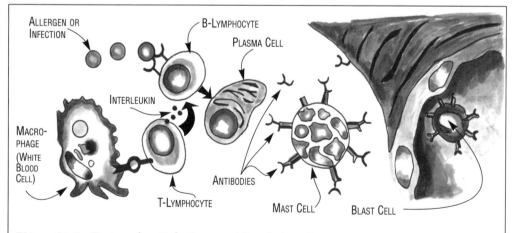

Figure 21-5: *Stages of an Infectious or Allergic Attack*
Allergies and infections stimulate the immune system to make antibodies. Some of these antibodies activate the immune system; others cause the basophils and mast cells to release histamine. From a natural medicine perspective, some of the antibodies produced can cross-react with the person's own tissues, causing a variety of autoimmune diseases.

had a perfectly healthy child and continues a healthy life.

JURGEN WITH RHEUMATOID ARTHRITIS

Jurgen was a feisty old German who was pretty suspect about natural medicine, but he came to Caring Medical on the insistence of his wife. He had aggressive rheumatoid arthritis with an elevated rheumatoid factor and was needing stronger and stronger pain medication. He received extensive testing and was found to have various food allergies and a mycoplasma infection. He was placed on an allergy elimination diet, nutriceutical products, and an antibiotic. Upon follow-up, he shouted, "This natural medicine stuff is for real! I am down from 3200 mg to 200 mg per day on the ibuprofen!" Within three months, he was rheumatoid factor negative. He continues in good health but does take some nutritional supplements for his joints.

DAREN WITH PEMPHIGUS VULGARIS

Daren was full of blisters. He was a dejected teenager, as pemphigus wreaked havoc on his body. He tested very high for an allergy to milk, and when confronted about his milk consumption, he answered, "I drink a half gallon per day. I thought milk was good for your bones!" Daren was an athletic star at his high school. Since the pemphigus hit, he was on steroid medication and a type of chemotherapy. Soon he was off all the medications, but he did miss his milk. Pemphigus, though, was not missed. It should be noted that because of the severity of his case, he did receive ozone therapy, which appeared to help resolve his condition quicker.

THE NATURAL MEDICINE APPROACH TO AUTOIMMUNE DISEASES

Natural medicine principles involve giving the body what it is missing, and removing from the body that which is harmful. Generally, with autoimmune diseases, the body is missing essential fatty acids and is hormone depleted. Thus, these items are supplemented. Because of the various hormones and medications with which

FIGURE 21-6: ORGANISMS THAT CAN BE FOUND IN THE BLOOD BY POLYMERASE CHAIN REACTION (PCR) TESTING

- Candida
- Chlamydia Pneumoniae
- Chlamydia Species
- Chlamydia Trachomatis
- Cytomegalovirus
- Epstein-Barr Virus
- Hepatitis A
- Hepatitis B
- Hepatitis C
- Herpes Type 1
- Herpes Type 2
- Herpes Type 6
- HIV-1
- Lyme Disease
- Mycoplasma Fermentans
- Mycoplasma Genitalium
- Mycoplasma Hominis
- Mycoplasma Orale
- Mycoplasma Pneumoniae
- Mycoplasma Species
- Ureaplasma Urealyticum
- Other Infectious Agents by Request

the person has been treated, people with autoimmune diseases often have various degrees of liver toxicity, systemic inflammation, and adrenal insufficiency that respond well to nutriceutical supplementation.*

To help the body stop producing autoantibodies, the person is placed on an allergy elimination diet. The offending foods to which the person is allergic are avoided for three months. At that time, the person should undergo provocation/neutralization allergy treatment to desensitize for the offending food. If no improvement is seen, then serial dilution testing and treatment is done for chemical and inhalant allergies. It is also possible to test and treat for sensitivities to one's own natural hormones—estrogen, progesterone, or serotonin.**

To determine if there is an offending organism related to the person's autoimmune disease, PCR testing for offending organisms in the blood is done (See **Figure 21-6**). This actually tests for the DNA of the organisms; and thus their presence in the person's blood. The treatment regime will

---

* For a complete list of the nutritional supplements (protocols) often used at Caring Medical to treat autoimmune diseases, please see www.benuts.com, or call 1-877-RX-BEULAH. Click on the autoimmune disease that you are interested in, and the various nutritionals used will be shown.

** For a complete explanation of provocation, neutralization, and serial dilution allergy testing and treatment, please see the Caring Medical web site at www.caringmedical.com.

then depend on which organism is found in the blood. For bacteria, an antibiotic is given; if a virus, antivirals; and for a fungus infection, antifungals. Some people desire to do more interventional natural medicine treatments such as photoluminescence (ultraviolet blood purification) and ozone therapy. An even more aggressive regime is Insulin Potentiation Therapy. In this treatment, the person is given ozone therapy for immune stimulation, followed by insulin to help potentiate the effect of the various medications to enter the cells or the central nervous system to help eradicate the organism.

IT IS NEVER TOO LATE TO START
JAN WITH RHEUMATOID ARTHRITIS

Jan is surely glad she started. Though her joints are severely deformed from rheumatoid arthritis, she decided to start on antibiotic therapy due to the presence of bacteria in her blood, along with her long list of supplements. She also started an aggressive exercise program upon the recommendation of Dr. Hauser. "She puts the rest of my clients to shame," exclaims Bob Gadja, a world-renown kinesiotherapist in Palatine, Illinois, who treats Jan. "She works out harder and longer than my football stars. Her abdominals are like rocks!" Jan is a testimony to making an ability out of a disability. She is active in the community and her church. She is someone who truly inspires and is inspired!

For the person who desires more information on relieving inflammatory arthritis and autoimmune diseases through natural medicine principles and anti-infection medications (such as antibiotics), please refer to the following sources:

- *There Is a Cure for Arthritis*, by Paavo Airola. (Parker Publishing Company, Qwar Nyack, NY, 1973)
- *Arthritis Can Be Cured,* by B. Aschner. (ARC Books, Inc., New York, NY, 1971)
- *Food Chemical Sensitivity*, by R. Buist. (Prism Press, San Leandro, Calif, 1986)
- *Rheumatoid Diseases Cured at Last,* by A. Di Fabio. (The Arthritis Trust of America, Franklin, Tenn, 1985)
- *Arthritis,* by A. Di Fabio. (The Arthritis Trust of America, Franklin, Tenn, 1997)

- *Skin Endpoint Titration,* by R. Mabry. (AAOA Monograph Series, Thieme Publishers, New York, NY, 1994)
- *The New Arthritis Breakthrough,* by H. Scammell. (M. Evans and Company, Inc., New York, NY, 1998)
- *Food Allergy,* by R. Trevino. (AAOA Monograph Series; Thieme Publishers, New York, NY, 1997)

Much of the above information is contained in a brochure that we wrote for our office, *Reversing Autoimmune Diseases with Natural Medicine.* There are numerous case reports of people's autoimmune diseases going into remission (the AMA does not permit the word *cure* to be used in medicine) by eliminating allergies and various infections. Many people with these low-level indolent infections who do not actually have autoimmune diseases, can feel just as poorly.

Because of the widespread use of PCR testing, it is now not only possible to document accurately and definitively that a person has a blood infection, but also to quantify it. Most of the time, the infections are not your run-of-the-mill bacteria such as staphylococcus or streptococcus, because these respond well to antibiotics. It is generally an atypical bacteria such as chlamydia or mycoplasma, a fungus such as candida, or viruses such as cytomegalovirus, herpes virus, or Epstein-Barr virus. These organisms are not sensitive to the typical penicillin or cephalosporin antibiotics that are routinely doled out to people.

Viral infections are especially difficult to cure, and modern medicine would even go so far as to say impossible to cure. Viruses incorporate into the cells as part of their life cycles. Various antiviral medications, like chemotherapy drugs, do not accumulate enough into the virus-infected cells to induce a cure. Thus, chronic hepatitis, herpes, and HIV infections are almost never cured, just controlled.

For the person who feels terrible and is found to have a chronic viral infection such as hepatitis C, the prognosis is grim. Slow progression to liver failure and then death is the outcome for many. A similar fate awaits someone with AIDS or HIV infection. Patient quality of life is generally diminished knowing the person has an incurable disease. Caring Medical sees a new case of herpes almost everyday because of recent exposure to the disease due to inappropriate social behavior. Some of these people test negative to herpes, and wow—are they happy. They know that when a person is diagnosed with herpes, it is herpes for life! Richer or poorer, sickness or in health, the herpes virus will always be there. That is—until IPT.

INSULIN POTENTIATION THERAPY— AN AGGRESSIVE ANTI-INFECTION TREATMENT

Insulin Potentiation Therapy is a method that can help potentiate the effects of medications such as antivirals, antifungals, and antibiotics. Since antivirals have a difficult time penetrating into cells, IPT is especially useful for conditions in which the microbe infiltrates the cells, such as viral diseases. Another significant fact is that many antivirals, antifungals, and antibiotics poorly penetrate the central nervous system, which can be corrected with IPT.

JOAN WITH LYME DISEASE AFFECTING THE NERVOUS SYSTEM

Joan struggled for years with a "disconnected" feeling in her head. She came to Caring Medical and was found to have adrenal insufficiency and hypoglycemia. After treatment, she felt less fatigue, but her mental fog and slight dizziness did not improve. PCR testing revealed Lyme disease, whereas her previous Lyme test (Western blot) was negative. She underwent many months of antibiotics without improvement in her mental fog symptoms. She agreed to undergo IPT to increase the antibiotic concentration in her central nervous system. She said after her second IPT, "This is the first time I am beginning to feel better." She has had four treatments thus far. She is working full time as a manager of a clothing store, recently moved, and again has an active life, much of which was possible because of IPT.

PEGGY WITH CHRONIC FATIGUE AND FIBROMYALGIA

Peggy came to Caring Medical from New York City for Prolotherapy. She had complete body aches and desired whole body Prolotherapy. She had several rounds of Prolotherapy, then Neural Therapy with only slight improvement in her pain. She was noted to have chronic Lyme disease and mycoplasma infection, which was being treated by an infectious disease doctor in New York City. She had received numerous rounds of oral and intravenous antibiotics prior to coming to Caring Medical. She was started on some antifungal medication after candida infection was found. She desired to try IPT since nothing else seemed to work. She received IPT using medications that treat Lyme disease and mycoplasma infection. She had a total of eight sessions and then tested negative for both organisms. Her energy and chronic pain diminished significantly.

SANDRA WITH MULTIPLE SCLEROSIS

Sandra was a long-time patient of Caring Medical who was being seen for chronic progressive multiple sclerosis. She had previously tried Avonex from her neurologist but was unable to tolerate it. Despite aggressive natural medicine, her multiple sclerosis continued to progress. She then underwent PCR testing and was found to have herpes in her blood. She was then given IPT with antiviral medications that cover herpes. She tolerated the treatment well, but one hour afterward experienced violent shaking with a temperature of 102.9, both indicative of Herxheimer's reaction, signifying that the microbe was being destroyed. Amazingly within a few hours after the treatment, she already noticed the strength in her arms returning.

The above case studies are just a few examples of why it is extremely important for anyone with a chronic disease to see a natural medicine specialist who understands chronic infections.

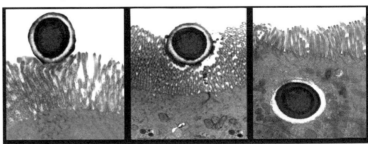

Pictures courtesy of Great Smokies Diagnostic Laboratory, Asheville, North Carolina.

Figure 21-7: Yeast Burrowing Through Intestinal Wall
Candida fungus infection is one of the causes of "Leaky Gut Syndrome." This ability of infectous organisms to translocate across the bowel wall in susceptible individuals can lead to autoimmune diseases and a host of other conditions.

Modern medicine does not recognize that microbes can traverse the bowel wall and infect the blood. Some people call this condition "leaky gut syndrome" (See **Figure 21-7**). The average physician does not realize that even commonly known infections such as mycoplasma can live intracellularly, and thus must be treated for longer periods of time. The usual and customary treatment regimes can and often do fail. When they do fail, the microbe still elicits an immune reaction, whereby the immune system fires off antibodies against it. These antibodies cause the person to be tired and achy, and if they are produced in sufficient amounts, an autoimmune disease can form. There are many reports that autoimmune diseases can have an infectious etiology.[2-11]

Perhaps the most commonly known chronic infection in natural medicine circles is *Candida albicans,* the cause of the common yeast infection. What women do not realize is that the infection grows in the digestive tract and makes its way to the vaginal area. If it can grow in the digestive tract of a woman, it can surely do the same in men. Candida can cause a myriad of symptoms, including carbohydrate craving, fatigue, malaise, and mental fog (See **Figure 21-8**). We believe most folks with fibromyalgia have candida infestation. The treatment is a low-carbohydrate diet and antifungal medications and herbs. This treatment regime can resurrect many a sick person from the "dead," but if he or she stops the antifungals, relapse occurs. The symptoms could recur for many reasons, but the one that makes the most sense is that the regular antifungal regime is not completely eradicating the organism. Perhaps in the future it will be IPT that finally gets these patients over the hump and over their candida.

SUMMARY

Modern medicine says that most chronic conditions such as autoimmune diseases have no known cause. Natural medicine practitioners are finding in these diseases that allergies, especially to foods, and various infections are the culprits. In susceptible individuals, the person's body makes autoantibodies against his or her own cells and tissues in addition to the antibodies against the allergen and/or food. When the person is put on a food allergy elimination diet and/or desensitized to the foods, inhalants, or chemicals that the person is mounting an immune reaction against, the symptoms of the chronic condition start to abate. Sometimes the production of the autoimmune antibody ceases.

Some infections such as herpes, HIV, Epstein-Barr, mycoplasma, Borrelia (Lyme disease), and cytomegalovirus are difficult to treat with medications because the organisms live intracellularly (inside the cell). The antiviral and antibiotic medications do not accumulate enough inside the cell to kill these organisms, so the disease often continues despite treatment. Because insulin helps these medications accumulate inside the cell, IPT is a viable option for patients with these conditions. If the infection affects the neurological system, such as in multiple sclerosis, polio, and Lou Gehrig disease, IPT should be a treatment to consider. Practitioners of IPT already have clients with these conditions who are improving, and some have recovered completely.

In the future, we hope that more patients will consider receiving IPT for previously thought "incurable" diseases. It is probable that if this occurs, the world will see many miracles happen because of IPT. ∎

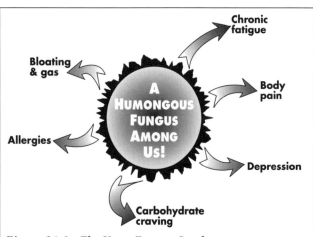

Figure 21-8: The Yeast Fungus Syndrome
The yeast fungus syndrome can mimic a lot of syndromes and conditions.

CHAPTER 22

The Other Potentiators, Including DMSO, Hyperthermia, Electrochemotherapy, Oxidative Therapy, and Nutrients

"THIS POTENTIATION MEANS THAT THESE DRUGS CAN BE USED IN SIGNIFICANTLY LOWER DOSES THAN THOSE USUALLY NEEDED TO OBTAIN A SATISFACTORY THERAPEUTIC RESPONSE; THUS THE DANGER OF SECONDARY TOXIC EFFECTS AND INTOLERANCE OF MEDICINES IS REDUCED."
—Dr. Jorge Garrido and Dr. Raul Lagos, Military Hospital in Santiago, Chile

In 1998, at a Prolotherapy conference in rural Illinois, Gustav A. Hemwall, M.D., was posed the question, "Why don't more doctors do Prolotherapy?" His answer was succinct and to the point: "It's too simple, just like the gospel." By many at the conference, Dr. Hemwall was considered the world expert in a technique that has relieved tens of thousands of their chronic pain complaints, yet it remains unknown for the many masses of people with pain. A similar analogy can be seen with Insulin Potentiation Therapy.

For over 70 years, the Donato Pérez García family of physicians have been curing people of chronic disabling diseases, like cancer, by utilizing something very simple, insulin. There is nothing high-tech about insulin. Insulin is remarkable, but it is "just" a natural hormone. The whole notion of IPT is that insulin potentiates the cancer-killing effects of chemotherapy. Surely something that is used to help cure cancer must be more sophisticated than this! Now if you tagged the chemotherapy drug to some fancy liposomal-based biotechnology-patented molecule, it would be on the front page of the *New York Times*. But talk about insulin: ho-hum. No matter how many books are written on Prolotherapy or Insulin Potentiation Therapy, it will be difficult for modern medicine to accept these therapies because they are just too simple.

WHAT IS A POTENTIATOR?

Stanley W. Jacob, M.D., wrote in *The Miracle of MSM,* "In practical terms, this means that the use of DMSO allows you to reduce the dosage of a therapeutic agent, such as chemo."[1] Ross loves quotes that are to the point. A potentiating agent is one that increases the effectiveness of another agent. **In regard to chemotherapy, a potentiator increases the kill power of the drug toward cancer cells.** Because of this ability, a lower dose of the medication is needed to get the same pharmacological effect.

Antibiotics work so well because they get to the site of the bacterial infection and kill the bacterium. Antiviral medication results are poor because they do not get inside the cell to kill the virus. Chemotherapy results are modest at best because the chemotherapy drugs do not get to the cancer cells in sufficient quantity to achieve a 100% kill. In regard to antiviral and chemotherapy medications, these are great virus and cancer cell killers in vitro (in the lab), respectively; the problem is that where it counts, in vivo (in the human body), they do not work. They work in the lab but not in the body. When a virus is exposed to an antiviral, it dies. When a cancer cell is exposed to chemotherapy, it is killed. All that is needed then is to get the antiviral into the cell that is infected or to get the chemotherapy drug to the cancer site. If this is accomplished, the success at getting rid of chronic viral infections and cancers will be greatly enhanced.

A potentiator can work by many different mechanisms to increase the effectiveness of a particular medication (See **Figure 22-1**). *In regard to chemotherapy, most potentiators work by increasing the concentration of the drug at the tumor site.* Any substance or process that does this will help cancer patients increase their chances of cure. It is for this reason that we often use multiple potentiators during a treatment at CCINMC. The main ones that can be incorporated during an IPT

FIGURE 22-1: MECHANISM OF ACTION OF MEDICATION POTENTIATORS

- ▪ ENHANCE CYTOKINE PRODUCTION
- ▪ IMPROVE PERMEABILITY ACROSS THE BLOOD-BRAIN BARRIER
- ▪ INCREASE CELL MEMBRANE PERMEABILITY
- ▪ INCREASE REACTIVE OXYGEN SPECIES
- ▪ INHIBIT ENZYME SYSTEMS
- ▪ RECRUIT CELLS INTO THE GROWTH PHASE OF THE CELL CYCLE
- ▪ REVERSE DISEASE PHYSIOLOGY
- ▪ STIMULATE THE IMMUNE SYSTEM

---

treatment include insulin (of course), DMSO, hyperthermia, electricity, biooxidants (including hydrogen peroxide), and ozone therapy, as well as simple nutrients such as selenium.

THE POTENTIATION OF CHEMOTHERAPY IS ESSENTIAL IN REDUCING SIDE EFFECTS

Before discussing the other potentiators (besides insulin), it is important to reiterate why potentiation of chemotherapy is needed. Modern medicine uses extremely high doses of chemotherapy because this is what is needed to get enough of the medication to the tumor site to have a chance at killing it. This is in stark contrast to the dose needed when giving IPT (**See Figure 22-2**).

Drug	Typical Dose Given*	IPT Dose
Cisplatin	150 MG	15 MG
5-Fluorouracil	1,500 MG	200 MG
Cyclophosphamide	1,500 MG	200 MG
Methotrexate	60 MG	10 MG
Doxorubicin	100 MG	10 MG

Figure 22-2: Comparison of Chemotherapy Doses between Traditional Allopathic Medicine and IPT

The reason it is imperative for cancer patients to know about the various potentiators of chemotherapy is so they can get the cancer-killing power of the medications at much lower doses. Potentiators have a dramatic effect on increasing the safety of the medications. The fear of every cancer patient is death by chemotherapy. Consider these actual e-mails sent to our friend, Steve Meyer who received a bone marrow transplant for mantle cell lymphoma.

> My experience with Cisplatin, part of ESHAP, was most unpleasant. It is the only thing I have taken that really did bad things to my head. It gave me trouble with vision, concentration, and reading and resulted in an uncharacteristic depression. Those effects went away in time, but I also sustained kidney damage, which remains and has ruled out some treatments since. (M.H.)

> My husband's treatment with fludarabine caused an acute reaction, which caused his body to destroy his own red blood cells (hemolysis). Therefore, the doctor does not want to use it again. He has proposed REPOCH; however, because he had maximum doxorubicin, he is afraid of the cardiac problems when going beyond the maximum dose. He has also proposed DHAP with possible neurologic toxicity. (J.R.)

The above scenarios are repeated across the country every day. If we were to walk into any oncology ward in a hospital, a good percentage of the people would be there due to the side effects of chemotherapy. **These side effects occur with chemotherapy because oncologists are not using potentiators with the chemotherapy. Without potentiators, extremely high, toxic doses of chemotherapy must be used to have any chance to get a little bit of the chemotherapy drug to the cancer site.** This is extremely sad because many potentiators are available to use with chemotherapy, from something as sophisticated as electrochemotherapy to simple compounds, such as selenium and insulin.

DMSO

DMSO stands for dimethyl sulfoxide. It is a solvent derived from coal, oil, and lignin, the intercellular cement of trees. DMSO is found in milk, fruits, vegetables, and grains and is even normally present in small quantities in the human body.[2] Yes, DMSO is a constituent normally found in the human body.

DMSO is a truly unique chemical, as demonstrated by both its physical and chemical properties. It is composed of two methyl atoms, a sulfur atom, and an oxygen atom stacked in the shape of a pyramid (**See Figure 22-3**). The sulfur pole has a strong negative charge, and the oxygen a positive charge; the

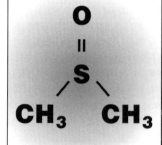

Figure 22-3: Chemical Structure of DMSO
Dimethyl sulfoxide is composed of two methyl (CH_3) groups, a sulfur atom, and an oxygen atom stacked in the shape of a pyramid.

---

* *Assuming a 150-lb man with cancer according to* The Cancer Chemotherapy Handbook *(Mosby Publishing, St. Louis, Mo, 1997).*

resulting electromagnetic-type force enables a DMSO molecule to attach to another—negative pole to positive pole—and form molecular chains.[3] DMSO as a solvent will dissolve most unsaturated and aromatic hydrocarbons, other organosulfur compounds, organic nitrogen compounds, and a number of inorganic salts. It also has a tremendous attraction for water, as shown by its ability to remove water from such common "drying" chemicals as potassium hydroxide, calcium chloride, and silica gel.[4] In probably unparalleled chemical compatibility, DMSO can readily mix with other solvents—water, alcohol, oils (lipids), and benzene. DMSO's solvent properties give it tremendous ability to transport substances through the skin, penetrate tissues and cell walls, and transport other substances with it.

DMSO is an organic sulfur compound widely used in alternative cancer treatment, particularly in biologic and metabolic therapies. A clear, colorless, viscous, and essentially odorless liquid, it is administered to patients by intravenous infusion, intramuscular injection, topical application, or oral solutions.[5,6]

DMSO is a respected, approved pharmaceutical agent in over 100 countries. Much of the research and publicity for DMSO was because of Stanley W. Jacob, M.D., of the Oregon Health Sciences University in Portland. DMSO as a therapeutic principle was first introduced to the scientific community in 1963 by a research team headed by Dr. Jacob. Dr. Jacob wrote in 1994 that,

> while DMSO has been called "the most controversial therapeutic advance of modern times," the "controversy" seems to be bureaucratic and economic rather than scientific. Over the past 30 years, more than 11,000 articles on the biologic implications of DMSO have appeared in the scientific literature. The results of these studies strongly support the view that DMSO may be the most significant new therapeutic principle presented to science in the last half of the 20th century.[7]

In 1978, it was approved by the FDA for the therapy of interstitial cystitis, a painful, disabling urinary bladder inflammation.

In the United States, DMSO is rarely used in modern medical therapeutics. This is extremely sad considering it has dozens of pharmacologic actions, including enhanced membrane transport.

(**See Figure 22-4.**) For the person with cancer, DMSO can be helpful for many reasons. It is an effective pain-reducing agent (analgesic), helping people get off morphine. It has bacteriostatic or antibiotic effects, reducing the risk of infections. It antagonizes platelet aggregation, which helps keep the blood thin. If a person has brain metastases or brain cancer, DMSO will help carry the chemotherapy drugs to the tumor site because it crosses the blood-brain barrier. It does have several "small" side effects, including making a person smell like garlic for a day or so after an infusion (some people think this should be considered a "big" side effect); as well as a localized skin rash (redness) if put on the skin; and occasional headaches, nausea, and dizziness.[6]

FIGURE 22-4: SOME OF THE PHARMACOLOGIC ACTIONS OF DMSO

- ANTAGONISM TO PLATELET AGGREGATION
- ANTI-INFLAMMATION
- BACTERIOSTASIS
- CELL DIFFERENTIATION
- CHOLINESTERASE INHIBITION
- CONNECTIVE TISSUE REPAIR
- CROSSES BLOOD-BRAIN BARRIER
- DIURESIS
- IMMUNE ENHANCEMENT
- MEMBRANE PENETRATION
- MEMBRANE TRANSPORT
- MUSCLE RELAXATION
- NERVE BLOCKAGE (ANALGESIA)
- POTENTIATION OF DRUGS
- VASODILATION

DMSO has tremendous solubility properties. In animal studies, when applied to the skin, it can be found within two hours in the following organs in decreasing order: spleen, stomach, lung, vitreous humor, thymus, brain, kidney, sclera, colon, heart, skeletal muscle, skin, liver, aorta, adrenal, lens of eye, and cartilage.[8,9] DMSO readily crosses most tissue membranes and has the ability to take chemicals and medications with it. Because of DMSO's unique chemistry, it has found use in a broad spectrum of medical conditions, including cancer; arthritis; cerebral edema; urinary tract disorders; osteomyelitis; burns; and musculoskeletal disorders such as sprains, strain injuries, and acute bursitis.[6]

DMSO AS A POTENTIATOR

Extremely low concentrations of DMSO (2% to 3%) have been shown to induce changes consistent with cell differentiation, such as increased cell doubling times. These changes have been observed in human melanoma, colon adenocarcinoma, and erythroid leukemic cell lines in vitro.[10,11] To investigate the potentiating effects of DMSO, Rodney F. Pommier, M.D., and associates at the Oregon Health Sciences University in Portland studied the cancer-killing effects of DMSO, chemotherapeutic drugs (Adriamycin, Vinblastine, 5-fluorouracil, Cisplatin), and the combination of both on five human tumor cell lines.[11] The five human tumor cell lines were Hep-2 (squamous cell carcinoma of the larynx), HEC-1A (adenocarcinoma of the endometrium), CAKI-1 (adenocarcinoma of the kidney), HT-29 (adenocarcinoma of the colon), and MCF-7 (adenocarcinoma of the breast). The mean percentage kill of MCF-7 cells with combinations of DMSO and antineoplastic agents is seen in **Figure 22-5.** The authors summarized the study as follows:

> Five human tumor reference cell lines were tested in vitro against 0 percent, five percent, and 10 percent DMSO; four antineoplastic agents; and combinations of five percent or 10 percent DMSO plus each antineoplastic agent. Synergistic cytotoxicity between DMSO and antineoplastic agents against each cell line were demonstrated. **We have concluded that delivery of standard doses of antineoplastic agents in five percent or 10 percent DMSO may be useful in the treatment of some tumors because of the marked increase in tumoricidal effect seen with some DMSO and drug combinations.** Alternatively, lower doses of antineoplastic agents might be delivered in DMSO, producing the same cytotoxic effect as a full dose of drug without DMSO but with less systemic toxicity.[11]

In another study by Dr. Pommier and associates, ovarian malignancies were harvested from 24 patients, and cytotoxicity testing was done against 10% DMSO alone, six antineoplastic agents alone (Adriamycin, anthracenedione, Cisplatin, 5-fluorouracil, methotrexate, and Vinblastine), and 10% DMSO plus each antineoplastic agent.[10] The mean percentage increase

FIGURE 22-5: MEAN PERCENT CELL KILL OF MCF-7 CELLS (ADENOCARCINOMA OF BREAST) WITH COMBINATIONS OF DIMETHYL SULFOXIDE (DMSO) AND ANTINEOPLASTIC AGENTS

DRUG & CONCENTRATION (μG/ML)	MEAN % CELL KILL		
	0% DMSO	5% DMSO	10% DMSO
ADRIAMYCIN			
0	0	9	47
0.1	8	18	54
1	20	17	66
10	91	91	94
VINBLASTINE			
0	0	0	40
0.05	13	7	39
0.5	50	48	57
5	88	100	100
50	100	100	100
5-Fluorouracil			
0	0	7	51
0.6	2	8	60
6	0	2	57
60	33	62	75
600	87	98	100
CISPLATIN			
0	0	9	54
0.2	3	42	70
2	39	47	75
20	78	80	88

As seen above, DMSO enhanced the cancer killing effects of Adriamycin, Vinblastine, 5-fluorouracil and Cisplatin. All of these agents are commonly used in clinical practice.

in cell kill for 10% DMSO plus various antineoplastics is seen in **Figure 22-6.** The authors concluded that "these results are strong evidence that true synergistic cytotoxicity against ovarian cancer occurs when antineoplastic agents are combined with 10% DMSO." They went on to say that

> DMSO (10%) is remarkably nontoxic in human trials and has been used in doses of 2-4 g/kg/day without appreciable side effects. We conclude that intraperitoneal delivery of antineoplastic agents in 10% DMSO may be useful in the treatment of ovarian cancer.[10]

It appears from other research that the potentiating effects of DMSO on chemotherapeutic drugs is because it increases the concentration of the medication in the blood and in the tumor.[12] In one animal study, the authors wrote,

---

FIGURE 22-6: MEAN PERCENTAGE INCREASE IN CELL KILL FOR 10% DMSO PLUS VARIOUS ANTINEOPLASTIC DRUGS

SYNERGISM	ADR	ANTH	CISP	5-FU	MTX	VINB
P ≤ 0.01	73	52	64	76	67	46

Adr = Adriamycin, Anth = Anthracenedione, CisP = Cisplatin, 5-FU = 5 Fluorouracil, MTX = Methotrexate, Vinb = Vinblastine

---

DMSO enhanced the cancer-killing effects of the chemotherapy drugs from 46% to 78%.

Orally ingested DMSO was found to cause a twofold increase in the concentration of labeled cyclophosphamide in plasma, brain, and liver tissues. This elevation persisted for approximately two to three hours but subsequently returned to the same level as that observed in water-fed rodents.[13]

It appears to work best when the DMSO is given at the same time as the chemotherapy drug. Just like insulin, DMSO's beneficial effects appear to last only a couple of hours after the compound gets into the system, making it a very safe agent.[13]

To see if the potentiating effects of DMSO caused a clinical improvement in cancer patient outcomes, Dr. Jorge Garrido and Dr. Raul Lagos at the Military Hospital in Santiago, Chile, treated 65 advanced cancer patients between 1969 and 1971. The protocol involved intravenous and intramuscular injections of DMSO, cyclophosphamide, and amino acids. In the discussion section, the authors noted:

> Innumerable clinical and experimental investigations have shown that DMSO potentiates and increases the therapeutic activity of corticosteroids, insulin, alkylating agents, antibiotics, anti-inflammatory and antirheumatic agents, pyrazolics, nitrates, digitalis-like compounds, and many others. This potentiation means that these drugs can be used in significantly lower doses than those usually needed to obtain a satisfactory therapeutic response; thus the danger of secondary toxic effects and intolerance of medicines is reduced.[14]

In most cases, the DMSO and cyclophosphamide were given intravenously daily or every two days. These physicians believed that low-dose, high-frequency treatment would be better for their sick cancer patients than the high-dose, low-frequency treatment that is typically done. Instead of giving a person 2,000 mg of cyclophosphamide, they gave only 150-200 mg/dose. Of interest is that this type of dosing is similar to what is done in IPT. Some of the results can be seen in **Figures 22-7A** and **22-7B**. The results are actually quite remarkable when one considers that 13 of the 15 inoperable breast cancer patients with metastases were induced to remission with the DMSO-cyclophosphamide potentiating therapy. Of the 65 patients, 44 achieved remission. The treatment was found to be very safe. As a side effect of the therapy, the authors did note that the synergism of DMSO-cyclophosphamide relieved pain, with the result that in many cases it was not necessary to use morphine.

DMSO AT CARING MEDICAL

We are strong proponents of IPT. As a matter of fact, the first patient treated with IPT at Caring Medical was given DMSO because of brain metastases, during which time the tumor shrank dramatically. We have used DMSO (in combination with other modalities) to treat scleroderma, chronic pain, multiple sclerosis, skin lesions, ulcers, circulatory disorders, and cancer. In regard to IPT, DMSO has a lot of pharmacological effects that make it an excellent agent for use during the treatment, the most important of which is that it helps with survival (**See Figure 22-8**). While morphine and other narcotics can be immunosuppressive (which is detrimental to the cancer patient), DMSO helps reverse some of the person's cancer physiology while providing pain relief. It can help patients get off these types of medications. At CCINMC, DMSO is often mixed in the syringe with the chemotherapeutic agent, as well as in the saline bag that is hung. Patients know they are loaded with DMSO when everyone avoids them like the plague. One particular patient from New York was asked never to fly a particular airline again because she still smelled like garlic 24 hours after her treatment was given—and stunk up the airplane on her way back

FIGURE 22-7A AND B: TREATMENT RESULTS

*Below are test results documenting the dramatic results on patients with cancer using DMSO with low-dose chemotherapy. **The results are remarkable!***

FIGURE 22-7A: Results of Treatments of Patients with Lymphomas

DIAGNOSIS	NUMBER OF CASES	SUBJECTIVE REMISSION	OBJECTIVE REMISSION
Hodgkin's Disease	8	8	7
Lymphosarcoma	10	10	10
Bone Sarcoma	3	3	3
Ewing's Tumor	1	1	1
Total	**22**	**22**	**21**

FIGURE 22-7B: Summary of Results of 26 Cases of Breast Cancer

DIAGNOSIS	NUMBER OF CASES	OBJECTIVE OR SUBJECTIVE REMISSION
Inoperable Breast Cancer with Metastasis	15	13
Recidivist Breast Cancer with Multiple Metastasis	11	10
Total	**26**	**23**

home after IPT treatment. For those who have sensitive sniffers, don't fret; generally the person cannot smell the DMSO—just everyone else.

HYPERTHERMIA

"FEVER IS THE STRUGGLE OF THE ORGANISM AGAINST ILLNESS; IT PURIFIES THE BODY LIKE A FIRE."

—HIPPOCRATES, (460-377 BC)

"How do you feel?" "I am feeling much better. I am starting to put on some weight and my appetite is much better." As the patient left the room, Steve Elsasser, M.D., explained to us that the person was receiving the "shake and bake" treatment for metastatic breast cancer. Over the course of the next year, we observed several patients in his natural medicine center receive a type of Coley toxin injection, which would cause their temperatures to hover around 105° for about two hours. Dr. Elsasser had many tumor regressions and cures with this approach. A New York physician, William B. Coley, M.D., in the 1920s found that certain infectious diseases, especially bacteria, when introduced into the body in the form of a sterilized vaccine, had a beneficial effect in cancer patients. Dr. Coley found his "toxins" could give the body's anti-cancer defenses a stimulus that would help the fight against the cancer cells. Dr. Coley reported a 41% complete cure in the cancer patients he treated.[15] Some of his data can be seen in **Figure 22-9**. Dr. Coley is credited with starting the field of immunotherapy, which involves trying to get the immune system to attack the cancer in a more fervent manner.

The above experience with Dr. Elsasser was our first exposure to the beneficial effect fever

FIGURE 22-8: SURVIVAL IN GASTRIC CANCER

As can be seen, patients given DMSO had increased survival over the control patients.

TIME (YEARS)	CONTROL N	% SURVIVAL	DMSO N	% SURVIVAL
0	55	100%	54	100%
1	33	60%	44	81.5%
2	22	40%	33	61.1%
3	15	27.3%	26	48.2%
4	6	11%	18	33.3%

N = Number of patients alive

Adapted from Awas S. Salim, University Department of Surgery, Medical City, Baghdad, Iraq, Chemotherapy, 38:135-144, 1992.

might have on cancer survival. Hyperthermia is the application of therapeutic heat to destroy or reduce cancer tumors. The rationale behind hyperthermia is that cancer cells are more heat sensitive than normal cells.[16] It is used at our center in Oak Park to potentiate the effects of chemotherapeutic medications, though it has many other beneficial effects and applications.

Traditionally, fever has been considered detrimental to the host. Fever, which means a body temperature above the usual range of normal, can have many different causes, including infection, exercise, and fever therapy (hyperthermia). (See **Figure 22-10**.) While extreme elevated temperatures definitely warrant antipyretic medications (ie, Tylenol to reduce the temperature), evidence is mounting that fever is a beneficial host response. Temperature elevation enhances certain functions of the immune system, particularly those involving the recognition, sensitization, and activation of mononuclear cells.[16] Furthermore, in vitro studies suggest that heated leukocytes pro

FIGURE 22-9: FIVE YEAR SURVIVAL RATES OF ADVANCED CANCER PATIENTS RECEIVING COLEY'S MIXED BACTERIAL VACCINE

TYPE OF CANCER	PERCENT SURVIVING FIVE YEARS AFTER TREATMENT
Inoperable Breast Cancer	65%
Inoperable Ovarian Cancer	69%
Osteosarcoma	90%
Soft Tissue Sarcomas	48%
Lymphomas	58%

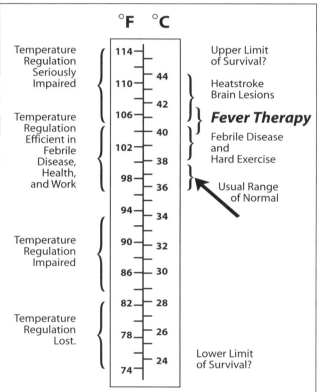

Figure 22-10: Body Temperatures under Different Conditions

During hyperthermia or fever therapy, the person's body temperature is raised to ~105°F.

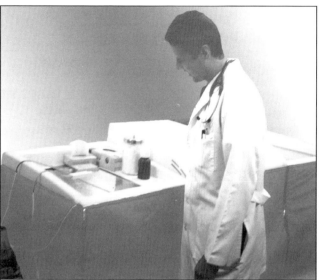

Figure 22-11: Garrett Swetlikoff, N.D., talks to one of his cancer patients, as she undergoes whole-body hyperthermia (WBH). Dr. Swetlikoff uses WBH as part of a comprehensive natural medicine approach to treat cancer at his clinic in Kelowna, British Columbia, Canada.

duce substances having both antimicrobial and anti-tumor activity.[17] The mononuclear and leukocyte cells are extremely important in the immune system aggressively fighting cancer.

If one goes on the Internet and researches various natural medicine cancer centers, it is obvious that many of them (eg, Germany) use whole body hyperthermia (WBH), the type of hyperthermia that increases the core body temperature. During the treatment, the heating of the body takes place through the noninvasive heating of the blood. Using a specific alloy that filters infrared rays, a special spectrum is created that allows the heat to pass through the skin without causing superficial burning. The WBH systems used today are totally computerized, allowing the treatment to be fully controlled by computer. The physician and clinical staff are able to continually observe the patient using the intensive care monitoring incorporated in the machine, including pulse, blood pressure, EKG (electrocardiogram), and oxygen content. The person's temperature is also monitored by various probes on and in the body. The person stays in the insulated "tent," sometimes called a whole-body cabin, for two to four hours. The person's temperature is typically raised to the 104-106°F range (See **Figure 22-11**).

Whole body hyperthermia has many beneficial effects, including enhanced immune system function, detoxification, and circulation (See **Figure 22-12**). Because of these wide-ranging effects, WBH is used for many different medical conditions, in addition to cancer (See **Figure 22-13**).

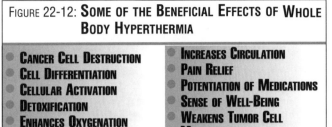

FIGURE 22-12: **SOME OF THE BENEFICIAL EFFECTS OF WHOLE BODY HYPERTHERMIA**

- CANCER CELL DESTRUCTION
- CELL DIFFERENTIATION
- CELLULAR ACTIVATION
- DETOXIFICATION
- ENHANCES OXYGENATION
- IMMUNE STIMULATION
- INCREASES CIRCULATION
- PAIN RELIEF
- POTENTIATION OF MEDICATIONS
- SENSE OF WELL-BEING
- WEAKENS TUMOR CELL MEMBRANES

FIGURE 22-13: **SOME OF THE CONDITIONS THAT WHOLE BODY HYPERTHERMIA HAS SUCCESSFULLY TREATED**

- Allergies
- Arthritis
- Autoimmune Diseases
- Cancer
- Cellulite
- Chronic Fatigue
- Chronic Pain
- Flu
- Gastrointestinal Disorders
- Infection
- Insomnia
- Menstrual Conditions
- Muscle Spasms
- Nervousness
- Obesity
- Osteoarthritis
- Toxicity
- Weak Immune System
- Wound Healing Impairment

PATHOPHYSIOLOGICAL MECHANISMS OF HYPERTHERMIA IN CANCER THERAPY

Increasing evidence supports the notion that malignant tumors can be damaged by a thermal dose (heat) that is not destructive to normal tissues. This preferential damage in tumors by hyperthermia is believed to be related to properties such as tumor blood flow, tissue oxygenation, pH distribution, and energy status.

Normal tissues respond to hyperthermia by increasing blood flow to dissipate the heat. For instance, heating at 45°C (113°F) causes a pronounced flow increase up to a factor of 15 in the skin and a factor of 10 in muscle. Blood flow in tumors, especially those that are rapidly growing, is very poor and sluggish when compared with that of normal tissues. At any given energy input (heat or fever), the temperature rises distinctly more in tumors than in normal tissues since the efficacy of heat dissipation in tumors is much reduced. The end result is that after hyperthermia, the blood flow in tumors is reduced, which is

in sharp contrast to normal tissue. This decreased blood flow causes a subsequent decrease in the cancer's oxygen consumption, pH, and energy production.[18,19] The combined effects can and often do end in tumor cell destruction (See **Figure 22-14**). For a localized prostate cancer, for example, localized hyperthermia can be used as a primary treatment, but most studies have confirmed that hyperthermia is best used as an adjunctive treatment alongside other cancer-killing modalities (See **Figure 22-15**).

Hyperthermia has another significant effect on cancer cell physiology—it increases microvascular permeability. On average, vascular wall permeability is three to 10 times higher in tumors than in the tissue of origin or in normal host tissues. Various studies have confirmed that hyperthermia, at temperatures used in clinical treatment, increases microvascular permeability of cancer cells by twofold.[20,21] This is one of the mechanisms by which WBH would be expected to potentiate the effects of chemotherapy.

Hyperthermia cytotoxicity is maximal in the S phase of the cell replication cycle (See **Figure**

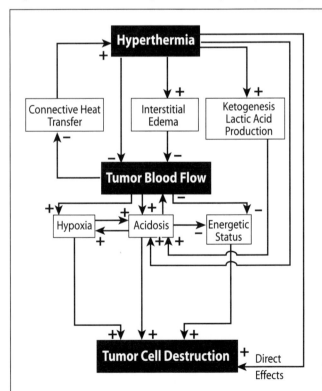

Figure 22-14: A Diagram Showing the Principles of Heat-Induced Tumor Cell Destruction

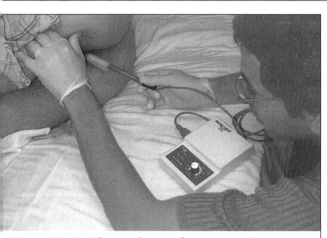

Figure 22-15: Thermotherapy for Prostate Cancer
Localized hyperthermia to the prostate is done while the person undergoes IPT. Both treatments help potentiate the effects of chemotherapy, aiding in the cancer patient's recovery.

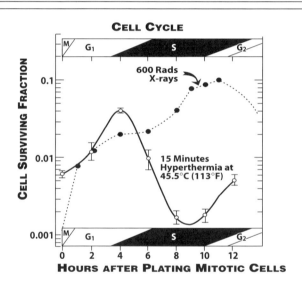

Figure 22-16: Hours after Plating Mitotic Cells
Sensitivity of cancerous cells during the growth cycle to heat or x-rays. Cancerous cells are most sensitive to heat during the S phase of the cell cycle.

22-16). Since insulin helps recruit cancer cells into the S phase of the cell cycle, it would make sense to give hyperthermia along with or after IPT. As we will see, many studies show that hyperthermia, like insulin, can potentiate the killing effects of chemotherapy. Hyperthermia has also been studied extensively to increase the tumor destruction effects of radiotherapy.[22]

HYPERTHERMIA POTENTIATES RADIOTHERAPY

Radiation therapy is one of the "big three" in cancer therapy, along with chemotherapy and surgery. There are many patients who are undergoing this therapy when they first consult with us at Caring Medical. The best approach would be to see a natural medicine specialist when first given the diagnosis of cancer, not when a person is in the middle of an already prescribed regime. For people undergoing radiation therapy to their tumor sites, we recommend the two "hyper" treatments: hyperoxygenating the blood and hyperthermizing it. Ozone and oxygen therapies, as discussed later in this chapter, can also potentiate the effects of radiation therapy.

To give an overview on the data showing that hyperthermia potentiates the effects of radiation, consider that the following research was done in the 1970s and 1980s:

- Public Health Service study found that for certain cancers producing tumors close to the skin, 75% of the tumors disappeared after combination therapy with hyperthermia and radiation, compared to 44% after radiation only.[23]

- Ned Hornback, M.D., of Indiana University treated 72 patients with advanced cancer. Complete remission was achieved in 92% of those given hyperthermia following radiation.[24] Dr. Hornback compared the results obtained in the treatment of advanced cervical cancer using radiation alone and using radiation combined with hyperthermia. Complete local control rates were 53% and 72%, respectively.[25]

- Ronald Scott, M.D., of Roswell Park Memorial Institute treated 59 patients with superficial malignancies using radiation alone or combined with hyperthermia. The complete tumor response at six months was 39% and 87%, respectively. By one year, nearly half of the tumors eliminated with radiation alone had recurred, while all the tumors given the combination treatment remained controlled.[26]

- A tabulation of worldwide results obtained in 2,330 patients by hyperthermic oncologists revealed at least a partial response in

67% of the patients treated with a combination of hyperthermia and radiation versus 33% of those treated with radiation alone.[27]

Because of the mounting research on the benefits of hyperthermia, the American Cancer Society removed hyperthermia from its unproven methods list in 1977; **in 1984, the technique was approved by the FDA as a medical procedure to treat cancer.**[6] Yet most cancer patients in the United States have never heard of hyperthermia, even though it is currently being used on tens of thousands of patients around the world each year.

The *American Cancer Society's Guide to Complementary and Alternative Cancer Methods* notes that **numerous laboratory and clinical studies have demonstrated that heat therapy can enhance the effectiveness of radiation therapy in local and regional tumor control and the effectiveness of chemotherapy in some cancers.**[28] It also noted that whole-body heat therapy is currently under investigation as a method to treat system-wide illnesses. A small, randomized clinical trial found that there were some positive effects of using the combination of whole-body heat therapy and melphalan (a chemotherapy drug), but more research is needed. The National Cancer Institute is currently sponsoring three Phase II clinical trials using whole-body heat therapy in combination with chemotherapy drugs in treating patients with advanced melanoma, advanced sarcoma, and metastatic and recurring lymphoma.[28] As you will soon see, the American Cancer Society forgot to mention all the other studies that show hyperthermia's effectiveness with cancer.

The story of hyperthermia and cancer therapy is fascinating. In one of the most prestigious cancer journals in the world, in a 1974 article entitled "Hyperthermia: Potential as an Anti-tumor Agent," the following was written in the abstract:

> Abundant laboratory and clinical evidence exists which demonstrates that tolerable levels of hyperthermia can regularly affect a delay in tumor growth, often a complete regression, and occasionally a permanent control of tumor. This means that in some tumors, aerobic and hypoxic cells are inactivated by the heat applied. Further, moderate hyperthermia is a potent sensitizer to ionizing radiation. The mechanisms of action of hyperthermia remains unknown; however, there is

prompt suppression of DNA, RNA, and protein synthesis, reduction of oxygen consumption, labilization of lysozymes, etc. Effect of heating is strongly correlated with temperature level: an increase in temperature by one degree C reduces time for a specified response by a factor of two. Application of local, regional, or systemic hyperthermia to the human cancer patient alone or in combination with radiation or certain drugs may be considered as an attractive potential therapy modality.[29]

There have been many other studies to show that hyperthermia (either local or systemic) potentiates the effects of radiation. In a large study coordinated by the UCLA School of Medicine, 1,170 adult cancer patients were followed. In this study, the author noted that tumor regressions were more frequent with combination thermoradiotherapy (60%) or thermochemotherapy (28%) than with hyperthermia alone (23%).[30] It should be noted that the patients in this study had advanced primary, recurrent, metastatic, or refractory solid cancer; the vast majority of whom had failed one or more prior therapies. In other nonrandomized Phase I and Phase II trials, it was shown that the combination of hyperthermia and radiation produced a twofold increase in the response rate over standard radiation alone.[31] In a German study, it is easy to see from **Figure 22-17** the improvement in clinical outcome when radiation therapy is combined with hyperthermia.[32] When combined with radiation therapy, hyperthermia can cause a significant clinical response,

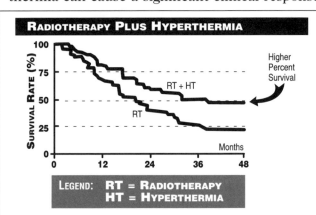

Figure 22-17: Comparison of Radiotherapy Alone with Radiotherapy Plus Hyperthermia in Locally Advanced Pelvic Tumors

In a prospective, randomized, multicenter trial, hyperthermia was shown to potentiate the cancer-killing effects of radiation therapy.

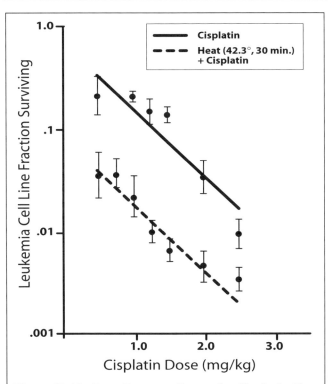

Figure 22-18: Dose-Response Curves for Cisplatin Alone (Solid Line) and Hyperthermia (30 min at 42.3°C) Followed Immediately by Cisplatin Administration (Broken Line) Against Leukemia Cell Line Fraction Survival

Hyperthermia significantly increased the cancer killing effects of cisplatin on this leukemia cell line.

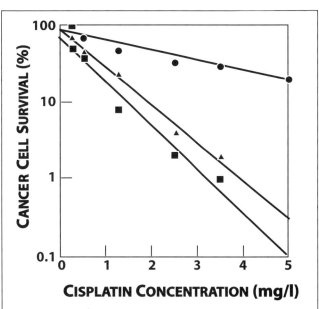

Figure 22-19: Survival of Cancer Cell Line Exposed to Cisplatin

Incubation with Cisplatin at 37°C (●), at 40°C (▲), and at 43°C (■). All curves were adjusted for the control values of 37°C, 40°C, and 43°C and were performed in triplicate at each temperature. This study showed that hyperthermia helped increase the chemotherapy drugs' concentration in the cancer cells—and subsequently had an enhanced cancer-killing effect.

even with difficult-to-treat cancers such as liver or pancreatic cancers.[33]

HYPERTHERMIA POTENTIATES CHEMOTHERAPY

Hyperthermia has been shown to be an effective agent for potentiating the effects of chemotherapy. Experimental data on the combined treatment of hyperthermia and Cisplatin treatment (chemotherapy) demonstrated improvement of its cytotoxic effect against experimental animal tumors.[34-36] In a study published in the *Journal of the National Cancer Institute,* hyperthermia prior to Cisplatin increased its cancer-killing effects by as much as two log kills. In practical terms, the fraction of cancer cells killed with a set amount of chemotherapy was 25%, but when the cells were heated to 42°C, the same amount of chemotherapy killed 99% of the cells[34] (See **Figure 22-18**). The study also showed that with the hyperthermia treatment, the drug uptake of the Cisplatin was greatly increased (72%) in the cancer cells. In another study, the combination of chemotherapy and hyperthermia was found to give an enhanced concentration of chemotherapy in the cancer cells in vitro by 3.4 and in vivo by 4.1.[37] In other words, hyperthermia increased the uptake of the chemotherapy by 400%! This study also showed that hyperthermia increased the depth of penetration of the chemotherapy drug by 1-2 mm, resulting in an additional aliquot of drug available to the tumor core. The real question is in survival. As can be seen by **Figure 22-19**, the higher the concentration of chemotherapy in the cancer cell, the greater the survival. The author concluded:

This study may have clinical relevance, since it has been demonstrated that intraperitoneal Cisplatin treatment could improve clinical responses in patients with ovarian cancer who failed to respond to systemic Cisplatin treatment. Further improvements in terms of therapeutic index might therefore be achieved by combining intraperitoneal treatment with regional hyperthermia. We demonstrated in our rat model that the drug-heat combination exposed peritoneal tumors to more Cisplatin than after Cisplatin treatment alone, resulting in higher intratumor platinum concentrations.[37]

This is one of the most important points about understanding IPT and other potentiating factors. They almost all work by increasing the chemotherapy drug's concentration in the cancer cells, thus potentiating their effects.

Hyperthermia has been shown to enhance the killing effects of many different chemotherapy agents, including ifosfamide, Adriamycin, Mitomycin, 5-fluorouracil, bleomycin, and cyclophosphamide[38-41] (See **Figures 22-20** to **22-23**). All one has to do is glance at these figures and realize that chemotherapy's cancer-killing effects are dramatically enhanced by slight elevations of body temperature. This makes sense when one looks at the data from these studies. G. Wiedemann and associates at the Medical University of Lubeck, Germany, found that the concentration of the activated drug (ifosfamide) within the first 60 minutes at 41°C exceeded by over twofold that at 37°C.[38] The bone marrow toxicity of the same drug dose did not significantly increase with body temperature. Amazing!

Hyperthermia, by increasing S phase cycle cell kill, enhancing cancer cell membrane permeability, and increasing cancer cell acidosis… improves the results when given with chemotherapy, compared to a person just utilizing chemotherapy alone. In addition, hyperthermia has been shown to protect normal cells from some of the damaging effects of chemotherapy.[42] Hyperthermia can also make a cancer cell sensitive to a chemotherapeutic drug that it previously had resisted.[43,44] This reversal of drug resistance appears to be because hyperthermia substantially increases the uptake of chemotherapy drugs into the cancer cells. It is for these and many other reasons that most chemotherapeutic agents have been shown to be potentiated by heat (See **Figure 22-24**).

Hyperthermia, alongside chemotherapy, can be a potent weapon against cancer. A multi-institutional clinical study on hyperthermia of many deep-seated and highly resistant tumors was done at seven institutions. A total of 177 people were studied in the trial; 81 (46%) received hyperthermia and chemotherapy. Complete

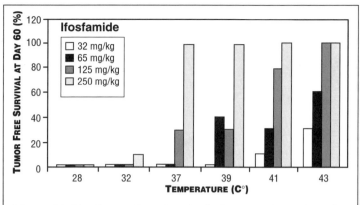

Figure 22-20: Tumor-Free Survival Time as a Function of Temperature and Chemotherapy Dose of Ifosfamide

Chemo-Thermotherapy—human MXI breast cancer xenographs in mice treated with heat and different doses of ifosfamide.

Adapted from Wiedemann, G. Local Hyperthermia enhances cyclophosphamide, Ifosfamide, and cis-diamminedichloroplatinum cytotoxicity on human derived breast carcinoma and sarcoma xenografts in nude mice. Journal of Cancer Research and Clinical Oncology. 1992:118:129-135

responses and partial responses were obtained in 80% of the cases with lung cancer, 39% with stomach cancer, 56% with liver cancer, 35% with pancreatic cancer, 71% with bladder cancer, 100% with primary rectal cancer, and 47% with recurrent rectal cancer.[45]

QUERCETIN AS HYPERTHERMIA POTENTIATOR

It appears that certain flavonoids—most notably quercetin—may potentiate the ability of hyperthermia to destroy tumor cells.[46] Quercetin inhibits intracellular synthesis of heat shock proteins, which protect cells against damage from heat.[47] Heat shock proteins are universally induced in human cells exposed to high temperatures. Inhibiting the

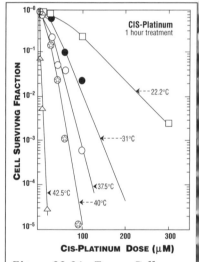

Figure 22-21: Tumor Cell Surviving Curve Treated with Heat and Cis-Platinum

Cis-Platinum is potentiated by heat. Cell survival data for V-79 Chinese hamster lung cells treated for one hour with Cis-Platinum under differing hyperthermia conditions.

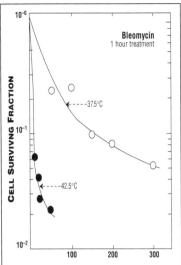

Figure 22-22: Tumor Cell Surviving Curve Treatment with Heat and Bleomycin

Bleomycin is potentiated by heat. Cell survival data for V-79 Chinese hamster lung cells treated for one hour with bleomycin under differing hyperthermia conditions.

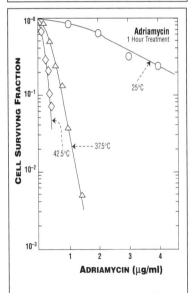

Figure 22-23: Tumor Cell Surviving Treatment with Heat and Adriamycin

Adriamycin is potentiated by heat. Cell survival data for V-79 Chinese hamster lung cells treated for one hour with adriamycin under differing hyperthermia conditions.

synthesis of these proteins increases the vulnerability of tumor cells to stress damage.[48] Quercetin can also inhibit lactic acid transport from some carcinoma cells.[49,50] By inhibiting lactic acid transport, quercetin may lower intracellular pH. Therefore, under heat stress, quercetin may inhibit proliferation of tumor cells by inhibiting heat shock protein synthesis and by reducing intracellular pH. In cervical carcinoma cells, quercetin did not induce cytotoxic effects at normal body temperature but did potentiate hyperthermia-induced cytotoxicity at 41°C. Quercetin is one of the herbal remedies that we prescribe. It is discussed a little later in this chapter.

SUMMARY

Compelling evidence exists that hyperthermia therapy as part of a multimodal treatment approach is a valuable tool that should be used more often in cancer therapies,

FIGURE 22-24: INTERACTION OF HEAT AND CHEMOTHERAPEUTIC AGENTS

POTENTIATED BY HEAT	UNAFFECTED BY HEAT
Adriamycin	Actinomycin
Bleomycin*	Cytarabine
BCNU*	Etoposide
Carboplatin*	Floxuridine
Cisplatin*	Hydroxyurea
Cyclophosphamide	Methotrexate
Dacarbazine	PALA
Epirubicin*	Vinblastine
Ifosfamide*	
Lomustine	
Melphalan*	
Mitomycin C*	
Mitoxantrone	
Nimustine	

*Verified in clinical studies

Most chemotherapy drugs appear to be potentiated by hyperthermia.

Adapted from Towle, L.R., Hyperthermia and drug resistance; Hyperthermia and Oncology, Vol. 4 Chemopotentiation by Hyperthermia. 1994, pp 9-20; Hager, E.D. Passive Hyperthermie; Komplementäre Onkologie 1997, 164-180.

either systemically, which involves the whole body, or locally, just around the tumor. It is clear that hyperthermia potentiates the effects of other traditional modalities that a cancer patient may undergo, including radiation therapy and chemotherapy. As such, it is a very beneficial adjunctive treatment with Insulin Potentiation Therapy.

ELECTROCHEMOTHERAPY

"OVER THE PAST 10 YEARS, ELECTROCHEMICAL THERAPY (ECT) HAS BEEN USED TO TREAT MORE THAN 7,000 CASES OF VARIOUS KINDS OF MALIGNANCY IN CHINA. THE TOTAL EFFECTIVE RATE OF ECT, WHEN APPLIED TO MALIGNANT TUMORS LISTED ABOVE IS 70 PERCENT. MOREOVER, ALL OF THESE TUMORS WERE TREATED IN THE MIDDLE AND LATE STAGES (STAGES III AND IV)."

—Dr. Yu-Ling Xin, China Japan Friendship Hospital, Beijing, China

Electro-chemotherapy (ECT) was developed in Europe by the Swedish professor Björn Nordenström and the Austrian doctor Rudolf Pekar. It is used in many cancer centers across Europe and Asia. (Most notably, ECT is used at China Japan Friendship Hospital in Beijing, China under the guidance of Professor Yu-Ling Xin (see **Figure 22-25**). Dr. Yu-Ling Xin was taught this therapy by Dr. Nordenström. The therapy

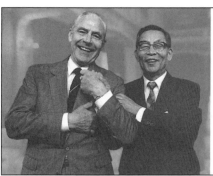

Figure 22-25: Dr. Björn Nordenström and Dr. Yu-Ling Xin at the First BCEC Symposium Held in Stockholm, Sweden, September 12-15, 1993.

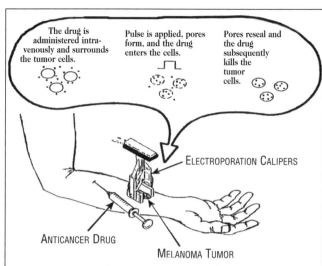

Figure 22-26: Schematic Diagram of the ECT Process and Treatment of Melanoma

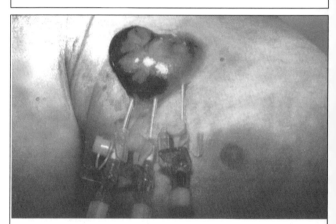

Figure 22-27: Electrochemotherapy to Lymph Node Metastases

employs galvanic electrical stimulation to treat tumors and skin cancers. An ECT session resembles an electroacupuncture treatment, in which small needles are placed into the skin. Using local anesthesia, the physician inserts a positively charged platinum, gold, or silver needle into the center of the tumor and places negatively charged needles around the tumor, no farther than 3 cm apart. Voltages of six to 15 volts are used, depending on tumor size. Tumors as large as five to 10 cm³ have been killed with ECT.

To enhance the cancer-killing power of ECT, small amounts of chemotherapy agents are sometimes applied to the skin and driven into the tumor by a kind of sweating effect of the electric current ("iontophoresis"). For skin cancers, current is passed between positively charged needles placed underneath the base of the tumor and a negatively charged skin patch commonly applied to the surface[51] (See **Figure 22-26**). The therapy can be given to superficial or deep cancers. For superficial cancers, the needle electrodes can be placed in the office. For deep cancers, the procedure should be done under x-ray guidance (See **Figure 22-27**).

ECT is known by several names, including electrocancer therapy, percutaneous galvanochemical therapy, and galvanic therapy, because it involves the use of high-intensity galvanic current to:

- Trigger electrobiological and electrochemical mechanisms to permanently destroy tumor tissue
- Stimulate the immune system
- Reverse resistance to conventional cancer therapies
- Potentiate the effects of chemo and radiotherapy[52]

It is suitable not only for superficial tumors but also for deep-seeded tumors and solid tumors. Tumors that can be reached by needle electrodes but are considered inoperable for reasons of esthetics or function but treatable by ECT are as follows:

- Breast cancer, especially recurrences subsequent to radiotherapy and chemotherapy
- Ear, nose, and throat tumors
- Skin tumors such as basal cell carcinoma, spindle cell carcinoma, and melanoma
- Skin metastases
- Soft tissue tumors
- Isolated organ metastases[52]

Like hyperthermia, ECT is a very powerful cancer tool that is underutilized in the United

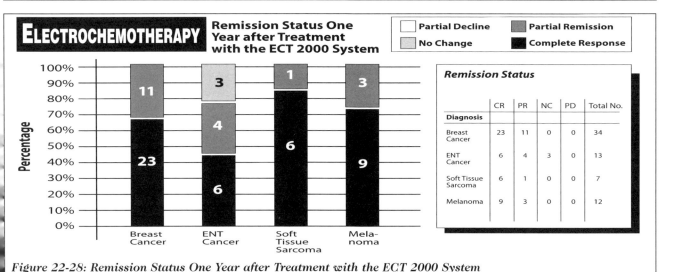

Figure 22-28: Remission Status One Year after Treatment with the ECT 2000 System
Data Adapted from Friedrich R. Dowes Klinik Stibeorg, Bad Aibling, Germany

States. One wonders why when the technique is very much based in science and the results with cancer have been outstanding. Consider the results of just one clinic utilizing the technique (See **Figure 22-28**). One has to remember that these are complete remission rates on tumors that are very advanced or recurrent. Imagine what the results would be in early stage cancers.

At the Fourth International Symposium on Biologically Closed Electric Circuits, Professor Yu-Ling Xin, the then chief of Thoracic Surgery at the China Japan Friendship Hospital in Beijing, China, explained the indications for the application of ECT:

> Electrochemical Therapy (ECT) is a method for treating tumors. Specially made platinum needles (electrodes) are inserted into the tumor mass. The needles are connected to an instrument that produces direct electric current. The direct current results in a process called "electrolysis," which occurs in the tumor mass. This electrolysis destroys the tumor cells.
>
> The voltage used in this procedure ranges from six to eight volts. The electrodes with a positive charge are called anodes; while electrodes carrying a negative charge are called cathodes. When electricity is sent through the system, the area surrounding the anode becomes strongly acidic (pH 1-2). The area surrounding the cathode becomes strongly basic (pH 12-14). It is this strong acidity and/or alkalinity that kills the tumor cells.

This treatment is simple and easily administered. There is no need for a surgical operation, and there are no side effects, such as those that occur as a result of radiation or chemotherapy. ECT has been shown to be safer, more effective, and less traumatic than other methods. In addition, recovery time is quick.

Over the past ten years, ECT has been used to treat more than 7,000 cases of various kinds of malignant tumors in China. There are approximately twenty-four kinds of malignant tumors. Examples of treatable visceral cancers are lung cancer, esphogeal cancer, liver cancer, throat cancer, cancer of the adrenal gland, rectal cancer, cervical cancer, prostate cancer, and tumors of the meningeal membrane. Examples of treatable superficial cancers include breast cancer; thyroid adenomas; cancer of the subaural glands, tumors of the maxillofacial region; cancer of the lip, tongue, and skin; and rhabdomyosarcoma.

The total effective rate of ECT, when applied to these malignant tumors is seventy percent (70%) (see **Figure 22-29**). Moreover, all of these tumors were treated in the middle and late stages (stages III and IV). Most of the cases were inoperable or not responsive to radiation and/or chemotherapy. To these patients, and especially to patients who have had recurrent tumors following surgery, ECT effectively relieves the patient's suffering and extends life expectancy. Of course, ECT is not a panacea that cures every case of malignant tumors.

FIGURE 22-29: EFFECTIVENESS OF 1,610 CASES OF MALIGNANT TUMORS TREATED WITH ELECTROCHEMICAL THERAPY

CR = Complete Response PR = Partial Response NC = No Change	Number of Cases	CR No.	%	PR No.	%	NC No.	%	PD No.	%	CR + PR No.	%
Esophageal Cancer	478	68	14.2	264	55.2	71	14.9	75	15.7	332	69.5
Lung Cancer	415	130	31.3	201	48.4	41	9.9	43	10.4	331	79.8
Liver Cancer	308	87	28.5	148	48.5	35	11.5	35	11.5	235	77.0
Breast Cancer	105	40	38.1	42	40.0	14	13.3	9	8.6	82	78.1
Skin Cancer	88	61	69.3	27	30.7	0	0	0	0	88	100.0
Thyroid Andenocarcinoma	66	40	60.6	21	31.8	5	7.6	0	0	61	92.4
Parathyroid Cancer	46	30	65.2	11	23.9	4	8.7	1	2.2	41	89.1
Melanoma	41	10	24.4	11	26.8	12	29.3	8	19.5	21	51.2
Cancer of Oral Cavity	35	13	37.1	14	40.0	5	14.3	3	8.6	27	77.1
Rhabdomyosarcoma	21	6	28.5	7	33.3	5	23.8	3	14.3	13	61.9
Prostate Cancer	10	4	40.0	4	40.0	2	20.0	0	0	8	80.0
Total:	**1,610**	**489**	**30.4**	**750**	**46.6**	**194**	**12.0**	**177**	**11.0**	**1,239**	**77.0**

These results come from using ECT by itself. Imagine combining this therapy with another powerful cancer remedy—IPT!

Electrochemotherapy is a technique that can be used to potentiate the effects of chemotherapeutic drugs because ECT is one of the most potent ways to increase cell membrane permeability to nutrients and medications. In one study, ECT was shown to enhance the cytotoxicity of the introduced substance by a factor of 2×10^5.[53] In other words, ECT potentiated its effects by a factor of 200,000. It specifically causes the cell membrane (in the area of the electric field) to undergo a remodeling process, characterized by the occurrence of permeation structures, sometimes called "pores," across which an exchange of substances is allowed. The opening of the membrane barrier is transient when the strength of the external electric field is adequately chosen. Such reversibility, an essential feature of the system, allows cell viability to be preserved if desired. It is this increase in permeability that causes ECT to significantly potentiate the effects of chemotherapy.

The first in vivo application using pulsed electric fields and a chemotherapeutic agent to treat tumors in animals was reported in 1987 by Motonori Okino of Yamaguchi University School of Medicine in Japan.[54,55] The tumors in all subject animals grew when treated with electrical stimulation or chemotherapy alone, but when used together, tumor size was decreased by 47% at the end of four days compared to controls. Results were reported only for single treatments. In subsequent studies, Okino and associates found that, apart from reductions in tumor volume, there was a substantial increase of 200% in longevity for the electrochemotherapy-treated animals compared with controls.[56] Another research group in Japan, headed by H. Kanesada, used various chemotherapy drugs, including cyclophosphamide, Mitomycin, and Cisplatin, and found that high-voltage stimulation potentiated the effects of chemotherapy by up to a factor of 10.[57]

Most of the systemic study of electrochemotherapy has been done by Luis Mir and his colleagues at the Gustave Roussy Institut in Paris, France. Their initial study compared the killing power of bleomycin (chemotherapy), electrical stimulation, and the combination (electrochemotherapy). The researchers noted:

> After electric pulse delivery, we observed a substantial reduction (about 700 times) in bleomycin concentration, which reduces cloning efficiency to 50% of controls (EC_{50}). Moreover, after electric field treatment, bleomycin was cytotoxic even at very low external concentrations (starting with 10^{-9} mol/l) with a steep dose response curve. The relative gain in toxicity depends on the survival level considered. We have observed that the external bleomycin concentration re-

quired to kill 90% of treated cells (i.e., EC_{10}) was reduced 650,000 times after electric field treatment—conditions that do not affect cell viability in the absence of the drug.[58]

This study was done on cell cultures. When actually tested on animals in vivo, electrical stimulation potentiated the effects of the bleomycin by a mere factor of 10,000![59] These studies are unbelievable if one contemplates the facts. By using high-voltage galvanic stimulation, the killing effects of the chemotherapy on the cancer cells can be increased by 10,000-fold! The later study also was significant in that the electrochemotherapy-treated animals were essentially free of any chemotherapy-related side effects, and a significant number of them were cured of their cancer.

They followed this work with further experiments on spontaneous mammary tumors in mice and showed 23 complete responses and 13 partial responses out of a total of 38 tumors treated with ECT. Most tumors shrunk significantly within two to three weeks.[60] Subsequently, they reported the use of low-dose interleukin-2 administered over a few days following ECT treatment leading to an increased rate of complete cures in mice.[61]

Electrical stimulation was also shown to significantly potentiate the effects of bleomycin on fibrosarcoma in mice.[62] Other researchers found a 700- and 200-fold increase, respectively, in the cytotoxicity of bleomycin and netropsin compared to controls when tumor cells were subjected to electrical stimulation along with the chemotherapy.[63] ECT for brain tumors (gliomas) in animal models has shown that with bleomycin as the anticancer drug, the survival of the animals is increased by 200%.[64]

It should be evident from the above studies that electric stimulation does potentiate the effects of chemotherapy in vitro (cells in culture) and in vivo in animals. But does it have the same effects on human cancers? Luis Mir and associates at the Gustave Roussy Institut went on to conduct the first clinical trial with ECT in patients with head and neck squamous cell carcinomas who had already undergone extensive radiation and chemotherapy.[65] Seven patients with 34 nodules located in the anterior cervical region or upper part of the thorax were treated with one sixth of the dose of bleomycin typically given in the course of conventional chemotherapy. The bleomycin was given intravenously, and the electric pulses were applied near and on the tumor sites three and a half minutes after the injection. The response was very encouraging, as 14 of the nodules underwent complete regression, nine a partial regression, and growth was retarded in another six. Side effects were minimal. There was no change in the pulse rate or blood pressure during treatment. Instantaneous muscle contractions, described as painless by the patients, occurred in the neck and shoulder, as the pulse was applied and disappeared immediately after the treatment. Slight local edema was present in most patients and disappeared in 12 to 48 hours. The authors noted that "No serious incident, either general or local, occurred in spite of the bad health status of most of our patients."

To some people, these results may not seem impressive—but they are, considering the fact that this was with only one ECT treatment. Contemplate what the authors noted:

> In all the cases the growth of the treated nodules was at least slowed down as compared with that of the neighboring nodules not submitted to the electrical pulses but exposed to the same bleomycin dose.

The research group from the Gustave Roussy Institut confirmed the above results with a continuation of the above study.[66] I (Ross) had the opportunity to meet and talk with one of the oncologists (Christian Domenge, M.D., February 2001, at the office of J. Le Coz, M.D., Paris, France) involved in the above studies at the Gustave Roussy Institut in Paris, and he was absolute that electrochemotherapy works; unfortunately, the funding for the studies ceased. The technique has caught on, though, and various centers use it in Europe. Some of them are getting spectacular results.

> **When actually tested on animals in vivo, electric stimulation potentiated the effects of the bleomycin by a mere factor of 10,000!**

SUMMARY

Electrochemotherapy employs the use of galvanic electrical stimulation to treat tumors and skin cancers. The electrical stimulation has a direct anti-tumor effect and can potentiate the effects of chemotherapy. Like other potentiators, the main effect of ECT is to enhance the uptake of the medications by the tumor cells, increasing their cancer-killing abilities. The procedure is well tolerated and is utilized in cancer centers across Europe.

Anyone desiring more information on Electrochemical Therapy, please contact:

INTERNATIONAL ASSOCIATION FOR
BIOLOGICALLY CLOSED ELECTRIC
CIRCUITS IN BIOMEDICINE
% CARL F. FIRLEY
VICE PRESIDENT AND SECRETARY GENERAL
4976 S. W. BIMINI CIRCLE SOUTH
PALM CITY, FLORIDA 34990
561-283-2180 • FAX: 561-283-2180
iabc@adelphia.net

BIOOXIDATIVE THERAPIES

"ALL OF THE CANCER CELLS SHOWED MARKED DOSE-DEPENDENT GROWTH INHIBITION IN OZONE 0.3 AND 0.5 ppm. THESE FINDINGS LEAD US TO BELIEVE THAT OZONE—WHETHER ALONE, IN COMBINATION WITH RADIATION THERAPY, OR IN CHEMOTHERAPY UTILIZING ELECTROPHILIC COMPOUNDS—MAY HAVE THERAPEUTIC VALUE FOR PATIENTS WITH CERTAIN TYPES OF LUNG CANCER.[89]"

—Frederick Sweet, Ming-Shian Kao, Song-Chiau D. Lee
Washington University School of Medicine

Hyperoxygenation therapy—also called oxymedicine, biooxidative therapy, oxidative therapy, and oxidology—is a method of cancer management based on the erroneous concept that cancer is caused by oxygen deficiency and can be cured by exposing cancer cells to more oxygen than they can tolerate. The most highly touted hyperoxygenating agents are hydrogen peroxide, germanium sesquioxide, and ozone. Although these compounds have been the subject of legitimate research, there is little or no evidence that they are effective for the treatment of any serious disease, and each has demonstrated potential for harm. **Therefore, the American Cancer Society recommends that individuals with cancer not seek treatment from individuals promoting any form of hyperoxygenation therapy as an alternative to proven medical modalities.[67]**

It is important for people to realize that much of what is written in this book is not the established standard of care. The American Cancer Society, for the most part, promotes surgery, radiation therapy, and high-dose chemotherapy (the big three). For the person who wants their endorsement for the care being received, do not seek out a doctor who does IPT and surely do not seek out one that uses ozone therapy. Fortunately, in our opinion, the patient of today questions the "wisdom" of the American Cancer Society and all such agencies that say cancer will be cured by the big three. After millions of deaths, side effects, and millions of hours of human suffering for people who have used these "scientifically-proven therapies," cancer patients and their friends, families, and colleagues are reading about safer, more natural therapies and are consulting with professionals who use them.

We first learned ozone therapy from Steven Elsasser, M.D., one of the premiere natural medicine physicians in the United States. We were fortunate to also learn from Raj Alwa and Dr. Ratha Alwa, M.D., at their clinic in Lake Geneva, WI. Dr. Alwa is one of the kindest and most competent doctors we know. She had to give up her medical license in Wisconsin because of her use of ozone, though she had harmed no one. She now has several thriving clinics in India, where ozone therapy is well accepted (See **Figure 22-30**). We also traveled to Duisburg, Germany, to work with the then president of the German Ozone Society, Gerd Wasser, M.D. (See **Color Insert**.) If ozone is as dangerous as the American Cancer Society says, then why does Dr. Wasser do house visits and treat patients in their homes with ozone therapy? Dr. Wasser told us during one of our visits in 1997, "If you use the technique the way I showed you, the risk to a patient is zero." Do we believe the risk of using ozone therapy is zero? No,

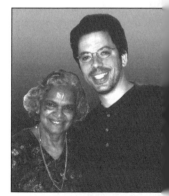

Figure 22-30: Dr. Hauser and One of His Ozone Teachers, Dr. Ratha Alwa
Dr. Alwa runs several clinics that use ozone in India, where this therapy is more accepted.

Figure 22-31: The White Cell or Somatic Cell

This diagram shows the effects of Hydrogen Peroxide on cellular metabolism.

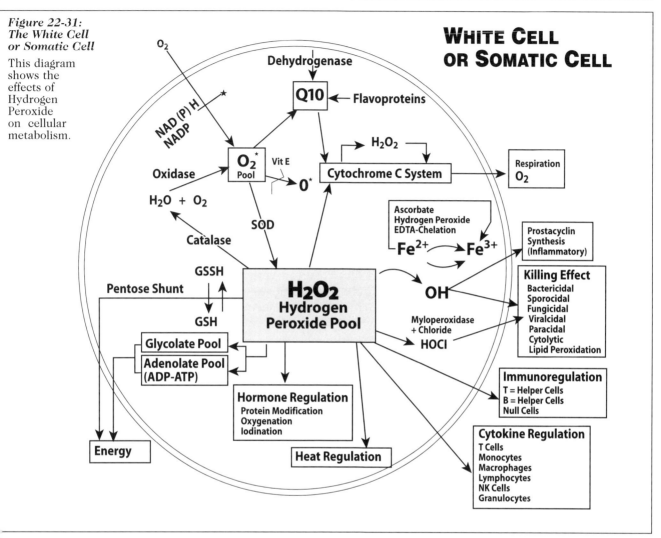

but it just about is, and it is hypocrisy for the American Cancer Society to push radiation therapy and high-dose chemotherapy and tell the public that ozone therapy and bio-oxidative therapies are dangerous and should not be used.

Caring Medical and Rehabilitation Services has over 10 years' experience using biooxidative therapies, including hydrogen peroxide, ozone therapy, and germanium. The medical potential for biooxidative therapies is based on the relationship of oxygen to human cells. Biooxidative therapies accelerate oxygen metabolism and stimulate the release of oxygen atoms from the bloodstream to the cells. When levels of oxygen increase, the potential for disease decreases. Although ozone and hydrogen peroxide are highly toxic in their purified states, they have been found to be safe and effective when diluted to

therapeutic levels for medical use.[68] For instance, according to Dr. Wasser in 1997, there are 10,000 medical professionals in Germany alone using ozone therapy in the treatment of human disease.

Biooxidative therapies involve the introduction of an oxidizing agent into the human body. Oxidation is the removal of electrons from a molecule, while oxygenation is the effective increase in the amount of oxygen and has nothing to do with electron transfer. Hydrogen peroxide is a powerful oxidizer critical in many reactions in the body, but it also separates into water and diatomic oxygen and serves as an oxygen source in the oxygenation of tissues (See **Figure 22-31**).

Hydrogen peroxide is a clear, colorless liquid that easily mixes with water. It is a compound made up of two hydrogen atoms and two oxygen atoms and is known chemically as H_2O_2.

Hydrogen peroxide is created in the atmosphere when ultraviolet light strikes oxygen in the presence of moisture. Ozone (O_3) is free oxygen (O_2) plus an extra atom of oxygen. When it comes into contact with water, this extra atom of oxygen splits off very easily. Water (H_2O) combines with the extra atom of oxygen and becomes hydrogen peroxide (H_2O_2).*

Both compounds, after being introduced into the body, increase the amount of free radicals that are formed. Though free radicals (highly reactive, unstable molecules with a free electron to give) have been suggested as the cause of many degenerative conditions, most people do not realize that it is the immune system's formation of free radicals, such as hydrogen peroxide, that allows immune system cells such as natural killer cells and macrophages to destroy cancer cells, viruses, bacteria, and fungi. Free radical formation is also the main mechanism by which chemotherapy kills cancer cells. Thus one would expect that biooxidative therapies would potentiate the effects of chemotherapy.

It is well known that the x-ray sensitivity of both normal and neoplastic tissue is greatly enhanced when irradiation is accomplished under increased oxygen tension.[69-72] Most of the studies showed that well-oxygenated tissue was generally two to three times as sensitive to radiation as less oxygenated tissue. For anoxic tissues (very poor oxygenation, which would include some cancer cells), sometimes twelve times as great a dose was required to produce a given degree of damage as when irradiated in an atmosphere of pure oxygen.[69,73] Thus, for patients undergoing radiation therapy, receiving biooxidative therapies prior to and after the radiation therapy should potentiate the killing effects of the radiation therapy on the cancer cells.

Starting in the early 1960s, research was begun to see if increased oxygen tension would potentiate the effects of chemotherapy. E. Krementz and associates from the Tulane University School of Medicine, New Orleans, LA, showed that increased oxygen tension potentiated the killing effects of alkylating agents (chemotherapy) on liver tumor cells by 30%.[74] In a subsequent study, they found that when the nitrogen mustard (chemotherapy) treatment was combined with increasing oxygen, tumor cell counts and the size of the tumor were reduced, and ultimately survival was significantly enhanced.[75] A. Smith, M.D., and researchers at the Surgical-Medical Research Institute at the University of Alberta in Canada found that infusions of hydrogen peroxide could increase survival when given with chemotherapy. The researchers noted: "These results demonstrate that hydrogen peroxide will potentiate the anti-tumor effect of TSPA on the Walker 256 carcinoma, presumably by raising the tumor oxygen tension."[76] N. Kaibara and colleagues at Kyushu University in Japan found that the combined treatment with Mitomycin and hydrogen peroxide resulted in a significant prolongation of survival times and a decrease in the viable tumor cell count as compared to those of Mitomycin alone.[77]

BIOOXIDATIVE TREATMENTS IN OUR OFFICE

Hydrogen peroxide is given via an intravenous drip. A 500-cc bag generally takes about two hours. Ozone therapy is given in the form of major autohemotherapy. During the treatment, about 100-150 cc of blood are removed from the body into a bottle, much like when a person donates blood. A similar amount of ozone gas is then mixed with the blood, and then the blood-ozone mixture is transfused back into the person (See **Figures 22-32 A-D**). One of these procedures is typically given before the IPT at our office.

If one studies the biochemical effects that take place with biooxidative therapies, it is clear that they should be part of a natural medicine cancer protocol. Some of the known scientific effects of ozone are as follows:**

- Activates cellular metabolism
- Modulates the immune system
- Regulates the antioxidative capacity of the biological system
- Activation of immunocompetent cells results in the physiological release of cytokines (interferons, interleukins)

---

* *Hydrogen peroxide and ozone therapy are utilized by natural medicine physicians around the world for a myriad of human diseases. For more information, please refer to www.caringmedical.com or read the Hauser's book on interventional natural medicine.*

** *As discussed in* The Use of Ozone in Medicine *by Renate Viebahn-Haensler (Karl F. Haug Publishers, Heidelberg, Germany, 1999).*

FIGURE 22-32 A-D: MAJOR AUTOHEMOTHERAPY OZONE THERAPY

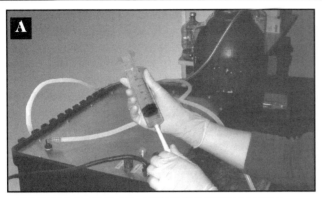
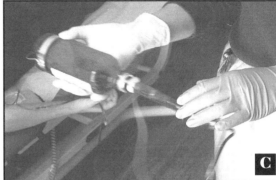
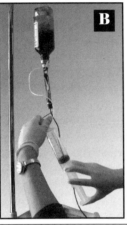
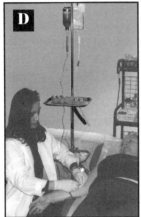

Figures 22-32 A-D:

A: Ozone gas is put into syringes.

B: Ozone gas is injected into a bottle with the patient's blood.

C: Ozone and blood is gently mixed together, causing the patient's blood to turn a bright red color.

D: The ozone-blood mixture is transfused back into the patient's body.

- Activates red blood cells to release oxygen
- Bactericidal
- Viricidal
- Destroys cancer cells
- Stimulates detoxification

Ozone is used to purify the water in many cities of the world, including Moscow, Helsinki, and Los Angeles. Obviously, ozone must have tremendous disinfectant, germicidal, and detoxifying abilities. What most people don't know is that ozone selectively inhibits the growth of human cancer cells. This was shown by researchers from the Washington University School of Medicine in St. Louis who conducted an experiment in which cancer cells and normal human cells were exposed to varying degrees of ozone.[89] All cancer cells including alveolar (lung) adenocarcinoma, breast adenocarcinoma, uterine carcinosarcoma, and endometrial carcinoma had significant growth inhibition with ozone therapy (see **Figure 22-33**). The study showed that all of the cancer cells showed marked dose-dependent growth inhibition in ozone at 0.3 and 0.5 ppm. There was no growth inhibition of the noncancerous lung cells at these ozone levels. At 0.8 ppm, the growth of the noncancerous cells was inhibited 50 percent, but all four types of cancer cells were inhibited more than 90 percent. The authors noted that at 0.5 ppm, **"all of the cancer cells had growth rates several times lower than that of the aged, noncancerous cells."** They concluded that "evidently, cancer cells are less able to compensate for the oxidative burden of ozone than normal cells. These findings lead us to believe that ozone—alone, in combination with radiation therapy, or in chemotherapy utilizing electrophilic compounds—may have therapeutic value for patients with certain forms of lung cancer."[89] The authors of this book would add that, perhaps these authors' conclusions are too narrow. More appropriately, it should have said "...may have therapeutic value for patients with cancer." What we have found is that it *does* have therapeutic value

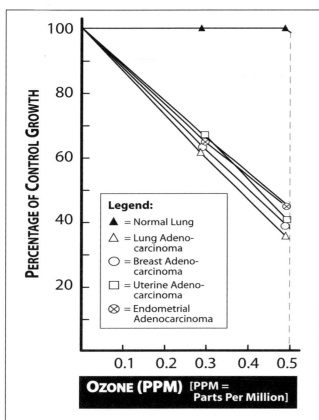

Figure 22-33: Inhibition by Ozone of Growth Malignant Cells in Culture
The percentage of growth inhibition is calculated by subtracting the percentage of growth from 100. The data are from cell counting on the eighth day of incubation. There is a nearly linear relationship between inhibition of growth of the cancer cells and increasing ozone levels.

for our patients with cancer, which is why it is included in this book.

The medical uses of ozone in medicine are many. For the person interested in this subject, please visit www.caringmedical.com.

NUTRIENTS AS POTENTIATORS

There is no arguing the fact that the cancer patient has little hope of survival without good nutrition. So it is no wonder that once the person has been given the diagnosis, family members, friends, colleagues at work, and anyone else who knows the patient either tell him or her what nutrients to take or purchase them for the patient. While the notion is good that nutrients are helpful to the body, it is best for the cancer patient to get assistance from a nutritionally oriented medical doctor.

Many cancer patients whom we have seen have been told by their oncologists to stop their vitamins and herbs because they will interfere with chemotherapy or radiation therapy. The thought is that cancer itself imparts an oxidative stress on the host organism, but administration of antineoplastic agents during cancer chemotherapy results in a much greater degree of oxidative stress than that which is induced by the cancer itself. This is illustrated by the elevation of lipid peroxidation products; the reduction of the total radical-trapping capacity of blood plasma; the marked reduction in plasma levels of antioxidants such as vitamin E, vitamin C, and beta carotene; and the marked reduction of tissue glutathione (GSH) levels that occurs during chemotherapy with essentially all chemotherapy drugs.[78,79] The main concern is whether dietary supplementation with antioxidants and other nutrients would interfere with the mechanism whereby antineoplastic agents are cytotoxic to cancer cells.

If one studies the mechanisms by which chemotherapy destroys cancer cells, it is generally not by the formation of reactive oxygen species, which could be inhibited by antioxidants. As has been alluded to already, most chemotherapy drugs work by altering DNA. The mechanisms by which they do this include inhibiting a key enzyme, cross-linking, alkylation, fragmentation, intercalation, and other means. Because of this fact, it is doubtful that antioxidants or other nutrients would inhibit chemotherapy effectiveness.

Another factor in deciding whether to take various nutritional products is the fact that most nutrients have some chemopreventive effect. In other words, people who have sufficient amounts of these vitamins and minerals have a lower incidence of cancer. As will be discussed later, many nutrients have anticancer effects themselves because they reverse some aspect of cancer physiology. These are additional reasons why one would expect nutrients to potentiate chemotherapy's effectiveness, not inhibit it.

To do a thorough job on the subject of nutrients and their interaction with chemotherapy would take a book all by itself. A colleague of ours, Davis W. Lamson, M.S., N.D. (we served on a board together), wrote a great article entitled "Antioxidants and Cancer Therapy II: Quick Reference Guide."[80] In this article, he has some wonderful tables that summarize some of the effects of various nutrients on the effects of chemotherapy. Nutrients that have been shown to have chemotherapy potentiating effects are depicted in **Figure 22-34**. Only a few of the actual studies are highlighted here. Dr. Lamson summarized the findings as, "The vast majority of in vivo and in vitro studies have shown enhanced effectiveness of standard cancer therapies or a neutral effect on drug action."[80]

Another wonderful review on nutrients and cancer chemotherapy was written by Kenneth A. Conklin.[81] A summary of the significant findings as they pertain to the potentiating qualities of various nutrients is given below.

VITAMIN E

Vitamin E, in vitro, has been shown to enhance the cytotoxic effect of several anticancer drugs, including 5-fluorouracil, doxorubicin, vincristine, dacarbazine, Cisplatin, and tamoxifen. (See **Figure 22-35**) Studies with laboratory animals have shown parenteral administration of vitamin E to enhance the anticancer effect of 5-fluorouracil and Cisplatin, although it had no apparent effect on the tumoricidal properties of doxorubicin.

VITAMIN C

In vitro studies with several tumor cell lines have shown vitamin C to enhance the cytotoxic activity of doxorubicin, Cisplatin, paclitaxel, dacarbazine, 5-fluorouracil, and bleomycin. Vitamin C has also been shown to increase drug accumulation and to partially reverse vincristine resistance of human non-small cell lung cancers. Animal studies have shown that vitamin C at 500 mg/kg and 1,000 mg/kg enhances the chemotherapeutic effect of cyclophosphamide, Vinblastine, 5-fluorouracil, procarbazine, carmustine, and doxorubicin.

FIGURE 22-34: NUTRIENTS THAT HAVE BEEN SHOWN TO HAVE CHEMOTHERAPY POTENTIATING EFFECTS

- Vitamin A
- Beta Carotene
- Vitamin C
- Coenzyme Q_{10}
- Vitamin D
- Vitamin E
- Genistein
- Ginseng
- Glutathione
- Melatonin
- N-Acetylcysteine
- Quercetin
- Selenium

FIGURE 22-35: EFFECT OF VITAMIN E IN COMBINATION WITH PHARMACOLOGICAL AGENTS ON NEUROBLASTOMA AND GLIOMA CELLS IN CULTURE

TREATMENTS	Cell Number (% of Untreated Control)	
	GLIOMA	NEUROBLASTOMA
5-FU	71	63
5-FU + Vitamin E	32	15
Adriamycin	36	42
Adriamycin + Vitamin E	22	12
Bleomycin	77	54
Bleomycin + Vitamin E	42	29
Vitamin E	50	53

Vitamin E in this study was shown to enhance the cancer-killing effects of various chemotherapeutic agents on these brain cancer cell lines.

Adapted from Vitamin E increases the growth inhibitory and differentiating effects of tumor therapeutic agents on neuroblastoma and glioma cells in culture, by K. Prasad, J. Edwards-Prasad, S. Ramanujam, and A. Sakamoto, Proceedings of the Society for Experimental Biology and Medicine, 1980, 164, pp. 158-163

BETA CAROTENE

Beta carotene has been shown to enhance the cytotoxicity of melphalan and BCNU on human squamous carcinoma cells and of Cisplatin and dacarbazine on melanoma cells. In mice with transplanted mammary carcinoma, beta carotene enhanced the anti-tumor effect of cyclophosphamide; and in mice transplanted with fibrosarcoma, beta carotene enhanced the anti-tumor effect of melphalan, carmustine, doxorubicin, and Etoposide.

GENISTEIN

Genistein has been shown to enhance the accumulation of Cisplatin and doxorubicin in accumulation-defective resistant cancer cells and to increase the accumulation of Cisplatin in non-resistant cancer cells.

QUERCETIN

Quercetin has been shown to enhance the cytotoxicity of several antineoplastic agents. In multidrug-resistant cancer cells, quercetin markedly enhanced the growth-inhibitory effects of doxorubicin. In drug-sensitive cells, quercetin has been shown to enhance the antiproliferative activity of Cisplatin, nitrogen mustard, busulfan, and cytosine arabinoside.

DOC, WHAT'S THE POINT?

In regard to cancer care, determining the best possible, least toxic regime is vital for a good outcome. Once the exact type of cancer and the aggressiveness of it is determined, a cancer program is developed. Hopefully for many cancer patients, this will include IPT. Because IPT doctors are nutritionally minded, it is probable that the person will be put on a nutrient/supplement program. We have developed our own products for cancer patients.* Many vitamins, herbs, and nutriceuticals have specific anticancer effects. In other words, they are natural chemotherapy. They have been shown, at least in vitro, to have cancer cell-killing effects. The three most common types of natural chemotherapy that we prescribe are high-dose quercetin, vitamin A, and vitamin D. Besides being natural chemotherapy, they are also potentiators of chemotherapy.

One of our favorite nutrients to prescribe is quercetin. It has potent anticancer effects, but it is also a potentiator. An in vitro study using human ovarian and endometrial cancer cell lines found that the addition of 0.01 to 10 mM quercetin caused a 1.5- to 30-fold potentiation of the cytotoxic effect of Cisplatin.[82] Many other supplements have been shown by studies to have equal potentiating effects. In one study, the researchers reported that the long-term cure rate for a transplanted adenocarcinoma of the breast increased from 0% to 90% by the addition of vitamin A (retinyl palmitate) or synthetic beta carotene when used in combination with radiation therapy or cyclophosphamide.[83] In regard to vitamin D, there are many studies that show it has anticancer effects, but it is also a potentiator. In one study done at the New Jersey Medical School in Newark, researchers showed that pretreating breast cancer cells with 1,25-dihydroxyvitamin D_3 or all-trans-retinoic acid lowered the threshold for cell killing by the chemotherapy agents Taxol and Adriamycin (See **Figure 22-36**).

It is important to note that during the IPT procedure, the physician may order a nutrient potentiator to be given to enhance the effectiveness of the IPT. For example, there have been numerous studies showing that glutathione, if given before Cisplatin, significantly decreases that drug's

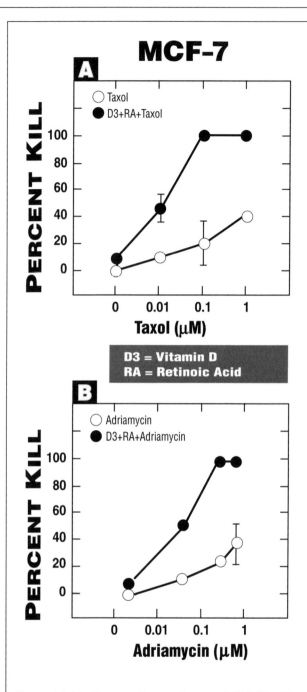

D3 = Vitamin D
RA = Retinoic Acid

Figure 22-36: Percent Breast Cancer Cell Kill with Chemotherapy Alone Compared to Chemotherapy Plus Vitamin D (D3) and Retinoic Acid (RA)

The nutrients significantly enhanced the cancer-killing effects of Adriamycin and Taxol, two common chemotherapy drugs for breast cancer. The control was not counted.

---

* *The complete cancer nutriceutical line that we use can be reviewed and ordered at www.benuts.com.*

neuro- and nephrotoxicity (nerve and kidney damage).[84,85] There are other studies that indicate that it also increases the Cisplatin cancer-killing effect.[86,87] In one of the studies, glutathione injected before the Cisplatin allowed 75% more of the drug to be given. In another study, the glutathione increased the response rate in patients by 50%. For these reasons, some doctors give some glutathione intravenously before giving Cisplatin during the IPT procedure.

Another agent that we commonly give during IPT is selenium. A recent study examined the additive or synergistic effect of selenium alone and in combination with standard anticancer drugs, Adriamycin (doxorubicin) and Taxol, on various tumor cells after 72 hours. Results demonstrated that breast, lung, small intestine, colon, and liver cancer cells showed an increase in apoptosis (cell death). The selenium also enhanced the chemotherapeutic effect of Taxol and doxorubicin on these cells.[88] The authors stated:

> In conclusion, selenium has a significant antineoplastic effect on breast, lung, liver, and small intestinal tumor cells. Supplementation of selenium enhanced the chemotherapeutic effect of Taxol and doxorubicin in these cells beyond that seen with the chemotherapeutic drugs used alone. **These in vitro studies on several cancer cell lines suggest a potential benefit of selenium-enhancement of anticancer effects on other systems, and therefore offer further relevance to clinical trials efforts.**

SUMMARY

IPT involves the use of insulin to potentiate the effects of medications such as chemotherapy drugs. Besides insulin, there are other potentiators, including DMSO, hyperthermia, electrochemotherapy, biooxidative therapies, and various nutrients (including selenium; glutathione; genistein; and vitamins A, C, D, and E). These agents can be used as part of the IPT regime to enhance the potentiating effect of the treatment.

The reason that potentiation is needed in regard to chemotherapy is that for adequate tumor kill to occur, a substantial amount of the drug must reach the tumor site. Using the conventional means of treatment, this means giving massive doses of chemotherapy that have horrific side effects, including bone marrow suppression, immune suppression, loss of hair, kidney damage, nerve damage, and a host of others. When IPT and/or other potentiators are given, research has shown that the cancer-killing effects of the chemotherapy are enhanced. This allows lower doses of chemotherapy to be given to get the same tumoricidal effects, which proportionally increases the safety of the procedure.

The science behind various potentiators is excellent, especially in regard to the most potent of the potentiators, insulin. By combining chemotherapy with potentiators, it is possible to have a powerful and effective method of treatment without the risk of grave side effects. This is bound to improve outcomes, and it is only a matter of time before the comprehensive approach to cancer therapy includes IPT. ■

Reversing cancer physiology— What is it? How to reverse it?

When talking with cancer patients, the concept of reversing cancer physiology is easy for them to grasp. There is generally a reason why a person's body allows a cancer to start and continue to grow. The process to correct this is called *reversing cancer physiology*. Let us say from the start that the primary method to reverse cancer physiology is to get rid of the cancer. So reversing cancer physiology starts with Insulin Potentiation Therapy.

The information that follows in the rest of the book will be new to most people. This information is the opinion of the authors— and we feel the science behind these beliefs is sound. Much of what is presented has been learned by practical experience in treating cancer patients the last ten years.

It is now possible in a doctor's office to document cancer physiology. The various tests that we use will be presented. It is just as easy to document that the person's cancer physiology has reversed to normal physiology after treatment by repeating the same tests. In other words, the material presented for the most part can be objectively found, treated, and corrected. What could be more scientific than that?

Cancer physiology in females starts with estradiol, so this is where we start the next sections because ladies are supposed to go first. . . ■

> **There is generally a reason why a person's body allows a cancer to start and continue to grow.**

CHAPTER 23

Estradiol: The Nemesis of the Female

"THE INCIDENCE OF BREAST CANCER HAS BEEN INCREASING AT AN ANNUAL RATE OF 1.2% SINCE 1940. SINCE 1940, BREAST CANCER MORTALITY HAS ALSO INCREASED."
—American Cancer Society

"SCIENTISTS SAY ESTROGEN BELONGS ON CANCER LIST."
—Headline in the New York Times, December 16, 2000

Reversing cancer physiology means not only stopping the physiology that is promoted by the cancer but also that which caused the cancer to grow in the first place. All cancers have causes. Discovering these causes may spare future generations from preventable cancer.[1] Though the American Cancer Society has done remarkable work at getting the word out that cigarette smoking causes cancer, they have not done as much to spread the word about another potent carcinogenic—iatrogenically given estradiol.

According to the *American Cancer Society Textbook of Clinical Oncology,* oral contraceptives, steroidal estrogens, and especially estradiol are carcinogenic. Using the exact nomenclature of the book: "Oral contraceptives and steroidal estrogens are chemicals and mixtures judged to be carcinogenic to humans by the International Agency for Research on Cancer, and estradiol is in a class of carcinogenic chemicals."[1-3] Hopefully this will help women realize that estradiol is a potentially dangerous substance. What most women do not realize is that estradiol is at least partly responsible for many of the conditions that plague women, such as dysmenorrhea, premenstrual syndrome (PMS), endometriosis, uterine fibroids, fibrocystic breast disease, migraine headaches, and chronic pelvic pain, not to mention conditions such as breast, cervical, ovarian, and uterine cancer (see **Figure 23-1**). In summary, one could say that a female's ultimate nemesis is not men, but estradiol.

NOT ALL ESTROGENS ARE CREATED EQUAL

Before describing the effects of estradiol, it is important to realize that not all estrogens are created equal. In the normal, nonpregnant female, estrogens are secreted in major quantities only by the ovaries. Only three estrogens are present in significant quantities in the plasma of the human

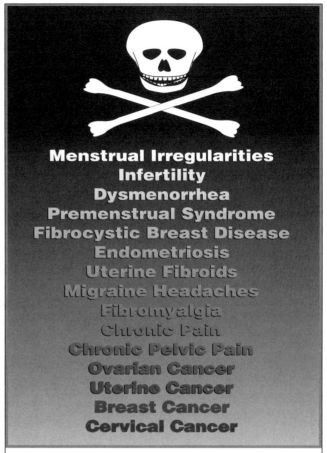

Figure 23-1: Conditions in Which Estradiol Has Been Implicated
This is the *who's who list* of female health disorders.

female: estradiol-17β (hereafter estradiol), estrone, and estriol (see **Figure 23-2**). The principal estrogen secreted by the ovaries is estradiol. The estrogenic potency of estradiol is 12 times that of estrone and 80 times that of estriol. Considering these relative potencies, one can see that the total estrogenic effect of estradiol is usually many times that of the others combined.

Physicians who practice natural medicine will often perform a comprehensive saliva hormone profile on patients with chronic diseases. This test measures the free fraction of hormone available to work and act on tissues, whereas blood tests measure total hormone levels, with the majority of it being bound up by proteins, especially sex hormone-binding globulin. So it is best

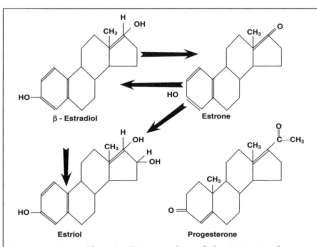

Figure 23-2: Chemical Formulas of the Principal Female Hormones
Most female medical conditions are caused by estradiol excess.

for a woman to find out her **biologically active hormone level** by testing the free fraction in the blood or doing a test for urine or salivary hormone levels. Inevitably for the chronically ill female patient, estradiol excess is found.

Estradiol excess has many physiological and biological effects (see **Figure 23-3**). Estradiol has been implicated in causing an increase in prolactin, aldosterone, insulin, histamine, and prostaglandin levels, while causing a decline in the liver's ability to detoxify and a decline of activity in endorphins, neurotransmitters, and B vitamins. These effects can cause women to suffer from acne and various skin lesions, constipation, allergies, moodiness, irritability, depression, water retention, chronic musculoskeletal aching, and severe menstrual cramps.[4,5] Perhaps even more importantly, these are the symptoms in such dreaded female conditions as dysmenorrhea, PMS, endometriosis, uterine fibroids, fibrocystic breast disease, migraine headaches, and chronic pelvic pain. Since estradiol excess causes the symptoms of these conditions, it makes sense to implicate it in the propagation of these conditions.

Figure 23-3: Estradiol Physiological Effects
. . . .

INCREASES:

Aldosterone	Histamine	Prolactin
Breast Stimulation	Insulin	Prostaglandin
Cervical Stimulation	Ovarian Stimulation	Uterine Stimulation

DECREASES:

Liver Detoxification Ability	B Vitamins	Neurotransmitter Activity

These facts are important because routinely when we question a woman with uterine, ovarian, breast, or cervical cancer, inevitably she gives a history of having one or more of the above conditions. Most women whom we see for breast cancer have had a long history of menstrual irregularities, used birth control, and have had treatments for such conditions as migraine headaches or endometriosis. These conditions, we believe, are all tied to the same physiology: estradiol excess. For the woman desiring to reduce her risk for female cancers, estradiol levels have to be decreased. If a woman wants to know if she has breast, uterine, or cervical cancer physiology, then the first question we would ask is, "Do you have a normal menstrual cycle?" Most women answer, "Yes, as long as I take oral contraceptive pills." Do you see the problem? A woman has estradiol excess causing PMS, painful periods (dysmenorrhea), or endometriosis, for which the gynecologist prescribes birth control pills. The doctor is felt to be a hero because the woman has no more PMS, painful periods, or endometriosis pain; unbeknownst to the patient, however, is that if the estradiol excess continues, there is increased risk of breast, uterine, ovarian, and cervical cancer.

"M.O.": STOMACH CANCER

On June 27, 2001, M.O. came to Caring Medical for IPT from a referral from a prominent natural medicine physician in New York. She was only 58 years old, but already had a major surgery because of a diagnosis of cervical cancer four years prior and now was faced with Stage 4 stomach cancer. She was not a surgical candidate because the cancer had spread.

This case is presented to talk about the importance of cancer physiology. We asked her if she was on any hormone replacement, though it was nowhere on the history sheet that she filled out. Then she "confessed" that she had been on Premarin for the last 15 years. We asked her if she had a history of yeast infections. She was wondering why we would ask such a strange question in a cancer consultation and admitted that she had fought yeast infections for years. We then explained cancer physiology to her. Because her cancer physiology was never dealt with during her first cancer crisis, she developed another cancer. Natural medicine is about reducing one's risk of cancer. For the woman with cancer or

FIGURE 23-4: CONTRAINDICATIONS TO THE USE OF ORAL CONTRACEPTIVES

ABSOLUTE	RELATIVE CONTRAINDICATIONS TO ESTROGEN	OTHER RELATIVE CONTRAINDICTIONS
Venous Thrombosis	Uterine Fibroids	Anovulation/Oligo-ovulation
Pulmonary Embolism	Lactation	Depression
Coronary Vascular Disease	Diabetes Mellitus	Severe Headaches
Cerebrovascular Accident	Sickle Cell Disease	(especially Vascular)
Current Pregnancy	Hypertension	Acne
Malignant Tumor: Breast, Endometrium, Ovary	Age 30+ and Cigarette Smoking	Severe Varicose Veins
Hepatic Tumor	Age 40+ and High Risk for Vascular Disease	
Abnormal Liver Function		

Notice that female cancers are a contraindication to OCP use. Why? *Because they cause them!*

desiring to reduce her risk of cancer, an in-depth review of estrogens, oral contraceptives, and the various female conditions related to estradiol excess is warranted. The case of M.O. is a perfect example of this. It is our contention that she has developed two separate cancers in part because of her excessive estrogen stimulation, in large measure caused by the Premarin she was taking under a doctor's prescription.

ORAL CONTRACEPTIVE PILLS— PLEASE, PLEASE, AVOID THEM

It is rare for a young female to come to our office without ever having been put on "the pill." It is amazing how many young females are on oral contraceptive pills (OCPs). Realize that when the doctor says OCP, he or she is really saying, "Take this estradiol because it will make you feel good." If that is not bad enough, various OCPs are now advertised on television for their "good-looking skin" benefits. Give us a break! If a woman wants to get her skin looking great, go to a good esthetician and stop eating junk food. Nothing could harm a woman's body quicker than estradiol capsules. OCPs inhibit a woman's own production of hormones, as well as ovulation, as these are some of the ways they prevent pregnancy. In other words, OCPs interfere with the female's hormonal makeup without doing anything to correct the problem. **No female problem is due to an oral contraceptive pill deficiency.** Just like no chronic pain is due to an ibuprofen deficiency.

All one has to do is look at the contraindications to taking OCPs and know that they are not good for you (see **Figure 23-4**). Some of the indications for not taking OCPs are as follows: history of clotting disorders, breast cancer, endometrial cancer, ovarian cancer, abnormal uterine bleeding, migraine headaches, liver disease, smoking, varicose veins, depression, high blood pressure, heart disease, kidney disease, breast feeding, or pregnancy.[6] The reason for some of these restrictions is because OCPs can cause the condition. Yes, OCPs can cause uterine bleeding, migraine headaches, liver disease, clotting disorders, and high blood pressure, as well as various cancers. We have personally taken care of females in their 30s who have had strokes while on OCPs, which were suspected as the cause of the stroke. In regard to the later, make no bones about it, OCPs thicken the blood. As will be discussed later, thick blood or coagulopathy is a significant part of cancer physiology.

Natural medicine seeks to correct the underlying problems so the patient truly becomes healed and never has to come back to the doctor's office. For females taking OCPs, the underlying hormone, nutrient, dietary, or structural problems that are causing their symptoms go unchecked. A better approach is to stop the OCPs and get a natural medicine evaluation and have the problem cured. **What most women do not realize is that the menstrual cycle is the greatest guide of a woman's health. A woman who has regular menstrual cycles without any PMS or cramping is most likely in excellent health. A woman should not know when her menstrual cycle is coming. Menstrual cramps, moodiness, irregularity, and bloating are completely abnormal.** The various female conditions will now be discussed, along with ways that the underlying conditions and symptoms can be eliminated.

THE FEMALE CONDITIONS
PREMENSTRUAL SYNDROME

PMS is a recurrent condition of women characterized by troublesome symptoms generally seven to 14 days before menstruation. The earliest symptoms usually involve varying combinations of fatigue, depression, painful breast swelling, lower abdominal bloating, and constipation. Later symptoms include increasing anxiety, irritability, hostility, painful menstrual cramps, craving for sweets, and binge eating. A sensation of fluid retention is frequently experienced during the two to three days before the flow. Weight gain and edema are particularly common and distressing. Premenstrual acne flair-ups and headaches may precede the flow by one or two days.[7]

For some women, this monthly experience is devastating. Trivial episodes, especially with men, become major confrontations. Impaired judgment and forgetfulness may be incapacitating. PMS is estimated to affect between 30% and 40% of menstruating women.

One of the most common findings in women with PMS is an elevated estradiol to progesterone ratio.[8-10] Most commonly, this derangement is caused by a combined estradiol excess and progesterone deficiency. An increase in the estradiol to progesterone ratio contributes to PMS symptoms and is illustrated in **Figure 23-5**. These physiological effects of elevated estradiol can account for PMS.

Amount Excreted in Micrograms per 24 hours			
	2/14/00	5/8/00	Postmenopausal Reference Range
Estrone	17.1	9.9	1-7
Estradiol	*143.8*	30.6	0-23
Estriol	7.3	18.0	0-30
Total Estrogens	*168.2*	58.5	0-60
Testosterone	13.0	20.7	5-35

Figure 23-6: Urinary Hormone Levels for K.M.
K. M. was placed on chasteberry, flax seed oil, and a high soy, high-fiber, low-refined carbohydrate diet. In less than three months her hormonal levels were completely changed, decreasing her estradiol levels by 70 percent.

NATURAL MEDICINE TREATMENT FOR PMS AND DYSMENORRHEA

Since estradiol excess is the root cause for these conditions, the first step in curing the condition is getting a comprehensive hormone analysis (either saliva or urine) that includes, at a minimum, all three estrogens, progesterone, DHEA, and testosterone. It is important to do the test on the day when the person's symptoms are at their worst. This will then provide an accurate picture of what needs to be done so that progress can easily be monitored.

Estradiol excess is believed to be primarily due to an overproduction of estrogen within the body, but it can also be due to a relative increase in estrogen due to low progesterone secretion by the corpus luteum (a woman not ovulating). The hormonal makeup of a woman can easily be manipulated by diet and herbal remedies, as shown by the case study of K.M. She had struggled with terrible PMS for years, which included such symptoms as painful menses, painful and tender breasts, and depression prior to menstruation. Unfortunately for her, she was forced to make a change because she had been recently diagnosed with breast cancer, which is the end result of estradiol excess. (We will talk more about this later.) By changing her diet to include more soy and fiber (vegetables), flax seed, fewer refined carbohydrates, and high-dose chasteberry, she decreased her estradiol levels by 70% in less than three months (see **Figure 23-6**). Of significance to her was the fact that her breast cancer marker

---

FIGURE 23-5: **PMS PATHOLOGY**

An increase in the estradiol to progesterone ratio causes various physiological effects that account for the symptoms of PMS.

PHYSIOLOGICAL EFFECT	SYMPTOM
● Impaired Liver Function	Gastrointestinal Symptoms: Constipation, Bloating
● Reduced Manufacture of Serotonin	Mood Swings, Irritability, Anxiety
● Decreased Action of Vitamin B6	Depression
● Increased Aldosterone Secretion	Bloating, Weight Gain
● Increased Prolactin Secretion	Breast Swelling, Tenderness

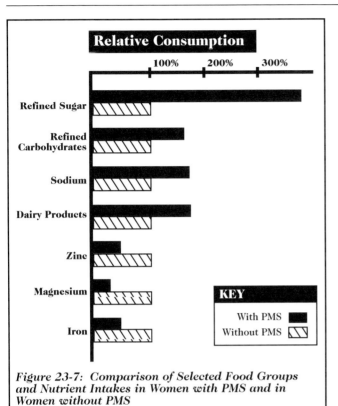

Figure 23-7: Comparison of Selected Food Groups and Nutrient Intakes in Women with PMS and in Women without PMS

CA 15-3 went from 39 (abnormal) to 17.3 (normal range). This is why covering up symptoms with OCPs is *dangerous;* your life could depend on it.

As indicated with K.M., the first step in reducing estradiol is for a woman to increase her intake of soy in the diet. Typically women are encouraged to eat one to three containers of tofu (16 oz. each) per week. Women have been shown to create a significant positive impact on their hormone levels and ratios by the inclusion of soy protein in their diets.[11,12] Besides increasing soy in the diet, simple carbohydrates must be reduced. **PMS patients consume 275% more refined sugar, 62% more refined carbohydrates, 78% more sodium, 79% more dairy products, 52% less zinc, 77% less magnesium, and 53% less iron than women without PMS.**[13] (see **Figure 23-7.**) In our office, women suffering from PMS are placed on the appropriate diet for their metabolic type in addition to the above recommendations, as well as the multivitamin/mineral supplement Supervits with

iron*—one of the few multivitamins that has twice as much magnesium as calcium. This happens to be exactly what these patients need.

To attack PMS and dysmenorrhea instead of women attacking other people because of rage and severe cramping, extra vitamin B_6 is needed. At daily doses of 200 mg to 600 mg, B_6 lowers serum estrogen and elevates serum progesterone levels.[14,15] We give patients vitamin B_6 in a highly assimilated form known as pyridoxal-5-phosphate. High estrogen levels have been implicated as a cause of depressed B_6 levels, which goes along with the conditions above. The active form of pyridoxine (B_6), pyridoxal-5-phosphate is a cofactor in the formation of the following neurotransmitters: dopamine, serotonin, and GABA.[14,16,17] Deficiencies of each of these neurotransmitters can cause many of the symptoms of PMS, particularly depression. If that does not make a woman with PMS just run out and start buying up all the B_6 she can get, then consider the fact that vitamin B_6 has been shown to have a similar effect as the drug bromocriptine in suppressing aldosterone.[14] Aldosterone is the hormone that helps the body retain sodium and thus water. Yes, women, that means no more bloating, or do you desire to be a bigger size each month?

From an herbal standpoint, the most potent of the estradiol-reducing herbs is *Vitex agnus-castus,* better known as chasteberry. It is given to reduce the estradiol/progesterone ratio. Specifically, it increases the production of lutenizing hormone and inhibits the release of follicle-stimulating hormone. This leads to an increased ratio of progesterone to estrogen with a corpus luteum-like hormone effect.[18-20] Chasteberry also inhibits the secretion of prolactin. In vitro studies demonstrate that certain constituents of chasteberry extract directly bind to dopamine receptors in the anterior pituitary gland. Dopamine is the physiological inhibitor of prolactin; thus it appears the dopaminergic effect of chasteberry results in an inhibition of prolactin synthesis and release.[21] For patients suffering from PMS and/or dysmenorrhea, one of the most useful products we have used with success is Menstrual Support, which contains a high concentration of *Vitex* standardized extract.* Various

---

* *All the products and supplements mentioned are available for purchase on-line at www.benuts.com or can be ordered by calling 1-877-RX-BEULAH (877-792-3852).*

studies have confirmed that to relieve the symptoms of PMS, *Vitex* is a woman's best friend.[22,23]

By changing one's diet and taking chasteberry and vitamin B_6, many of the etiological bases for PMS and dysmenorrhea will be corrected. If a repeat urinary or salivary hormone profile does not show a correction of the high estradiol/ progesterone ratio, then additional measures must be taken by the patient. These could include taking some low-dose thyroid hormone, iodine (Lugol's solution), calcium D-glucarate, diindolylmethane, or indole-3-carbinol (cruciferous vegetables). We have had success with all of these to help reverse estradiol excess physiology.

CHRONIC PELVIC PAIN—
GET READY FOR THE LAPAROSCOPY

As noted above, it is very easy for a woman to take ibuprofen to relieve menstrual cramps or chronic pelvic pain. If a family doctor cannot relieve a woman's pain with NSAIDs (nonsteroidal anti-inflammatory drugs), then an ultrasound of the pelvis is done. Inevitably, this will show endometriosis and/or a uterine fibroid. To the attending physician's delight, he can announce, "Alas, I have found your problem," and soon the woman is off to a gynecologist for laproscopic surgery.

Modern medicine often just chases findings and does not get at the root cause of the condition; this is quite evident by the surgical management of such conditions as endometriosis and uterine fibroids. As a side note, Caring Medical has never had a patient with these conditions ever have a laparoscopy; these conditions are easily managed with nutritional therapies. All this talk about PMS, fibroids, and other female disorders can get depressing, so how about a nice poem? (see **Figure 23-8**.)

ENDOMETRIOSIS

Endometriosis is a condition in which endometrial tissue is outside the uterine cavity. It is reported to affect 7% to 50% of menstruating women.

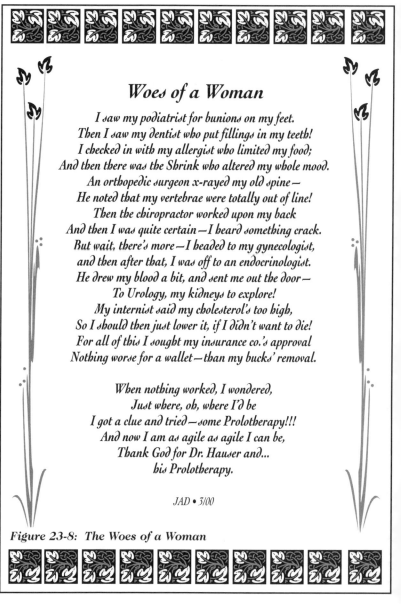

Woes of a Woman

I saw my podiatrist for bunions on my feet.
Then I saw my dentist who put fillings in my teeth!
I checked in with my allergist who limited my food;
And then there was the Shrink who altered my whole mood.
An orthopedic surgeon x-rayed my old spine—
He noted that my vertebrae were totally out of line!
Then the chiropractor worked upon my back
And then I was quite certain—I heard something crack.
But wait, there's more—I headed to my gynecologist,
and then after that, I was off to an endocrinologist.
He drew my blood a bit, and sent me out the door—
To Urology, my kidneys to explore!
My internist said my cholesterol's too high,
So I should then just lower it, if I didn't want to die!
For all of this I sought my insurance co.'s approval
Nothing worse for a wallet—than my bucks' removal.

When nothing worked, I wondered,
Just where, oh, where I'd be
I got a clue and tried—some Prolotherapy!!!
And now I am as agile as agile I can be,
Thank God for Dr. Hauser and...
his Prolotherapy.

JAD • 3/00

Figure 23-8: The Woes of a Woman

Characteristically, endometriosis occurs in high-achieving, nulliparous women with a type A personality. Generally, endometriosis is initiated in the third decade of life, becomes clinically apparent in the 30s, and regresses after menopause.[7,24]

Endometriosis is often blamed for unexplained infertility, dysmenorrhea, or dysparenunia (painful intercourse). Other symptoms of the condition include low back pain; rectal discomfort; and chronic, nonspecific pelvic pain. The interesting fact is that even with extensive endometriosis, pain may not be a significant clinical entity.[25] On the other hand, incapacitating dysmenorrhea and pelvic pain may be associated with minimal amounts of endometriosis. To quote the premier textbook of endocrinology, *"Thus, the degree of endometriotic involvement and spread bears no constant relationship to the presence or absence of subjective discomfort."*[26] In other words, it is impossible to blame pain on endometriosis just because it is there.

Unfortunately, the vast majority of women in the United States are told that they need a definitive diagnosis for their symptoms of pelvic pain, so laproscopic visualization of the pelvis is carried out, and the extent of the endometriosis is staged according to the classification (minimal, mild, moderate, severe) established by the American Fertility Society.[27]

To treat the condition, endometrial tissue is fried or burned, and various body parts of the female are removed, including the ovaries and uterus. If endometriosis is everywhere, the woman is placed on a medication such as Lupron that causes premature menopause. That means women in their 20s start having hot flashes. The amazing fact is that even with these drastic measures, the recurrence rates for endometriosis range from 37% to 74%, depending on the extent of disease.[28,29] Several studies have shown that with hysterectomy alone, the risk of recurrent pain is increased by a factor of 6.1 and risk of reoperation by a factor of 8.1.[30-32] According to a physician teaching journal, "It is thus prudent to tell patients that surgery will not necessarily cure

their disease."[33] To all of this we say…there must be a better way.

Endometriosis is commonly blamed for causing chronic pelvic pain. It is easy to see the reason for this when one considers the most common sites in which endometriosis occurs. Endometriosis occurs most commonly in the ovaries, on the broad ligament, on the peritoneal surfaces, on the posterior cervix, and in the rectovaginal septum (see **Figure 23-9**). A woman has pelvic or back pain, and there is some funny density on ultrasound or bluish-looking thing in the pelvis on laparoscopy, so it is easy to see why endometriosis is blamed for the complaint.

As noted above, women with severe endometriosis can have no complaints or be filled with endometriosis and have only mild symptoms. Because of these facts, it seems likely that something **besides** the endometriosis is causing the woman's pain. Further evidence of this is the fact that 30% to 40% of women with endometriosis are infertile, when in many instances the endometriosis does not appear to be interfering with normal reproductive processes. Sperm ascension, ovulation, and ovum pickup and transport can all take place with endometriosis.[34] Thus, **even infertility is most likely not from the endometriosis itself but from the condition that caused it to develop in the first place, which is estradiol excess.** In regard to the pain experienced, the most likely culprit is either the nerves to the pelvic organs and/or the ligaments that support the pelvis. Before explaining how Neural Therapy and Prolotherapy can be used to treat endometriosis pain symptoms, another condition that causes women to undergo surgical procedures must be discussed—uterinefibroids.

UTERINE FIBROIDS

Uterine leiomyomas (fibroids) are smooth muscle tumors of the uterus (see **Figure 23-10**). Twenty percent of women develop uterine fibroids by 40 years of age, and they constitute the most common indication for major surgery in women.[7] As in endometriosis and for that matter breast lumps, the conventional medical treatment is to cut them out, even though almost all cases of fibroids are benign (less than 0.5% of fibroids become cancerous). However, it may be somewhat challenging just to remove the fibroid, so physicians often convince women that removing

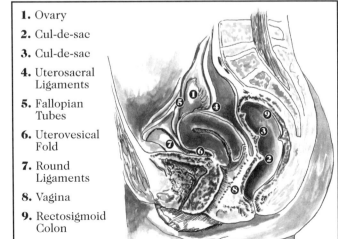

1. Ovary
2. Cul-de-sac
3. Cul-de-sac
4. Uterosacral Ligaments
5. Fallopian Tubes
6. Uterovesical Fold
7. Round Ligaments
8. Vagina
9. Rectosigmoid Colon

Figure 23-9: Common Sites of Endometriosis in Decreasing Order of Frequency

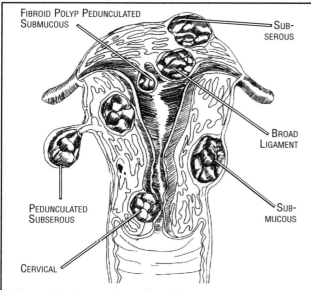

FIBROID POLYP PEDUNCULATED
SUBMUCOUS

SUB-
SEROUS

BROAD
LIGAMENT

PEDUNCULATED
SUBSEROUS

SUB-
MUCOUS

CERVICAL

Figure 23-10: Uterine Fibroids
Uterine Fibroids are non-cancerous tumors that can grow anywhere on the inner muscular wall or the outside of the uterus.

the whole uterus is the best option. So prevalent are hysterectomies now that it is currently the second most common surgical procedure performed on women in the United States. There are now a whopping 750,000 hysterectomies per year.[35] Of the female surgeries, it is surpassed only by cesarean section. The sad fact is that many of these hysterectomies are performed on women in their 20s and 30s who have no children.

In addition to the loss of childbearing ability and the emotional trauma of such surgery, recovery from a hysterectomy takes an average of one year. Further, studies show that for a 35-year-old woman who has had a hysterectomy, the risk of heart attack or angina increases seven times. Premenopausal women who have a hysterectomy without ovary removal begin menopause typically five years earlier because one of the long-term effects of the surgery is **accelerated aging of the ovaries**. This may be due to the fact that the blood supply to the ovaries is compromised by removal of the uterus.[35]

Most women do not realize that **the majority of uterine fibroids are asymptomatic**.[36] Occasionally, the patient may become aware of a lower abdominal mass if it protrudes above the symphysis pubis, but this is rare. Quite often, the development of discomfort comes on insidiously, and the symptoms are difficult for a patient to

define. She may complain of pelvic pressure, congestion, bloating, or a feeling of heaviness in the lower abdomen. As with endometriosis, menorrhagia and infertility are associated with it.[37] But just because a woman has a uterine fibroid does not mean her infertility is from it. Most likely, the fibroid has nothing to do with it, but the condition of estradiol excess that led to the fibroid has **everything** to do with it. Surgery is not needed; natural medicine is needed to lower estrogen levels.

Unequivocally, uterine fibroids are distinctly estrogen dependent.[7] They rarely develop before menarche and seldom develop or enlarge beyond menopause, unless stimulated by exogenous estrogens. **Fibroids can enlarge with amazing speed, especially during pregnancy or when exposed to oral contraceptives containing high doses of estrogens (almost all of them).** Women with uterine fibroids have a fourfold increased rate of developing endometrial cancer (another condition promoted by estradiol).[38]

Women around the country are learning of these dismal facts and are seeking alternatives to laproscopic surgeries or hysterectomies. They are realizing that by getting at the root cause of these conditions, disease stabilization or regression is possible. This could only occur because of the true healing effects of natural medicine.

WOMEN: IT IS EITHER NATURAL MEDICINE OR SURGERY—THE CHOICE IS YOURS

Once a physician mentions the words *fibroid* or *endometriosis* to a woman, it is only a matter of time before surgery is "entertained" (see **Figure 23-11**). The typical scenario is that a woman has menstrual cramps, diagnosed as dysmenorrhea, and NSAIDs are prescribed. These help for a time, but because the underlying estrogen dominance is not treated, various other symptomatology occurs, such as irritability, moodiness, and bloating, so she is diagnosed with PMS, and a stronger NSAID is prescribed. Eventually, these do not help, and a pelvic or transvaginal ultrasound is ordered. A hazy structure is seen by the ovary or uterus, and a "look and see" laparoscopy is advised. "It might be cancer" are the woman's immediate thoughts, so she relents. If endometriosis is found, various laproscopic laser surgeries are performed, and the woman is placed on OCPs and/or Lupron, which

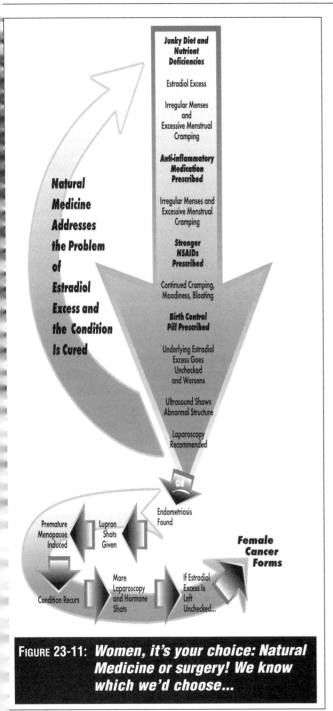

FIGURE 23-11: *Women, it's your choice: Natural Medicine or surgery! We know which we'd choose...*

Labels within figure:

Junky Diet and Nutrient Deficiencies

Estradiol Excess

Irregular Menses and Excessive Menstrual Cramping

Anti-inflammatory Medication Prescribed

Irregular Menses and Excessive Menstrual Cramping

Stronger NSAIDs Prescribed

Continued Cramping, Moodiness, Bloating

Birth Control Pill Prescribed

Underlying Estradiol Excess Goes Unchecked and Worsens

Ultrasound Shows Abnormal Structure

Laparoscopy Recommended

OR

Endometriosis Found

Female Cancer Forms

Premature Menopause Induced

Lupron Shots Given

Condition Recurs

More Laparoscopy and Hormone Shots

If Estradiol Excess Is Left Unchecked...

Natural Medicine Addresses the Problem of Estradiol Excess and the Condition Is Cured

---

state is never addressed, which increases her risk of such female cancers as breast and uterine cancer. So the patient loses a uterus but gains breast cancer. This is why we advocate a better solution, and this comes from natural medicine.

DOES NATURAL MEDICINE REALLY WORK? I HAVE ENDOMETRIOSIS AND UTERINE FIBROIDS!

It is interesting to watch the responses of women when they are told that there are alternatives to surgery for endometriosis and uterine fibroids. "Come on, does natural medicine really work?" "I have a tumor you know." "If this is so good, why doesn't every doctor do it?" "Yeah, but the surgery is already scheduled." Well, if the surgery is already scheduled, and you want to have it, go for it; don't let us stop you! A good example of the struggles that women have with the tumor issue is Lana.

Lana is Russian born and was very open to natural medicine. She had heard about Neural Therapy shrinking fibroids and desired that treatment. Apparently her fibroid was the size of a 12-week-old fetus, which is usually the size when the doctor starts talking operation. She was 42 years old and was told that the fibroid was the cause of her excessive menstrual bleeding.

We evaluated her and explained the procedure to her. Basically, she would receive two shots into and around some of the nerves that supply the ovaries, uterus, and pelvic organs (see **Figure 23-12**). She would know she was better by her menstrual cycle being better. She agreed to the injections and within about one minute the procedure was over. She then exclaimed, "That's it?" I (Ross) said, "Yep, that's it!" We agreed to meet after her next menstrual cycle.

About one month later, she came in and boldly demanded, "I want some more Neural Therapy!" We asked how her menstrual cycle was this month, and she calmly and quietly said "fine." "What do you mean, fine! That's great!" we exclaimed. We explained to her that she may not need any more treatments, as sometimes just a single Neural Therapy session was needed. However, she would not leave the office without getting another treatment, because she wanted thefibroid shrunk.

Lana came in for two more Neural Therapy sessions; each time she explained how her menstrual cycle was completely normal but wanted

---

induces a premature menopause state. If a uterine fibroid is seen, then a hysterectomy is recommended. Unfortunately, the recurrence rate for many of these surgeries is quite high, so in the end a lot of money is spent, along with the pain and disability suffered. **The most tragic aspect of this scenario is that the woman's estrogen dominant**

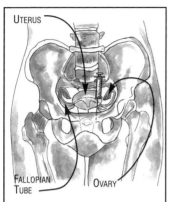

Figure 23-12: Neural Therapy for Pelvic Disorders

This treatment involves just two injections into and around the pelvic sympathetic nerves. Treatment like this is used for disorders such as pelvic pain, endometriosis, uterine fibroids, dysmenorrhea, and dysmenorrhagia.

the "tumor" gone. Regardless of our words that the "tumor" may have had nothing to do with the bleeding and that her underlying condition most likely abated with the Neural Therapy, she would not listen. To ease her mind, we put her on a Chinese herbal remedy that has been shown to shrink fibroid tumors. After several months on this, she had a repeat ultrasound that showed a 25% reduction. Though she still has the fibroids and no more symptoms, this confirms the fact that the fibroids were not causing her original problem. More than likely, however, she will come back demanding more Neural Therapy treatments because some of the fibroid "tumor" is still there.

Lana is a fantastic, nice person. We do not in any way want to be disrespectful to her, but when a doctor tells a woman that she has a "mass" or "tumor," the normal instinct is for the person to want to get it out. The fact is that most female masses, including breast cysts, ovarian cysts, endometriomas, and uterine fibroids, often have nothing to do with the symptoms from which the woman is suffering. Besides even if they did, a better approach than removing these structures would be to **remove the cause of why they formed in the first place.** We encourage women to get out of the box and consider natural medicine. For women like Lana who do not enjoy the knife treatment, interventional natural medicine is the way to go. The first step is dietary and nutriceutical changes as discussed previously, of which K.F. can surely testify that you can "natural medicine your fibroids away!"

FIBROID FINISHED, FINALLY—CASE OF K.F.

K.F. is a classic example of what was shown in **Figure 23-11.** Upon getting her menstrual cycle as a teenager, she began having terrible menstrual cramps. This was treated with NSAIDs, which progressed to stronger and stronger NSAIDs. Her symptoms worsened to include severe premenstrual tension, more painful menses that were prolonged, painful/tender breasts, vaginal discharge, and a significant depressed feeling before menstruation each month. She was then diagnosed with PMS. She was prescribed various medications, including antidepressants. She had tried numerous pain medications, including very strong narcotics, but her chronic pelvic pain continued and seemed to spread to the rest of her body. She was subsequently diagnosed with fibromyalgia.

She underwent a pelvic ultrasound that showed some "tumors," so she felt obliged to have a laparoscopy. During the laparoscopy, a lot of endometriosis was found. She eventually had numerous laparoscopies that removed some of the endometriosis via frying and laser. Unfortunately for K.F., these treatments did not decrease her symptoms, which now included infertility. In 1993, she underwent a laparotomy with a partial colon resection, which was said to be necessitated by her horrible case of endometriosis. She had another pelvic surgery prior to seeing us—a hernia repair caused by a weakening of the tissues from the surgery done in 1993.

By the time she saw us, she had suffered with chronic pelvic and back pain for 20 years, a "hormone" problem for 20 years, chronic fatigue for six years, and a long history for such things as insomnia, infertility, depression, sinus infections, gastrointestinal problems, difficulty losing weight, and uterine fibroids. This case is real and most likely pertains to you or someone you know. She was placed on a complex carbohydrate diet with lots of vegetables and protein. She was also tested for food allergies and placed on an allergy elimination diet. Her diet also consisted of a lot of tofu. She was given nutriceuticals to take, including chasteberry and flax seed oil. Neural Therapy to the pelvic area was also done. When she had her ultrasound a couple months later, a uterine fibroid could not even be seen. According to her, the gynecologist said, "Well, I'm not exactly sure what happened, but your fibroid has shrunk." K.F. knew exactly what happened, and it was not surgery. Natural medicine is powerful; uterine fibroids are no match for it.

FIBROCYSTIC BREAST DISEASE— AGAIN, TOO MUCH ESTRADIOL

Fibrocystic breast disease is the most common breast disease and is clinically apparent in about 50% of women.[7] A tremendous percentage of women have this condition, which is totally abnormal. Clinically, the cystic lesions are usually multiple and bilateral and are characterized by pain and tenderness, particularly premenstrually. The disease usually occurs in the premenopausal years with a cessation of symptoms postmenopausally, unless exogenous estrogens are administered.

The condition is believed to be due to a relative or absolute decrease in the production of progesterone or an increase in the amount of estrogen. **Estrogen promotes the growth of mammary ducts and the periductal stroma.** Patients with fibrocystic breast disease improve dramatically during pregnancy and lactation because of the large amount of progesterone produced by the corpus luteum and the placenta and the increased production of estriol, which blocks the hyperplastic changes produced by estradiol and estrone.[7] Any female medical condition that is worsened by estradiol is generally improved by progesterone, as they have opposing actions (see **Figure 23-13**). This is one of the reasons natural progesterone is used so freely by natural medicine practitioners. Fibrocystic breast disease is best treated by measures that lower estradiol levels, as discussed previously.

Sometimes women are given the diagnosis of mastalgia. Mastalgia is a fancy medical term for breast pain for which we have no clue as to its origin. Mastalgia is one of those hidden complaints that women have but do not talk about. Breast pain is not something women routinely bring up at the dinner table. In fact, mastalgia is quite common. When questioned directly, 45% of working women reported mild breast pain and 21% complained of severe breast pain.[39] Breast pain is the most common complaint for which women with breast symptoms present to the primary care physician.[40]

FIGURE 23-13: THE OPPOSING ACTIONS OF ESTROGEN AND PROGESTERONE

ESTROGEN EFFECTS	PROGESTERONE EFFECTS
Creates proliferative endometrium	Maintains secretory endometrium
Breast stimulation	Protects against breast fibrocysts
Increased body fat	Helps use fat for energy
Salt and fluid retention	Natural diuretic
Depression and headaches	Natural antidepressant
Interferes with thyroid hormone	Facilitates thyroid hormone
Increased blood clotting	Normalizes blood clotting
Decreases libido	Restores libido
Impairs blood sugar	Normalizes blood sugar levels
Loss of zinc and retention of copper	Normalizes zinc and copper levels
Reduced oxygen levels in all cells	Restores proper cell oxygen levels
Increased risk of endometrial cancer	Prevents endometrial cancer
Increased risk of breast cancer	Helps prevent breast cancer
Slightly restrains osteoclast function	Stimulates osteoblast bone building
Reduces vascular tone	Necessary for survival of embryo
	Precursor of corticosterone production

Figure 23-13: The Effects of Estrogen and Progesterone
These hormones are complete opposites. Typically, most women with chronic illnesses have too much estrogen and too little progesterone.

Typical medical treatments for nondescript breast pain range from hormone manipulation (with menopause-inducing drugs) to various surgeries, including removing part of the breasts. A method of lowering estradiol that is especially helpful in fibrocystic breast disease is administering iodine in the form of supersaturated potassium iodine or Lugol's solution. Iodine is needed by the body for proper thyroid function, so thyroid hormone levels should also be checked. For some women, the problem is not cysts in the breasts but breast pain, coming from a musculoskeletal structure such as the ribs or sternum. Natural medicine solutions are the best options, including Prolotherapy (see **Figure 23-14**). (A complete discussion on the musculoskeletal conditions in women is explored in *The Woman's Guide to Curing Her Chronic Pain,* available from Beulah Land Press at www.benuts.com.)

THE MENOPAUSE MYTH...ESTROGEN

Menopause is that time in a woman's life when the ovaries stop ovulating and producing hormones, which causes a drastic decline in hormone levels. This occurs in American women generally around the age of 50.[41] This decline in hormone levels causes a variety of symptoms, including irregular menses, hot flashes, insomnia, nervousness, irritability, depression, and osteoporosis. Because of these well-known symptoms, especially the hot

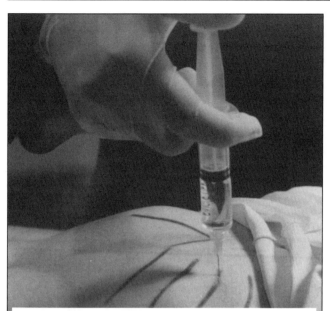

Figure 23-14: Prolotherapy of the Rib-Sternal Junction
This treatment is effective at eliminating musculoskeletal causes of chest and breast pain.

flashes and osteoporosis, women have been fed the menopause myth that estrogen is necessary to reverse these symptoms.

What most women do not know is the blood production rates of their hormones before and after menopause. As can be seen in **Figure 23-15**, *all hormone production levels decline except estrogens, which actually increase in menopause.*[42] The reason for this is the conversion of male hormones made by the adrenal gland to estrogens. The interesting fact is that this conversion is more efficient the greater the percentage of body fat on a woman. So just from this information, it does not make a lot of sense to give postmenopausal women estrogen. *The*

Physician's Desk Reference lists estradiol as one of the components of Premarin. Most people know that estradiol is the most widely used hormone in postmenopausal women, which is 100% estrogen but 100% of the wrong kind of estrogen. So do you see why we are 100% opposed to this? Okay, enough with the 100% stuff.

"But doctor, if I don't use estrogen, I'm going to get osteoporosis, and what about my hot flashes?" It is true that estrogen builds bone and gets rid of hot flashes. **The menopause myth is that women believe that estrogen is the only hormone that reduces hot flashes and osteoporosis, which is simply not true.**

Hot flashes, for instance, are abolished by treatment with either estrogen, progesterone, or androgens. It has even been shown that placebos eliminate hot flashes.[41] Various other nutriceuticals have been shown to reduce hot flashes, including flax seed oil, soy, flavonoids, gamma-oryzanol, boron, and progesterone.[43] For the woman with hot flashes, the first step is to eat a high-protein, high-vegetable diet. No more ice cream, cookies, and other forms of sugar. No pasta and bread either! I know I seem ornery, so let's have a cartoon (see **Figure 23-16**). The next step would be to take some herbal supplements that have the above nutritionals in them. The ones we carry include Menstrual Support, Female Age Well, and Premensulator. The names could be better, but they work. Consider also adding some soy to your diet. If this does not work, start using progesterone cream, preferably under the care of a natural medicine doctor. If estrogen is needed, an estriol cream can be prescribed.

FEMALE CANCERS: THE END RESULT OF TOO MUCH ESTRADIOL

Some of our patients have succumbed to laparoscopies and hysterectomies in the past. A few patients have seen a long-term benefit, but for the majority of them, the benefits were only temporary. Most of the time, these surgeries *temporarily* help symptoms such as excessive bleeding or cramping, but they do nothing about correcting the underlying estradiol excess. Unfortunately, if left unchecked,

FIGURE 23-15: BLOOD PRODUCTION RATES OF HORMONES		
	REPRODUCTION AGE	**POST-MENOPAUSAL**
ANDROSTENEDIONE	2-3 mg/day	0.5-1.0 mg/day
DEHYDROEPIANDROSTERONE	6-8 mg/day	1.5-4.0 mg/day
DHEA-SULFATE	8-16 mg/day	4-9 mg/day
TESTOSTERONE	0.23-0.25 mg/day	0.05-0.1 mg/day
ESTROGEN	0.350 mg/day	0.45 mg/day

Only the production of estrogen increases with menopause, yet this is the hormone most prescribed. Is it any wonder why female cancers are so prevalent in women during their menopausal years?

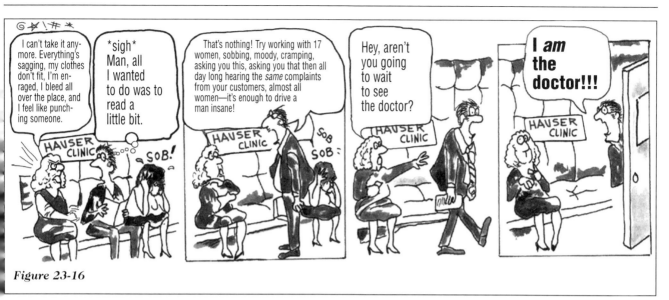

Figure 23-16

some will ultimately be diagnosed with breast, cervical, ovarian, or uterine cancer. *The facts support this, as breast carcinoma is the most common malignancy in women in North America and Western Europe, and a woman's most common cancer death.* Despite advances in treatment, only modest improvements in survival have been achieved.[44] This makes one think that perhaps the reason survival has not improved is because the underlying problem, specifically prolonged estradiol excess, is not being addressed in these women.

Each year, about 200,000 women will be newly diagnosed with breast cancer, and the numbers just keep rising. The sad fact is that long-term follow-up studies of women treated for clinically evident breast cancer by local treatment alone have indicated that excess mortality from metastatic disease persists for over 30 years (see **Figures 23-17A** and **B**). From a number of such studies, it appears that of women with clinically apparent breast cancer treated only with local surgery and/or radiotherapy, less than 30% can expect freedom from relapse during their lifetime.[45-47] These statistics do not even take into account endometrial (uterine) cancer, which is the most common gynecological malignancy, or ovarian cancer, which causes the most deaths from any gynecological malignancy, in excess of 24,000 per year in the United States. Of note is that endometrial cancer is uncommon below the age of 40, with a peak incidence of about 70 years; a full one third of breast cancers occur in those

age 70 or older, with its greatest prevalence occurring at 55 years.[44]

Let's think about it…cancer of the breast is the most common cancer affecting females, and it is their most common cancer death. Supposedly its cause is unknown, but it is almost unheard of in men who also have breasts, making a hormonal relationship very likely. Epidemiological and other scientific evidence definitely points in this direction.

Everyone agrees that cancer is a multifactorial disease, but the evidence implicating excess estrogen and/or prolonged estrogen exposure is great for female cancer (see **Figure 23-18**). Korenman and colleagues[48] suggest that unopposed estrogen action is a major risk factor for breast cancer, based on five premises:

1. Human breast cancer is induced by carcinogens in a susceptible (ie, a hormone-primed) mammary gland.

2. Unopposed estrogenic stimulation favors tumor induction.

3. There is a long latency between tumor induction and clinical disease.

4. The duration of the estrogen window is proportional to breast cancer risk.

5. Inducibility declines with establishment of normal ovulatory menses and becomes very low during pregnancy.

It appears that OCP use is a risk for breast cancer when used either before the first full-term

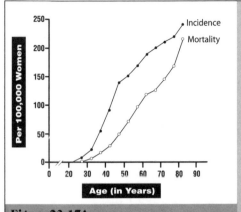

Figure 23-17A:
Age-specific incidence rate (1982) and mortality rate (1985) for breast cancer in the United Kingdom.

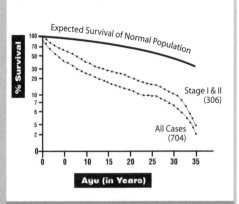

Figure 23-17B:
Long-term survival of 704 patients with metastatic breast cancer.

FIGURE 23-17A AND 17B:

Notice the high mortality rates from breast cancer for over 30 years, suggesting that the underlying problem with these patients is not being addressed—even with prior surgery and radiotherapy they had.

pregnancy or before age 25.[49,50] Again, this is because many OCPs have an estradiol derivative. When the amount of free estradiol is measured in the blood, a significantly higher level is found in those who have breast cancer.[51] This is similar to the data that we see in our breast cancer patients at Caring Medical. Specifically, we look at salivary/urinary hormone levels because these are free and not bound to sex hormone-binding globulin, which is the protein in the blood that binds estradiol. For anyone interested in female cancer risk, we look at the estrogen quotient, which is the total estriol divided by estrone plus estradiol in a 24-hour urine collection (see **Figure 23-19**).

A typical result would be like the one we found in Jane Blumberg, one of our natural medicine zealots who wanted to treat her breast cancer naturally. We think she was shocked when we started testing her for cancer physiology. From her initial estrogen quotient, it was clear that she had a lot of work to do (see **Figure 23-20A**). This test result was even after she had been taking a lot of herbal supplements. This is another example of a case where it is imperative that a cancer patient be under the care of a natural medicine doctor (preferably one that practices IPT). Herbal supplements to treat physiology should be prescribed and, as such, should be monitored by a natural medicine physician.

Since the reader is familiar with Betty Jo Davis, the person whose case was discussed in **Chapter 17**, one can see her estrogen quotient study in **Figure 23-20B**. As one can see, it is very similar to Jane

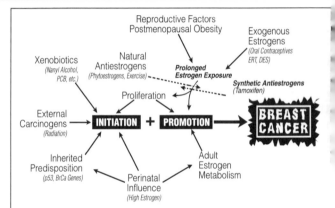

Figure 23-18: Interactions Between Estrogens and Other Factors in the Development of Breast Cancer
Notice that the *primary* factor in the genesis of breast cancer is estrogen.

$$\text{Estrogen Quotient} = \frac{\text{Estriol}}{\text{Estrone} + \text{Estradiol}} \quad \text{Normal} > 1.0$$

Figure 23-19: Estrogen Quotient
The estrogen quotient is inversely related to breast cancer risk. The higher the Estrogen Quotient (thus, lower estadiol levels), the lower the risk.

Blumberg's results. Both women had breast cancer and, obviously, based on the test results, still had cancer physiology upon coming to Caring Medical.

The reader will be interested to know that one of the major studies on the estrogen quotient was from the University of Nebraska School of Medicine with collaboration from the Boston University School of Medicine and Harvard Medical School

STEROID	Concentration in μg/24hr		
ESTRONE	6.5	ESTROGEN QUOTIENT =	0.08 L
ESTRADIOL	40.0		
ESTRIOL	3.5	$\dfrac{Estriol}{Estrone + Estradiol}$ NORMAL:> 1.0	
TOTAL ESTROGENS	50.0		

			Reference Range	
			Male	Female
TESTOSTERONE	58.50	H	20 - 200	5 - 35
PROGESTERONE	1.50		1 - 3 non-luteal	1 - 3
			luteal	1 - 6

ADULT REFERENCE RANGE FOR ESTROGENS IN μg/24hr

Figure 23-20A: Estrogen Measurement Quotient of Jane Blumberg
Her high estradiol levels compared to the other estrogens was the reason for her low estrogen quotient.

MERIDIAN VALLEY LABORATORY

515 West Harrison St. Ste. 9
KENT, WA 98032
253-859-8700

COMPREHENSIVE HORMONE PROFILE

Patient: Betty Jo Davis

Accession Number:

Sex: F Age: n/g
Dr./Clinic: Ross Hauser

Total Volume:	1800	ml
Creatinine:	0.7	gm/24hr
Normal	0.5 - 2.0	gm/24hr

Date Collected:
Date Received:
Date Reported:

If Creatinine Value is outside normal range, results may be affected.

STEROID	Amount Excreted in μg/24hr			Adult Reference Range	
		Phase	Day	Female	Male
ESTRONE	7.2	Luteal	17 - 26	3.0 - 52	
		Follicular	27 - 11	2.0 - 39	
		Mid Cycle	12 - 16	11.0 - 46	
		Post Menopausal		1.0 - 7.0	
					3 - 8
ESTRADIOL	61.2 H	Luteal	17 - 26	1.0 - 27	
		Follicular	27 - 11	1.0 - 23	
		Mid Cycle	12 - 16	4.0 - 45	
		Post Menopausal		0 - 23	
					0 - 23
ESTRIOL	5.9	Luteal	17 - 26	9.0 - 60	
		Follicular	27 - 11	3.0 - 48	
		Mid Cycle	12 - 16	20 - 130	
		Post Menopausal		0 - 30	
					12 - 26
TOTAL ESTROGENS	74.3	Luteal	17 - 26	13 - 139	
		Follicular	27 - 11	7.0 - 110	
		Mid Cycle	12 - 16	38 - 221	
		Post Menopausal		0 - 60	15 - 57
ESTROGEN QUOTIENT =	0.09 L	Estriol / (Estrone + Estradiol)=		> 1.0	N/A
				Female	Male
TESTOSTERONE	7.65			5 - 35	20 - 200
PROGESTERONE	3.60	Non-luteal		1 - 3	1 - 3
		Luteal		1 - 6	

Figure 23-20B: Estrogen Measurement Quotient for Betty Jo Davis
One can see the similarities between her test results and those of Jane Blumberg. Both women had breast cancer and obvious cancer physiology.

published in the *Journal of the American Medical Association* in 1966.[52] This study involved 146 urine samples from healthy fertile and infertile premenopausal and post-menopausal women and 182 specimens from breast cancer patients. The results showed that in healthy premenopausal women, the mean estrogen quotient was 1.5, whereas in the breast cancer patients, it was 0.6. Similarly lower levels were found in the postmenopausal breast cancer patients compared to the healthy women. The study also found that women with breast cancer secreted significantly more total urinary estrogens than healthy women.

Realize this study was done in the 1960s, yet estradiol continues to be the main hormone given to women. In the discussion section of this study, the author notes:

> **Temporary regression of endocrine dependent mammary (and endometrial) cancer metastases would be expected, following correction of an *endocrine imbalance* which contributed to carcinogenesis. Besides estriol and its epimers, testosterone, hydrocortisone, and progesterone experimentally impede estradiol uterotropic activity. Removal by oophorectomy (ovary removal) of the major and perhaps only site of estradiol synthesis in the female has long been found effective in palliation of breast cancer.[52]**

The data suggest that competition may exist at the molecular level for a limited number of enzyme attachment sites between estradiol and various impeded estrogens. All estrogens are not created equal, and if a woman needs an estrogen, please pick estriol.

As we discussed earlier, a woman's hormonal makeup can be changed. Estradiol levels can be

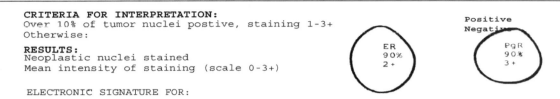

```
CRITERIA FOR INTERPRETATION:                               Positive
Over 10% of tumor nuclei postive, staining 1-3+            Negati
Otherwise:
                                                    ER            PgR
RESULTS:                                            90%           90%
Neoplastic nuclei stained                           2 +           3 +
Mean intensity of staining (scale 0-3+)

ELECTRONIC SIGNATURE FOR:
```

Figure 23-21: Pathology Report Showing That Vanessa's Breast Cancer Is Estrogen Receptor Positive

decreased by a lower hydrogenated (vegetable) oil consumption as well as increasing one's fiber content in the diet.[53, 54] We have also found that it is necessary for a woman to eliminate refined carbohydrates, including white flour, grains, sugar, and fruit juice. To enhance the estrogen quotient, various nutriceuticals are given, including flax seed, chasteberry, and soy. A good example of this is a current patient of ours, Vanessa.

CASE STUDY OF VANESSA B. WITH BREAST CANCER

Caring Medical is used to seeing clients from all over the country, and Vanessa B. came a long way to get to Oak Park, IL. She came partly because she is a 43-year-old widow raising three children on a bus driver's salary who had been recommended to undergo a prolonged course of high-dose chemotherapy for her breast cancer diagnosis. She literally could not do it with all of her life responsibilities. Her breast lumpectomy and lymph node biopsies showed a grade II infiltrating ductal carcinoma with lymph node involvement. The DNA index showed a potential doubling time of 19 days, signifying an aggressive tumor. Of particular interest to us was the fact that the cancer was estrogen positive (see **Figure 23-21**). Prior to coming to us, her physician drew a blood estrogen level, which was high at 370. One of the tests done in our office was a 24-hour urinary hormone profile. The results are shown in **Figure 23-22**, both before and after starting on a nutriceutical program.

FIGURE 23-22: RESULTS FROM A 24-HOUR URINARY PROFILE FOR VANESSA B.

HORMONE LEVEL	BEFORE	AFTER
DHEA	.06 (L)	1.14
Estrogen quotient	.97 (L)	2.62
Testosterone	31.50	44.06

L = Low

Her estrogen quotient definitely improved, as well as her anabolic (male) hormone levels. The

tests were done only four months apart as evidence that it is possible to change a person's hormonal milieu in a very short period of time. So what did (and is) Vanessa taking? Nothing more than we have discussed, including high-dose chasteberry, flax seed oil, potassium iodide, DHEA, and natural thyroid hormone. Vanessa is also eating according to her metabolic type, which includes a high amount of soy products. In May 2001, her oncologist did a complete workup, and all of her cancer markers and x-ray studies were completely normal. Will they stay completely normal? Only time will tell, but if she stays on her nutriceutical program and receives close follow-up in regard to her hormonal makeup, the likelihood of success is great. To further interest you, **Figure 23-23** is a section of her balancing body chemistry questionnaire from our office. Hopefully never again will you think of PMS and dysmenorrhea as not having much significance. In Vanessa's case, they were the clue that something major was brewing...and that something major was breast cancer. Is Vanessa happy? Consider reading the letter that Vanessa wrote to us (see **Chapter 28**).

For the woman who is still not convinced of the harm of estradiol, let's take brief look at endometrial cancer.

> Chronic stimulation of the endometrium by estrogens, without the differentiating effects of progestins, is the primary etiological factor associated with the development of hyperplasia and subsequent progression to adenocarcinoma (cancer). Both endogenous (anovulation) and exogenous (hormonal therapy) sources of unopposed estrogen increase the risk of endometrial adenocarcinoma...this cause and effect relation is widely accepted....[44] (see **Figure 23-24**.)

This quote is from one of the main textbooks on the etiologic basis for female cancers. We'll continue:

CANCER: THE ENEMY

Terrorism dominates the news today. Not as well covered in the news is another kind of terrorism that kills 1,516 Americans every day. The terror is called "cancer."

Jane Seymour and James Keach

The National Foundation for Alternative Medicine

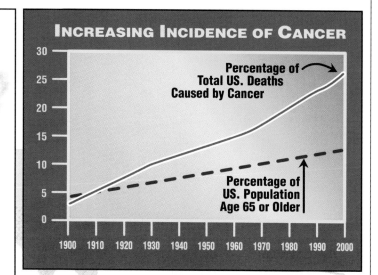

INCREASING INCIDENCE OF CANCER

Percentage of Total US. Deaths Caused by Cancer

Percentage of US. Population Age 65 or Older

PET Scan Showing Metastatic Cancer

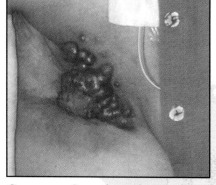

Lung Tumor

Melanoma Eroding Knee Cap

Cancerous Growth on the Skin

Cancer Cells

```
Collected: 05/17/2001 11:00    Ordering Dr: HAUSER,ROSS MD

CA19-9              H  11000
                       Reference range: <37
                       Unit: U/ML
                       PERFORMED AT SKBL
                       (NOTE)
```

Blood Cancer Marker—Highly Elevated

BREAST CANCER...WOMENS' NUMBER 1 CANCER KILLER

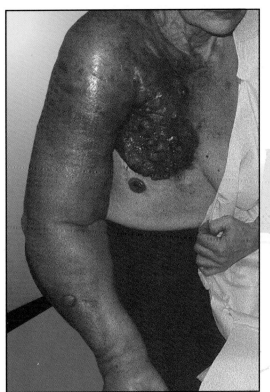

The Face of Breast Cancer

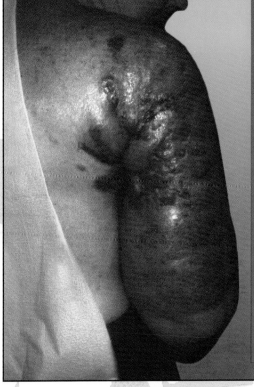

The Devastating Effects of Breast Cancer

Consider five women ostensibly with the same breast lesion—a 1.5 cm invasive ductal breast carcinoma. Each has adjacent in-situ ductal changes and one axillary lymph node involvement, but no other recognized tumor. Although the odds of their being alive at any given time can be predicted, we cannot be more precise about their future courses. We simply do not know whether, when, or where "Metastases" will occur.

The Lancet, 1994;34:734-735

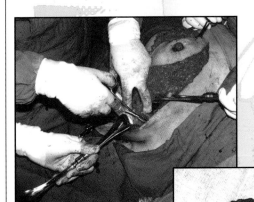

A Mastectomy

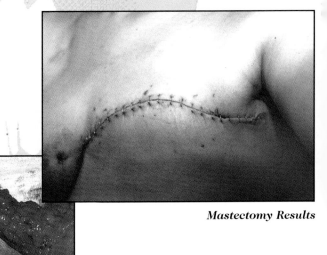

Mastectomy Results

A Breast after a Mastectomy

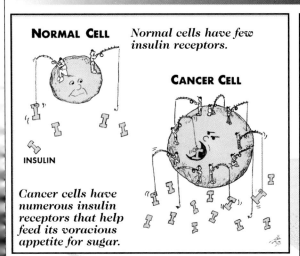

NORMAL CELL

Normal cells have few insulin receptors.

CANCER CELL

INSULIN

Cancer cells have numerous insulin receptors that help feed its voracious appetite for sugar.

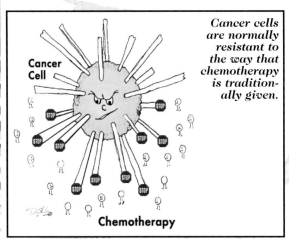

Cancer Cell

Cancer cells are normally resistant to the way that chemotherapy is tradition-ally given.

STOP

Chemotherapy

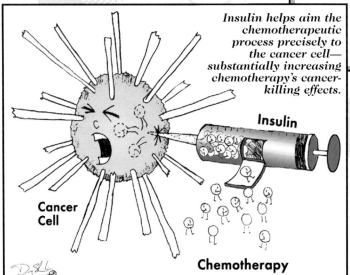

Insulin helps aim the chemotherapeutic process precisely to the cancer cell—substantially increasing chemotherapy's cancer-killing effects.

Insulin

Cancer Cell

Chemotherapy

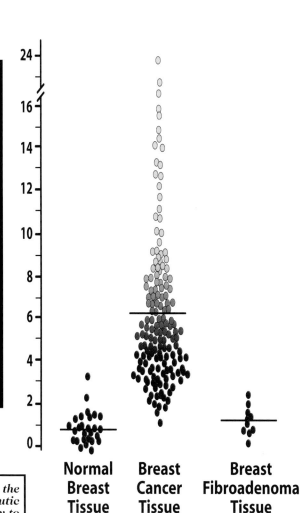

Insulin Receptor (ng/0.1 mg Protein)

Normal Breast Tissue

Breast Cancer Tissue

Breast Fibroadenoma Tissue

Scientific studies have shown that breast cancer cells have many more insulin receptors than normal breast tissue or benign breast tumors.

CANCER'S FIERCEST FOE: INSULIN POTENTIATION THERAPY

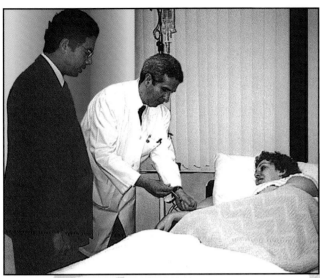

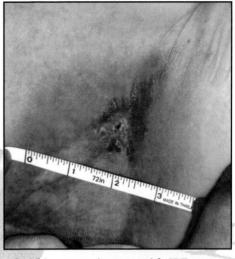

The skin tumor is gone with IPT. (Note the "Before" pictures previously shown.)

Dr. Donato Pérez García, the most experienced practitioner of IPT, demonstrates the technique to Ross A. Hauser, M.D., at Dr. Pérez' clinic in Tijuana, Mexico.

Below is the last paragraph of a letter that Dan Weigand sent to our office. We hope his message that IPT can help heal a person with cancer starts resonating throughout the world.

> I concluded the ten weeks of IPT treatment in early June. I then had another series of tests done. I returned to Caring Medical on June 22, 2000 to review the tests. No cancer was showing on the tests. I give praise and thanks to the Lord for my healing. I thank the many people who prayed for me. And finally I thank Dr. Hauser whom God is using in a mighty way. I would urge people to take charge of their own health and to seek alternative healing whenever possible.
>
> Dan Weigand
> Oak Lawn, Il.

In the treatment of the sick person, the physician must be free to use a new diagnostic and therapeutic measure, if in his or her judgment it offers hope of saving life, re-establishing health or alleviating suffering.

Declaration of Helsinki
World Medical Association

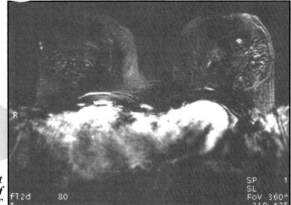

MRI of Breast Shows Absence of Tumor after IPT

Another woman saved her breast and life with IPT.

```
IMPRESSION:
1. Negative PET scan. The hypermetabolic
   activity in the left breast is no longer
   visualized.
```

IPT: THE PIONEERS

Dr. Donato Pérez García (Donato 1) with his wife Irene Bellon de Pérez meet the Archbishop of Mexico, after a nun was cured of Polio because of IPT, Circa 1950.

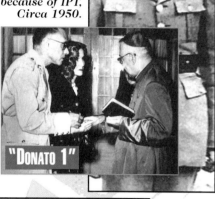

"DONATO 1"

Donato Pérez García, M.D. (Donato 1, 1891-1971). Discoverer and developer of IPT. Practiced IPT from 1928-1971 in Mexico City. Demonstrated and patented IPT in the United States in 1939. He successfully treated many serious diseases using IPT, including cancer, infections, and many other kinds of chronic diseases.

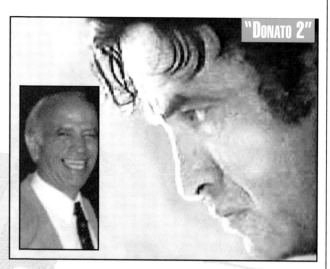

"DONATO 2"

Donato Pérez García y Bellon, M.D. (Donato 2, 1930-2000). He practiced IPT from 1956 to 2000 in Mexico, having learned it from his father. He treated a wide range of cancers, infectious diseases, arthritis, and many other conditions. He then passed on the technique to his son.

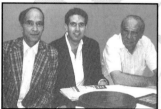

Dr. Donato Pérez García y Bellon (Donato 2), Dr. Donato Pérez García (Donato 3), and Mr. R. Munguia visit in May of 1987.

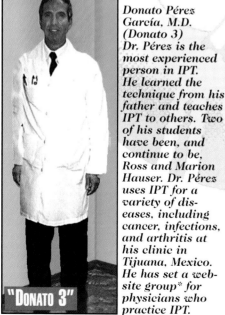

"DONATO 3"

Donato Pérez García, M.D. (Donato 3) Dr. Pérez is the most experienced person in IPT. He learned the technique from his father and teaches IPT to others. Two of his students have been, and continue to be, Ross and Marion Hauser. Dr. Pérez uses IPT for a variety of diseases, including cancer, infections, and arthritis at his clinic in Tijuana, Mexico. He has set a website group* for physicians who practice IPT.

* iptdoctors@yahoogroups.com.

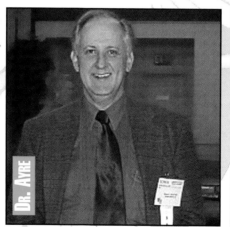

DR. AYRE

Steven G. Ayre, M.D., brought the practice of IPT to the United States and did much of the scientific research validating it. He actively promotes IPT around the country via lectures and training seminars. He currently practices IPT in his Burr Ridge, Illinois office.

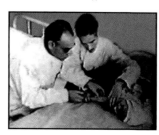

Donato 1 and Donato 2 treating a patient with IPT.

DEDICATION

We gratefully acknowledge the pioneering effort and dedication of Donato Pérez García, Sr., M.D. (1896-1971) who first conceived of, and developed this treatment protocol, called "Insulin Potentiation Therapy" (IPT). This man's son and grandson—Dr.'s Donato Pérez García-Bellon, Sr. and Jr., are also due tremendous gratitude for the many years of their own effort in carrying on with this work under the most trying circumstances that are the lot of all innovators in medicine. Finally, we thank Steven G. Ayre, M.D., for his scientific interpretations and publications on IPT that have served to make this valuable medical therapy accessible to the larger medical community. He has personally taught us the technique and then subsequently we received additional training from Dr. Donato Pérez García Jr. Thank-you both for helping us help our cancer patients with this effective and powerful treatment.

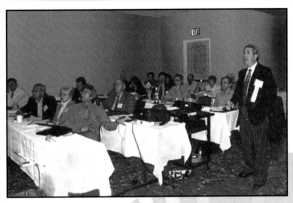

Dr. Donato Pérez García explains the technique of IPT to a group of physicians at an IPT training seminar.

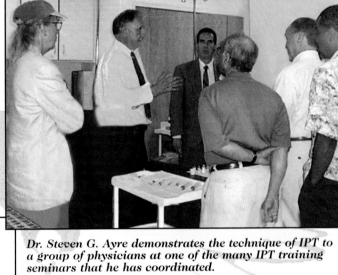

Dr. Steven G. Ayre demonstrates the technique of IPT to a group of physicians at one of the many IPT training seminars that he has coordinated.

Chris Duffield, Ph.D., www.IPTQ.org website creator. He calls IPT "the second discovery of insulin"™. Chris has done an amazing job with this website, donating many hours to create and manage the site.

Many physicians are joining the crusade to get IPT accepted into the mainstream of cancer care. Leading the charge are Steven G. Ayre, M.D., and Donato Pérez García, M.D.

INSULIN POTENTIATION THERAPY COLLABORATIVE GROUP

We the undersigned, jointly affirm Insulin Potentiation Therapy (IPT) as represented in U.S. patent #5155096 and presented at the International Oxidative Medical Association conference, February 21-22, 2001, as well as at major national and international scientific meetings, published in the peer-reviewed medical literature, to be a safe and rational medical therapy, supported with over 60 years of positive clinical outcomes.

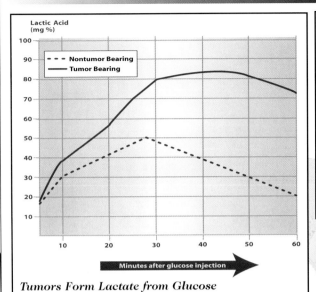

Lactic Acid (mg %)

- - - Nontumor Bearing
— Tumor Bearing

Minutes after glucose injection

Tumors Form Lactate from Glucose

NORMAL PHYSIOLOGY VERSUS CANCER PHYSIOLOGY

BIOCHEMICAL PARAMETER	PHYSIOLOGY		
	CANCER	NORMAL	SOURCE
BLOOD pH	ALKALOSIS	NORMAL	STURROCK/1913[2]
GLYCOLYSIS	HIGH	NORMAL	CORI/1925[3]
LACTIC ACIDOSIS	PRESENT	ABSENT	WARBURG/1926[4]
CELL pH	ACID	NORMAL	HARDE/1927[5]
ENERGY PRODUCTION	ANAEROBIC	AEROBIC	WARBURG/1930[6]
CARBOHYDRATES FEED TUMORS?	YES	NO	GOLDFEDER/1933[7]
CARBOHYDRATE TOLERANCE	DECREASED	INCREASED	JACKSON/1934[1]
CELL pH DECREASED WITH GLUCOSE?	YES	NO	KAHLER/1943[8]

In cancer patients, the changes seen in carbohydrate metabolism are an increase in glucose production and development of insulin resistance. Combined, they tend toward a state of glucose intolerance. Tumor cells may act as a glucose drain...

Clinical Oncology Cancer Textbook, published 2001, American Cancer Society

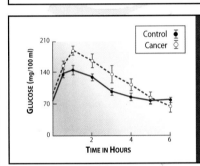

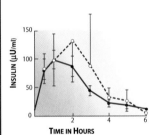

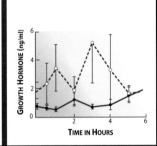

Control ●
Cancer ○

Blood levels high in glucose, insulin, and Growth Hormone are some of the basic elements of cancer physiology.

Coagulopathy is commonly found in cancer patients.

PLATELET AGGREGATION TESTING

Patient:

Physician: Dr. Hauser

Accession # 081101-03

Note: In analysis of data, it is important to consider **1.** Primary Diagnosis, **2.** Medications which may influence test results, and **3.** remember, that no single test result should ever be considered.

Scoring Guide
1. = Excellent **2.** = Good **3.** = Average
4. = Poor **5.** = Abnormal

DATE	PRE TX	POST TX	ADP	EPIN	COLL	THROM	COMMENTS
08/11/01	X		3	1	4	5	*The thrombin response reflects increased rate for clot formation. Review antioxidants, essential fatty acids in view of collagen response.*

High estradiol levels are one of the main "feeders" of female cancers

STEROID	Concentration in µg/24hr		
ESTRONE	17.1	**ESTROGEN QUOTIENT =**	0.05 L
ESTRADIOL	143.8 H	$\dfrac{\text{Estriol}}{\text{Estrone + Estradiol}}$	**NORMAL:> 1.0**
ESTRIOL	7.3		
TOTAL ESTROGENS	168.2	**Reference Range**	

REVERSING CANCER PHYSIOLOGY WITH NATURAL MEDICINE

The female lymphatic system. Since the breast is full of lymphatics, natural medicine physicians advocate no bra or limited time wearing a bra as this device has been shown to significantly increase breast cancer incidence.

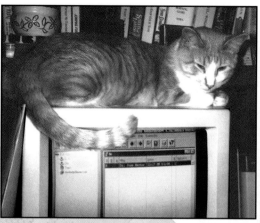

Squeaky, our cat, illustrates the proper activity for cancer patients to be pursuing—rest. To have a tumor go into remission using natural medicine, much rest is needed. Thanks, Squeaky, for that illustration.

Reversing Cancer Physiology through IPT and Natural Medicine

1. Balance the biophysical and biochemical systems of the cells of the body.

2. Detoxify the cells and the body by allowing the transport of toxins out of the cells.

3. Increase the effectiveness of medications (potentiating) by enhancing their transport into cells.

Donato Pérez García, M.D. (Donato 1), description of the mechanisms by which he surmised Insulin Cellular Therapy produced its healing effects.

Some of the nutrients in foods (such as broccoli) include indole-3-carbinol and diindolyl-methane. These help reverse cancer physiology by manipulating the estrogen metabolism.

THE HAUSER DIET FOOD PYRAMID

Fruits, Complex Carbohydrates, Whole Grains: 0-2 Servings

Fats, Oils: Nuts, Seeds, Cod Liver Oil — 1-3 Servings

Vegetables: Legumes, Brocolli, Cauliflower, Beans, Spinach — 2-4 Servings

Protein: Tofu, Soy, Fish, Poultry, Meat, Eggs — 3-5 Servings

Our web site is www.benuts.com. There, our patients can access Beulah Land's high-quality pharmacy-grade nutritional supplements, offering over 500 items.

Orders for Beulah Land Nutritionals come from all over the world. Many of the products that we carry for connective tissue healing, chronic pain, sports injury healing, and in regard to reversing cancer physiology—were formulated by Ross A. Hauser, M.D.

Benuts
Be Nuts for Your Health!

BEULAH LAND NUTRITIONALS
WWW.BENUTS.COM
MEDICAL ARTS BUILDING • 715 LAKE ST., STE. 706, OAK PARK IL 60301 • 708.848.7789 • FAX 708.848.0978

...giving hope where there was none before...

There are only two ways to live your life. One as though nothing is a miracle. The other is as though everything is a miracle.
—Albert Einstein

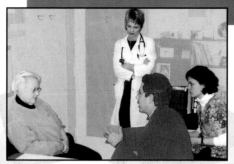

The most important aspect of healing is whether the doctor is funny or not. Here, it is evident that his joke is bombing...

Mary Lou Dagiou, R.N., gives Ozone Therapy to an IPT patient.

Caring Medical & Rehabilitation Services
g Cancer & Interventional Natural Medicine Ce

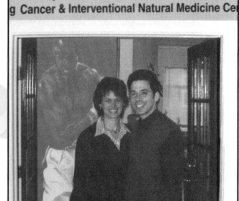

Ross and Marion Hauser stand in front of the Caring Cancer and Interventional Natural Medicine Clinic door.

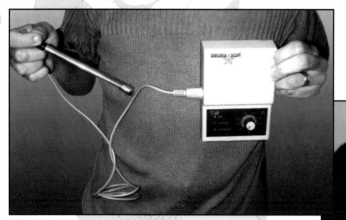

This is the hyperthermia unit used in conjunction with IPT for Prostate Cancer.

Jeri Halla, R.N., administers IPT on Betty Jo Davis. After 10 sessions, her breast tumor was gone per MRI scan.

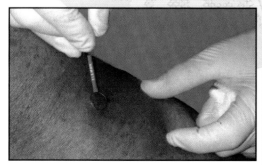

Radiofrequency removal of a skin lesion. The pathology came back non-Hodgkin's lymphoma.

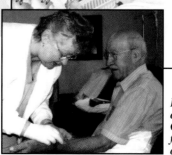

Patsy Holian gets a patient ready for Chelation Therapy for a circulation disorder.

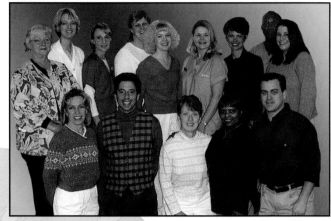
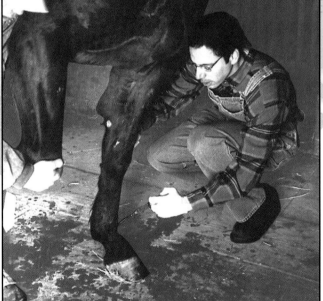

LEARNING NATURAL MEDICINE FROM EXPERTS AROUND THE WORLD

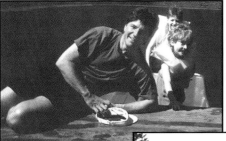

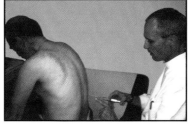

Lorenz Fisher, M.D., Neural Therapy, Switzerland. Dr. Fisher has incredible technique with the needle. Ouch! He sticks six inch needles where no needle has gone before. We have taught courses with him and dined with his great family.

We have had some wonderful teachers that have given of their time and energy to show us interventional natural methods to help people regain their health.

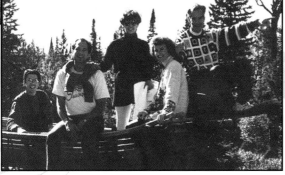

Doug Kaufmann, Nutritionist, Texas, explained to us the fungus etiology of many conditions. He is shown here with his two strapping boys. We had a wonderful day of fishing together that day. He has a national cable television show now on Family Net called "Your Health."

Steven Elsasser, M.D., Natural Medicine Specialist, Illinois. He is on the far right. He took us under his wing when we first started Caring Medical. He was decades ahead of his time. Among the things he taught us included allergy testing, herbal medicine, ozone therapy, and the business side of medicine. We did teach him something, Prolotherapy.

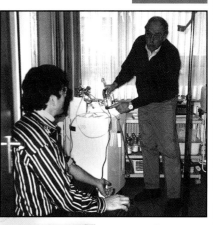

Gerd Wasser, M.D., Ozone Therapy, Germany. Dr. Wasser, the then-president of the German Ozone Society, treats a very jet-lagged Dr. Hauser with Ozone Therapy at his clinic in Bad Meinberg Germany. Remember the German way is the right way!

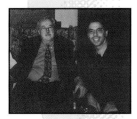

Jurgen Huneke, M.D., Neural Therapy, Germany. We had to get a picture of Dr. Huneke socializing, because he is great at it. Anyone who goes to his seminars knows that the real seminar doesn't start until the wee hours of the night over German beer. He is still the president of the International Neural Therapy Society. Be careful, his wife loves champagne and will up her handicap in golf to win a bottle during a golf match!

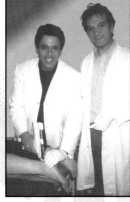

Jacque Le Coz, M.D., Mesotherapy, France. Dr. Le Coz has written many of the books on Mesotherapy and treats athletes from the French National Team. Mesotherapy is great for cellulite, ladies.

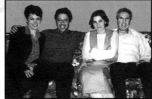

Donato Pérez García, M.D., Insulin Potentiation Therapy, Mexico. As you would expect, Dr. Pérez has a wonderful home, family, and wife. He is a tremendously caring doctor and any cancer patient would be in good hands under his care. For us, he is a great role model of the ideals of a physician.

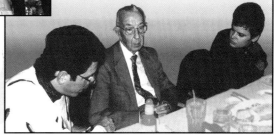

Gustav A. Hemwall, M.D., Prolotherapy, Illinois. The doctor who taught us kindness and bedside manner. Dr. Hemwall was considered the world expert in Prolotherapy. We worked with him for several years until his retirement. Little did he know when he said "You can do whatever you want," that we would progress to working with cancer and IPT. Shown here is our interview of him for our book. Prolo Your Sports Injuries Away! We were shocked to learn that just two days later he had a stroke and soon afterwards died.

PASTOR PETER BLAKEMORE: OUR INSPIRATION

For us, cancer therapy is very personal. With every cancer patient that crosses our path, we see a little bit of Pastor Peter. He was our confidant, pastor, and friend. We miss him terribly.

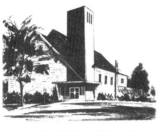

YOU ARE WELCOME AT HARRISON STREET BIBLE CHURCH

Harrison and Taylor · Oak Park, Illinois

John H. Blakemore - Peter J. Blakemore, Pastors

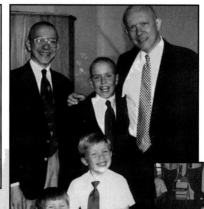

Pastor Peter's oldest boys Peter (tallest) and Andrew shaved their heads to ease the discomfort for Pastor Peter while he went bald from the high dose chemotherapy. Also in the picture are Ryan and John (the smallest).

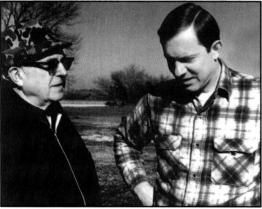

This grandfather clock was given to Marion and Ross by Marla, Peter's wife, shortly after his death. The inscription on the inside says "Presented to Ross and Marion, August 27, 1995, the day of Peter Blakemore's death." This was Pastor Peter and Marla's idea because—for the last year of his life—we put our lives on hold to try and save his life. We have been there, and know what it's like to see your very best friend die. We wish we would have known about IPT then. This clock sits in the middle of our house and is a constant reminder to us to live the Godly Christian life that Pastor Peter lived and taught.

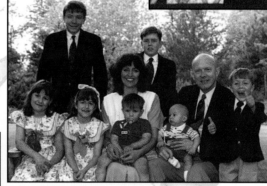

The gang at Harrison Street Bible Church. Notice Ross and Marion in the front row, and Pastor Peter and Marla in the second.

Pastor Peter had a lot to live for. His seven children and Marla are our adopted family. They are all precious to us.

A healthy Pastor Peter with his dad, Pastor John Blakemore on the farm in southern Illinois. Because of the influence of these two men, Ross and Marion started a Christian charity natural medicine clinic in rural Illinois called Beulah Land Natural Medicine Clinic. Marla Blakemore is on the board of that ministry.

Too many friends and family experience what we did with Pastor Peter— a funeral. His life and experience with cancer motivate us. We are sure he would die if it meant that others would live. Perhaps that is what God intended.

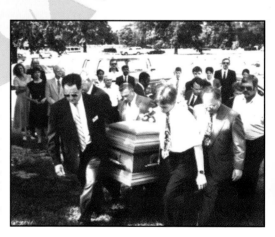

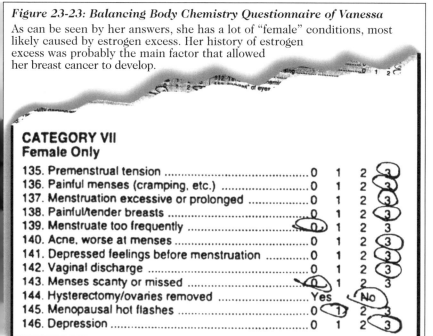

Figure 23-23: Balancing Body Chemistry Questionnaire of Vanessa
As can be seen by her answers, she has a lot of "female" conditions, most likely caused by estrogen excess. Her history of estrogen excess was probably the main factor that allowed her breast cancer to develop.

CATEGORY VII
Female Only

135. Premenstrual tension 0 1 2 (3)
136. Painful menses (cramping, etc.) 0 1 2 (3)
137. Menstruation excessive or prolonged 0 1 2 (3)
138. Painful/tender breasts 0 1 2 (3)
139. Menstruate too frequently ....(0) 1 2 3
140. Acne, worse at menses 0 1 2 (3)
141. Depressed feelings before menstruation 0 1 2 (3)
142. Vaginal discharge 0 1 2 (3)
143. Menses scanty or missed ....(0) 1 2 3
144. Hysterectomy/ovaries removed ....Yes (No)
145. Menopausal hot flashes 0 (1) 2 3
146. Depression 0 1 2 (3)

A clear-cut and relatively simple hormonal involvement in endometrial carcinogenesis has been established from epidemiological, laboratory, and clinical data: estrogens promote carcinogenesis and progestins counteract that effect.[44] (see Figure 23-25.)

Notice that estrogens clearly increase a woman's risk of endometrial cancer, and progesterone decreases it. Progesterone has many effects, but perhaps its most significant one is that it increases the catabolism of estradiol and thus decreases a woman's cancer risk.

ACTION PLAN FOR REDUCING CANCER RISK AND BEATING FEMALE CANCERS

1. Take dysmenorrhea and PMS seriously.

2. Get under the care of a natural medicine physician.

3. Do a comprehensive hormone profile, checking the free fraction of estradiol and the estrogen quotient at least yearly.

4. Do not take any synthetic hormone product where the primary active ingredient is estradiol.

5. If hormones are needed, take estriol, progesterone, testosterone, or DHEA only if these levels are low on the above tests.

6. Eat according to your metabolic type.

7. Increase the amount of soy protein in the diet.

8. Eat plenty of vegetables.

9. Substantially cut back on the amount of refined carbohydrates consumed.

10. Take a standardized high potency chasteberry nutriceutical.

11. Add some iodine to your diet or supplement regime.

12. Consume ground flax seed and cold- pressed flax seed oil.

13. Get on a complete natural medicine program that can include liver detoxification, colon cleansing, amalgam removal, nutrient absorption analysis, and others.

14. Exercise as much as possible.

15. Have a positive mental attitude. Dr. Hauser always says, "A negative thought has a negative effect on your body. A positive thought has a positive effect on your body."

16. Determine to develop a strong faith in God.

17. Read the Bible daily and do other activities that increase faith in God.

18. Follow the golden rule: Do unto others as you would like them to do unto you.

FIGURE 23-24: RISK FACTORS IN THE DEVELOPMENT OF ENDOMETRIAL CARCINOMA

CHARACTERISTIC	RISK RATIO
Obesity > 50 lb	10
Unopposed estrogen	9.5
Obesity > 30 lb	3
Diabetes	2.8
Late menopause	2.4
Nulliparity	2
Hypertension	1.5

Estradiol is a major culprit in the development of uterine cancer.

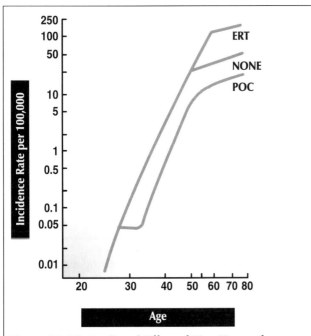

Figure 23-25: Predicted Effect of Five Years of Progesterone Oral Contraceptive (POC) or Estrogen Replacement Therapy (ERT) on Endometrial Cancer

If a woman wants to develop endometrial cancer, taking estradiol is a good place to start.

Adapted from Biology of Female Cancers *by S. Langdon, W. Miller, and A. Berchuck, page 190, © 1997, CRC Press, Boca Raton, FL*

19. Read the rest of this chapter on how to aid the body in breaking down estradiol by taking calcium D-glucarate, indole-3 carbinol, and diindolylmethane.

20. If cancer has developed, get IPT.

SURGEONS ARE GOOD, BUT NOT THAT GOOD

Prior to learning IPT, we would treat cancer patients with the usual and customary natural medicine remedies, proper diet, herbs, some intravenous Laetrile, ozone therapy—you know, the standard stuff. The best candidate for that type of treatment was a woman with breast cancer who had clear surgical margins. Such patients generally did great with natural medicine, but even in the best-case scenario, we were still relying on the surgeon to remove the tumor. Natural medicine in that scenario would reverse the cancer physiology, and the woman would often stay cancer free. When a couple of our patients had cancer recurrences, even while under strict natural medicine programs, we got a wake-up call that the conservative approach really should be an

aggressive approach. For us, this meant giving cancer patients IPT.

For many cancers, surgery is still the best approach to reduce the majority of the cancer. For stage 1 breast cancer (localized), the 5-year survival rate with a radical mastectomy is only 80%, and the 10-year survival rate is 62%.[55] If the biopsy specimen from the radical mastectomy showed lymph node involvement, then the five-year survival rate is 36%, and the 10-year survival rate is 22%. The absolute five year survival rate in patients generally treated under radical mastectomy is 50-55%. If all patients with breast cancer are included, five year survival rates are about 38%, and as many as 25% are found to be beyond the operable stage at the time of first examination.[56] The criteria of inoperability for breast cancer vary, but the factors considered to be contraindications to radical mastectomy because of a recurrence rate of nearly 100% are as follows:[57]

- Extensive edema of skin over the breast
- Satellite nodules in the skin over the breast
- Intercostal or parasternal tumor nodules
- Edema of the arm
- Supraclavicular metastases (biopsy proven)
- Inflammatory carcinoma
- Distant metastases
- Two or more of the following: skin ulceration, edema of the skin of limited extent (less than one third of breast), fixation of tumor to chest wall, axillary nodes with >1-in diameters and biopsy proven to be invaded, or fixation of axillary nodes to skin or the deep structures of the axilla

If one wants to know why traditional oncologists are so quick to offer chemotherapy to breast cancer patients, the above statistics are the reasons. Oncologists know that even with the most aggressive breast removal techniques, 50% of breast cancers recur. This is the reason *all* women with breast cancer are recommended to get systemic treatment. We agree with oncologists on this point, but the systemic treatment we recommend is IPT. One of the main reasons we can confidently recommend IPT versus traditional chemotherapy for breast cancer is because if one looks at the 10-year survival rate with high-dose chemotherapy for breast cancer, it is modest at best. Directly quoting the *American Cancer Society Textbook of Clinical Oncology,* "At the end of 10 years, the survival of patients with positive lymph nodes who are given adjuvant systemic therapy will be about 10% better than that of patients not given this therapy."[58] One of the largest research projects on this topic comparing no postoperative chemotherapy versus 12 cycles of CMF (cyclophosphamide, methotrexate, and 5-fluorouracil) showed a 10-year relapse-free survival of 31.4% versus 43.4% and an overall survival of 47.3% versus 55.2%.[59] For such a modest gain in survival, it is our opinion that women with female cancers would be best serviced by systemic treatments that reverse cancer physiology and make chemotherapy more effective. IPT is the best approach for the breast cancer patient.

Some women will say, "You ain't giving me any chemotherapy, even if it is small doses like IPT; I'll get radiation therapy." This may sound like a good option, but this is a false notion. As one can see from **Figure 23-26,** radiation therapy does not significantly alter eight-year survival rates.[60, 61]

Breast cancer, like any other cancer, is not a foe to be taken lightly. Consider this statement made by the American Cancer Society: "It is the most common cancer among women. The incidence of breast cancer has been increasing at an annual rate of 1.2% since 1940. Since 1940, breast cancer mortality has also increased."[58]

If one looks at the natural history and biology of breast cancer, some insight can be gained in regard to appropriate treatment. The following statement is taken directly from the *American Cancer Society Textbook of Clinical Oncology:*

> Some breast cancers will double in size within a *few days,* while others will take >200 days. *The average doubling time for human breast cancers is estimated at about 100 days.* Cancers can be readily palpated in the breast when they reach a diameter of approximately 1 cm. A "sphere" of this size contains approximately one billion cells, which is the result of 30 doublings of a single cell. Assuming that a preclinical breast mass grows logarithmically with a doubling time of 100 days, it would require *10 years* to reach a point where it could be diagnosed. Although it is unlikely that metastases occur during the first 20 doublings, some breast cancers metastasize soon after that point, and the probability of metastases increases

steadily the longer the breast cancer grows before detection. Most patients with a diagnosis of breast cancer have likely had the disease for five to 10 years prior to diagnosis, and a substantial percentage will have had well-established metastases for several years even if these cannot be detected on physical examination, x-rays, bone scans, or magnetic resonance imaging (MRI).[58]

The news media are good at highlighting the latest breast cancer breakthrough, which is almost always another chemotherapy medication. They then show a patient who did well with Herceptin or whatever drug being highlighted. What they do not tell is the fact that the overwhelming majority of women with metastatic breast cancer die of the disease. *The Biology of Female Cancers* notes:

> Adjuvant therapy for breast cancer is well-established, but current data suggest that it may cure at most 20 to 30% of women with operable breast cancer. Despite the almost

---

FIGURE 23-26: EFFECTS OF MASTECTOMY, LUMPECTOMY, AND LUMPECTOMY PLUS RADIOTHERAPY ON EIGHT-YEAR SURVIVAL*

Radiation therapy does not significantly alter the eight-year survival of breast cancer patients.

	NODE NEGATIVE	NODE POSITIVE[†]
DISEASE-FREE SURVIVAL[‡]		
Total Mastectomy	66	45
Lumpectomy	61▲[‡]	42
Lumpectomy + Radiotherapy	66	47
DISTANT-DISEASE-FREE SURVIVAL[‡]		
Total Mastectomy	74	51
Lumpectomy	70**	49
Lumpectomy + Radiotherapy	71	53
OVERALL SURVIVAL		
Total Mastectomy	79	60
Lumpectomy	77	60
Lumpectomy + Radiotherapy	83	68

* Results from the National Surgical Adjuvant Breast Project (NSABP) trial B-06; all patients also had axillary node dissection.

† All node-positive patients received adjuvant chemotherapy.

‡ An initial local failure within the breast is not counted as an event if patient is free of recurrence in skin and distant sites at end of follow-up period.

▲ P= .05 vs mastectomy

**P= .03 vs mastectomy (other differences not statistically significant)

universal application of systemic treatment to women with metastatic disease, *none are cured by this approach.* It is clear, therefore, that current treatments are inadequate, and an understanding of the biology of the disease may allow more effective treatments to be designed and tested.[44]

In other words, reverse cancer physiology to improve outcomes.

We hope the above highlighted facts put a chill into the hearts of women and men who have women as significant others. This last statement is really the reason why we specifically wrote this chapter. We have said very little about IPT thus far. For most cancers, prior to the cancer being diagnosed, the person has had cancer physiology for years, possibly decades. Routine medical visits giving a person a clean bill of health do not check for cancer physiology. Much of the information in this chapter—and for that matter, this book—is not known by a most oncologists, or at least he or she does not tell it to patients. It is for this reason that a person with cancer needs to see a doctor who treats cancer with IPT and is familiar with the principles of natural medicine. It is imperative that all people be checked for cancer physiology but especially women, as female cancers are killers waiting for their next victim.

Most people are generally familiar with the various risk factors for female cancers, including obesity and a high fat diet. Anyone doing some cancer research has seen the tables that show the risk factors for developing various female cancers, including breast and endometrial cancer (see **Figure 23-27**). We agree with these lists, but other risk factors are excluded because they are not politically correct; however, since I (Ross) am a politically incorrect kind of guy, I am going to tell you about them. This is another reason to see a doctor who does IPT because such physicians are generally politically incorrect—they desire to do what is best for the patient, not what is best for the AMA.

THE BRA AND BREAST CANCER STUDY

The Bra and Breast Cancer Study began in May 1991 and ended in November 1993. The research was headed by Sydney Ross Singer and Soma Grismaijer and involved interviewing approximately 400 women with breast cancer in each of five major cities across the United States:

San Francisco, Denver, Phoenix, Dallas, and New York City. A total of 2,056 women diagnosed with breast cancer were interviewed. In each city, they also interviewed approximately 500 women, for a total of 2,674, who had no known diagnosis of breast cancer. They were asked many lifestyle questions, all of which can be researched in their book *Dressed to Kill.* The results of their research can be seen visually in **Figures 23-28** and **23-29.** Their findings are astonishing:[62]

FIGURE 23-27: RISK FACTORS FOR DEVELOPING BREAST CANCER

- Increasing Age
- Hereditary Factors
  Familial
  Genetic
- Prior history of breast cancer
  In situ
  Invasive
- Benign breast disease
  Atypical hyperplasia
- Endogenous endocrine factors
  Age at menarche
  Age at menopause
  Age at first pregnancy
- Exogenous endocrine factors
  Postmenopausal estrogen replacement
- Oral contraceptives
- Environmental factors
  Region of birth
  Diet
  Alcohol

The risk factors are similar for other female cancers.

> Breast cancer risk is decreased by 19-fold if a bra is worn for less than 12 hours per day compared with the general standard population.

> Women who wear bras for over 12 hours daily, but not to sleep, have a 24-fold greater chance of developing breast cancer compared to women who remove their bras after 12 hours.

> Women who go braless throughout the day have a 24-fold reduction in breast cancer compared with the standard general population.

> Breast feeding affords a 3.5-fold protection against breast cancer.

> Women who wear their bras all the time (24 hours/day) have a 113-fold increase in breast cancer incidence when compared with women who wear their bras less than 12 hours daily.

➤ Wearing a bra all the time is associated with a 125-fold greater incidence of breast cancer than wearing no bra at all.

To put the numbers in perspective, a comparison with lung cancer is in order. Lung cancer is 10 to 30 times more common in smokers than in nonsmokers. In the Bra and Breast Cancer Study, women who wear bras 24 hours a day have a 125-fold greater chance of getting breast cancer than women who do not wear bras at all and a 113-fold greater chance of getting breast cancer than women who wear bras for less than 12 hours daily. **This is anywhere from four to 12 times greater in significance than the connection between cigarette smoking and lung cancer!** In this study, 99% of the women in the cancer group said they had worn their bras 12 hours or more per day. Surely, bra wearing is a significant risk for a woman getting breast cancer, but it is one of many cancer risk factors that are not mentioned in the press, by the AMA, or by the American Cancer Society. On page 171 of their book, the authors state they contacted representatives of the National Cancer Institute, the American Cancer Society, the President's Cancer Panel, the American Women's Medical Association, the National Organization for Women, the Women's Research and Education Institute, the National Women's Health Network, and the National Women's Health Resource Center. In the words of the authors,

> None responded. Not even the women's groups. None. Whom can you trust when culture is the biggest enemy of your health? Can you trust your culture's leading authorities? Can you trust your culture's government? Can you trust your culture's private industry?[62]

These are more reasons for a person with cancer to seek out the best natural medicine specialist one can find.

The researchers in the Bra and Breast Cancer Study feel the bra causes lymphatic congestion in the area. As one can see from **Figures 23-30A** and **23-30B,** the breast is a very lymphatic organ. Most lymphatic vessels of the breast lead to the axillary (underarm) lymph nodes. Women who want to enhance the size appearance of their breasts use bras that are very constricting so as to push their breasts upward. These tight-fitting bras constrict the lymph flow out of the breast, causing toxicity

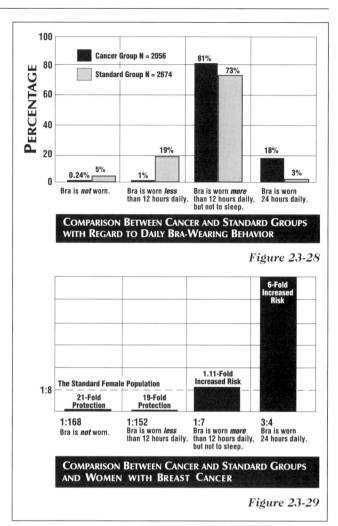

Figure 23-28

Figure 23-29

buildup within the breast and ultimately increasing a woman's risk of breast cancer.

The researchers urge women to feel comfortable with their own bodies. Society says bigger is better. A woman's body is her own. She should not let society dictate what her body should look like. To decrease her risk of breast cancer, a bra should not be worn. If some support is used, it should be as nonconstricting as possible. There were some "healthy" trends that we should have followed from the 1960s. I (Ross) will make no more comments on this subject. I am a male, married, and work with 17 women on a daily basis. I have learned that women are often the smarter, superior sex in many regards. Enough said.

SOY—ANOTHER BREAST CANCER REDUCER

Female breast cancer is rare in much of Asia, but it has been the most common cause of cancer

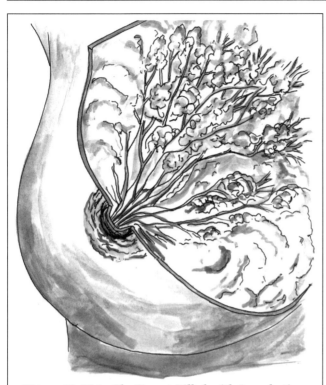

Figure 23-30A: The Breast Filled with Lymphatics

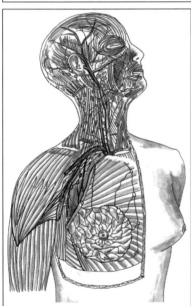

Figure 23-30B:
The lymphatic drainage from the breast extends into the axilla and neck.

greater urinary isoflavone concentrations have reduced risk and rates of breast cancer.[64,65] Some of the soy isoflavones, such as daidzein and genistein, have been shown to have anticancer effects.[66]

Numerous human and animal studies have confirmed that high soy food consumption is associated with a lower incidence of breast cancer. There are several mechanisms by which soy foods reduce risk:[67,68]

- Isoflavonoids bind to estradiol receptor sites, thereby making them less available to estradiol and xenoestrogens.
- Many isoflavonoids and phenols are antioxidants.
- Many isoflavonoids and phenols are used by liver enzymes to metabolize estradiol to estrone and ultimately to estriol.

Recently, soy has suffered some bad press because some studies have shown that it proliferates estrogen-sensitive tissues and thus could stimulate instead of protect against breast or uterine cancer.[69,70] Consider the facts in **Figure 23-31** concerning the estrogen potencies of estradiol versus the soy isoflavones genistein and daidzein as reported by the Third International Congress on Phytomedicine in Munich, Germany, October 2000. The relative estrogenic potencies of the phytoestrogens compared to estradiol are 1:1,200 for genistein and 1:7,500 for daidzein.[71] In addition, a high soy diet has been shown to decrease estradiol levels by 25%.[72] This can be explained with an analogy. If a man is punching a woman in the jaw with all of his force, the impact would be mighty. If the woman blocks the punch with her raised fists, she still feels the blow, but it does no damage to her (see **Figures 23-32A** and **23-32B**). Since her raised fist still hit her face and she felt a blow does not mean that her actions were for naught. The man belting the unprotected female represents estradiol. The raised fists represent soy isoflavones that block the massive stimulatory effect of estradiol, so the end result is a lot of estrogen blockade. (For more

death in North America and most of Europe.[63] Many have suspected that Asian women have such a low rate of breast cancer because of their consumption of soy. Even the American Cancer Society includes soy and the phytoestrogens (plant-based estrogens) on their cancer protective list.[58]

Soy contains isoflavones, which are phytoestrogens or plant-based substances that bind to estrogen receptors. Studies have shown that those women who consume high quantities of isoflavone-rich soy products and have

FIGURE 23-31: ESTROGEN POTENCIES OF ESTRADIOL VERSUS SOY ISOFLAVONES ON ESTROGEN RECEPTORS		
RELATIVE BINDING	**ErA**	**ErB**
Estradiol	100	100
Genistein	4	87
Daidzein	0.1	0.5

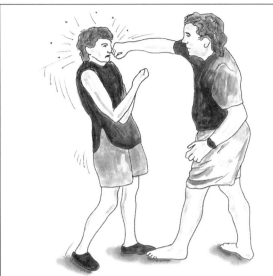

Figure 23-32A: This is how estradiol stimulates female organs, such as the breast and uterus. Just like this woman being punched by the man—it's got to hurt.

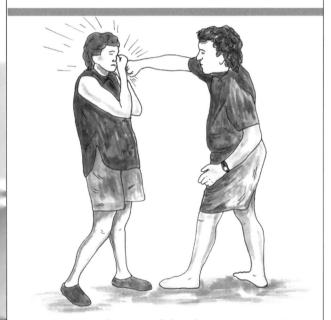

Figure 23-32B: The woman's hands represent soy. Soy helps block the potential massive stimulation by estradiol of female organs like the breast, much in the same way that this woman's hands are blocking the man's punch. She'll still feel it—but not nearly as much.

information on the cancer-fighting effects of soy isoflavones, please see **Chapter 29.**)

ABORTION AND LACK OF LACTATION— OTHER BREAST CANCER RISK FACTORS

It is currently politically correct to have an abortion. No big deal; get the blob out of you. For a time, it was politically correct to avoid breast-feeding, but now the federal government has completely reversed this thinking to the point that the surgeon general is writing a report on the benefits of breast-feeding.

There is strong evidence that lactation reduces the risk of breast cancer. A study published in the prestigious *New England Journal of Medicine* concluded: "As compared with parous women who did not lactate, the relative risk of breast cancer among women who first lactated at less than 20 years of age and breast-fed their infants for a total of six months was .54." [73]

It is doubtful in the twenty-first century that we will see many moms under 20 breast-feeding their children for six months or more. A more typical response for a pregnant teenager is to get an abortion. One of the risks for the woman who has an abortion is breast cancer. An increased risk of breast cancer in women who have had an induced abortion has been reported in 13 out of 14 studies on white, African American, and Asian American women. There has been an association found in 27 out of 33 studies worldwide, dating back to 1957. The only published American study specifically funded by the National Cancer Institute to investigate the abortion/breast cancer link found a statistically significant risk increase of 50% in women overall who had any abortions, an increase of more than 100% in women who had an abortion before age 18 or after age 30, an increase of 80% in women with a family history of breast cancer who had any abortions, and an incalculably high risk increase in women with a family history of breast cancer who had an abortion before age 18. [74] If the studies are reviewed in total, the vast majority show that abortion increases the risk of breast cancer from 30% to 100%, though a few show the risk as high as 400%. [75]

The action plan, then, is to meet a nice fellow, get married, and then have kids. If a woman gets pregnant before marriage, have the baby and breast-feed him or her for six months. If that is not feasible, give the newborn up for adoption.

Is abortion personal to me? You bet! My wife Marion is adopted. She was born before abortion was legal. If abortion had been legal at the time of her birth, she would have had an over 50% chance of being killed. If my wife had not been born, I would not have met her, and I probably would not be doing anything I am doing now. No natural medicine, no Prolotherapy, and certainly no IPT. The very fact that you are reading this book that could save your life or the life of your loved one is because my wife was not killed before birth. She was given up for adoption. She grew up in a great home, met a great guy, and has helped me write some great books. I shudder to think how many Marions have been killed through "legalized" abortion.

FLAX SEED: A WOMAN'S BEST FRIEND

If a dog is man's best friend, then surely flax seed and flax seed oil should be a woman's best friend. Flax seed is the most significant source of plant lignans, one of the main classes of estrogenic compounds in plants called phytoestrogens.[118] When consumed, the primary plant lignans, secoisolariciresinol and matairesinol, are converted by the human gut bacteria into the mammalian lignans, enterodiol and enterolactone, which are diphenolic compounds having a structural similarity to estradiol.[111, 112] (see **Figure 23-33.**) Flax seed and its isolated lignans have been shown to possess numerous chemoprotective effects. Flax seed has been shown to reduce the early risk markers for and incidence of breast and colon carcinogenesis in animal models and to help normalize menstrual cycle length in premenopausal women.[112,114] Enterolactone and enterodiol, the lignans (a type of plant estrogen) excreted in response to flax seed consumption have also been shown to reduce early markers for and incidence of mammary carcinogenesis in animal models, decrease cell proliferation, increase concentrations of sex hormone-binding globulin, and inhibit the activity of three enzymes (aromatase, 5α-reductase, and 17β-hydroxysteroid dehydrogenase) that play key roles in sex hormone metabolism.[115-117] Flax seed oil, which contains α-linolenic acid has also been shown to reduce mammary tumor growth and mammary tumorigenesis.[118]

Some of the cancer preventive effects of flax seed may be mediated through its influence on endogenous sex hormone production, metabolism, and biological activity. As has been presented, there is overwhelming evidence that estradiol increases breast cancer risk. Recent research has shown that the metabolites of estradiol have different biological activities, and these may play a role in the etiology of breast cancer. Of particular interest are the primary metabolites 2-hydroxyestrogen and 16α-hydroxyestrone, which are formed from estrone by two irreversible, mutually exclusive hydroxylation pathways.[119] (see **Figure 23-34.**)

The 16α metabolite has significant estrogenic activity and thus is associated with an increased risk for breast cancer, whereas the 2-hydroxy pathway is protective against breast cancer.[120,121] On the basis of these findings, the ratio of 2-hydroxylated to the 16α-hydroxylated estrogen metabolites, the 2/16α ratio, has been used as a biomarker for breast cancer risk, with an increase in the ratio considered protective.[122] Recent studies showing a significant decrease in this ratio in women with breast cancer further support this hypothesis.[123, 124]

Several human studies have investigated whether dietary components can alter the 2/16α ratio. A high-protein and a low-fat diet were shown to increase the ratio, as well as the consumption of broccoli and indole-3-carbinol, a compound found in cruciferous vegetables (discussed later).[125, 127] Another way that a woman can significantly affect this ratio is by increasing the amount of flax seed consumed in her diet. This was shown by a study in which postmenopausal women were given their normal diets plus varying degrees of ground flax seed (0, 5, or 10 g/day).[128] The study found that flax seed supplementation significantly increased urinary 2-hydroxy estrogen excretion and the urinary 2/16α hydroxy estrogen ratio in a linear dose-response fashion (see **Figure 23-35**). The authors noted that

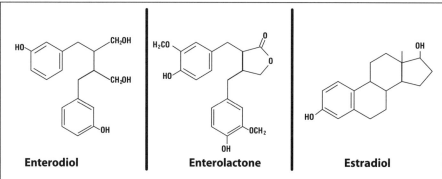

Enterodiol   **Enterolactone**   **Estradiol**

Figure 23-33: Mammalian Lignans: Enterodiol, Enterolactone, and Estradiol

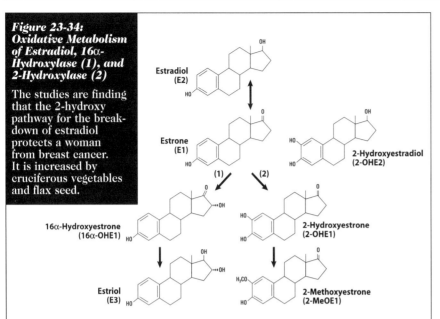

Figure 23-34: Oxidative Metabolism of Estradiol, 16α-Hydroxylase (1), and 2-Hydroxylase (2)

The studies are finding that the 2-hydroxy pathway for the breakdown of estradiol protects a woman from breast cancer. It is increased by cruciferous vegetables and flax seed.

"these results suggest that flax seed may have chemoprotective (cancer-preventing) effects in postmenopausal women. In a follow-up study, the researchers showed that flax seed, but not wheat bran, was able to significantly increase the urinary 2/16α ratio.[129] The reason stated was:

> Although lignans are present in other plant foods, such as legumes, whole cereals, fruits, and vegetables, flax seed is by far the most significant source. By weight, mammalian lignan production from flax seed meal is 120 times higher than most legumes, over 180 times higher than most whole cereals, and over 260 times higher than most fruits and vegetables. Therefore, it is very difficult for an individual to obtain the quantity of lignans supplied by 10 grams of flax seed by consuming other foods.

For these and many other reasons it is obvious that it is appropriate to say that flax seed should be a woman's best friend.

RESIST PREMARIN AND ESTRADIOL-BASED HORMONES

The last discussion in this chapter gets back to the fact that estradiol is the nemesis of female cancers. When a woman comes to Caring Medical for cancer prevention or treatment, part of reversing cancer physiology is evaluating and treating estradiol dominance. This is done by stopping estradiol consumption, reducing estradiol levels by diet and herbal supplementation, and blocking estradiol receptors via medications or herbal supplements. When we explain this, women will often stop us before we even finish speaking, "Doctor, my cancer was not estrogen receptor positive." "I do not have breast cancer." "The oncologist said Premarin doesn't affect lung cancer." "How else am I going to stop the hot flashes?" Let me (Ross) say right off the bat that it is my contention that estradiol has a negative healing effect for a woman with *any type of cancer*. There is ample evidence that estradiol stimulates the growth of certain female cancers, regardless of estrogen receptor status.[76] **Specifically in regard to breast cancer, one study showed that estradiol increased the proliferation of estrogen receptor-positive breast cancer cells by 213% and estrogen receptor-negative tumors by 233%.**[77] Estradiol is bad for almost all female cancer patients. It is that

FIGURE 23-35: URINARY 2-OHESTROGEN, 16α-OHE1, AND 2/16α-OHE1 RATIO DURING EACH FEEDING PERIOD

In this study, flax seed consumption significantly increased the production of the 2-hydroxy metabolites of estradiol.

		FLAX SEED	
	CONTROL	**5 GRAMS**	**10 GRAMS**
2-OHEstrogen, μg/24 hours	10.72	12.09	14.39*▲†
16α-OHE1, μg/24 hours	2.67	2.60	2.97
2/16α-OHE1 ratio	4.02	4.64	4.85‡ **

a: Values are geometric means with 95% confidence intervals in parentheses. 2-OHEstrogen, 2-hydroxyestrogen; 16α-OHE1, 16α-hydroxyestrone, 2/16α-OHE1 ratio, ratio of 2-hydroxylated to 16α–hydroxylated estrogen metabolites.

b: Statistical significance is as follows: significantly different from 5 grams flax seed ($p < 0.05$); ▲ , significantly different from control ($p < 0.0005$); † , linear trend between control, 5 grams flax seed, and 10 grams flax seed ($p < 0.0005$, $r^2 = 0.815$); ‡, significantly different from control ($p < 0.05$); **, linear trend between control, 5 grams flax seed, and 10 grams flax seed ($p < 0.05$, $r^2 = 0.769$). g = grams

FIG. 23-36: THE TOP ELEVEN PRESCRIPTION DRUGS IN 1999

RANK	PRODUCT
1	Premarin Tabs
2	Synthroid
3	Lipitor
4	Prilosec
5	Norvasc
6	Prozac
7	Claritin
8	Zithromax Z-Pak
9	Zoloft
10	Glucophage
11	Prempro

The number one and eleven drugs each have Premarin in them and the estradiol that comes with it.

plain and simple. We are laying down the groundwork for this, but this is not a statement that will be endorsed by any big medical society. Few people have written as much against estradiol as we have in our various natural medicine books. We consider ourselves as somewhat experts on the topic because of all of the papers we have reviewed on the subject. In this chapter, it has been our purpose to give you only a *small sampling* on the topic of estradiol.

IMPORTANT POINT #1:
PREMARIN INCREASES ESTRADIOL LEVELS

Premarin is the #1 prescription drug in the United States (see **Figure 23-36**). Premarin is pregnant mare urine (horse urine); this is where the name came from. In a study in 1980, Premarin given to women was found to increase their estradiol levels by over 350%[78] (see **Figure 23-37**). The authors concluded:

> In view of the prolonged presence of equilin and the possible association between treatment with conjugated equine estrogens and endometrial cancer, it is suggested that equilin-containing compounds should not be given for more than 12 months.

Most physicians give young women estradiol-containing birth control pills or post-menopausal estradiol-containing hormone replacement for *decades*.

Many alternative health providers are concerned about the cancer risk with prescription drug hormone therapy. One of the most knowledgeable on this subject is our friend and colleague Gail Gelsinger, R.N. She runs a natural medicine practice in association with Frank Noonan, M.D., in Ephrata and Robesonia, PA. She described some of her concerns in a letter. (See **Figure 23-38**.) Most natural medicine specialists believe that hormone levels should be checked, and hormone supplementation should be without estradiol, or with as little as possible.

IMPORTANT POINT #2:
THE ESTRADIOL 16α-HYDROXYLATION CONNECTION

The metabolism of estradiol, the ovarian estrogen, is primarily oxidative. There is an initial oxidation to estrone, which in turn, is oxidized principally via two alternative pathways: 2 hydroxylation, which leads to the nonestrogenic metabolites 2-hydroxyestrone and 2-methoxyestrone, and 16α-hydroxylation, which leads to the highly estrogenic metabolites 16α-hydroxyestrone and estriol. Thus, the total estrogenic impact of a given amount of secreted estradiol depends on the relative magnitude of the 2-hydroxylation (nonestrogenic) and 16α-hydroxylation (estrogenic) pathways. This relative magnitude is quite constant under most biologic circumstances, except the 2-hydroxylation/16α-hydroxylation ratio is increased in hyperthyroidism and decreased in hypothyroidism.[79] This is one of the reasons that checking thyroid function is a part of a good natural medicine evaluation for cancer physiology and cancer prevention.

In 1966, Zumoff and colleagues reported that men with breast cancer showed markedly increased 16α-hydroxylation of estradiol; then in 1971, they found the same association in women.[80,81]

FIGURE 23-37: SERUM ESTROGEN LEVELS OF WOMEN ON PREMARIN THERAPY

Premarin significantly increases a woman's estradiol levels—increasing the risk of female cancers.

	WEEKS ON PREMARIN THERAPY			
STEROID	0	3	7	11
Estradiol (pmol/l)	180	314	304	633
Estrone	167	569	633	655

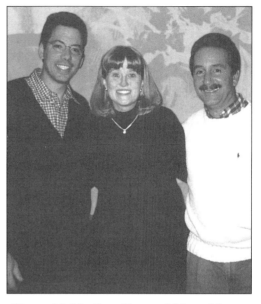

Figure 23-38: Ross Hauser, M.D., with Friends and Colleagues Gail Gelsinger, R.N., and Frank Noonan, M.D.

IPT helped save Gail's father who was diagnosed with lymphoma.

Dr. Frank C. Noonan

The Lincoln Building
1248 West Main Street • Ephrata, PA 17522
(717) 733-1736

FAMILY PRACTICE

May 14, 2001

Ross Hauser, MD - Sent Via Fax

Dear Dr Hauser:

There are approximately 20 million women experiencing menopause today and 60 million will reach menopause by the year 2010.

Because of the many symptoms which accompany menopause, it can be a stressful time for women. Many will take traditional hormone replacement therapy; however, in recent years there have been general concerns about the relationship of these medications to cancer. In particular, concerns have been raised concerning ovarian cancer and, although less well-documented, breast cancer. Recently a medical journal reported that ovarian cancer is twice as likely in women taking prescription drug hormone therapy (i.e. Premarin, Provera and Prempro)

With this in mind, I began a serious study of hormonal care. I realized that the hormones offered to women are either synthetic or made from horse urine and do not match our biological estrogen structure. In addition, blood testing may not be a true representation of hormonal status.

Today, after years of study, we are able to offer a complete natural approach to menopause. Our hormonal care includes accurate hormonal value testing, natural bioidentical hormones and complete patient care follow-ups. Our new video will be available in the near future and we will certainly send you a copy.

I would like to take this opportunity to thank you for the years of nutritional networking which has helped us to provide our patients with conscientious and quality care. I am very grateful for my friendship with both you and Marion.

Yours truly,

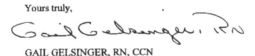

GAIL GELSINGER, RN, CCN

Subsequent researchers confirmed their findings and greatly expanded the study of 16α-hydroxylation in breast cancer with the following findings:[82, 83]

- Increased 16α-hydroxylation was confirmed in women with breast cancer.
- Increased 16α-hydroxylation was found in women at familial high risk for breast cancer.
- Increased 16α-hydroxylation was found in mouse strains with a high incidence of breast cancer; the degree of increase paralleled the degree of risk in different strains.
- Elevated 16α-hydroxylation in mice appeared to be inherited as an autosomal dominant.
- The presence of murine mammary tumor virus was associated with elevated 16α-hydroxylation; introduction of virus into animals without it raised hydroxylation, and deletion of virus from animals containing it lowered hydroxylation.
- 16α-hydroxyestrone was found to be genotoxic in vitro to breast epithelial cells and induces atypical proliferation.
- Dietary addition of indole-3-carbinol, which has the effect of decreasing the oxidation of estradiol to its 16α-hydroxy metabolites, largely prevented breast cancer in mice with a high incidence of spontaneous cancer.

IMPORTANT POINT #3:
ESTRADIOL AND 16α-HYDROXY METABOLITES CAN BE DECREASED WITH DIET AND HERBAL SUPPLEMENTS

Epidemiological studies have long suggested that obesity is associated with increased risk

FIGURE 23-39: THE EFFECTS OF VLF (10%) HFI (35-45 GD) DIET ON ESTROGENS AND MENSTRUAL FUNCTION

	CONTROL (30% AHA)	MONTH 2 (VLF/HF DIET)	LEGEND:
Menstrual Cycle Length, *days*	28.2 ± 3.4	25.8 ± 5.2	**VLF:** Very Low Fat Diet
Follicular Phase, *days*	15.8 ± 4.2	13.4 ± 4.1	
Luteal phase, *days*	12.3 ± 3.0	12.4 ± 3.0	
Estradiol (follicular), *pg/mL*	73.4 ± 16.7	54.8 ± 29.9*	**HF:** High Fiber
Estradiol (luteal), *pg/mL*	193 ± 86	151 ± 70*	
Estrone (follicular), *pg/mL*	73.4 ± 27	59.4 ± 23.7*	**AHA:** American Heart Association
Estrone (luteal), *pg/mL*	86.7 ± 35	71.4 ± 32.9*	

No significant effects on estrone sulfate and SHBG.
*Significantly different from 30% AHA diet $p < 0.05$

Effects of a low-fat diet fed ad libtum on estrogens and menstrual function. Many hormones are affected by such a diet; in this study the levels of the female hormones (estradiol and estrone) involved in breast tumorigenesis were reduced by about 25% in both the follicular and luteal phases of the cycle. AHA—American Heart Association; HF—high fiber; SHBG—sex hormone-binding globulin; VLF—very low fat diet.

for many different types of cancers, including endometrial and breast cancer. One of the reasons for this is that obesity has a powerful effect of decreasing 2-hydroxylation, resulting in increased availability of biologically active estrogens.[84] Obesity is also associated with insulin resistance, and the American Cancer Society acknowledges that cancer patients have impaired insulin sensitivity. Glucose intolerance is documented by hyperglycemia and delayed clearance of blood glucose in cancer patients after oral or intravenous glucose administration.[58] These are some of the reasons that the best diet for many cancer patients may be a high-protein, low-glycemic index diet. High-protein diets have been shown to increase 2-hydroxylation as compared to high-carbohydrate or high-fat diets. They also help resolve glucose intolerance and insulin resistance.[85]

The most common diet recommended for breast cancer patients is one that is low in fat. A very low-fat diet has the effect of lowering estradiol levels (see **Figure 23-39**). One has to remember that any diet that keeps a person's percentage of body fat down will lower estradiol levels. A low-calorie, high-protein, low-carbohydrate, or low-fat diet will do this. The safest diet for a breast cancer patient is going to be one that is free of simple carbohydrates (breads, pastas, sugar) and high in vegetables. Adding protein in the form of fish and tofu would also help reverse breast cancer physiology.

One of the most famous women who treated her breast cancer with natural means is Lorraine Day, M.D. She is an avid proponent of natural means, and we highly recommend her tape "Cancer Doesn't Scare Me Anymore," which is available at 1-800-574-2437. She sent us a nice letter as well as her principles for overcoming cancer (see **Figure 23-40**).

We agree with the principles that Lorraine Day has laid out. She lives in sunny California, and typically people who live in warmer climates need more carbohydrates than others. We would include more protein in the diets of our cancer patients than she would, but her principles are nonetheless excellent. She is truly an inspiration to us and to the cancer patients she helps get on the natural health path.

High-protein diets have the effect of lowering blood glucose levels. One interesting study involved injecting animals with an aggressive strain of breast cancer then feeding them diets that would result in either hypoglycemia, normoglycemia, or hyperglycemia. There was a dose-dependent response in which the lower the blood glucose, the greater the survival at 70 days[86] (refer back to **Figure 11-10**).

CASE OF CINDY, BREAST CANCER

To illustrate the dramatic effects diet can have on breast cancer, consider the case of Cindy. She was originally diagnosed with breast cancer in November 1995. She underwent a mastectomy and radiation therapy. She suffered a recurrence of the cancer in November 1999, with additional radiation. Again, she was not doing anything to reverse her cancer physiology. She saw Doug Kaufmann, a nutritionist on television, and started on a high-protein, low-carbohydrate diet, and she asked us to prescribe some antifungal medicine. He is one of the experts on the etiology of

God's Health Plan An Educational Resource Only by Lorraine Day, M.D.

Figure 23-40

N NUTRITION

- Fruit, vegetables, grains in their most natural form (raw whenever possible and organically grown whenever possible—grown without pesticides). No meat or poultry (it's all full of pesticides, hormones, and disease). No fish (all the streams and lakes are polluted). I don't eat anything that has ever had a face on it.

- No dairy products (they're full of the same pollutants that meat is). Rice Dream, a brand of rice milk available at the healthfood store is a pleasant and tasty substitute.

- No sugar, no sugar substitutes. A total of a teaspoon of honey per day can be used.

- A minimal amount of salt.

- No soda, no coffee, tea, or any caffeinated beverages.

- Carrot/apple juice: I drink eight glasses of a mixture of carrot and apple juice per day.

- Juice is made fresh in my juicer.

- To four of these juices, I add one heaping tablespoon of Barleygreen.

- I also take two tablespoons of liquid Kyolic (odor-free garlic) for my immune system and two tablespoons of acidophilus each day. Both are available at the health foodstore.

LORRAINE J. DAY, M.D.

Dear Dr Hauser,
Thanks for your note
Here is my plan. It has
become a way of life. I
will always eat and live
this way.
Sincerely,
Lorraine Day MD.

E EXERCISE

- 30 to 60 minutes of aerobic exercise per day. Walking is best.

W WATER

- I drink 12 to 15 glasses of distilled water per day, in addition to drinking my carrot juice.

- The body loses 10 glasses of water per day from perspiration, breathing (your breath IS moist) food digestion and assimilation and other losses. 10 glasses per day is necessary just to stay even. A person must have normally functioning kidneys to drink this much water. For every ten glasses of water I drink, I make sure that I take in a total of one half teaspoon of salt. When the body loses water, it also loses salt and the salt must be replaced to keep the water in the body.

- Adequate water intake is absolutely mandatory for proper elimination.

S SUN

- I make sure I get 30 minutes of sun per day—but not at the hottest time of the day. Morning sun is best. The sun's rays are healing and cause certain important chemical reactions to occur in the body, including the conversion of Vitamin D.

T TEMPERANCE

- No caffeine, alcohol, smoking, street drugs, or medicinal drugs. No strong spices, no sugar, or sugar substitutes.

A AIR

- At least 30 minutes of fresh air and deep breathing per day. Three of these requirements (exercise, sun, and fresh air) can be accomplished by a 30-60 minute walk outdoors per day.

R REST

- Adequate rest every day. At least eight hours of sleep at night, going to bed by 10:00 or 10:30 P.M. Also naps during the day if required.

T TRUST IN GOD

- This is the most important part of the whole plan. God has been my physician. He is the only one who knows exactly what is wrong with me and exactly how to make me well. I pray three times a day, study my Bible, and ask for God's direction in every aspect of my life including my (his) health plan. I read the healing promises in the Bible daily. Stress must be removed from a sick person's life in order to get well. If there is stress on the job or stress at home, between husband and wife or any other area of the family, then those areas of stress must be dealt with by taking it to the Lord. Stress is one of the biggest killers. Holding anger or resentment is also a killer. It turns on the one who is angry and destroys him or her. It must be let go.

- Two other requirements for healing are an attitude of gratitude (being thankful for what we have) and Benevolence (doing things for others who cannot pay you back). Get outside of yourself and think about others.

This is the plan I used to get well from invasive breast cancer that had spread to my underlying pectoralis muscle and to the lymph nodes under my arm. I had a lumpectomy but refused a mastectomy. I refused removal of the lymph nodes, I refused chemotherapy and radiation. The surgeon could not remove all the cancer but with this plan, the cancer is gone from my underlying muscle, and my lymph nodes have returned to normal. I am well, with no evidence of cancer. I do not and cannot guarantee in any way that this plan will work for anyone else. But I believe in it completely.

cancer from fungus infestation. Her results were very demonstrable (**Figure 23-41**). Cindy is still being followed as a patient, and as long as her cancer markers go down, nothing else will have to be done. Diet can be powerful medicine.

FIGURE 23-41: CANCER MARKER RESULTS FOR CINDY AFTER STARTING ON ANTIFUNGAL MEDICATION AND A HIGH-PROTEIN DIET

CANCER MARKER	OCT., 2000	JAN. '01	APRIL '01	SEPT. '01
CA 27-29	120	107	77	65

The natural approach to reducing estradiol levels starts with a low-glycemic index diet that includes lots of high-fiber vegetables and low-fat protein sources. The next step is to take supplements that help decrease the body's ability to make estradiol and then help it break down into nonestrogenic metabolites such as 2-hydroxyestrone. The main supplements for this, in addition to flax seed, are indole-3-carbinol, diindolylmethane, calcium D-glucarate, and chrysin. These are some of the supplements that we recommend to a breast cancer patient, and, for that matter, cancer patients in general, which are discussed in **Chapter 28.**

Indole-3-carbinol is a compound naturally found in cruciferous vegetables, such as cabbage, broccoli, bok choy, brussel sprouts, cauliflower, cress, kale, mustard, radish, horseradish, turnip, rutabaga, and kohlrabi. When these cruciferous vegetables are crushed, chewed, or exposed to an acid environment, like that of the stomach, indole-3-carbinol is changed into another indole called diindolylmethane (see **Figure 23-42**). These two substances have the following effects:[87-89]

➤ Reduce the activity of estrogen receptors in the body.

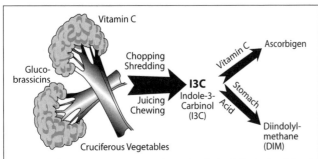

Figure 23-42: The Process by Which Indole-3-Carbinol and Its Derivatives Are Formed from Cruciferous Vegetables

➤ Promote "selective cell death," which helps the body's removal of malformed and/or damaged cells.

➤ Encourage the beneficial metabolism of estradiol in the body.

The main effect of these substances is to increase the 2-hydroxylation of estradiol. Most studies show that it can increase the 2-hydroxylation of estradiol by 50%[90-92] (see **Figure 23-43**). Specifically, it increases the 2/16α-hydroxyestrone ratio in urine.[93] This ratio is one of the measurements that we often get in a 24-hour urine collection when evaluating a female patient for cancer physiology (see **Figure 23-44**). It is interesting to note that the relationship between breast cancer risk factors and the 2/16α ratio (see **Figure 23-45**). Taking indole-3-carbinol or diindolylmethane has the net effect of lowering the estrogenic stimulation in women, thereby resolving one aspect of female cancer physiology. It should be noted that consuming cruciferous vegetables is a good idea, but it would take more than two pounds of raw broccoli per day to significantly improve the ratio. This is why a supplement containing diindolylmethane and indole-3-carbinol is recommended.*

Indole-3-carbinol is a potent anticancer compound. Sharma and associates found that indole-3-carbinol was a potent anticancer compound that has many of the same effects as tamoxifen[94] (see **Figure 23-46**). Like tamoxifen, it interrupts the cell cycle. In studies from the University of California, indole-3-carbinol inhibited the growth of estrogen receptor-positive breast cancer cells by 90% compared to Tamoxifen's 60%. In estrogen receptor-negative cells, indole-3-carbinol stopped the synthesis of DNA for new cells by about 50%, whereas tamoxifen had no significant effect.[95,96]

If that is not reason enough for a woman to take indole-3-carbinol or diindolylmethane, consider the fact that indole-3-carbinol has also been shown to help overcome multidrug resistance to chemotherapy.[97] It was also found to cause regression of cervical carcinoma in situ in eight of 17 patients.[98]

Chrysin is a flavonoid isolated from *Passiflora* (passion flower) that has been shown to

* The nutriceuticals we use can be seen and purchased at www.benuts.com, or 1-877-RX-BEULAH (877-792-3852).

FIGURE 23-43: SUMMARY OF URINARY ESTROGENS BEFORE AND AFTER INDOLE-3-CARBINOL (I3C) TREATMENT

METABOLITE*	BEFORE I3C MEAN	AFTER I3C MEAN	CHANGE OVER PRE-I3C VALUES [◊] (95% CONFIDENCE INTERVAL)	P [‡]
20HE1	0.958	1.698	0.91	.011
20HE2	0.650	1.327	2.31	.30
40HE1	0.156	0.211	0.75	.25
2METE2	0.340	0.301	-0.08	.44
17-EPI	0.260	0.169	-0.14	.53
16-EPI	0.305	0.244	0.04	.89
E2	0.545	0.362	-0.28	.016
E1	1.507	1.083	-0.26	.008
E3	1.201	0.654	-0.37	.014
16αOHE1	0.360	0.183	-0.45	<.001
15αOHE1	0.026	0.020	-0.20	.018
16βOHE1	0.183	0.096	-0.17	.55
16OXO	0.229	0.100	-0.49	<.001
SUM**	6.72	6.45	-0.03	.34

I3C caused a significant decrease in the amounts of estradiol and its 16α metabolites, while raising 2-hydroxylation metabolites, which would theoretically decrease a women's risk of cancer.

* All metabolites expressed as nanomoles/millimoles creatinine: 20HE1 = 2-hydroxyestrone; 20HE2 = 2-hydroxyestradiol; 40HE1 = 4-hydroxyestrone; 2METE1 = 2-methoxyestrone; 17-EPI = 17-epiestriol; 16-EPI = 16-epiestriol; E2 = estradiol; E1 = estrone; E3 = estriol; 16αOHE1 = 16α-hydroxyestrone; 15αOHE1 = 15α-hydroxyestrone; 16βOHE1 = 16β-hydroxyestrone; 16OXO = 16-oxoestradiol.

[◊] Mean percent change/100.

[‡] P values for mean percent increase (decrease) over pre-13C values.

** Total measured urinary estrogens.

Adapted from Changes in Levels of Urinary Estrogen Metabolites after Oral Indole-3-Carbinol Treatment in Humans, by J. Michnovics, H. Adlercreutz, H.L. Bradlow, Journal of the National Cancer Institute, 1997, Vol. 89, No. 10.

inhibit the transformation of testosterone to estradiol.[93] The enzyme responsible for this transformation is aromatase. Another aromatase inhibitor used at Caring Medical in breast cancer patients is quercetin, a bioflavonoid. Medications such as Femara and Arimidex are used for breast cancer treatment and are aromatase inhibitors. For the woman being treated for breast cancer at Caring Medical, it is typical to be put on an aromatase inhibitor.

It should be noted that in postmenopausal women, estrogen is largely derived from the extraglandular conversion of adrenal androgens, and the rate and degree of this conversion increases with body weight.[99] The heavier a woman is, the more estradiol that will be formed from testosterone because of the enzyme aromatase.[100] It appears that some breast cancers themselves display aromatase activity, which converts androgens into estrogens.[101] Thus, aromatase inhibition is a very logical method of estrogen deprivation, particularly in the postmenopausal woman, since it can potentially inhibit synthesis of estrogen both within and beyond the breast (see **Figure 23-47**).

Test	Result	Abnormal Result	Normal Range
2-Hydroxy (E1+E2+E3)	2.69 ng/ml	Low	Premenopausal: 4–100 ng/mL Postmenopausal: 1–20 ng/mL
16α - Hydroxyestrone	7.43 ng/ml		Premenopausal: 2 - 40 ng/mL Postmenopausal: 0.6 - 10 ng/mL
2/16α Ratio	0.362	Low	0.6–6.0 Premenopausal Mean 2.3 Postmenopausal Mean 2.0

Figure 23-44: Determination of Urinary 2/16α Ratio in a Cancer Patient at Caring Medical
This is one of the tests that is done to check estrogen physiology in female cancer patients. The low 2-Hydroxyestrogen level and low 2/16α ratio documented this aspect of cancer physiology in this individual. She is now on a natural medicine regime to reverse this physiology.

Breast Cancer Risk		2/16α Ratio
Heredity	⬆	⬇
Obesity	⬆	⬇
Thinness	⬇	⬆
Smoking	⬇	⬆
High-Fat Diet	⬆	⬇
High Protein Diet	⬇	⬆
Fish Oil Diet	⬇	⬆
Exercise	⬇	⬆
Cruciferous Vegetables	⬇	⬆
Indole-3-Carbinole	⬇	⬆
Dioxin	⬇	⬆
Flax Seed	⬇	⬆

Figure 23-45: For every condition or item above, breast cancer risk is increased or decreased. Notably for each one, we see the opposite effect on the 2/16α hydroxyestrone ratio.

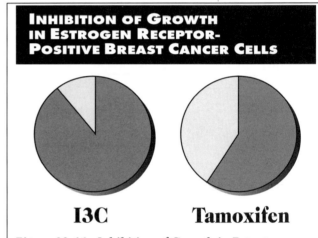

INHIBITION OF GROWTH IN ESTROGEN RECEPTOR-POSITIVE BREAST CANCER CELLS

I3C **Tamoxifen**

Figure 23-46: Inhibition of Growth in Estrogen Receptor-Positive Breast Cancer Cells

Indole-3-carbinol, like tamoxifen, interrupts the breast cancer cell cycle. The shaded area indicates the percentage of estrogen receptor inhibition in breast cancer cells.

Adapted from Life Expansion Magazine, *October 1999*

Calcium D-glucarate is an effective cancer-inhibiting supplement, particularly in hormonally-driven cancers, such as breast and endometrial cancer. Calcium D-glucarate is the calcium salt of D-glucaric acid, a naturally occurring substance found in humans and many plants that is an important detoxifying agent because of its effects on glucuronidation. Bean sprouts, apples, grapefruits, and cruciferous vegetables contain approximately 350 mg/100 grams Lettuce and grapes only provide 10 mg/100 grams.[39]

Calcium D-glucarate works by metabolizing an excess of estrogen in the body. Normally, estrogen is metabolized in the liver, and the body rids itself of estrogen by passing it through the liver, where it hooks onto a conjugate called glucuronic acid and passes out with the stool. This process, called glucuronidation, is the way the body detoxifies and cleans house. Glucuronidation converts toxins, carcinogens, and steroids to glucuronide-bound products that can be excreted harmlessly through the biliary or urinary tract. The enzyme beta-glucuronidase can potentially deconjugate these bound carcinogens, but glucuronic acid prevents this from occurring.

Several animal models of human breast cancer have yielded promising results. Rats who were continued on calcium D-glucarate after tumor

METABOLISM OF SELECTED ESTROGENS

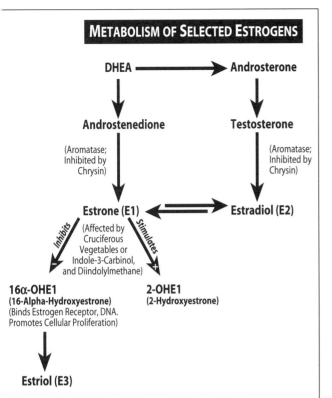

Figure 23-47: Metabolism of Selected Estrogens
Estrogen metabolism can be altered significantly by eating cruciferous vegetables and taking supplements such as indole-3-carbinol or chrysin.

POSSIBLE CAUSES OF BREAST CANCER

Genetic Factors
Early onset of menstruation
Pregnancy late in life or not at all
Late menopause
Shorter menstrual cycles

Environmental Factors
Xenoestrogens (synthetic compounds that mimic estrogen)
Pesticides, herbicides, halogenated compounds, etc.
Lack of sunlight
Power lines, electric blankets, radiation, etc.

Iatrogenic (Doctor Induced)
Oral contraceptives
Body weight (the more overweight, the more the risk)
Exercise level (Women who exercise have a reduced rate.)
Alcohol and coffee consumption

Dietary Factors
Increased saturated fat
Decreased antioxidants
Decreased dietary fiber
Decreased alpha-linolenic acid and omega-3 fatty acids
Decreased dietary "phytoestrogens"

Figure 23-48: Possible Causes of Breast Cancer
Adapted from M. Murray, Breast Cancer: Update on a Growing Epidemic, Natural Medicine Journal, 1999: 2:1-266

induction had already occurred actually experienced a decrease in tumor volume of approximately 73%. There was a 50% decrease in beta-gluconidase activity and a 23% reduction in serum estradiol.[40] This shows that calcium D-glucarate reduces serum estrogen levels, which in turn inhibits some types of breast cancer. In addition to preventing breast cancer (as well as other hormone-related cancers), calcium D-glucarate can inhibit the recurrence of cancer and be part of a protocol for the treatment of cancer.[67,102] In animals, calcium D-glucarate can inhibit cancers of the colon, lung, liver, skin, and urinary bladder.[103]

THE NATURAL MEDICINE ACTION PLAN TO DECREASE ESTRADIOL

1. Do not take estradiol-containing hormone replacement in the form of Premarin, oral contraceptive pills, or postmenopausal hormone replacement.

2. Decrease sugar, grain, and pasta consumption.

3. Decrease fat in the diet.

4. Increase fiber-containing foods in the diet, such as vegetables.

5. Increase low-fat protein sources in the diet, such as soy and fish.

6. Make ground flax seed and flax seed oil a significant part of the diet.

7. Consume as many cruciferous vegetables as possible.

8. Eat a high-soy diet.

9. Take a supplement of chasteberry and vitamin B_6.

10. Take a soy isoflavonoid supplement.

11. Take indole-3-carbinol and/or diindolylmethane.

12. Supplement with chrysin and quercetin.

13. Use the nutriceutical calcium D-glucarate.

For the woman with cancer, this approach is a good start. Knowing the possible causes of breast cancer and eliminating those factors is the next best step (see **Figure 23-48**). It is always a good idea to test urinary hormones for 2/16α ratios and the estrogen quotient before and after an aggressive dietary and herbal program. In addition, it is also necessary to start a cancer treatment plan that is safe but has demonstrative results. This is why we recommend IPT.

INSULIN POTENTIATION THERAPY— CANCER THERAPY OF THE NEW MILLENNIUM

We do not want to leave you with the feeling that if you have a big cancerous mass in your breast, all you need to do is the above. Every medical treatment has its place and that means surgery, radiation, and high-dose chemotherapy. For the woman who desires to go outside the box, like Vanessa, for cancer therapy, then Caring Medical is a good place to start (or another center that uses IPT in the treatment of cancer). Just to make sure you have learned what you need to about IPT, let's review information about IPT that is in a brochure from our office.

HOW DOES IPT WORK?

During IPT, a small dose of insulin is given to the patient to induce a state of low blood sugar (hypoglycemia). When the patient begins to have symptoms such as a feeling of lightheadedness and weakness (hypoglycemic symptoms), low doses of traditional chemotherapy are given by intravenous push. When insulin is given, the cancer cells are fooled into thinking they are going to be fed food, when in reality they are going to be destroyed by chemotherapy. The doses of chemotherapy used during IPT are one tenth to one fourth the traditional doses given during high-dose chemotherapy; therefore, the side effects are minimal. Patients are given immune-stimulating treatments along with the IPT, thereby allowing the patients with solid tumors to get many of the cancer-killing effects of traditional chemotherapy without as many negative side effects.

IPT takes advantage of several characteristics of cancer cells. Research has shown that some solid tumors have more insulin receptors than normal cells.[104-106] Insulin also causes some cancer

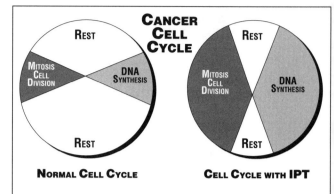

CANCER CELL CYCLE

NORMAL CELL CYCLE — REST, DNA SYNTHESIS, REST, MITOSIS CELL DIVISION

CELL CYCLE WITH IPT — REST, DNA SYNTHESIS, REST, MITOSIS CELL DIVISION

Figure 23-49: Insulin and the Cancer Cell Cycle
During rest periods, cancer cells are impenetrable by chemotherapy. *Note:* with IPT, the cell rest periods become shorter, and the times (during mitosis and DNA synthesis) that the cells can be affected by chemotherapy are greatly enhanced. Because the cancer cells are more easily penetrated, the amount of chemotherapy required to kill them is significantly reduced.

cells to go into the proliferative growth phase, at which time chemotherapy can work more effectively.[107] (see **Figure 23-49**). In many instances, less than 10% of the cells that make up the tumor are proliferating (growing) at any point in time. The remaining 90% of cells, therefore, are not susceptible to most chemotherapy agents because chemotherapy works primarily during this proliferative growth phase of DNA synthesis.[108] This is one explanation why some patients respond to IPT even when they have failed other cancer treatments (see **Figure 23-50**). In regard to breast cancer, insulin has been shown to enhance the recruitment of human breast cancer cells into the S phase from 14% to 42% with continuous stimulation for many hours versus a 14% to 21% increase with a one-hour pulse stimulation.[109]

HOW DO I KNOW IF IPT IS RIGHT FOR ME OR SOMEONE I LOVE?

IPT is most successful if used as a first-line treatment. In other words, it works best if the patient has not already received traditional high-dose chemotherapy and/or radiation therapy. That is not to say that you would not be a candidate if you have received these things. Each case is evaluated on an individual basis. It is always prudent to obtain several opinions when considering cancer treatment options before starting anything. When reviewing treatment options, we hope you will consider coming to the place where *"The care of the patient begins with Caring..."* ®

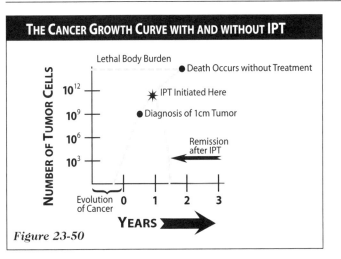

THE CANCER GROWTH CURVE WITH AND WITHOUT IPT

Figure 23-50

CAN I RECEIVE NATURAL MEDICINE THERAPIES ALONG WITH TRADITIONAL RADIATION THERAPY OR CHEMOTHERAPY?

Radiation therapy and high-dose chemotherapy generally cause side effects such as immune suppression and stress to such organs as the heart, liver, and kidneys. To reduce these side effects, some people utilize natural remedies in conjunction with traditional radiation or chemotherapy with varying degrees of success. In general, Caring Medical has tremendous success in helping patients get through these therapies with minimal side effects. This is accomplished through various nutritional therapies and enzyme supplementation, as well as herbal nutriceuticals for the liver, kidney, heart, and immune system as needed.

HOW WILL I BE MONITORED WHILE UNDERGOING NATURAL MEDICINE TREATMENTS?

This is perhaps the most important question of all. Depending on the type of cancer, various monitoring methods are available, including traditional cancer blood markers (PSA, CA 19-9, CEA, and CA-125), CT scans, bone scans, and biopsies. Caring Medical also uses various laboratories that utilize very sensitive cancer markers, including the AMAS test, as well as other blood markers for very specific kinds of cancers. Because Caring Medical is a natural medicine clinic, nutritional markers are also utilized, including pH, protein levels, enzyme analysis, weight, energy level, cholesterol level, and other specific protocols that relate to a the body's overall metabolism.

HOW DO I GET STARTED ON OBTAINING A NATURAL MEDICINE OPINION ABOUT MY CANCER?

Caring Medical and Rehabilitation Services is conveniently located just 10 minutes from downtown Chicago in the beautiful suburb of Oak Park, Illinois.

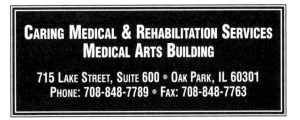

See our web site at www.caringmedical.com, www.iptcancer.com, and www.IPTQ.org, which is designed and maintained by Chris Duffield, Ph.D., whose knowledge and zeal for this therapy is truly admirable.*

SUMMARY

Women need to be aware of the unique hormonal milieu of their bodies compared to men. When women have health problems, it is generally because of estradiol excess, not men. This estrogen can be in the form of endogenous estrogens (own body production) or exogenous estrogens (OCPs or hormone replacement after menopause). Women are realizing that the central cause of such conditions as dysmenorrhea, PMS, endometriosis, uterine fibroids, and fibrocystic breast disease is estradiol excess. If this underlying cause is not dealt with, uterine and breast cancer can result. That is why having laparoscopies and various surgeries for these conditions is not the best option; the underlying estrogen excess continues. By changing one's diet to include more soy protein and fewer refined carbohydrates combined with such nutriceuticals as flax seed, chasteberry, pyridoxal-5-phosphate, essential fatty acids, and others, these chronic conditions can be reversed because estradiol levels are depressed. This improves the estrogen quotient, which is the amount of estriol divided by the amount of estradiol plus estrone in a 24-hour urine collection. The higher the estrogen quotient, the lower a woman's risk is for breast cancer.

---

* *On the web site www.IPTQ.org is contact information on physicians trained in IPT. Many of them also practce natural medicine.*

The metabolism of estradiol involves 2- and 16α-hydroxylation. The lower the 2/16α hydroxylation ratio, the greater the risk for a woman getting breast cancer. Cruciferous vegetables contain the compound indole-3-carbinol and increase 2-hydroxylation, reducing a woman's risk of breast cancer. Indole-3-carbinol is converted to diindolylmethane in the body. Another powerful supplement to reduce estradiol levels in the body is calcium D-glucarate, another substance found in cruciferous vegetables. This substance acts by increasing glucuronidation and inhibiting beta-glucuronidase, which assists in the metabolism of estradiol, decreasing its levels. In animal studies, calcium D-glucarate reduced cancer recurrences and inhibited cancer formation.

Breast cancer, as well as the other female cancers, is a growing epidemic. It is currently estimated that one out of eight women in the United States will develop breast cancer at some time during her life. There are many possible causes of breast cancer, but the most obvious one appears to be excess estradiol.[110] The way for a woman with cancer to reverse her cancer physiology starts with treating the cancer and lowering her estradiol levels.

For the woman who already has breast cancer, one of the treatment options available is IPT, which utilizes insulin's ability to increase cell membrane permeability to enhance the uptake of various substances or medications into the cells to make them more effective for treatment. Since some cancers have more insulin receptors than normal cells, insulin can be used to potentiate the effects of medications such as chemotherapy drugs. Thus, only one tenth to one fourth the normal dose of these medications is needed to effectively treat the cancer, thereby minimizing side effects.

All of the female conditions generally start with a woman having menstrual cramps, a condition known as dysmenorrhea. If the underlying estradiol excess is not corrected, this condition progresses to PMS and onward to endometriosis, uterine fibroids, and potential breast and uterine cancer. This is why natural medicine physicians attack the hormonal milieu problem first. If this problem is not addressed, the end result could be breast, uterine, or cervical cancer. By reducing estradiol levels with diet and herbal remedies, female cancer physiology is reversed, and so is the risk of these hormone-sensitive cancers. ■

CHAPTER 24

The Ten Myths of Cancer and "Modern" Cancer Therapy

"A MYTH IS SOMETHING THAT WILL NEVER BE TRUE NO MATTER HOW MANY PEOPLE BELIEVE IT."
- Ross A. Hauser, M.D.

Most people seek alternative health providers because the allopathic treatment they tried was not effective. This is not an optimal circumstance, as alternative cancer therapies, like IPT, work best when they are given as the *first-line therapy*. If this is done, this is often the *only* treatment that will be needed.

Cancer patients seek out traditional oncologists because they, like their oncologists, and believe the ten myths of cancer and modern cancer therapy. Perhaps an even worse scenario is when someone searches on the Internet and reads something about an herb and then uses it as the sole treatment for cancer. This is no way to handle a life-threatening disease. When the tumor continues to grow, the person then seeks out an experienced alternative health provider. Again this is not the optimum because a very large tumor with metastases is much harder to treat than a localized cancer. We often say to patients and staff in the office, "It is *easy* to shrink tumors; it is *hard* to cure cancer." The main reason it is hard is because people come to us and other IPT physicians after they have had other very toxic regimes at the hands of their oncologist. These treatments can destroy the person's immune system and organ systems beyond repair. Thus, it is important for the cancer patient to understand the ten myths of cancer and modern cancer therapy, so appropriate treatments can be utilized.

MYTH #1: CANCER IS A TUMOR MASS

Most cancer patients and oncologists think of cancer as a tumor, a mass of defiant cells. Thus treatment is directed at removing it, radiating it, or chemo-ing it. Sometimes this regime is effective at eliminating all of the cancer cells for a time, only to have the cancer recur, often at a distant site. This indicates that the tumor mass is only able to form because the body allows it. The truth of the matter is that **cancer is a systemic deterioration of the body's biochemistry, which in the end causes cancer physiology.** In simplis-

tic terms, the difference between normal and cancer physiology can be viewed as shown in **Figure 24-1**. It is easy to see that cancer physiology is, for the most part, the opposite of normal physiology.

TRUTH: *Cancer is a systemic condition, not a localized one.*

FIGURE 24-1: DIFFERENCES BETWEEN NORMAL PHYSIOLOGY AND CANCER PHYSIOLOGY

	CANCER	NORMAL
Blood pH	Alkaline	Normal
Tumor Site pH	Acid	Normal
Blood Platelets	Sticky	Normal
Energy Production	Anaerobic	Aerobic
Angiogenesis	High	Low
Apoptosis	Low	High
Blood Coagulation	High	Low
Cell-to-Cell Adhesion	High	Low
Collagenase Activity	High	Low
Differentiation	Low	High
Female Estrogen	High	Normal
Glucose Consumption	High	Low

MYTH #2: CANCER IS AN ACUTE ILLNESS

Because cancer patients and oncologists see cancer as an emergent, acute problem that involves a destructive, localized mass of cells that are going to kill the body, surgery, radiation therapy, and high-dose chemotherapy are recommended to kill *the thing*. It is not uncommon for an IPT physician to get calls from patients *after* they have had a first chemotherapy treatment because they feel like death, whereas prior to the treatment they felt fine, full of life. Such patients had chemotherapy because the cancer was presented as acute, and therapy needed to be started *immediately*. No one bothered to tell the patients that they probably had been forming the cancer for years, possibly decades, and that the only recent development was that it was *discovered*.

Cancer patients need to realize that most cancers take years to develop. The person has had and maintained cancer physiology for years. It is best to take some time, pray, and seek out the opinion of several physicians, especially one who does IPT, before a treatment regime is started. It took most people years to develop cancer; it is okay to take some time to start therapy.*

TRUTH: *Cancer is a chronic condition.*

MYTH #3: SURGERY IS THE ANSWER

It is amazing to us how many people have surgery for their cancers and think they are fine. "See, doctor, the margins were clear, and they can't find any more cancer." The "they can't find any more cancer" just means that the CT scan, mammogram, or some other x-ray was okay. The person often has not had a comprehensive panel of cancer markers and certainly was not checked by his or her oncologist for cancer physiology. Recently, we saw a male patient who had surgery for melanoma who gave us the above history. We then did blood tests for various cancer markers and cancer physiology. It was evident from the tests that the person was far from cancer free. Shortly thereafter, a mass appeared on his testicle that was found to be melanoma.

Surgery is effective at removing the tumor mass. That is it. Many cancers recur when surgery is the only treatment option a person uses because it does not kill cells that are not in the tumor mass, and, of course, surgery does not reverse cancer physiology.

TRUTH: *Surgery alone is not the answer for cancer cure.*

MYTH #4: CANCER CAN BE KILLED BY THE MAGIC BULLET

Let's face it folks, there is no magic bullet. About every week, there is some story about a pharmaceutical company that has a *new improved* cancer drug. The press runs some stories on it, the success stories are told, and then it does not pan out. Recent medications that have gone this route are Herceptin and Taxol for breast cancer. Do they work in some patients? Of course, but when they came out, we were all led to believe that the cure for breast cancer had arrived. Herceptin could selectively attack cells that contained the Her-2 protein—the magic bullet myth.

We now hear very little about Herceptin. If one reads the side effect profile, it is far from a selective magic bullet. It can kill all right, much more than cancer cells.

Another reason the magic bullet will never appear is because a tumor mass is made up of a *heterogeneous* mix of cancer cells. In other words, when a person is found to have a lung cancer mass with metastases in the liver, the cells on the outside of the lung mass may be different from the ones on the inside of the mass, which also may be different from the cells of the liver metastases. They are all lung cancer cells, but the antigens on the cell surface, their individual biochemistry, may make some of the cells more receptive to kill by the immune system and various chemotherapy medications. This is why a person may get some tumor regression of one cancerous lesion with high-dose chemotherapy but another one grows. High-dose chemotherapy too often relies on just one or two medications. This is in contrast to when a patient undergoes IPT. Often three to five different chemotherapy medications are used (in low doses) so as to affect the whole population of cancer cells in the patient.

TRUTH: *Cancer can be killed by IPT and reversing cancer physiology.*

> No one bothered to tell the cancer patient that he or she probably had been forming the cancer for years—possibly decades—and that the only *recent* development was that their cancer was *discovered*.

---

* *For the person with impending central nervous dysfunction that affects the brain or spinal cord, immediate treatment is necessary. There are other circumstances that need immediate attention, but the vast majority of patients can take some time to start therapy.*

MYTH #5: THE ONCOLOGIST KNOWS THE BEST TREATMENT

The AMA and American Cancer Society have done a good job of making the message clear: *If you have cancer, you need an oncologist because the oncologist knows the best treatment.* It is true that oncologists treat cancer patients and thus know a lot about cancer. Their primary treatment recommendation is, however, high-dose chemotherapy. It is a known fact that most patients are not cured of cancer by high-dose chemotherapy, so the best that the greatest oncologist has to offer is not that good by the above statement.

We do recommend that all of our cancer patients seek out the best oncologist they can find for a consultation. A cancer patient should know all of the treatment options, including high-dose chemotherapy. The specialist who is an expert on high-dose chemotherapy is, of course, the oncologist. If the options are really researched, it will become clear to the cancer patient that high-dose chemotherapy does not have a high success rate. An alternative will need to be chosen, which often should be IPT.

TRUTH: *The oncologist knows the best high-dose chemotherapy treatment for a particular cancer.*

MYTH #6: THE ONLY TREATMENT OPTION IS HIGH-DOSE CHEMOTHERAPY

Many patients succumb to high-dose chemotherapy because they are told by their oncologists that it is the only option they have. Nothing could be further from the truth! The earth is a big place! Surely there must be other options! High-dose chemotherapy does have its successes, but it has far more failures. There are times such as with acute leukemias and lymphomas (especially those in blast crises) where we recommend high-dose chemotherapy. There are other cancers such as testicular cancer (the now famous Lance Armstrong case) where high-dose chemotherapy has a reasonable success rate. For the majority of other cases, the person has many more treatment options than he or she is told. Treatments such as IPT need to be used before immunosuppressive treatments such as high-dose chemotherapy.

TRUTH: *High-dose chemotherapy should often be the last treatment option.*

MYTH #7: THERE IS A 70 PERCENT CHANCE OF SUCCESS

Cancer patients receive high-dose chemotherapy for various reasons, but the one that they believe is that it is going to work. Most commonly, they are told, "There is a 70% chance of success." The patient hears, "There is a 70% chance you will get cured of your cancer." What the oncologist means is that "there is a 70% chance of tumor response or shrinkage." In reality, the average high-dose chemotherapy regime given to cancer patients with solid tumors only has a 5% chance of inducing a cure for the person. Most people would not accept hair loss, vomiting, helplessness, and months of feeling terrible if there was only a 5% chance of "success."

TRUTH: *There is a 5% chance of solid tumor cure with high-dose chemotherapy.*

MYTH #8: NUTRITIONAL PRODUCTS INTERFERE WITH THE EFFECTIVENESS OF CHEMOTHERAPY

We cannot tell you how often patients have told us their oncologists do not want them taking any nutritional products while undergoing chemotherapy because it will interfere with its effectiveness. The truth is you do not need the antioxidants to make the therapy ineffective; high-dose chemotherapy *itself* is ineffective at curing cancer. The sad part about statements made about natural medicine products and techniques by oncologists is that they know nothing about them nor do they call physicians who recommend them to their mutual patients. **We have never had even one oncologist call us!** Yet many of our patients are seeing an oncologist (to get labs and CT scans covered by insurance) and take supplements we have recommended. We have had x-ray technicians and physicians look at the scans and be amazed that the person's "untreatable cancer" was significantly shrunk and ask the patient "What did you do?", but never call us— the people responsible for the therapy.

If one researches herbal supplements and antioxidants that have been studied in cancer patients receiving chemotherapy, the overwhelming majority have been found to do at least one of the following:

- Enhance survival
- Decrease side effects
- Potentiate the killing effects of the chemotherapy
- Make patients feel better

What we would like to know is, which one of these effects, shown scientifically, is the one the oncologist finds objectionable?

TRUTH: *Nutritional products increase the effectiveness and decrease the side effects of chemotherapy.**

MYTH #9: EAT WHATEVER YOU WANT

Nutrition and natural remedies are commonly put down by oncologists as having no connection with outcomes or, worse yet, as experimental or investigational. Since when has eating vegetables or taking vitamins been "experimental"? By the way, who is investigating all of these natural remedies? Surely not the American Cancer Society.

You are what you eat. If a person eats sweets, chips, and fried foods, besides growing a bigger belly, a tumor will most likely grow. The high carb American diet is why close to one in two Americans will get cancer in their lifetime. Once diagnosed with cancer, a person's diet and lifestyle should never be the same. If it stays the same, so does cancer physiology and the likelihood of tumor recurrence.

TRUTH: *Eat whatever you want if you want your cancer to grow or recur.*

MYTH #10: INSULIN POTENTIATION THERAPY IS EXPERIMENTAL

"My oncologist told me that he never heard of Insulin Potentiation Therapy, so it must be experimental." Unfortunately for the cancer patient, he or she does not realize that most cancer treatments are experimental because pharmaceutical companies are still looking for the magic bullet. New and improved drugs are developed because the old and current methods of treating cancer patients are not working. The so-called scientific-based medicine shows that high-dose chemotherapy shrinks tumors but very few prove that it cures cancer. If a person receives a treatment that is 5% effective at "curing" the problem, surely the treatment is experimental.

Another thing that shows that the typical regimes of chemotherapy are experimental is the fact that the regimes for the various cancers are continually changing because of new, scientific discoveries. When one looks at the results, they are anything but impressive. The changes occur because the current scientific regime does not work. Contrast this to the so-called experimental Insulin Potentiation Therapy that has been used for treating cancer for over 50 years with little modification. The central technique of using insulin to potentiate the effects of low-dose chemotherapy remains the same. Most of the medications used are generic and are used because they work when combined with insulin as part of IPT. All they needed to be was *potentiated*.

TRUTH: *High-dose chemotherapy is experimental.*

ALTERNATIVE MEDICINE MYTHS

It would not be entirely fair to end this chapter here because there are some myths that pertain to the way alternative health providers view cancer and cancer therapy. We write of these because we have seen (or heard of) too many patients die because some alternative healer told them or wrote about the miraculous healing powers of some herbal product that they thought was going to cure them of their cancer.

MYTH: CANCER IS AN IMMUNODEFICIENCY DISEASE

When the average person is diagnosed with cancer, he or she still looks and feels pretty good. The person generally gives a history of not being sick, not getting infections, working full time, having good energy, but having an odd pain. The odd pain is diagnosed as cancer. In other words, when first diagnosed, the average cancer patient has no signs of having a suppressed immune system. Yet almost every alternative remedy for cancer is for immune strengthening. **The bottom line with cancer is that the immune system is not**

---

* *Nutritional products should be prescribed by a natural medicine physician who is familiar with the cancer patient's case. There are some drug, vitamin, and herb interactions that are negative.*

recognizing the cancer as it should. This is why there is a mad rush to get cancer vaccines FDA approved. The main objective of a cancer vaccine is to help the immune system fight the cancer by *recognizing* it as cancer.

Sure, there are some cancer patients who have an immunodeficiency problem, but this is generally because they are not eating and are malnourished. For the person receiving high-dose chemotherapy, immunostimulatory herbs are good, but using them to kill cancer cells and bypassing effective treatments like IPT is not wise. Direct cancer-killing therapies such as IPT are needed because a person with cancer has an immune system that is not alarmed about a cancer growing so it does not fight it as strongly as it should. In such a situation, a powerful, effective, cancer-killing therapy is needed. Patients around the globe are realizing this is IPT.

TRUTH: *Cancer is partly an immunosurveillance problem.*

MYTH: HERBAL MEDICINE CAN CURE METASTATIC CANCER

As a natural medicine physician running one of the largest natural medicine centers in the world, I (Ross) know that herbal medicine can cure. Almost every day I hear of herbal medicine miracles. People travel from around the globe to see us and the natural medicine staff at Caring Medical. It is not that we are so great; it is that natural medicine is great!

In all of our years of going to conferences and treating patients, we have not seen evidence of a single patient cured of metastatic cancer (solid tumors) who used herbal medicine alone. We are sure that a patient or a few of those patients are out there, but the cancer patient should beware: **Herbal medicine cannot cure metastatic cancer.** It may shrink it for a while, but do not play Russian roulette with your life. Do not put your hope in something your friend heard about. Make sure you are under the care of a physician who treats a lot of cancer, preferably a doctor who does IPT. Herbal medicine can help, and there are lots of patients who have had allopathic treatment and herbal medicine and been cured. But herbal medicine alone cannot cure metastatic cancer in the overwhelming majority of cases.

TRUTH: *Herbal medicine can help treat metastatic cancer.*

MYTH: ALLOPATHIC MEDICINE IS OF THE DEVIL

We have had the opportunity to treat many natural medicine zealots who believe allopathic medicine is of the devil. They will have nothing to do with a person who practices AMA-sanctioned medicine, even if they are recommended by a natural medicine doctor. The correct position, as in most situations, is to avoid extremism. There are times when surgery, radiation, and/or high-dose chemotherapy are needed. Allopathic medicine is not of the devil but ignorance perhaps.

TRUTH: *Allopathic medicine has its place.*

MYTH: ALL CHEMOTHERAPY IS BAD

Because of the high failure rates of high-dose chemotherapy at curing cancer, chemotherapy is not what people want to treat their cancer. The problem comes in when someone is an appropriate IPT candidate and will not get the therapy because it involves chemotherapy. The feeling is that "all chemotherapy is bad." When confronted with such a patient, we simply ask, "Do you want something that kills cancer cells, yes or no?" If the answer is yes, then you want chemotherapy because that is what the word means, "cancer killing." If you do not want your cancer killed, then do not come here. Because insulin and other therapies can potentiate the effects of chemotherapy, the dosages used are lower and so are the side effects. So in the armamentarium of cancer therapies, there is a place for chemotherapy, mostly in the hands of a physician utilizing IPT.

TRUTH: *All chemotherapy has its place.*

MYTH: IF I HAD CANCER, I WOULDN'T GET CHEMOTHERAPY

No explanation is needed. Everybody talks big when they are healthy. When you are sick, you do what you have to do to get healthy. In the form of IPT, chemotherapy works.

TRUTH: *If you had cancer, you would do what was needed to be done to live.*

MYTH: CANCER PATIENTS SHOULD JUICE

Many cancer patients have excessively high blood insulin levels, which makes them more prone to getting cancers. Insulin has a stimulatory effect on cancer that can be used to make the cancer cells more *receptive* to chemotherapy, one basis for IPT. For the person desiring to decrease cancer growth between IPT treatments, or to prevent cancers from forming, insulin levels need to be lowered. Juicing, because of the massive amounts of carbohydrates, will cause insulin levels to rise. Juice does contain a lot of nutrients, but if it involves a lot of fruit juices, juicing surely will not be in the cancer patient's best interest.

Vegetable juicing has its place and often can help a person detoxify. Again, in all the conferences we have attended, cancer patients we have treated, and colleagues with whom we have talked, we do not know of a single person who has seen his or her metastatic cancer go into remission with juicing and herbal medicine alone.

The vast majority of alternative health providers who treat cancer patients put them on a strict vegetarian diet. From a science point of view as it relates to insulin, this is not the correct approach. This does not mean the person should eat bacon at every meal, but a much lower carbohydrate diet than juicing is needed if high insulin levels are part of the person's cancer physiology.

For the person who has low insulin levels when diagnosed with cancer or who wants a program for cancer prevention, it may be appropriate to be a vegetarian and drink vegetable juices. The best way to find out is via a glucose-insulin tolerance test and metabolic typing. This approach will help determine the appropriate diet based on various tests and questionnaires the person fills out.

To say one diet fits all patients and all cancers is naive and untrue. For the cancer patient with low insulin levels, a high blood pH (alkaline), and low urine pH (acidic), a juicing type diet would be appropriate. If the person with cancer had the exact opposite physiology, then a high-protein, low-carbohydrate diet would be needed.

TRUTH: *Cancer patients should eat according to their metabolic type.*

DON'T FORGET CANCER MONITORING

There are many things that people believe, and no matter how many times or with whatever strength they believe them, they will never be true. One of the common myths that people believe is that there is no way to monitor cancer except by some x-ray study. The next couple of chapters will deal with the various blood tests that are used by natural medicine physicians to monitor cancer and cancer physiology.

MYTH: THERE ARE NO BLOOD TESTS TO MONITOR MY PARTICULAR CANCER

TRUTH: *There are many blood tests to check for cancer and cancer physiology.* ■

To find out about these, you are going to have to read the next chapter...

CHAPTER 25

Natural Medicine Cancer Monitoring—It Could Save Your Life

As the United States gets caught up with the rest of the world in the utilization of nutrition and natural medicine techniques in the prevention and treatment of human diseases, patients with even serious conditions such as cancer are open to its alluring promises. "The cure for all cancers," "this herb changed my life," and various other claims are easy to come by for anyone enlisting the various Internet search engines or browsing the alternative medicine section of any bookstore. Natural medicine or an herb can change a life and possibly even help a person with cancer, but curing all cancers is doubtful at best, probably unlikely, and assuredly misleading. Remember, you are hearing this from us, some of the leaders in natural medicine in the United States and people who utilize natural remedies to treat patients with cancer.

Cancer is not something to treat half-heartedly. Anyone coming to Caring Medical for cancer therapy or prevention will initially be told about appropriate cancer monitoring. This is because natural medicine cancer monitoring most assuredly could save the person's life. If the person is not monitored effectively, it is probable that the cancer will return or spread; if the cancer is watched closely by appropriate natural medicine techniques and markers, then aggressive measures can be taken when needed. This will help save the person's life. *The person who goes by how he or she feels will most likely be another cancer statistic because improvement in health is a poor measure of cancer regression.*

Most assuredly the person who stops sugar and grains and eats more vegetables, drinks juices, and takes herbs is going to feel better. While the person feels better, the cancer can be growing and infiltrating more organs. A healthy diet and proper nutritional supplements help the body organs function better but do not in any way make the immune system destroy cancer cells. On the contrary, the various vitamins and nutrients that a person is taking to be healthy could, in fact, be *feeding* the cancer. It is only by appropriate objective monitoring that a person would know if his or her particular cancer was arresting (stop growing) or going into remission (shrinking).

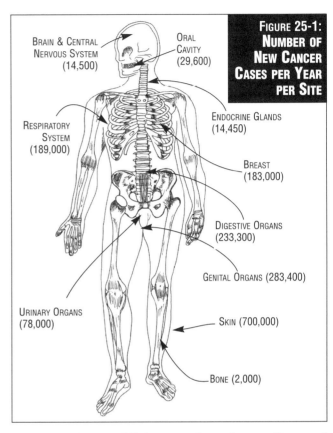

FIGURE 25-1: NUMBER OF NEW CANCER CASES PER YEAR PER SITE

BRAIN & CENTRAL NERVOUS SYSTEM (14,500)

ORAL CAVITY (29,600)

RESPIRATORY SYSTEM (189,000)

ENDOCRINE GLANDS (14,450)

BREAST (183,000)

DIGESTIVE ORGANS (233,300)

GENITAL ORGANS (283,400)

URINARY ORGANS (78,000)

SKIN (700,000)

BONE (2,000)

From **Figure 25-1**, it is clear that millions of people are struggling with cancer. **Figure 25-2** shows that for many of these, the struggle will end in death. Cancer is continuing and increasing its toll on human life. The numbers are staggering, and there appears to be no end in sight. The traditional treatments of surgery, radiation, and high-dose chemotherapy are not working for many people with cancer, and, thus, they seek alternatives when these have failed. As more and more information becomes available via the Internet, many people with cancer are now using alternative methods as first-line therapies because of the dismal results of traditional treatments with certain types of cancers, especially those with metastases. This is exciting in one sense because it will give alternative medicine a chance to show what works and what does not work; the problem occurs when patients become their own doctors and do not closely monitor their progress on the particular regime that they are trying. Because of

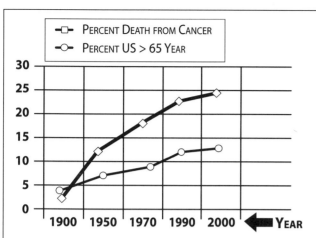

Figure 25-2: *Increasing Incidence of Cancer in America* (*Not Totally Due to Our Aging Population*)

In 1900, 3% of deaths in America were from cancer. Today, that number is 24% and climbing. The percentage of Americans over age 65 has increased from 4% to 12%.

Adapted from Universal Almanac, *p. 225 Andrews, Kansas City, 1989. Also* Cancer Journal for Clinicians, *Vol. 50, No. 1, Jan. 2000*

all of these factors, it is imperative that a person with cancer be under the guidance of a physician familiar with effective and sensitive cancer monitoring. If this is done, it will be evident very quickly whether the particular treatment is working or not working and then appropriate recommendations or changes can be made in the regime.

Another aspect of the importance of sensitive cancer monitoring is the fact that the ability for a patient to be cured of a malignant disease is, in general, a function of tumor size, location, and cell biology. The early diagnosis of small, localized tumors that are amenable to surgical resection confers the best prognosis. Since early diagnosis and smaller tumor burdens are the best predictors of cure for many tumors, the issue of when and how to screen asymptomatic individuals for malignancy is an important one. Again, how a person feels is a poor sign as to the presence or absence of cancer. It is for this reason that sensitive markers be used for tumor screening and response to therapy.

In malignant disease, there is aberrant expression of a number of genes. Many of the products of these genes, including hormones, enzymes, immunoglobulins, and a variety of other proteins, may be secreted by the tumor cell. If there is sufficient secretion (dependent on the tumor burden and the secretory capacity of each cell) without rapid metabolic degradation, the secreted

protein may be detectable in the serum (blood). These proteins or biomarkers are potentially useful for screening populations, early detection of patients with suspected disease, assessing tumor burden and prognosis, assessing response to therapy, and evaluating early recurrence. Currently available radioimmunoassays can often detect minute amounts (nanograms) of the marker substance. All of the marker proteins, however, are products of normal cells and may be present in small amounts in normal serum. Furthermore, the levels of some marker proteins may also increase with inflammation. The more common traditional tumor markers can be seen in **Figure 25-3**.

FIGURE 25-3: COMMON BLOOD CANCER MARKER TESTS

MARKER	TUMOR TYPES
Alpha Fetoprotein	Hepatoma, testicular cancer
AMAS Test	Nonspecific for carcinomas
CA 125 (cancer antigen)	Ovarian and other epithelial cancers
CA 19-9, 15-3	Breast, ovarian, and other carcinomas
CEA (carcinoembryonic antigen)	Gastrointestinal, breast, lung, and ovarian cancers
HCG (human chorionic gonadotropin)	Testicular cancer, choriocarcinoma
PSA	Prostate cancer

If someone has a particular cancer and the tumor marker is elevated, then this may be a good measure to use in monitoring the response to treatment. It is always a good idea to test the blood for these traditional markers because often their cost is minimal; in some instances, they can give the information that is sought. Problems occur because in some people with extensive metastatic disease, the traditional tumor marker may be negative, whereas in a benign condition, it may be markedly elevated. Some examples of patients currently being treated at Caring Medical will make this clearer.

CANCER MARKER CASE STUDIES
NORM—PROSTATE CANCER

Norm came to Caring Medical on January 20, 1998, for a nutritional consultation concerning his prostate cancer. He was diagnosed by biopsy in December 1997. He was a Gleason grade 3. His PSA level at the time of the initial consultation was 14.7. He did not desire hormone therapy, surgery, or other traditional remedies. He was interested in seeing if he could control the condition with nutritional remedies.

His initial workup at Caring Laboratory Services showed multiple mineral deficiencies as well as elevated testosterone and dihydrotestosterone levels, which were felt to be feeding the cancer. He also had some abnormalities with his pH, as his system was *too alkaline*. His metabolic type was more carnivore, and the protein was increased in his diet. In addition, he was started on an aggressive herbal program that included supplements to thin his blood, balance his pHs, strengthen his adrenal glands, and decrease his dihydrotestosterone levels.

Norm has been faithful with his nutritional regime, and his PSAs (normal is 0 to 4) have been as follows:

DATE	PSA
2/9/98	6.4
5/4/98	9.3
6/10/98	6.29
10/22/98	7.3
3/17/99	4.0
1/27/00	4.6

This is a good case to show that cancer can be arrested with a strict nutritional regime. He recently sent us a picture of himself with his dog. With the card was a small note: For the new book—how to live…get a good doctor and a good dog (See **Figure 25-4**).

JOAN—BREAST CANCER MASS

Joan is a beautiful 46-year-old who came to Caring Medical on March 26, 1999, because of a recurrence of left breast carcinoma. She stated, "I am not doing any more chemotherapy!" In 1996, she was first diagnosed with stage IIB cancer and underwent a lumpectomy with node dissection, followed by three months of traditional chemotherapy (six sessions of cyclophosphamide, methotrexate, and 5-fluorouracil). Her cancer was classified as a large, moderately differentiated, ductal carcinoma in situ and was estrogen receptor-positive. Five of the ten lymph nodes removed in 1996 were positive for cancer.

Upon review of her medical records, she was noted to have a left breast mass per ultrasound that was 30 mm × 25 mm near the 12 o'clock position. Biopsy of the mass confirmed that it was a recurrence of her diffuse infiltrating ductoral carcinoma (grade 2 of 3) with changes consistent with lymphatic infiltration. Joan was not going to

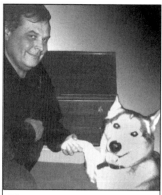

Figure 25-4: Norm and His Good Dog

How to live long? Get a good doctor and a good dog.

do conventional therapy, so she came to Caring Medical for cancer treatment and nutritional consultation. She was recommended to undergo IPT but because of previous bad experience with chemotherapy, she refused and desired to do comprehensive natural medicine.

She underwent comprehensive blood testing of her cancer markers, which showed a positive AMAS test and an elevated CA 15-3. She was also found to have a low estrogen quotient at 0.22 [estriol/(estrone + estradiol) in the urine] and significant nutrient deficiencies and bowel dysbiosis (bad organisms in her stools). She was ready to try an aggressive natural medicine approach.

Joan was asked to increase her intake of genistein with a concentrated soy supplement. She was also placed on an appropriate vegetarian diet appropriate for her metabolic type. Her nutriceutical program was designed to help thin her blood, balance the pH, correct her high estradiol in relationship to estriol, as well as clean her colon. From a hormone standpoint, she was placed on DHEA and testosterone. She was also given high-dose vitamin D, which helps with the differentiation of cancer cells and acts like a "natural" chemotherapeutic agent by stopping rapidly reproducing cells.

Because of the expense of the AMAS test and diagnostic tests, follow-up tests were limited. We used the CA 15-3 (normal is 0 to 30) to monitor her breast cancer. The results are as follows:

DATE	CA 15-3
11/26/99	39
5/19/00	29.1

She continued to have a left breast mass, but it was noticeably softer and less dense for some time. In addition to the above, she wore a magnet on the area as prescribed. If cost was not an issue, she would definitely have the 24-hour urine collection for estrogen quotient redone, as her cancer is estrogen driven. She refused to take estrogen blockers (such as tamoxifen or Arimidex). As a side note, she has suffered from uterine bleeding since age 14, and an ultrasound of her pelvis showed a large fibroid on the uterus and ovarian cysts—all consistent with a physiology that is estrogen dominant.

How is her breast tumor doing? She has had multiple ultrasounds and agreed to get an MRI of the breast on September 12, 2000, which showed that the mass is $32 \times 30 \times 20$ mm, so its size has not changed in the last two years with nutritional therapies. Joan during this time lived a very full and vibrant life as evidenced by her huge smile when she comes to the office, though she made this doctor nervous as h*ll.

Early in 2001, she came in complaining that her breast was heavier. This is usually a sign that the cancer is growing. On physical examination, it was clear that this was the case. We had a tearful time together, and I (Ross) explained that she needed *today* to do something more aggressive. She chose to have a mastectomy. She came in for one IPT treatment, then we lost her to follow-up. It is a very sad case, and it is presented for that reason. It was probable from the beginning that she would need to do something more aggressive. She had a phenomenal immune system and appeared to be in perfect health. If she wanted to do modeling, she could. But even after her mastectomy with nonclear margins, Joan continues to avoid the inevitable—she needs aggressive systemic treatment. In her case, the best option would be IPT.

JANICE—NEWLY DIAGNOSED BREAST CANCER

Starting on July 20, 1998, Caring Medical would never be the same. On this day, Janice walked into the office. She already had a massive accumulation of knowledge about all the conventional and nonconventional treatments concerning breast cancer. Her condition was diagnosed via a right breast sterotactic core biopsy on July 1, 1998, which showed invasive ductal carcinoma grade III.

On the initial consultation, we made it clear to Janice that if she was to treat her cancer nutritionally, then she needed to try and find a blood marker for the cancer. We also informed her that despite advances in natural medicine, the best treatment option to quickly decrease tumor load and increase survival was surgery (this was our pre-IPT days). Below is a summary of her initial tests results:

JANICE' RESULTS:				
AMAS	CA 15-3	CEA	CA 27-9	CA 19-9
—	12	0.4	9.0	5.7

NORMAL RESULTS:	*NORMAL VALUES OF THE CANCER MARKERS*			
AMAS	CA 15-3	CEA	CA 7-9	CA 19-9
0-99	0-30	0-5	0-37	

Janice did decide to undergo a mastectomy, which was performed on August 7, 1998. The pathological report showed that seven of 17 lymph nodes were positive for cancer. Her tumor measured 1.8 cm and was both estrogen and progesterone positive. She was placed on tamoxifen by her oncologist. She refused postoperative chemotherapy and decided to use natural medicine instead.

Upon the initial natural medicine testing, it was found that she also had a low estrogen quotient at 0.15 (normal is over 1.0). She was then placed on a high vegetation, soy diet along with chasteberry and other nutritional supplements to reverse this. Because she was starting natural medicine after the surgery, another round of cancer markers was drawn and then redrawn as necessary. **See Figure 25-5** for a summary of Janice's test results.

From Janice's test results, one can see that the only test that was an appropriate marker of her breast cancer was the AMAS. Throughout most of her clinical course, she has had some low-level type of cancer activity that most likely relates to her high estrogen secretion. Interestingly, when her AMAS value jumped on June 26, 2000, it was because she had stopped taking poly-MVA and her oral Laetrile. In our office, we check thiocyanate levels to ensure people are absorbing their Laetrile, and her level was 0; she then confessed she was not taking it.

As a side note, all of her CT scans and mammograms have been fine—no evidence of tumor. Her initial estrogen quotient was the lowest we had seen at 0.08, and a follow-up urinary estrogen

DATE	AMAS	CA 15-3	CEA
8/27/98	188 (H)	13.0	0.6
10/27/98		12.0	0.7
11/6/98	127 (H)		
1/22/99	139 (H)		
6/1/99		6.0	0.5
6/16/99	8		
9/7/99		6.0	0.6
9/29/99	106 (H)		
1/21/00	52		
6/26/00	145 (H)		
10/5/00		5.0	0.5
11/30/00	107 (H)		

H = High

Figure 25-5: Janice's Test Results

quotient on August 8, 2000, was still low at 0.55 but a vast improvement from her initial test. To help improve estrogen quotient, she ate a high soy diet and took various supplements, including soy isoflavones, as well as a concentrated extract of chasteberry, flax seed oil capsules, and an estrogenic blocker, Femara.

AMAS TEST

The AMAS test measures serum levels of AMA or antimalignin antibody. AMA is the antibody to malignin, a 10,000 dalton polypeptide that has been found to be present in most malignant cells, regardless of cell type or location. Unlike tests such as CEA, which measure less well-defined antigens whose serum levels tend to be inconsistent but elevated late in the disease, the AMAS test measures a well-defined antibody whose serum levels rise early in the course of the disease. In some cases, the AMAS test has been positive (elevated) early, i.e., one to 19 months before clinical detection.

The AMAS test is a very nonspecific test for cancer activity. It is elevated in almost all types of cancers. For sera determined within 24 hours of being drawn, the false-positive and false-negative rates are less than 1% (specificity and sensitivity greater than 99%); for stored sera, false positives are 5%, and false negatives 7%.

The AMAS test can be used as a screening test for the presence of cancerous cells in the body. It can also be used to determine prognosis as a neg-

ative test in the face of obvious cancer carries a poor prognosis. A negative AMAS test with known cancer signifies a poor immune response to the cancer and thus the poorer prognosis.

OTHER PROGNOSTIC INDICATORS

Besides cancer markers, other prognostic indicators are used at CCINMC. For cancer patients in general, increases in body weight, lean body mass, albumin level (protein levels), and cholesterol carry a better prognosis. Maintaining or increasing body weight, especially protein stores signified by an increase in serum albumin, means the body is in the healing mode. This is one of the reasons testosterone is given to patients at CCINMC. Having a normal or elevated cholesterol is often a sign that the liver is functioning well. Also, if body chemistry values such as liver and kidney function tests are normal, along with white blood cells being normal, there is a more favorable prognosis.

CANCER MONITORING AT CCINMC

Besides monitoring the above prognostic indicators on at least a monthly or bimonthly basis for active patients, CCINMC believes in aggressive cancer marker monitoring. This would include blood tests for C-reactive protein and erythrocyte sedimentation rate, both signs of systemic inflammation. These values are elevated with cancer and typically go down when tumor regression is occurring. If a person is receiving IPT, the blood cancer markers are typically checked after every six IPT treatments. Tumor shrinkage generally starts to occur between the fourth and sixth treatment. (See **Figure 25-6**.) If after 12 IPT treatments the blood cancer markers, CT scans, other x-ray studies, and PET scans are within normal limits, the person is presumed cancer-free, and the IPT sessions are stopped. Regarding cancer monitoring, once the person is in remission, it is recommended that every three months during the first year, a CEA, CA 125, CA 15-3, and AMAS test are given, depending, of course, on the type of cancer. After the first year, these are done twice yearly for two years and then yearly thereafter. A person with a diagnosis of cancer, even if remission has occurred, should get at least yearly cancer marker monitoring.

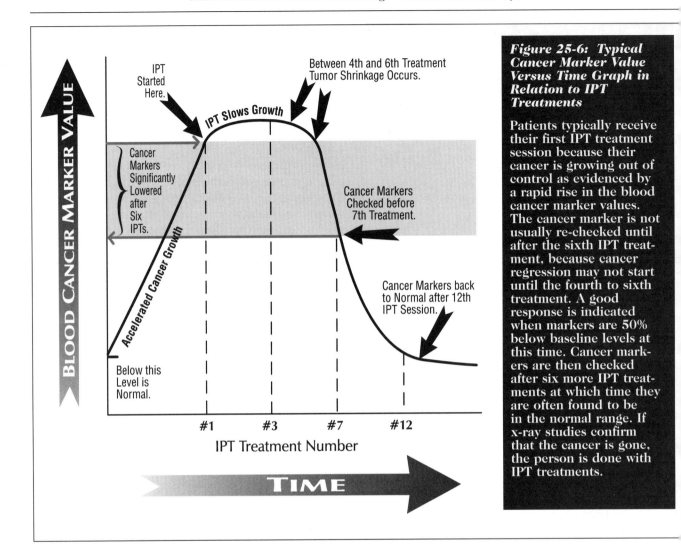

Figure 25-6: Typical Cancer Marker Value Versus Time Graph in Relation to IPT Treatments

Patients typically receive their first IPT treatment session because their cancer is growing out of control as evidenced by a rapid rise in the blood cancer marker values. The cancer marker is not usually re-checked until after the sixth IPT treatment, because cancer regression may not start until the fourth to sixth treatment. A good response is indicated when markers are 50% below baseline levels at this time. Cancer markers are then checked after six more IPT treatments at which time they are often found to be in the normal range. If x-ray studies confirm that the cancer is gone, the person is done with IPT treatments.

SUMMARY

Battling cancer is a matter of life or death. It is important that the proper approach of monitoring of the cancer be done. CT scans, biopsies, and various other x-ray studies have their place but do not forget to get comprehensive blood cancer marker tests. They could save your life. ∎

CHAPTER 26

Understanding Cancer Physiology: The Key to Success

"BUT EVERY DOCTOR WHO HAS A CANCER PATIENT MUST RETHINK HIS ATTITUDE TOWARD THE DISEASE. HE MUST RECOGNIZE THAT THERE IS A NEED FOR A PROPERLY COORDINATED COOPERATION BETWEEN THE CLASSIC METHODS AND THE CONCEPT THAT CANCER, FROM THE VERY OUTSET, IS A DISEASE OF THE WHOLE BODY."
–Josef Issels, M.D.

Josef Issels, M.D., was a holistically minded doctor before holistic medicine was cool. In the articles written about him, it is said that he cured cancer but not just any cancer. He cured advanced, recurrent cancer—cancer that had laughed at radiation and thrived on chemotherapy. He is the founder of the Issels vaccine, which some cancer patients use with success. We really appreciate what he wrote in his book, *Cancer: A Second Opinion:*[1]

> In 1956 I formulated a set of rules for my medical staff, putting into writing principles I had long adhered to. They are:
>
> 1. Never promise a cure to anybody.
> 2. In dealing with prognosis, tell a patient or his/her responsible relatives that the first step is to arrest the tumor.
> 3. That will prolong life.
> 4. The next step is to try and make the tumor regress.
> 5. That will bring a further prolonging of life.
> 6. The patient should be told that the eventual medical aim is to try and reach the stage where the tumor disappears completely.
> 7. Time itself is another factor. Patients should be told that cure is a matter of time—in their case five years free of disease, the statistical yardstick used to measure cure rates.
> 8. Our aim is to try and achieve that situation. But we can make no promises. And we never talk to "cure" but "remission."
> 9. We always talk with the knowledge that positive treatment can be offered. That is much more precise and beneficial.
>
> By following these rules no doctor should fall under suspicion of offering false hope—a charge that is frequently leveled at those of us who argue more can be offered in the treatment of cancer than is generally available in conventional medical circles today.

We think it is fair to say that doctors who utilize IPT adhere to the principles laid out by Dr. Issel. The cancer patient reading this book should not go away with the feeling that IPT is the cure for all cancers. But it is a step in the right direction. It can help many people become cured of their cancers, but on the way, there will be many who will not get cured. By combining IPT with natural medicine treatments, at least the individual's quality of life will be improved, and this is what we believe Dr. Issels was saying. More holistically minded treatments help a person's quality of life and often prolong life. He could not guarantee a cure and neither can we.

Cancer is not an immunodeficiency disease. We know this sounds contradictory to what most people believe about cancer, but it is true. We would say the primary reason why natural remedies fail to help cancer patients is because they are aimed at stimulating the cancer patient's immune system. Since cancer is not an immunodeficiency disease, the remedy or therapy does not work. Consequently, understanding cancer physiology is the key to success.

The fact that cancer is not an immunodeficiency disease has been known for decades. R. T. Prehn, M.D., summarized the role of the immune system and cancer as follows:

> Most and perhaps all neoplasms arouse an immune response in their hosts. Unfortunately, this response is seldom effective in limiting tumor growth. Immunologic surveillance, as originally conceived, probably does not exist. The early weak response to nascent tumors stimulates rather than inhibits their growth. A truly tumor-limiting reaction occurs only in exceptional tumor systems, and then it is relatively late and ineffectual. Immunity may be of great importance in limiting the activity of oncogenic viruses, but is probably seldom the determiner of whether or not an already transformed cell gives rise to a lethal cancer.[2]

"I don't want to go to him; he's not an oncologist." "Dr. Hauser, what does he know about cancer?" Patients explain to me all the reasons why their relatives tell them not to come to Caring Medical, but if the cancer patient does come, there is one statement that generally swings him or her over to natural medicine. **Your oncologist is doing nothing to reverse your cancer physiology; this is in the realm of the natural medicine specialist.** In this chapter, we will explain how cancer forms and what cancer physiology is. The next couple of chapters will expound on various aspects of this.

Cancer is not a rogue mature cell that has gone crazy and revolted against the body. This is a critical statement that needs to be understood. Another falsity is that cancer cells proliferate rapidly. The opposite is actually true. **Most neoplastic cells do not cycle faster than their normal counterparts.** For example, 40 kg of gastrointestinal cells and 10 kg of white blood cells are produced annually by the average human. This is a prodigious effort in cell replication when we consider that the fetus in utero requires nine months to achieve 4 kg of weight. In contrast, a patient may die harboring a tumor of less than 5 kg that took several years to develop. **It is often the changes in the person's physiology that kills, not the tumor mass itself**—another reason that understanding cancer physiology is the key to successful treatment.

Tumors increase in size not because the tumor cell cycle is faster than normal cells but because so many tumor cells are cycling. The key to successful therapy is how to keep the mass of tumor cells cycling down. High-dose chemotherapy has the side effects it does because it destroys both normal and malignant cells. Destruction of normal white blood cells and gastrointestinal cells may result in infection, bleeding, nausea, and diarrhea. The traditional oncologist cycles the chemotherapy because normal cells recover faster from the destruction than cancer cells. This is one of the reasons that IPT makes so much sense because it helps target the chemotherapy so lower doses of the medication are needed, which also leads to a much lower incidence of side effects.

Patients who just use natural remedies are often relying primarily on herbs or a natural therapy's ability to improve the immune system and to eradicate the cancer. Unfortunately, just strengthening the immune system will not do it. The person needs some therapy with direct cancer-killing effects. By giving IPT, which directly kills tumor cells, the quantity of tumor cells growing is decreased.

Cancer often starts when the person is exposed to a carcinogen, such as cigarette smoke. **Figure 26-1** shows the differences under a microscope between normal lung tissue and two types of lung cancer. One can easily see the

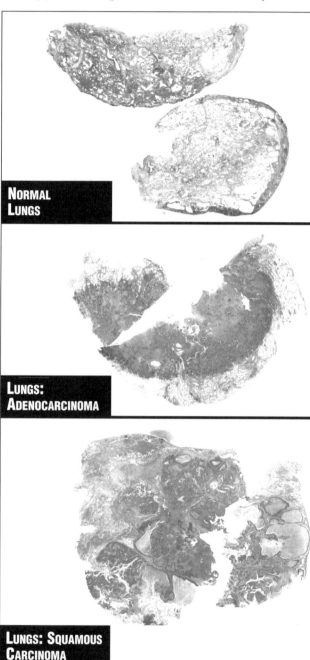

NORMAL LUNGS

LUNGS: ADENOCARCINOMA

LUNGS: SQUAMOUS CARCINOMA

Figure 26-1: Photograph of Three Different Slices of Lung—Indicating Various Lung Pathologies

To diagnose the type of cancer, part of the tissue must be examined by a pathologist under a microscope.

FIGURE 26-2: TNM DEFINITIONS

PRIMARY TUMOR

Tx	Primary tumor cannot be assessed
T0	No evidence of primary tumor
Tis	Carcinoma in situ; intraductal carcinoma, lobular carcinoma in situ, or Paget's disease of the nipple with no tumor
T1	Tumor 2 cm or less in greatest dimension
T1a	0.5 cm or smaller
T1b	More than 0.5 cm, but not more than 1 cm in greatest dimension
T1c	More than 1 cm, but not more than 2 cm in greatest dimension
T2	Tumor more than 2 cm but not more than 5 cm in greatest dimension
T3	Tumor more than 5 cm in greatest dimension
T4	Tumor of any size with direct extension to chest wall or skin
T4a	Extension to chest wall
T4b	Edema (including peau d'orange), ulceration of the skin of the breast, or satellite skin nodules confined to the same breast
T4c	Both (T4a and T4b)
T4d	Inflammatory carcinoma (see definition in text)

REGIONAL LYMPH NODE INVOLVEMENT

Clinical

Nx	Regional lymph nodes cannot be assessed (e.g., previously removed)
N0	No regional lymph node metastasis
N1	Metastasis to movable ipsilateral axillary node(s)
N2	Metastasis to ipsilateral axillary lymph node(s) fixed to one another or to other structures
N3	Metastasis to ipsilateral internal mammary lymph node(s)

Pathologic

pNx	Regional lymph node metastasis cannot be assessed
pN0	No regional lymph node metastasis
pN1	Metastasis to movable ipsilateral axillary node(s)
pN1a	Only micrometastasis (none larger than 0.2 cm)
pN1b	Metastasis to lymph node(s), any larger than 0.2 cm
pN1bi	Metastasis in one to three lymph nodes, any more than 0.2 cm in greatest dimension
pN1bii	Metastasis to four or more lymph nodes, any more than 0.2 cm and all less than 2 cm in greater dimension
pN1biii	Extension of tumor beyond the capsule of a lymph node metastasis less than 2 cm in greatest dimension
pN1biv	Metastasis to a lymph node 2 cm or more in greatest dimension
pN2	Metastasis to ipsilateral axillary lymph nodes that are fixed to one another or to other structures
pN3	Metastasis to ipsilateral internal mammary lymph node(s)

DISTANT METASTASES

Mx	Presence of distinct metastasis cannot be assessed
M0	No distant metastasis
M1	Distant metastasis (including metastasis to ipsilateral supraclavicular node(s)

STAGE GROUPING

Stage 0	Tis, N0, M0
Stage I	T1, N0, M0
Stage IIA	T0, N1, M0
	T1, N1,† M0
	T2, N0, M0
Stage IIB	T2, N1, M0
	T3, N0, M0
Stage IIIA	T0, N2, M0
	T1, N2, M0
	T2, N2, M0
	T3, N1, M0
	T3, N2, M0
Stage IIIB	T3, any N, M0
	Any T, N3, M0
Stage IV	Any T, any N, M1

* Definitions for classifying the primary tumor (T) are the same for clinical and pathologic classification. If the measurement is made by physical examination, the examiner should use T1, T2, or T3. If other measurements, such as mammographic or pathologic, are used, the examiner can use the subsets of T1.

† The prognosis of patients with N1a is similar to that of patients with pN0.

Adapted from Boal Cancer Principles and Practice of Oncology, 5th edition, Lippincott-Raven, © 1997

difference in the cells. This pathologic difference is how the diagnosis of cancer is made by biopsy and surgical specimens.

Since malignant tumors have the intrinsic ability to kill the host unless they are removed, they are often removed. Even patients who come for an IPT consultation are often told that the primary tumor should be removed to decrease the tumor load. **The smaller the tumor burden, the more likelihood of inducing a complete remission with IPT.** The latter reason is what causes modern medicine to suggest surgery as the first-line option for cancer care.

The process of finding out how much tumor is present is called *tumor grading. Tumor grading* is an indication of the degree of malignancy and correlates to a degree with prognosis. Tumor staging describes the size of the primary lesion, the degree of invasion, and the presence of lymph node involvement and metastases. Staging also plays a role in establishing prognosis. Grading, or the degree of anaplasia (abnormality of how the cells look under a microscope), is assessed from

1 to 4, with 4 the most malignant. Each cancer is staged slightly differently. In regard to breast cancer, the system can be quite complex, as is seen in **Figure 26-2**.

The stage and grade of cancer is important in making treatment recommendations. The person with cancer must realize, however, that there are numerous factors to consider, including the DNA content (ploidy), S phase fraction, estrogen receptor status, and many other factors (See **Figure 26-3**). It is for these reasons that a patient needs to provide any physician giving recommendations copies of his or her x-rays, CT scans, MRI reports, biopsy/surgical reports, and any pathology reports that were done on the cancer tissue.

The more localized a tumor, the greater the likelihood of a successful outcome. Any tumor that is outside the boundaries of the surgical biopsy, such as in the lymph tissue, blood, or another organ, necessitates some type of systemic therapy in order to produce a successful outcome. When a metastasis is found (secondary tumor), it is almost always multiple and therefore not amenable to

FIGURE 26-3: SOME FACTORS THAT ARE KNOWN TO INFLUENCE THE PROGNOSIS OF BREAST CANCER

Time Dependent
Tumor size
Axillary node status
Systemic micro- and macrometastases

Histopathological
Histological type
Cytological and nuclear grade
Lympho-vascular invasion

Markers of Proliferation
DNA content (ploidy)
S-phase fraction
Monoclonal antibodies
Ki67, KiSi, MIB-1

Markers of Apoptosis
bel-2

Growth Factors, Oncogenes, and Receptors
Estrogen receptor
Progesterone receptor
Epidermal growth-factor receptor
erb-B2 protein
H-ras protein
c-myc protein
p21
pS2
Heat-shock proteins

Growth-Suppressor Genes
p53

Factors for Invasion and Metastasis
Proteinases
Cathepsin-D
Stromelysin-3
Tenascin
Laminin receptors
Angiogenesis factor (bFGF)
nm 23 gene product

Adapted from Biology of Female Cancer, *CRC Press, Boca Raton, FL, 1997*

surgery or irradiation. For these people, IPT or high-dose chemotherapy is the only hope for obtaining a cure.

When a person is found to have cancer and metastases, he or she is in shock. "I couldn't believe it; I had almost no symptoms." The reason a person has almost no symptoms with cancer is because tremendous reserves have been built into most of the organ systems. For example, an otherwise healthy adult can survive with one half of a healthy kidney. After removal of one kidney, the other undergoes hypertrophy (growth), which compensates to a degree for the loss of tissue. A person can survive easily with a single functioning lung. In the case of the liver, generally about 75% of it has to be destroyed before there is no turning back. An animal can survive after removal of two thirds of its liver; over the course of a week, it can regenerate the lost tissue.[3]

There are times, however, when traditional treatments such as surgery or irradiation are needed to help survival. Cancers and cancer metastases can block vital organs or ducts of the digestive tract, stopping the body's ability to process food. If the intestines or a liver bile duct are completely blocked, this is a medical emergency and either surgery must be performed to keep the duct open, for instance, by placing a stent in it, or irradiation must be done to shrink the tumor. Another emergency is when a cancer is growing in the central nervous system, such as in the brain. The cancer can easily destroy vital brain centers by increasing intracranial pressure. Again, in such a situation, some emergency-type treatment such as radiation therapy and high-dose Decadron (steroid) are often given.

Other life-threatening situations that Caring Medical takes very seriously are yeast, fungi, and bacterial infections in cancer patients. These are often the cause of death for many cancer patients who have the wasting syndrome of cancer called cachexia. Cachexia results from the starvation and debilitation of the patient by cancer. The person is wasted, weak, and incapable of mounting a good immune reaction. This syndrome is an immunodeficiency problem. It is for this reason that antifungal and antibiotic medications are often given with IPT. It is very dangerous for a cancer patient to get an infection, so in many respects it is prophylactic. If a person has cachexia, then aggressive nutrition, sometimes via a G-tube (stomach) or J-tube (intestine), is needed if the person is not eating. Once a person's nutritional status improves, as evidenced by weight gain, increased appetite, and improvement in albumin blood levels, the immune system returns and the risk of infection drops dramatically.

At this point, it is much more likely the person could tolerate aggressive IPT. If a person is cachetic when starting IPT, it may be given only once every two to three weeks, instead of the customary once or twice per week.

Tumors are generally named according to the tissue or organ in which they originate, then a suffix is added to denote whether the tumor is benign or malignant (See **Figure 26-4**). The suffix *-oma* literally means "a tumor of" and is construed to mean a benign tumor. Accordingly, a fibroma is a benign tumor of fibrous connective tissue. A lipoma, chondroma, and neuroma are benign tumors of fat, cartilage, and neural tissue, respectively. An adenoma is a benign tumor of glands. Benign tumors are generally slow growing and do not have the metastatic potential of malignant tumors.

Three suffixes identify malignant tumors: *-carcinoma, -sarcoma,* and *-blastoma.* The suffix *-carcinoma* implies a malignant tumor of epithelial origin. For example, *carcinoma* of the lung signifies a malignant tumor derived from epithelium of the lung. Adenocarcinoma of the breast signifies a malignant glandular epithelial tumor of the breast. Squamous cell carcinoma of the skin is a malignant tumor of squamous epithelium of the skin. *Sarcoma* is the designation given to malignant tumors of connective tissue. For example, osteo-sarcoma is a malignant tumor of bone-forming cells. Finally, a group of highly malignant childhood tumors is denoted by the suffix *-blastoma.* These include neuroblastoma, originating in the neuroblasts of the adrenal medulla; retinoblastoma, originating in the retina of the eye; and nephroblastoma, originating in embryonic cells of the kidney.

To really understand cancer physiology, the concept of differentiation must be explained. The term refers to the acquisition of the mature phenotype of cells. It is how embryonic or baby cells grow up to be mature cells. In the embryo, there are three germ (primitive) layers, from which the various organs derive (See **Figure 26-5**). Ectodermal tissue, for example, has the genetic potential to create skin, brain, breast, and sweat gland tissue. The process by which it forms this mature tissue is termed *differentiation*. One must realize, however, that the differentiation process of cells continues throughout a person's life. There is a continual turnover of cells in the human body, with the "old" cells being destroyed and the "young" ones maturing. In a variety of tissues such as the colon, intestines, skin, testis, bronchus, bladder, and bone marrow, tissue renewal is mediated by a population of precisely controlled stem cells. These stem cells are undifferentiated, much like the germ cells discussed above. These undifferentiated stem cells are genetically programmed to differentiate into various adult cell populations (See **Figure 26-6**). Examples of this include blood stem cells that give rise to red blood cells, white blood cells, and platelets and skin stem cells that give rise to the various types of skin cells.

It is now known that the majority of cancers begin when normal stem cells are altered. When given the appropriate environment, these initiated cells will express the malignant phenotype. **Malignant stem cells derived from normal stem cells are undifferenti-**

FIGURE 26-4: CHART OF THE NOMENCLATURE OF CANCER

Origin	Benign	Malignant
Epithelial Endothelial	Adenoma of liver, salivary gland, colon, kidney, breast	Adenocarcinoma of liver salivary gland, colon, kidney, breast
Mesenchymal Connective Tissue	Lipoma Fibroma Chondroma	Liposarcoma Fibrosarcoma Chondrosarcoma
		Neuroblastoma Retinoblastoma Nephroblastoma
Germinal Tumors	Teratoma	Teratocarcinoma Embryonal carcinoma Seminoma
Other		Hepatoma synovioma Melanoma Leukemia

Cancers are often named based on the tissue of origin of the cancer.

FIGURE 26-5: THREE GERM LAYERS AND THE TISSUES DERIVED FROM THEM

EMBRYONIC ORIGIN	ADULT DERIVATIVE
ECTODERM	SKIN
	BRAIN
	BREAST
	SWEAT GLANDS
MESODERM	FIBROUS TISSUE (CONNECTIVE)
	CARTILAGE
	BONE
	MUSCLE
ENDODERM	GUT
	LIVER
	LUNG
	PANCREAS

ated from the outset and bear close resemblance to their normal counterparts.[4,5] Another interesting fact is that if the malignant stem cells differentiate, they always express the appropriate determined phenotype. For example, a breast stem cell that turns malignant always differentiates into breast cancer.

When a cancer is staged, the pathologist is trying to figure out exactly how closely the cancer cells resemble their normal counterparts. If the cancer cell is very dissimilar and has not differentiated, it is called anaplastic, which carries a worse prognosis. Because many of the very aggressive tumors are anaplastic, some oncologists view cancer cells as having a block in differentiation.

It is now accepted unequivocally that some cancer cells can differentiate into terminally differentiated benign, if not normal, cells, whereas others display abortive differentiation. Some display so little differentiation that it is almost impossible to identify the tissue involved and make a diagnosis.

It is now known that even anaplastic cells of cancer have the potential for differentiation, although they may not express it, which rein-

HEMATOPOIESIS

Figure 26-6: Hematopoiesis Chart Depicting a Generalized Version of Blood Cell Lineages

With hematopoiesis, stem cells become blood cells. All the cells of the body come from stem cells.

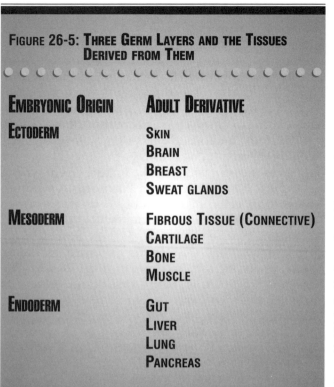

forces the idea that carcinogenesis does not alter the original histiotypic determination of the cells (how they look under the microscope when mature); **it superimposes the malignant phenotype on them.** One of the natural methods of treating cancer is designed to give cancer stem cells an opportunity to differentiate into benign or more normal cells. Cancer cells can only express the normal (nonmalignant) phenotype when placed in the appropriate environment. Substances such as DMSO, vitamin D, butyrate, daidzein, and quercetin help do this.

If a person does not get the malignant stem cells to differentiate, eventually a mass of malignant cells will form. One of the distinguishing features of these malignant cells is that they have lost the capacity for *apoptosis. Apoptosis* is a type of naturally occurring cell death that occurs in healthy tissues. Apoptosis plays many important roles, including eradicating redundant or "old" cell types, removing embryonic tissues to generate the morphology of the adult, balancing the proliferation of renewing tissues to regulate tissue mass, selecting clones during lymphocyte maturation, and removing genetically damaged cells to prevent oncogenesis (cancer forming).[6-8]

The precise control of apoptosis, that is, its regularity, predictability, and localized nature, leads to the notion of an intracellular, genetically programmed pathway that kills a cell from within and protects surrounding cells from the presumed lethal hit inside the cell. Hence the term *programmed cell death* is synonymous with apoptosis. There are known natural substances such as DMSO, genistein, quercetin, and retinoic acid that have been shown to cause a dose-dependent induction of apoptosis in human tumor cell lines. (These are covered in **Chapter 30.**) These substances by way of their ability to induce apoptosis have been shown to at least kill cancer cells in vitro. They are generally given as part of our comprehensive natural medicine program.

Selective apoptosis is generally by "suicide" of the cell from within. However, extracellular substances, such as tumor necrosis factor and monoclonal antibodies against T and B cells, have been shown to trigger apoptosis, as has extracellular hydrogen peroxide.[9,10] This is one of the reasons why hydrogen peroxide and ozone therapy (which raises tumor necrosis factor) are used as part of the IPT protocol at CCINMC. In summary, apoptosis can occur from extracellular factors to which all cells in the vicinity are exposed, but to which only a handful respond. This indicates that apoptosis can be "murder" as well as suicide.

As long as the tumor cells remain localized, there is an enhanced chance of cure. Once the tumor metastasizes, the tumor load starts increasing exponentially, and prognosis is decreased. Thus, understanding the mechanisms of metastases and preventing or curbing them will enhance survival.

It may shock people to know that metastases are not random events. They are distinct events that occur in the metastastic cascade (**See Figure 26-7**). Because metastases occur through an orderly process, disruption of any of the events in the cascade, at least in theory, decreases the chances of disseminated cancer.[11,12]

FIGURE 26-7: EVENTS IN THE METASTATIC CASCADE

★ DISRUPTION IN THE BASEMENT MEMBRANE

★ CELL DETACHMENT (SEPARATION)

★ CELL MOTILITY

★ INVASION

★ PENETRATION OF THE VASCULAR SYSTEM

★ CIRCULATING CANCER CELLS

★ ARREST (STASIS)

★ EXTRAVASATION AND PROLIFERATION

Metastases are a very orderly event.

Most malignancies are carcinomas, which are tumors of epithelial cells. Epithelial cells are supported by basement membranes, which separate epithelial cells from the vasculature. Blood capillaries and lymphatic vessels are not found in epithelia, and epithelial cells must derive their sustenance and oxygen from underlying vascularized connective tissues (See **Figure 26-8**). Thus, basement membranes must be disrupted if carcinoma cells are to gain access to vessels (blood and lymphatic) for subsequent dissemination and formation of metastases.

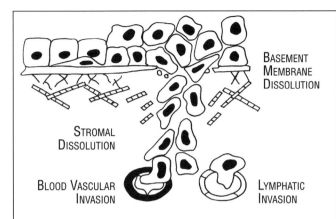

Figure 26-8: Destruction of the Basement Membrane
Metastases start with destruction of the basement membrane and invasion into the blood vasculature and lymphatic system.

BASEMENT MEMBRANE DISSOLUTION

STROMAL DISSOLUTION

BLOOD VASCULAR INVASION

LYMPHATIC INVASION

Basement membranes are made up of Type IV collagen. Destruction of the basement membrane by Type IV collagenase is a common feature of malignancy.[13,14] Collagenases in the body are met-alloproteinases, which are enzymes that require a metal ion for activity. If collagenolytic activity is important in invasion of the basement membrane by cancer cells, then inhibiting the degradation of collagen would impede invasion and metastasis. Metalloproteinases require various metals to function. There is a lot of research going on in regard to metalloproteinase inhibitors. There have been some early successes in helping to retard metastases from forming when metalloproteinase inhibitors are given.[15] The one that we use in our office is tetramolybdate, which binds copper. There are several anecdotal reports of chelation therapy with EDTA and DMPS helping cancer patient survival. Both of these agents are known to bind heavy metals, which is probably the mechanism of how cancer survival is helped by these agents. EDTA is a known inhibitor collagenase[16]—another mechanism in which EDTA chelation therapy could theoretically help cancer patients. Similarly, excess cysteine inhibits both cell detachment and the enzymatic activity of Type I collagenase.[16] This is a basis for using high-dose glutathione in cancer patients. Intravenous glutathione is sometimes given with the IPT treatment.

The next step in the metastatic cascade is cell detachment. Cancer cells have reduced cohesiveness. Ordinarily, normal cells do not separate from their cohorts in a tissue; they stay in place. Cancer cells, however, exhibit a deficiency in cohesiveness, and this loss is essential in the metastatic cascade.[17,18] Normal cells are not easily torn apart, whereas cancer cells separate easily.[19]

Substances that help increase cancer cell cohesiveness would then interrupt the metastatic cascade. It has been observed that EDTA inhibits tumor cell dissociation—another mechanism of action in which EDTA would be expected to help cancer survival. EDTA also decreases platelet stickiness—another way it helps reverse cancer physiology.

Enhanced cell motility is another property of malignant cells. The higher the cell motility in some cancers, the greater the propensity to metastasize. It has been shown in animal studies that cells that have a high cell motility also have a high metastatic competence that is related to the anaerobic capability of the cells themselves.[20-22] This is one mechanism of action of natural remedies that specifically inhibits cancer cell physiology. By inhibiting anaerobic metabolism, cancer cells are inhibited, whereas normal cell physiology is not. This topic is discussed in detail later, but some discussion is warranted now. A high-carbohydrate, sugar-laced diet favors anaerobic metabolism. This causes a person to have very high insulin levels, which are a setup for cancer. Once a person decreases his or her carbohydrate intake, the body goes to a more aerobic metabolism. In a woman, lowering one's estradiol levels will have the same effects. Some of the substances that we use in our office to assist aerobic metabolism are given in **Figure 26-9**. Thus, it is apparent that one of the mechanisms to correct cancer physiology is blocking lactate dehydrogenase and pushing metabolism toward the aerobic side (See **Figure 26-10**). One of the best ways to do this is with aerobic exercise. If someone has the reserve to do it, then maintaining an exercise program is a good idea. We are also quick to prescribe oxygen for our cancer patients. For weak, debilitated cancer patients, some extra oxygen in the air they breathe can do wonders.

FIGURE 26-9: SUBSTANCES THAT ASSIST IN AEROBIC METABOLISM

SUBSTANCE	MECHANISM OF ACTION
ADENOSINE MONOPHOSPHATE (AMP)	PRECURSOR TO ATP (ADENOSINE TRIPHOSPHATE), AEROBIC ENERGY SOURCE
LAURIC ACID	DECREASES LACTIC ACIDOSIS
L-CARNITINE	DECREASES LACTIC ACIDOSIS
MALIC ACID	INHIBITS LACTATE DEHYDROGENASE
NADH (REDUCED NICOTINAMIDE ADENINE DINUCLEOTIDE)	INHIBITS LACTATE DEHYDROGENASE
OZONE	HELPS RED BLOOD CELLS RELEASE OXYGEN
QUERCETIN	INHIBITS LACTATE DEHYDROGENASE

Another method to affect cancer cell motility is by inhibiting the cytoplasmic microtubule complex that is involved in the movement of cancer cells. The chemotherapeutic agents Vinblastine and vincristine depolymerize microtubules and thus inhibit invasion. Adriamycin, a commonly used medication in IPT, also inhibits tumor cell invasion.[23] For some patients at CCINMC, colchicine is prescribed, as it is a well-known microtubule inhibitor commonly used for gout.

Carcinoma cells that have detached from the primary tumor mass, have penetrated the basement membrane, and exhibit motility, now come in contact with connective tissues. This is crucial for the advancing cancer cell because it must get a new blood supply from the capillaries in the connective tissues. One of the methods that

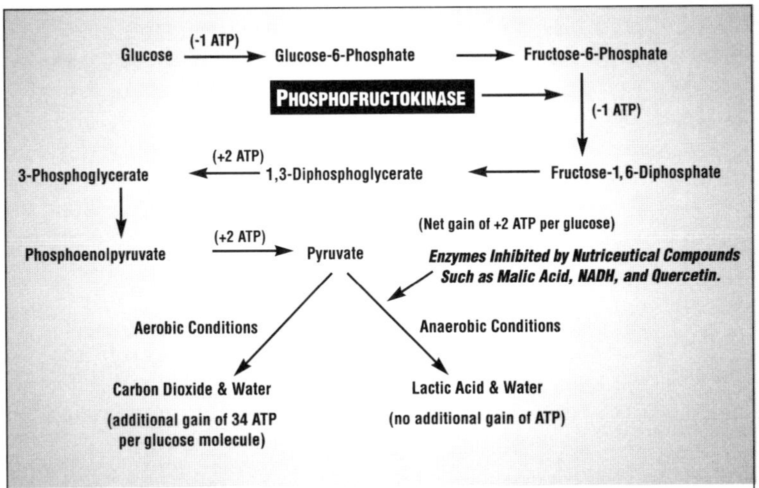

Figure 26-10: The Breakdown of Glucose for Energy
Aerobic metabolism produces much more energy per glucose molecule (36 ATPs) compared to anaerobic metabolism (2 ATPs). Cancer physiology is more anaerobic. Nutritional supplements can help push the physiology toward the aerobic side...

human breast neoplasms, as well as other human malignancies, gain access to the capillaries is by the secretion of Type I collagenase, which degrades Type I collagen, a principal component of the intercellular matrix of connective tissue.[24] Neoplastic cells gain access to small vessels by digesting an opening in the outside wall of the vessel through which they migrate to the lumen. Fortunately, most cancer cells that are exposed to the blood circulation are destroyed or damaged. This is the primary reason cancer cells are not found in the blood of all cancer patients.

Although the circulatory system is a hostile environment for cancer cells, if the cells survive (and some obviously do), they may grow in the vasculature and be swept away to anatomically distant sites. Cancer cells in the circulation adhere to each other and to lymphocytes and platelets, forming emboli. A fibrin-containing thrombus (blood clot) forms, which stabilizes the embolus, increasing the likelihood of cancer cell survival in the circulation. The importance of these microemboli should not be overlooked, as patients on blood-thinning medications, such as Coumadin, have increased survival. Presumably the efficacy of the anticoagulant derives from the dissolution of the clot, resulting in exposure of the cancer cells to the circulation, hastening their death.[25-27] For this reason, interventional natural medicine specialists will use blood-thinning agents such as heparin, Coumadin, or natural substances such as vitamin E, garlic, and essential fatty acids in patients with cancer. We feel so strongly about this that the next chapter is on this topic.

The final stage of the metastatic cascade is the extravasation and growth of the metastases. Extravasation from the blood into the capillaries requires the cancer cell to transgress the basement membrane of the capillary. At this point, the cancer cells are restricted in growth to a lump of 0.5 to 1 mm in diameter due to the limited nutrient supply available by diffusion from the blood. Without angiogenesis, the center of the tumor cell colony becomes necrotic.[28] Angiogenesis is the formation of new blood vessels by the cancer cell mass. Various agents have been shown to successfully inhibit angiogenesis, including genistein, cartilage extracts, interferon-alfa, glutathione, vitamin A, and vitamin D.[29] In regard to a comprehensive natural medicine approach to cancer, along with IPT, we have patients receive interferon-alfa shots (low-dose, immune stimulant), high-dose vitamin A and D, and glutathione when appropriate.

It is evident from this discussion on the process of cancer formation and metastases that **there is nothing a metastatic cell can do that is not a routine task for normal cells.** Thus the inappropriate behavior of cancer cells does not derive from cell properties that develop de novo but is probably related to the expression of otherwise normal cell attributes at an inappropriate time or place. For instance, the condition of endometriosis involves normal endometrial tissue outside the uterus in such structures as the ovaries, uterine tubes, uterine ligaments, and other places. It continues to grow and live outside its normal location. The main treatment for it is surgery and stopping the secretion of the normal female hormones estrogen and progesterone for a time period. At menopause, the condition abates.

This information is important because two thirds of cancer patients have metastases at the time of diagnosis. If by preventive measures we could decrease this figure, the survival rate from cancer would be enhanced greatly; also, if we can decrease the likelihood of future metastases while a person is undergoing an aggressive treatment, such as IPT, the odds of survival will be increased. Though this is important, it is still the goal of successful cancer therapy to concentrate on the primary tumor. This is the "hub" of the cancer and utilizes various methods to steal "food" from the body and elude cancer detection.

Unfortunately, even in the new millennium, people are of the mind-set that a "magic bullet" or medication will be found to treat cancer, primarily as a result of the successes in the antibiotic treatment of infectious diseases. This concept was well explained in a *New England Journal of Medicine* paper on cancer by George Weber, M.D.[30]

> The success in the treatment of infectious diseases is in contrast to the failure in the therapy of most neoplastic disorders. On the average, 50 percent of patients with cancer die of the disease, even if the best therapeutic modalities are applied. Few, if any, infectious diseases still have a 50 percent mortal-

ity after early, appropriate chemotherapy (drug therapy).

> The main differences are that in neoplasia, the cells to be destroyed are not foreign but those of the host, the immunologic processes do not appear to have the same dramatic role as in infectious diseases, the growth fraction is variable, and **total** kill of the cancer cells is probably necessary. The low growth fraction in many of the common solid tumors makes treatment particularly difficult. As pointed out by Frei and Zubrod the pharmacologic sensitivity of human tumors is related to the growth rate and growth fraction: the rapidly growing tumors with the largest growth fraction are the most sensitive to chemotherapy. Selective chemotherapy is available for many infectious diseases, and combination chemotherapy is avoided if a therapeutic alternative exists. In successful treatment of human neoplasia, combination chemotherapy, with expertly designed pharmacology, is essential; curative results have been achieved in 10 of approximately 100 neoplastic disorders in man.

It is important for everyone involved in cancer therapy to understand the success rates of traditional allopathic therapy. The following is a good summary and is taken from the Pezcoller Prize lecture given by Maurice Tubiana at the European Congress of Oncology and subsequently printed in the *European Journal of Cancer*.[31]

> The contribution of local control in the cure of cancer remains a matter of crucial importance. At diagnosis approximately 70% of patients with cancer have no detectable distant metastasis and over half of them are cured by loco-regional treatment only. In western Europe and the USA, out of 100 patients with cancer, approximately 22% are cured by surgery, 18% by radiotherapy (alone or associated with other agents in a combination in which radiotherapy has the prominent role) and 5% by chemotherapy (alone or in combination but with the leading role to chemotherapy). Since the use of combination treatments is becoming of increasing importance, these figures are tentative.

> Suit has stressed that one third of patients who die do so as a consequence of failure to control loco-regional diseases. This is particularly the case in patients with head and neck, gynaecological, genito-urinary and gastrointestinal

cancer, bone and soft tissue sarcomas, and tumours of the central nervous system. Hence, one of the main potential sources of progress is to improve loco-regional control. However, since approximately half the patients whose death is caused by local extension have occult metastases at the time of initial treatment, the potential benefit related to an improvement in local control amounts to only 8-10% of patients. Nevertheless about half of the progress in the cure rate which can be expected in the next two decades will result from advances in local treatment and the other half from advances in systemic treatment. These two fields of research are not competitive but complementary.

Thus,

- Local control of cancer is important, but will not be the cure for cancer.

- The person relying on local treatments only for his or her cancer is taking a very big chance of recurrence.

- Modern systemic high-dose chemotherapy has a very poor success rate in 90% of cancers.

- Allopathic state-of-the-art oncology has essentially no good systemic treatments for cancer in the way they are currently administered.

The premise for people with cancer and those treating them is to understand cancer physiology because this is one of the keys to successful treatment.

Most people understand that, in general, cancer cells grow at a much more rapid rate than normal cells. This is most evident by measuring the amount of DNA synthesis versus its breakdown in cancer cells. The key enzymes involved in DNA synthesis increase in activity manifold, whereas there is a decrease in the catabolic enzyme activity in parallel with tumor growth rate.[30] The absolute values of the various enzyme activities can easily be contrasted, comparing the cells of a normal liver with those of a liver tumor. The tumor cells show a tremendous increase in activity.[31] These studies support the notion that there is a definite, significant difference in the activities of these enzymes between cancer cells and normal cells. In regard to DNA synthesis, the best medications to stop the enzyme activity

involved in this are chemotherapy drugs. The mechanism of action of many chemotherapeutic agents is by inhibiting the various enzymes involved in DNA synthesis, as has already been discussed. The only problem is that the medications are not targeted in traditional high-dose chemotherapy. They are targeted to a large degree by Insulin Potentiation Therapy, which is the rationale for the success of IPT compared to traditional chemotherapy. See the contrast of the two in **Figure 26-11**.

IPT uses the differences in DNA synthesis between cancer cells and normal cells and then potentiates the effects because of the insulin given. There are other methods that should also be used by the cancer patient to take advantage of other ways in which cancer cells differ from normal cells, and these form the basis of reversing cancer physiology.

FIGURE 26-11: A COMPARISON OF TRADITIONAL CHEMOTHERAPY AND IPT

	TRADITIONAL CHEMOTHERAPY	IPT
ENERGY LEVEL	TERRIBLE	GREAT
EXPERIENCE	LIKE HELL	LIKE HEAVEN
FREQUENCY	LOW (GIVEN EVERY 3 TO 4 WEEKS)	HIGH (GIVEN ONCE TO TWICE/WEEK)
HAIR	LOST	KEPT
HOW THEY FEEL DURING	WORSE	BETTER
IMMUNE SYSTEM	SUPPRESSED	STIMULATED
MENTAL STATUS	DEPRESSED/FATIGUED	ENCOURAGED
SIDE EFFECTS	HIGH	LOW
SUCCESS	POOR	HIGH

CANCER PHYSIOLOGY VERSUS NORMAL CELL PHYSIOLOGY

In simplistic terms, **Figure 26-12** shows the differences between normal and cancer cell physiology. Some of the differences between normal and cancer physiology have already been explained, but further detail is needed to understand the natural and synthetic remedies that are available to reverse cancer physiology.

DIFFERENTIATION

Cancer cells form from stem cells that do not differentiate or mature normally. Stem cells are capable of both self-renewal (self-replacement) and clonal expansion and, therefore, appear immortal.

FIGURE 26-12: DIFFERENCES BETWEEN NORMAL CELLS AND CANCER CELLS

	Normal	Cancer
Differentiation	Cells mature	Cells stop maturing
Apoptosis	Cells die	Cells don't die
Platelets/fibrin	Normal	Sticky
Angiogenesis	Very little	A lot
Metabolism	Aerobic	Anaerobic
Energy source	Oxygen	Sugar
pH	Normal	Acid at site, alkaline in blood
Cells	Repel one another	Adhesion (stick) to each other

Under normal circumstances, stem cells act as a source of new cells during tissue repair. Under cancerous conditions, the proliferation of stem cells is unchecked. Furthermore, their daughter cells do not fully differentiate or acquire the functions of more mature cells. If they did differentiate, their ability to proliferate would be reduced.

Stem cells are present in high numbers in tissues that constantly renew their population, such as bone marrow and the intestinal lining. Bone marrow cells have a turnover rate of approximately five days, as opposed to several years for some vascular cells.[32]

One of the ways tumor cells can be classified is by their level of differentiation. Tumor grade indicates the degree of differentiation in the tumor as a whole. Tumors that are poorly differentiated generally grow faster and are assigned a higher grade. The opposite is true for tumors that are well differentiated. If tumor cells do not differentiate, the tumor is called anablastic (literally, not formed). These tumors are especially lethal.

The progression of some malignancies is thought to be due to a block in differentiation. Agents that induce differentiation may be useful in treating these malignancies. A number of natural agents demonstrate the ability to induce differentiation in human leukemia, melanoma, colon carcinoma, bladder carcinoma, brain cancer, as well as in a variety of animal cell lines. When these cells are exposed to differentiating agents, they can develop into normal cells and lose their ability to proliferate. Natural agents that induce differentiation are listed in **Figure 26-13**. Many of these agents are used at Caring Medical for our cancer patients. Two of the more common

agents are high-dose vitamin A (or its derivatives) and vitamin D. In addition, high-dose intravenous DMSO is utilized because it induces differentiation in a wide range of human neoplastic cell lines in vitro (See **Figure 26-14**). DMSO crosses the blood-brain barrier and cell membranes and can potentiate the effects of chemotherapy, making it an excellent adjunctive treatment with IPT.

FIGURE 26-13: NATURAL AGENTS THAT INDUCE DIFFERENTIATION IN VITRO

BERBERINE	CHAN SU	BUTYRIC ACID
BROMELAIN	CYTOKINES	DAIDZEIN
TRYPSIN	DOCOSAHEXAENOIC ACID	
CHYMOTRYPSIN	NIU BANG ZI	
DING XIANG	LING ZHI	RETINOIC ACID
VITAMIN D_3	DMSO	QUERCETIN

The concept of "once a cancer cell, always a cancer cell" is just not true. This is because a tumor is a dynamic system composed of malignant stem cells and their well-differentiated and benign progeny, admixed to form a caricature of the tissue of origin. Malignant stem cells are responsive to environmental controls and are derived from normal stem cells by a process equivalent to a postembyronic differentiation. Thus, neoplasms have their origin in the process of tissue maintenance and renewal.[29] According to G. Barry Pierce from the Department of Pathology at the University of Colorado Medical

FIGURE 26-14: CELL LINES THAT DIFFERENTIATE IN RESPONSE TO DMSO IN VITRO

CELL LINE

◆ HUMAN PROMYELOCYTIC LEUKEMIA (HL-60)

◆ HUMAN HEPATOMA (PLC/PRF/5) AND HUMAN HEPATOBLASTOMA (HEP G2)

◆ HUMAN OVARIAN CARCINOMA (AMOC-2)

◆ HUMAN RHABDOMYOSARCOMA (A-673, RD, AND A-204)

◆ CULTURED HUMAN T LYMPHOMA

◆ HUMAN NEUROBLASTOMA (SH-SY5Y)

◆ SIX HUMAN GLIOMA CELL LINES

◆ HUMAN MELANOMA (MM96E)

DMSO also helps transport substances into cells and across the blood-brain barrier, making it an excellent adjunctive treatment with IPT.

PROLIFERATION OF MALIGNANT STEM CELLS

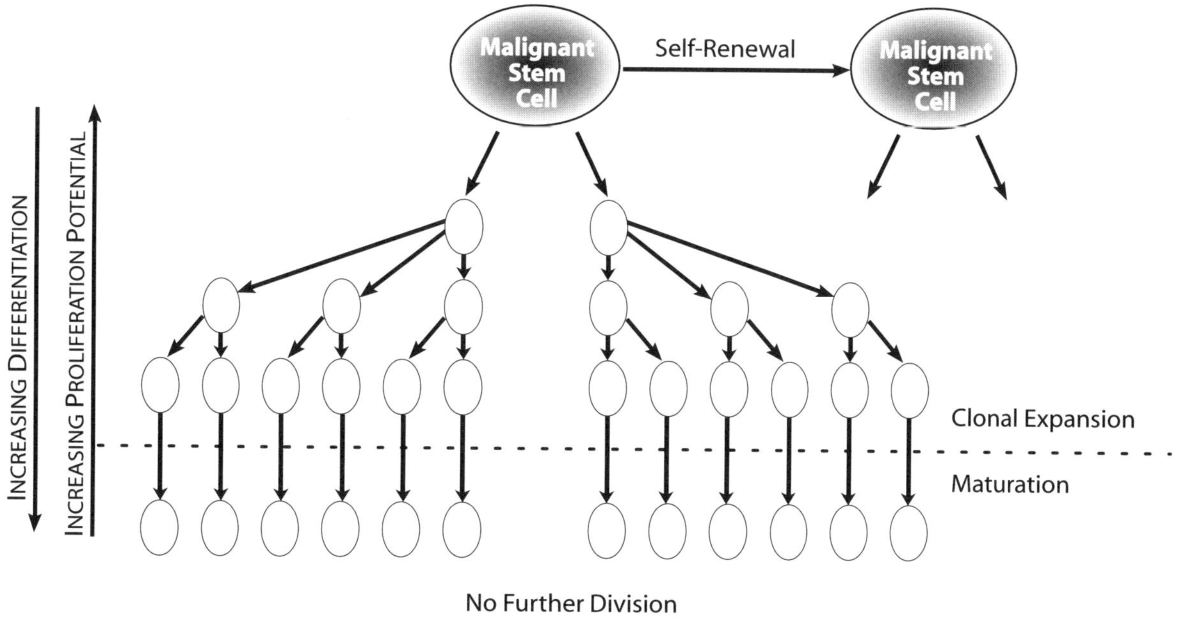

Figure 26-15: Proliferation of Malignant Stem Cells
Inducing malignant stem cells to differentiate makes them less aggressive. In certain situations they can become benign cells.

School, in research supported in part by the American Cancer Society and the National Institutes of Health:

> On the basis of experiments employing cloning, isotope tracer, and electron-microscopic techniques, the premise has been established that stem cells of malignant tumors differentiate, an observation compatible with the idea that the target in carcinogenesis is the normal stem cell of the particular tissue, and that the lesion produced by carcinogenesis is a change in the controls governing the expression of differentiation by malignant stem cells.[33]

These facts suggest that we can induce differentiation in the cancer cells to form less aggressive cancer or benign cells (See **Figure 26-15**).

APOPTOSIS

Uncontrolled cell proliferation is the hallmark of cancer. The goal of cytotoxic chemotherapy has always been to produce tumor cell necrosis.

There is another way in which tumor cells die, apoptosis. Cancer cells have lost the ability to die at the same rate as normal cells. There are normal cells in the body that proliferate rapidly, such as those that line the stomach or accommodate bone marrow. In contrast to cancer cells, however, these cells have a limited life span, so under normal conditions the numbers of these cells do not continue to grow, only repopulate.

Apoptosis or programmed cell death is a genetically controlled response for cells to commit suicide. Programmed cell death occurs during normal development and differentiation. Each mature cell of the body has a normal life span; for the red blood cell, this is 120 days. By day 121, the old red blood cell is replaced by a new one. In cancer cells, no such programmed cell death occurs, which leads to cancer cells being called "immortal." The goal of reversing cancer physiology is to cause them to die or induce apoptosis. Apoptosis is in many respects, tied to differentiation, because if a cancer cell differentiates, it will in some measure "regain" the ability to die.

Many of the same natural agents that induce differentiation also induce apoptosis. This includes DMSO, quercetin, retinoic acid, and vitamin D_3. Other agents that have been found to induce apoptosis in cancer cell lines include mistletoe (a common cancer remedy in Europe), genistein, and the Chinese herbal formula xiao chai hu tang.[32] One must remember that most of the studies done on cancer cells are in vitro (in the laboratory), not in vivo (in the human body). Many of the natural agents do have potent cancer-killing effects in vitro. Researchers at the Prefectural University of Medicine in Kamigyo-ku, Kyoto, Japan, showed that quercetin, a flavonoid found in many plants, markedly inhibited the growth of human gastric cancer cells[34] (See **Figure 26-16**). Another potent natural inducer of apoptosis is genistein, an isoflavone found in legumes. Researchers at the Department of Clinical Chemistry, the University of Helsinki, Finland, showed significant effects in suppressing the proliferation of liver cancer cells.[35]

The obvious question in regard to apoptosis is how come the cancer cell does not differentiate or die a normal programmed cell death? It appears that two of the main factors that cause cancer cells to grow and subsequently be resistant to apoptosis are insulin and IGF-1 (insulin-like growth factor). As can be seen in **Figure 26-17**, for the cancer cell to go through the cell cycle, various types of growth factors are required, including insulin and IGF-1.[36,37] M. Resnicoff and associates at Thomas Jefferson University in Philadelphia conducted several studies and found that **there was a direct correlation on the amount of IGF-1 receptors on cancer cells and their ability to resist apoptosis.**[38-40]

Evidence is rapidly accumulating that the IGF-1 activated by its ligands plays a crucial role in cell proliferation in at least three different ways: **(A)** it is mitogenic; **(B)** it is required in several types of malignancies for the establishment and maintenance of the transformed phenotype and for tumorigenesis; and **(C)** it protects tumor cells from apoptosis, both in vitro and in vivo.[38]

Cancer uses these IGF-1 receptors to protect itself, and IPT physicians use them to bomb the cancer with targeted chemotherapy. By giving insulin, which cross-reacts with the IGF-1 receptor, the cancer cell is fooled into thinking it is growth time, but low-dose chemotherapy is then given. While the IPT is working, funeral arrangements are made for the cancer cells. This is another reason why understanding cancer physiology is one of the keys to success.

BLOOD COAGULOPATHY: THE MEANS BY WHICH CANCER PHYSIOLOGY INDUCES ANGIOGENESIS

The blood-clotting cascade system is necessary for survival. It is the way we stop bleeding when we cut ourselves. The essential feature of blood clotting is the formation of many interlocking strands of fibers (fibrin) that form a strong, stable network that prevents the further leakage of blood. If, however, the body forms too much fibrin, excessive clotting will occur, which can have a damaging effect on circulation. The process by which a blood clot is dissolved is fibrinolysis. A healthy circulatory system then has a fine balance between the amount of blood clotting (coagulation) and blood clot dissolving (fibrinolysis).

Numerous authors have reported reduced fibrinolysis in humans with neoplastic diseases.[41-43] The end result is an accumulation of fibrin sufficient to produce a provisional fibrin stroma surrounding the tumor.

The fibrin stroma provides a structure that physically supports the tumor. In the early stage

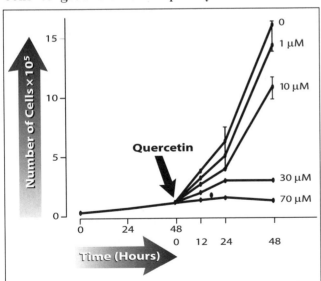

Figure 26-16: *Effects of Quercetin on the Growth of Gastric Cancer Cells*

Various concentrations of quercetin were added on the second day after inoculation of the cells. The values represent means ± SD. The arrow indicates when quercetin was added. The study showed that quercetin had a potent effect by decreasing growth of these cancer cells.

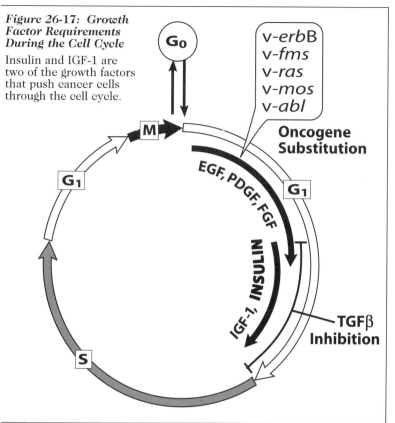

Figure 26-17: Growth Factor Requirements During the Cell Cycle

Insulin and IGF-1 are two of the growth factors that push cancer cells through the cell cycle.

the immune system and thus is not detected as a tumor by the immune system (i.e., natural killer cells). When tumors are prepared for in vitro assays against drugs, they are routinely treated with proteolytic enzymes (eg, pepsin or chymotrypsin) that dissolve the protein coat, exposing the tumor cell surface to the drug. Thus, the in vivo existence of a coat on the tumor surface may explain why some drugs have little or no effect in vivo, while the same drugs are active in vitro.[50]

Fibrinolysis is diminished in cancer patients, but it still exists. Up to 90% of fibrinogen (the precursor of fibrin) may be degraded immediately. Research suggests that fibrin degradation products appear to play a significant role in angiogenesis. In normal wound healing, once fibrinolysis is complete, angiogenesis stops. However, in the case of a tumor, inflammation continues, as does fibrin production and degradation. Therefore, angiogenesis is continuous in tumors.[44]

Angiogenesis is the means by which the cancer continues to grow. By increasing new blood vessel formation, the cancer has an unlimited food supply, as long as the host is alive. Thus, fibrin formation and systemic inflammation are important because they are the means by which tumor-associated angiogenesis is propagated.

The best approach to stop angiogenesis in cancer patients is not by taking shark cartilage but by stopping the *reason* for the angiogenesis. The first step would be to take natural supplements that either stop fibrin formation or stimulate fibrinolysis. Once fibrinolysis is complete, angiogenesis stops.

In documenting cancer physiology, Caring Medical routinely does blood tests to measure coagulation parameters in cancer patients. Some of the more common tests done are discussed in the next chapter, as well as how to reverse the coagulopathy that occurs with cancer physiology.

New blood vessel formation needs to be slowed in a cancer patient because tumor angiogenesis permits metastasis. Briefly, for metastases to form, the tumor cells must gain access to the vasculature, survive in the circulation, arrest in the

of tumor growth, the fibrin stroma encases individual tumor cells or clumps of tumor cells. The stroma in some tumors can comprise up to 90% of a tumor's mass.[44,45]

This accumulation of fibrin, in and around the tumor, appears to be important for tumor survival against the immune system and medical treatments. In vitro and in vivo studies have shown that warfarin (Coumadin), a blood thinner that prevents the red or fibrin part of a blood clot, increased the efficacy in which chemotherapy was cytotoxic to tumor cell lines, thus enhancing cancer patient survival.[46-48] Increased survival was also shown when the formation of the white or platelet thrombus was decreased by giving cancer patients dipyridamole.[49]

There has been speculation as to why there is an increase in coagulation. The situation with cancer might be akin to pregnancy, in which the placenta contains a layer of fibrin (Nitabuch's layer) that presents as "self" to the immune system. **This fibrin "coat" that the tumor puts on may be the mechanism by which it goes undetected by the immune system.** By using host proteins to make a fibrin shield, the coated tumor appears as "self" to

microvasculature of the target organ, exit from this vasculature, grow in the target organ, and induce angiogenesis. Angiogenesis is necessary at the beginning as well as at the end of this cascade of events[51,52] (See **Figure 26-18**). The clinical significance of this can be seen when one considers that the number of microvessels in a cancer mass correlates to the percentage chance of having metastasis (See **Figure 26-19**). In invasive breast cancer, there is a significant, direct correlation between the highest density of microvessels in a histological section and the occurrence of metastases.

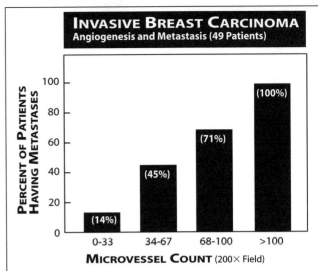

Figure 26-19: Invasive Breast Carcinoma
Metastatic disease among 49 patients in relation to microvessel count in progressive increments. The incidence of metastatic disease increases as vessel counts in the primary tumor increase, reaching 100% among patients with counts above 100 per $200 \times$ field.

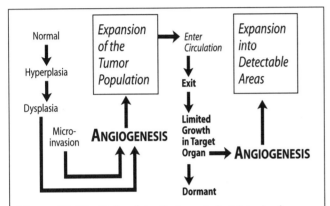

Figure 26-18: Role of Angiogenesis in Metastasis
In this diagram, angiogenesis occurs at the beginning of the metastatic cascade. It permits expansion of the tumor population, and it permits tumor cells to enter the circulation. Angiogenesis may also occur at the end of the metastatic cascade, where it permits expansion of the metastatic implant. A metastatic implant that is not angiogenic may remain as undetectable micrometastasis. Lack of angiogenic activity may be one cause of tumor dormancy.

It appears that tumor growth is angiogenesis dependent. One study showed a 400% increase in vascular density in tumors over normal tissue.[53] Some cancers cannot grow greater than 1-2 mm in diameter unless there is a proliferation of new blood vessel formation.[54,55] Once new blood vessels have formed, the cancer may enter a phase of rapid growth, including metastases. The endothelial cells that line the myriad of new blood vessels secrete growth factors, including FGF (fibroblastic growth factor), PDGF (platelet-derived growth factor), IGF-1, prostaglandins, cytokines such as the interleukins IL-1 and IL-6, and GM-CSF (granulocyte-macrophage colony-stimulating factor), which augment tumor growth and further angiogenesis.[55]

The scenario in which growth factors prostaglandins, and cytokines stimulate angiogenesis is complex, and an in-depth review is beyond the scope of this book, but simple approaches can be taken to reverse this aspect of cancer physiology. Recent research has shown that prostaglandins are involved in the formation of tumor angiogenesis.[56,57] The enzyme that catalyzes the committed step in the synthesis of prostaglandins is cyclooxygenase. This enzyme can be easily blocked by various natural and synthetic medications. Some of these are being used by traditional oncologists for their cancer patients, including anti-inflammatory medications.

Some of the growth factors, such as FGF and IGF-1 that induce angiogenesis, can be secreted by the tumor itself. Thus, decreasing these depends on killing the cancer, which is where IPT comes in. Others such as PDGF are secreted by platelets. Platelets are important in cancer because platelet aggregation is an important mechanism that allows metastasis. Activated platelets are sticky and enhance the adhesion of tumor cells to the endothelial lining. Tumors promote platelet aggregation by stimulating the production of thromboxane and/or by inhibiting the production of prostacyclin.

Possible Results of Reversing Cancer Physiology

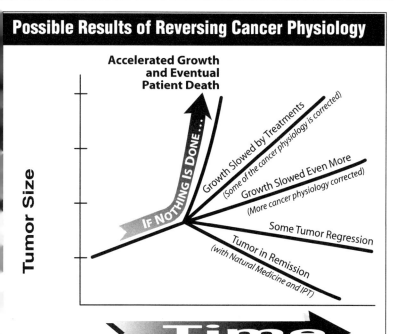

Figure 26-20: *Some Possible Results of Reversing Cancer Physiology*

The general response to reversing cancer physiology with natural medicine is a substantial slowing of tumor growth. If the treatment plan corrects enough of the cancer physiology, some tumor regression is possible. For complete tumor regression, generally an aggressive treatment, such as IPT, is needed.

GOALS OF REVERSING CANCER CELL PHYSIOLOGY

The obvious goal of reversing cancer cell physiology is tumor regression and cure. The varied effectiveness of this can be seen in **Figure 26-20.** When all the mechanisms of tumor survival have been removed, then a cancer cure is obtained. This is why most doctors who do natural medicine and/or IPT use a comprehensive approach to cancer therapy. IPT is used as the main treatment to kill the cancer cells, but other interventional techniques such as intravenous DMSO, ozone therapy, chelation, diet, and nutritional supplementation are given to affect the other variables of cancer survival. ■

There are various tests that can be done in the blood, including fibrinogen, fibrinogen split products, platelet aggregation study, and platelet levels. From our experience, when an individual's platelet counts start rising, it is likely that the cancer is spreading. Cancer physiology is evident by an elevated fibrinogen and platelet aggregation study. Fortunately, there are numerous natural agents that inhibit platelet aggregation and thus reverse this aspect of cancer physiology, as we will see in the next chapter...we have to do something to keep your interest.

CHAPTER 27

The Cancer Clotting Coat

THE FIBRIN COAT, IN TURN, CAUSES NEOPLASTIC CELLS NOT TO BE RECOGNIZED BY THE IMMUNOLOGICAL SYSTEM AND THUS MAKES THEM IMMUNE TO THE ATTACK BY THE NATURAL KILLER CELLS.

–L.G. Egyud and B. Lipinski, Medical Hypothesis, 1991

I (Ross) have spent much of the last 10 years studying the physiology of cancer. My motivation came from my mother and mother-in-law who had breast cancer; my pastor and friend who died at the age of 42 from immunoblastic lymphoma; and the matriarch of my family, my grandmother Eve Groobman who died from colon cancer. Currently, my aunt Karen is struggling for her life from colon cancer. Cancer has hit me personally, and almost every day I see it in the eyes of my patients.

Most of the cancer patients whom I see have very strong immune systems. They do not get colds and are very seldom sick and when tested, their immune systems are found to be within normal limits. The obvious question then to ask is, "How does the cancer escape immune detection and destruction?"

In most cases, stimulation of the immune system is insufficient therapy to cause tumor regression. Immune system stimulation is helpful to overcome cancer after radiation therapy or chemotherapy, but in and of itself, it cannot cause tumor regression. In studying cancer's ability to escape immune detection, the model that most correlates with it is the fetus in the placenta. As it turns out, the mechanism by which a human embryo is protected from rejection by the mother's immune system is similar to that which occurs with cancer. The amniotic fluid has a substantial amount of fibronectin, which protects the baby. Fibronectin is a large glycoprotein that binds to collagen near the cleavage site for collagenase. The "normal" fibronectin plays an important role in the adhesion of cells to the extracellular matrix. It is also involved in cell migration, by providing a binding site for cells, and thus helping them to steer their way through the extracellular matrix.[1] The fibronectin from amniotic fluid contains an irreversible inhibitor of collagenase.[2] Collagenase is an enzyme that degrades collagen and allows the penetration of substances into the extracellular matrix. Obviously, it would be harmful to the baby if the mother's immune system gained access to the baby and attacked it, so the amniotic fluid contains a collagenase inhibitor from fibronectin.

In regard to cancer, tumors are contained by a protein coat that is composed primarily of fibronectin.[3] Unlike normal fibronectin, this fibrin type is resistant to fibrinolysis (breakdown of fibrin). This unusual resistance of fibrin deposits in cancer tissue to fibrinolysis has been reported by several authors.[4,5] This is one way in which cancer

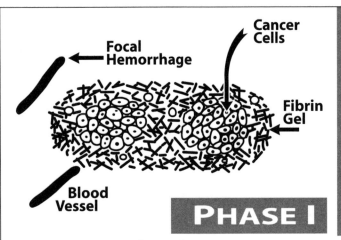
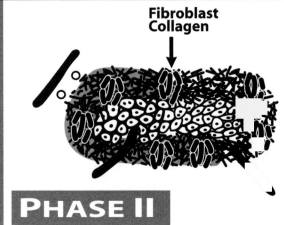

Figure 27-1: Cancer Clotting Coat
Cancers, by forming fibrin gel coats, can wall themselves off from immune attacks.

avoids immune detection. Cancers very early in their development can form a fibrin gel coat. When fibroblasts deposit some collagen in it, it provides a great shield against immune attack (See **Figure 27-1**). We call this fibrin-protein barrier the cancer clotting coat. Of interest is the fact that a woman's uterus is also loaded with a type of fibrin that is resistant to fibrinolytic degradation. It is believed that the fibrin deposits form a barrier against destruction by the mother's immune system.[6,7] It is likely that this fibrin gel is what allows a cancer to grow and eventually metastasize without an immune system attack and destruction (See **Figure 27-2**).

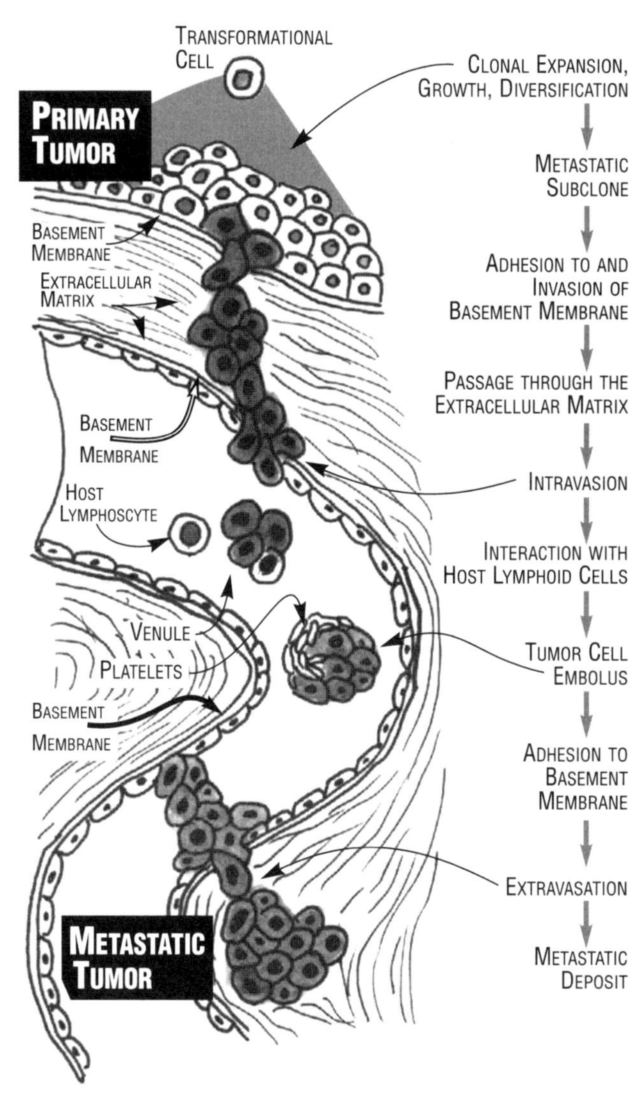

To better understand the cancer clotting coat, it will be necessary to look at the normal blood clotting cascade system. Once a blood vessel starts leaking, there are various events that occur to stop the further leakage of blood. The first four events occur within seconds and depend on platelet aggregation. The platelets strongly adhere to the collagen that was broken up to cause the leakage in the first place. The end result is a platelet plug. The platelets in the plug release substances that assist in the formation of thrombin, which activates the blood coagulation system. The essential feature of blood clotting is the formation of many interlocking strands of fibers (fibrin), forming a strong stable network that stops the blood loss (See **Figure 27-3**).

The cancer clotting coat is composed of some type of fibrinlike substance that is resistant to the normal fibrin degradation processes that occur in the body. This is part of the physiology that occurs with malignancy. This abnormal blood clotting is easy to document by platelet aggregation and immune system activation of coagulation testing. In platelet aggregation studies, a person's platelets are subjected to collagen, thrombin, ADP (adenosine diphosphate), and epinephrine; the majority of cancer patients show abnormal agglutination (See **Figure 27-4**). In the immune system activation of the coagulation cascade, the various levels of coagulation factors are monitored, including tissue factor (a procoagulant), which is often elevated. These tests document that the person with cancer has blood that clots too much or is too thick. (In the unsophisticated lingo of Dr. Hauser, "Ma'am, your blood has the consistency of split pea soup.")

Figure 27-2: Cascade of Events Leading to Metastasis
The tumor cell embolism evades immune system attack because of the cancer clotting coat.

FIGURE 27-3: THE NORMAL BLOOD CLOTTING SEQUENCE OF EVENTS IN A SMALL BLOOD VESSEL

1. Initial Constriction of the Damaged Vessel

2. Sticking Together of the Injured Endothelium

3. Clumping of Platelets to Form a Plug

4. Facilitation of the Initial Vasoconstriction

5. Blood Coagulation, ie, Formation of a Fibrin Clot

6. Retraction of the Clot

It is clear in some tumor lines that the cancer very quickly walls itself off with a cancer clotting coat, sometimes producing a complete fibrin gel within days.[8] The fibrin gel is replaced by a fibrin stroma filled with connective tissue components,

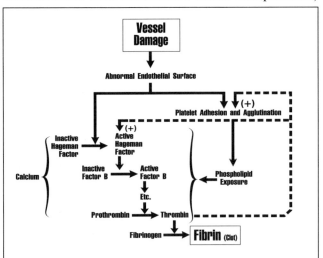

Figure 27-4: Summary of the Blood Clotting Mechanism

The dashed line indicates the positive feedback effect of thrombin on platelet adhesion. The end result of this process is a fibrin clot.

including collagen. As already stated, this cancer clotting coat enables the cancer to escape immune detection. It also has other important duties that help ensure cancer survival. This fibrin stroma provides a structure that physically supports the tumor, but perhaps even more importantly, this fibrin stroma appears to be the single most important precondition for angiogenesis[9,10] (new blood vessel formation). Studies show that the removal of fibrin through fibrinolysis terminates angiogenesis.[11]

There is obviously a practical reason to study blood coagulation in cancer patients. The literature documents that cancer patients experience an increased incidence of thombotic episodes (clotting episodes such as leg or lung blood clots) compared to the normal population or to noncancer hospitalized patients.[12] In particular, patients with adenocarcinomas, including those with breast cancer, have a relatively high incidence of such episodes.[13] It also appears that a cancer patient's clotting profile becomes even worse with high-dose chemotherapy.[14] It has also been documented that the more procoagulant the serum in a cancer cell line, the more virulent the cancer. Numerous other researchers have reported reduced fibrinolysis in people with cancer.[15-17]

FIGURE 27-5: CLOTTING SYSTEM ANALYSIS DURING DIFFERENT CYCLES OF CHEMOTHERAPY

The coagulation cascade is activiated by high-dose chemotherapy. This just enhances the cancer physiology that is already present.

CLOTTING FACTORS	BASAL VALUES	FIRST CYCLE‡ FIFTH DAY	SECOND CYCLE‡ (5TH DAY)
DD (ng/ml)	167.8	107.2*	92.4*
PAP (µg/ml)	0.9	0.7	0.7*
FAP (µg/ml)	3.1	2.8	3.0
FBG (mg/dl)	415.2	339.3†	337.4†
TAT (ng/ml)	2.9	3.8*	5.4*
PT (second)	11.0	10.6†	10.7*
APTT (second)	39.7	34.8†	35.3†
AT-III (%)	110.1	94.9	108.4

*$P < 0.05$ compared to basal values. †$P < 0.01$ compared to basal values.
‡Values are from the fifth day of chemotherapy. Values are expressed as mean.

LEGEND:

TAT = Thrombin-antithrombin III complex
PT = Prothrombin Time
APTT = Activated Partial Thromboplastin Time
AT-III = Antithrombin III
DD = D-dimer
PAP = Plasmin-α_2-Antiplasmin Complex

FDP = Fibrin Degradation Product
FBG = Fibrinogen
SCLC = Small Cell Lung Cancer
Non-SCLC = Non-Small Cell Lung Cancer
NV = Normal Values

An increased incidence of thrombosis or blood clot formation has long been recognized in malignancy.[12,18] The frequency of such a complication ranges from 5% to 10%, compared to an incidence of 0.1% in the general population.[19] By this alone, it is clear that cancer is a "procoagulant state." What most people do not realize is that high-dose chemotherapy also produces a "procoagulant state."[14] **So for the person receiving high-dose chemotherapy, the treatment itself is contributing to his or her cancer physiology.**

As a side note, it is common for patients with cancer, especially lymphomas, to be given corticosteroids. There has been a very well-established association between steroid therapy and thromboembolic complications.[20] This is one of the reasons why, whenever possible, physicians who utilize IPT do not typically administer steroids and use low-dose versus high-dose chemotherapy.

BLOOD COAGULATION AND ANTICOAGULATION

To further hammer this point home, consider just one study. Researchers at the Mie University School of Medicine in Tsu City, Japan, studied the blood coagulation parameters of 25 lung cancer patients before and after high-dose chemothera-

py.[21] D-dimer, plasmin-α-antiplasmin complex, fibrin degradation products, fibrinogen, antithrombin III, thrombin-antithrombin III complex, prothrombin time, and activated partial thromboplastin time were the parameters measured. Thirteen patients had stage IV cancer, 13 had non-small cell lung cancer, and 12 had small cell lung cancer. The patients were treated with cisplatin, Mitomycin, vindesine, and/or Etoposide. The study found a significant reduction in the plasma concentration of the fibrinolytic activity markers D-dimer and plasmin-α-antiplasmin complex following the administration of chemotherapeutic drugs. There was also a significant shortening of prothrombin and partial thromboplastic times and a significant elevation of the thrombin generation marker (See **Figure 27-5**). The authors concluded:

> These results show that relatively higher levels of coagulation activation and a lower fibrinolytic activity occur during cytotoxic drug therapy compared with basal values.... The results of this investigation suggest that an imbalance of the coagulation-fibrinolysis system might be a contributing factor in the pathogenesis of thrombotic complications during chemotherapy.

"Nearly all patients with cancer manifest laboratory evidence of hypercoagulability, and some develop clinical thromboembolic disease." These are not the words of Ross Hauser, but of F. R. Rickles of the Division of Hematology-Oncology from the University of Connecticut School of Medicine as published in *Cancer and Metastasis Reviews*.[22] This altered coagulability is noted throughout the oncology literature but is not being utilized clinically by the majority of oncologists to help patients reverse their cancer physiology. This abnormal clotting is so significant that some have noted that it is a more accurate measure than mammography when contemplating a biopsy on a breast lesion. In other words, having abnormal blood clotting was more diagnostic of a cancer on biopsy than an abnormal mammogram[23] (See **Figure 27-6**). This is not to say that women should not get mammograms, but it does say **that everyone with cancer should consider testing of blood coagulation parameters.**

The practical side of this discussion is to document that the person with cancer has "thick

---

FIGURE 27-6: COMPARISON OF MAMMOGRAPHY AND RECALCIFICATION TIMES OF THE ENDOTOXIN-INCUBATED SAMPLE (RTE) AS SCREENING TESTS FOR BREAST CANCER

This study showed that abnormal blood clotting was a better indicator than mammography in distinguishing benign from cancerous lesions.

	NONADVANCED CANCER	BENIGN BREAST DISEASE
MAMMOGRAPHY*		
Cancer positive	12	53
Cancer negative	11	15
TOTAL	23	68
RTE†		
≤ 4.4	23	37
≥ 4.4	0	31
TOTAL	23	68

*Sensitivity = 12/23 = 52% (Cl$_{95}$ = 31% to 73%) and specificity = 15/68 = 22% (Cl$_{95}$ = 13% to 34%). Predictive value of a positive test result = 12/65 = 18% (Cl$_{95}$ = 10% to 30%). Predictive value of a negative test result = 15/26 = 58% (Cl$_{95}$ = 37% to 77%).

†Sensitivity = 23/23 = 100% (Cl$_{95}$ lower limit = 85%) and specificity = 31/68 = 46% (Cl$_{95}$ = 33% to 58%). Predictive value of a positive test result = 23/60 = 38% (Cl$_{95}$ = 26% to 52%). Predictive value of a negative test result = 31/31 = 100% (Cl$_{95}$ = lower limit = 89%).

FIGURE 27-7: NATURAL AGENTS AND THEIR MECHANISMS OF ACTION FOR THINNING THE BLOOD*

Agents That Inhibit Fibrin Production or Stimulate Fibrinolysis:
- Garlic
- Artemisia
- Bromelain
- Cayenne Pepper
- Curcumin
- Dan Shen
- Hong Hua

Agents That Inhibit Increased Vascular Permeability:
- Horse Chestnut
- Dong Gui
- Butcher's Broom

Agents That Reduce Platelet Aggregation:
- Grape Seed Extract
- Coleus Forskohii
- Tocotrienols
- Ginger

* Adapted from J. Boik, Cancer and Natural Medicine. *Princeton, Minn: Oregon Medical Press; 1996:26-28.*

blood" that can be reversed with anticoagulation medications, diet, and herbal remedies. There are many different mechanisms with which to "thin" the cancer patient's blood. As can be seen from **Figure 27-7,** there are numerous medications and natural substances that can be used to inhibit tumor procoagulation. For practicality, the most common natural agents that we use are natural vitamin E (must be mixed tocopherols), pycnogenol, (grape seed extract), protease enzymes, coleus forskohlii, tocotrienols, and horse chestnut. If a person is able to stomach an essential oil, this is prescribed. We really like cod liver oil, but many of our patients do not. For patients with aggressive cancers, we have no problem getting them on Coumadin, an anticoagulation medication. The person is always monitored via blood tests to make sure the blood coagulopathy is correcting.

Anticoagulation, or blood thinning is commonly used in modern allopathic medicine as a means to treat such conditions as pulmonary embolism (blood clot in the lungs), and deep vein thrombosis (leg clot). It also is used to prevent blood clots from forming during or after surgery, or in heart conditions such as atrial fibrillation. The main mechanism by which blood thinning is accomplished is to block the vitamin K-dependent clotting factors by

the use of warfarin or Coumadin. This medication is generally taken at night before the person goes to bed. The level of anticoagulation is checked by drawing a blood sample for prothrombin time or the international normalized ratio. Studies on giving Coumadin to cancer patients have shown promising results. It has been clearly demonstrated that some of the procoagulant physiology of cancer can be reversed with Coumadin.[22] Various other studies have shown that Coumadin when given with chemotherapy increases survival for patients with lung and colon cancer when compared to survival with just chemotherapy alone.[25,26] If survival is enhanced with the use of Coumadin, it only makes sense that the anticoagulant must somehow be helping the penetration of the chemotherapy to the tumor cells. We believe that the fibrin-gel or cancer clotting coat that a cancer has surrounding it not only limits the immune surveillance system from killing it but also chemotherapy. Thus, for chemotherapy to work at its maximum ability, it is necessary to diminish the cancer clotting coat and the procoagulation physiology. It is for this reason that Coumadin is sometimes used by physicians to enhance (at least theoretically) the cancer-killing effects of IPT.

Another method used by modern allopathic medicine to "thin" the blood is by inhibiting platelet stickiness. This is done by various medications, including aspirin and dipyridamole. These medications are commonly prescribed for such conditions as coronary artery disease, peripheral vascular disease, and other circulatory disorders. It has been shown that for many conditions of excessive blood clotting, taking aspirin or another platelet inhibitor enhances survival. It would make sense that the same would occur for cancer.

In 1985, E. H. Rhodes of St. Hileir and Kingman Hospital in Surrey, United Kingdom, published in *Lancet* that stage III and stage IV patients with melanoma were being maintained on 300 mg of dipyridamole.[27] At five years, none of the stage III cancer patients had died, and the survival of stage IV patients was 77%. The expected survival of stage IV patients was 32%. One wonders how a simple medication can have such a profound effect. One explanation can be found in the research published in *Cancer Research* in March 1999, where it was demonstrated with three different tumor cell lines in mice that tumor cells can activate platelet aggregation and that platelet aggregates deactivate cytotoxic natural killer cells, preventing them from killing cancer cells. Whatever the mechanism, the benefits far outweigh the risks for a cancer patient to take some type of agent to inhibit platelet aggregation.

I (Ross) was intrigued recently when my friend Steve Meyer, who had a bone marrow transplant for mantle cell lymphoma, was placed on a NSAID to help reduce his risk of cancer recurrence. More and more research is coming out that these types of medications (ibuprofen, Vioxx, Celebrex) have chemopreventive potential against various cancers, including breast and colon.[28-30]

NSAIDs are medications that interfere with the body's ability to generate eicosanoids or prostaglandins that are involved in the coagulation and inflammatory cascades of the body. Some believe that one of the enzymes that is blocked by these medications, most notably cyclooxygenase-2, is required for angiogenesis to occur.[30] By blocking this enzyme, medications such as Vioxx and Celebrex are helping stop angiogenesis and, thus, tumor formation.

BLOOD CLOTTING COMPARISON BETWEEN NORMAL AND CANCER CELLS

When a blood clot forms, normally the body's anti-coagulation cascade is stimulated. The fibrin network of the blood clot is dissolved via the process of fibinolysis. In cancer patients, this fibrinolytic activity in the blood is inhibited.[31] Various explanations for this include an increased concentration of sulhydryl (-SH) groups and arginine-rich peptides in tumor tissue.[32] (See **Figure 27-8**). Whatever the mechanism, it is probable that the fibrin coat causes neoplastic cells not to be recognized by the immunological system and thus makes them immune to the attack by the natural killer cells.[33] This is just another reason why cancer patients should do everything they can to thin their blood.

HEAVY METALS AND BLOOD CLOTTING

There are many different reasons that blood clots excessively. Natural medicine doctors are continually faced with patients with poor circulation due to some factor causing an excessive amount of blood clotting. The most common rea-

COMPARISON OF CERTAIN CHARACTERISTIC FEATURES OF NORMAL AND CANCER CELLS

CHARACTERISTIC FEATURES	NORMAL CELL	CANCER CELL
Cellular Proliferation	controlled	accelerated
Oxidant status	normal	decreased
Free alpha-ketoaldehyde	high	low
Arginine content	moderate	increased
Concentration of -SH	low	high
Membrane Transglutaminse activity	low	high
Fibrinolytic system activity	active	inhibited
Fibrinogen cell-surface coat	absent	present

Figure 27-8
Cancer cells are able to inhibit fibrinolytic activity that would dissolve their fibrin coat. Because of this, they are able to avoid immune detection.

son for this is a diet high in saturated fat and sugar. Thus when the cancer patient starts on a high-protein (low-fat), low-carbohydrate diet (rich in vegetables), this will have a positive effect on the blood clotting parameters.

Another common cause of excessive blood clotting is infection. It is common when the bowels are tested in cancer patients to find intestinal dysbiosis or the growth of many potentially harmful organisms such as parasites, fungi, or abnormal bacteria. This is treated by giving the person soil-based organisms such as acidophilus and bifidus, as well as medications directed toward the organism(s) in question. The most common medications we use are antifungals.

An often overlooked cause of procoagulant activity is heavy metals. In one study, it was found that mercury caused a 56-fold increase in the rate of thrombin formation when platelets were subjected to it.[34] Some cancer clinics in other countries insist on cancer patients having their mercury fillings removed if they are to be treated. Heavy metal toxicity causing coagulopathy would be one indication for chelation therapy. Chelation therapy involves the intravenous injection of an amino acid derivative, such as DMPS (for mercury), or EDTA (for lead). These few examples are mentioned to note that coagulation problems can be quite complex and require a comprehensive natural medicine approach.

SUMMARY

Cancers are able to elude immune detection by many different mechanisms. One of them is probably the cancer clotting coat. This is comprised of a fibrin network of collagen that surrounds the tumor cells. Fibrin is the normal end product of blood clotting. Cancer physiology often involves blood coagulopathy. It is common to find in a cancer patient that markers for excessive blood clotting (coagulopathy) are high. Common tests to show this are platelet aggregation studies, as well as fibrinogen levels, thrombin-antithrombin III complex, and others. (See **Figure 27-9**.) Many cancer patients are treated with high-dose chemotherapy, which worsens the excessive coagulopathy, thus worsening their cancer physiology. Studies have shown that cancer patients who thin their blood with medications such as Coumadin and dipyridamole have better outcomes. There are many different methods to decrease blood coagulopathies, including nutriceutical products, for example, cod liver oil, garlic, curcumin, horse chestnut, bromelain, pycnogenol, vitamin E, and many others. It is best to have blood coagulation parameters checked before and after some type of anticoagulation therapy has been started to see if it has been corrected. If it has been corrected, this should have a positive impact on the outcome of other treatments the cancer patient requires. ∎

AMSCOT MEDICAL LABS. INC.
4125 Hamilton-Middletown Rd., Hamilton, OH 45011
PHONE (513) 737-4801 FAX (513) 737-4803

PLATELET AGGREGATION TESTING

PATIENT: ACCESSION #

PHYSICIAN: **DR. HAUSER**

NOTE: IN ANALYSIS OF DATA IT IS IMPORTANT TO CONSIDER (1) PRIMARY DIAGNOSIS (2) MEDICATIONS WHICH MAY INFLUENCE TEST RESULTS AND (3) REMEMBER THAT NO SINGLE TEST RESULT SHOULD EVER BE CONSIDERED IN ISOLATION AND SHOULD BE REVIEWED WITH RESPECT TO CLINICAL STATUS.

SCORING GUIDE
1 = EXCELLENT 2 = GOOD 3 = AVERAGE
4 = POOR 5 = ABNORMAL

DATE	PRE TX	POST TX	ADP	EPIN	COLL	THROM	COMMENTS
06/09/99	X		3	1	3	5	THE THROMBIN RESPONSE REFLECTS INCREASE RATE FOR CLOT FORMATION.

TEST	RESULTS (SECS)	NORMAL RANGE	FLAG	COMMENTS
PT - PRE TX		11 - 15		
APTT - PRE TX		16 - 31		
INR - PRE TX				
PT - POST TX		11 - 15		
APTT - POST TX		16 - 31		
INR - POST TX				

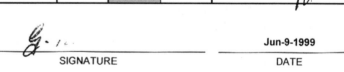
ABNORMAL RESULT

_____
SIGNATURE

Jun-9-1999
DATE

Figure 27-9: Abnormal Platelet Aggregation Study
This is a common finding in cancer patients, as cancer physiology causes the blood to clot excessively.

CHAPTER 28

Warning: Herbs Are No Substitute for an IPT Physician

"THE GREAT DELUGE OF MODERN CHEMOTHERAPY IS ABOUT TO WASH AWAY THE PLANT AND VEGETABLE DEBRIS."

-Morris Fishbein, M.D., quoted in 1927, written while he was Former Editor of the Journal of the American Medical Association

ZEALOUSNESS VERSUS IGNORANCE

Zealousness is no substitute for ignorance. Morris Fishbein, M.D., long-time editor of the *Journal of the American Medical Association*, was an ardent enemy of natural remedies. We doubt he researched them or used them, yet he wrote vehemently against them. Likewise, there are natural medicine zealots who take a few garlic pills and think this will cure the lump on the side of their neck. There is nothing that makes doctors sicker in the stomach than seeing someone die of a treatable disease. *Cancer is definitely a treatable disease,* but it is not curable when a person has had surgery, chemotherapy, radiation, more chemotherapy and is jaundiced. The time to start IPT in the treatment of cancer is now! Natural medicine or alternative medicine should not be a last resort. The cancer patient should use conventional medicine as a last resort but only on the advice of a physician who treats cancer patients. Let me repeat: Zealousness is no substitute for ignorance. The following cases will illustrate the point.

C.J.: FAMOUS BLACK BEAUTY QUEEN—BREAST CANCER

C.J. was referred to us by her chiropractor because of a mass on her breast. When she lifted up her shirt to show Ross the mass, he couldn't believe it. Her left breast was filled with a fungating mass that made it two to three times the size of the other one. What was even worse, was that she had been treating it with herbs and herbal wraps for over a year on the advice of her significant other.

We had some special times together over the next month. As I (Ross) was thinking about her in the doctor's lounge of the local hospital, they announced over CNN that she had died. Marion and I attended her memorial service. Prior to the cancer ravaging her body, she was a well-known beauty queen. What a loss. I wondered, "Why did she not get *appropriate* help earlier? What was she thinking?"

V.K.: SOAP OPERA STAR—OVARIAN CANCER

V.K. was also referred to us by a chiropractor. She had some lumps in her groin. She was feeling tired. She knew about these lumps for months. When I felt them, I knew immediately they were cancerous. Computed tomography (CT) scans showed ovarian cancer with metastases in the lymph nodes and liver. I immediately recommended that she stop working and get treatment. She told me that she had worked her whole life for her current role. She was one of the few black leads on a soap opera, and if the studio knew she had cancer, they would write her out of the script. She left to go back to Hollywood. I read about her death a few months later.

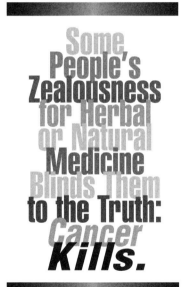

J.C.: NATURAL MEDICINE FANATIC—ABDOMINAL CANCER

J.C. came to see us on his own accord. He noticed about six months earlier that he had a vague abdominal pain. He tried every herbal thing he could think of and then decided to see a natural medicine specialist. He was convinced he had an enzyme deficiency. When taking his history on May 4, 2001, it was clear that something aggressive was going on. He was having tremendous difficulty swallowing food and had a lot of stomach pain. I (Ross) explained that I was a natural medicine specialist, but first and foremost I am a medical doctor. I insisted that he have cancer markers drawn and see a gastroenterologist for an endoscopy. He refused and thought it ridiculous when I spoke to him, but before leaving the office, he decided to go ahead with the cancer markers. I called him with his CA 19-9 level, which was markedly elevated (See **Figure 28-1**). He agreed,

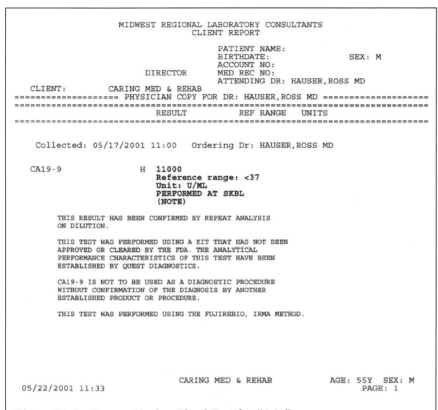

```
              MIDWEST REGIONAL LABORATORY CONSULTANTS
                          CLIENT REPORT
                                 PATIENT NAME:
                                 BIRTHDATE:                SEX: M
                                 ACCOUNT NO:
                    DIRECTOR      MED REC NO:
                                 ATTENDING DR: HAUSER,ROSS MD
       CLIENT:       CARING MED & REHAB
       =================== PHYSICIAN COPY FOR DR: HAUSER,ROSS MD ===================
       ================================================================================
                        RESULT        REF RANGE    UNITS
       ================================================================================


       Collected: 05/17/2001 11:00   Ordering Dr: HAUSER,ROSS MD


       CA19-9              H  11000
                              Reference range: <37
                              Unit: U/ML
                              PERFORMED AT SKBL
                              (NOTE)

            THIS RESULT HAS BEEN CONFIRMED BY REPEAT ANALYSIS
            ON DILUTION.

            THIS TEST WAS PERFORMED USING A KIT THAT HAS NOT BEEN
            APPROVED OR CLEARED BY THE FDA. THE ANALYTICAL
            PERFORMANCE CHARACTERISTICS OF THIS TEST HAVE BEEN
            ESTABLISHED BY QUEST DIAGNOSTICS.

            CA19-9 IS NOT TO BE USED AS A DIAGNOSTIC PROCEDURE
            WITHOUT CONFIRMATION OF THE DIAGNOSIS BY ANOTHER
            ESTABLISHED PRODUCT OR PROCEDURE.

            THIS TEST WAS PERFORMED USING THE FUJIREBIO, IRMA METHOD.




                           CARING MED & REHAB        AGE: 55Y  SEX: M
       05/22/2001 11:33                               PAGE: 1
```

Figure 28-1: *Cancer Marker Blood Test for "J.C."*
As can be seen, a normal CA 19-9 level is under 37. J.C.'s level was 11,000—indicating cancer.

breast in 1999. Her cancer had metastasized to the lymph nodes, but she had no other treatment except some herbal remedies. Now she has a swollen left armpit with palpable lymph nodes. Guess what? She now has Stage 4 breast cancer. She is going to need a lot more powerful treatments than the herbs she is taking. I am grateful she wrote to me, but she needed to see me immediately after her diagnosis was made, not after two years of letting her cancer grow. Do I think she still can be cured of her cancer? Yes, but it will take a lot more work and IPT treatments than if she had come originally. Zealousness for natural medicine is no excuse for ignorance. Cancer kills.

NATURAL MEDICINE IS MEDICINE

Jenifer Van De Pol joined Caring Medical in January 2001. She is an excellent clinician. She is trained as a physician assistant, but her love is natural medicine. She worked in a health foodstore for five years before receiving her formal medical training. When we were discussing what to put on her business card, I (Ross) told her to put natural medicine specialist. That is what she did because that is what she is. So it is with me. I am a medical doctor, but my heart and soul is in natural medicine. I am a natural medicine specialist.

Being a natural medicine specialist does not mean that I eat tofu for every meal, am a vegetarian, and picket the American Medical Association (AMA). It means that first and foremost I obey the first rule of medicine: "Thou shalt do no harm!" I desire to treat illness with the least invasive method that will be effective. For most chronic diseases, the least invasive method includes dietary changes, exercise, ample rest, and vitamins and minerals. If a procedure is needed, I choose to use methods such as Prolotherapy, Neural Therapy, mesotherapy, chelation therapy, photoluminescence, ozone therapy, intravenous

though hesitantly, to get a CT scan. I explained it was a matter of life or death. "How much is it going to cost? I don't have insurance." I received a call from my lab a few days later that J.C. wanted a hepatitis test because he was turning yellow. I explained again that it was most likely a cancer, but he wanted a hepatitis blood test. I called him immediately when I received the results of his CT scan that showed abdominal cancer. When I suggested a surgical consultation, he said, "Surgery costs a lot of money." He went on and on about this. I set up an appointment with a surgeon I trust to see if J.C. was a surgical candidate. I recommended Insulin Potentiation Therapy (IPT) to him. Do I think he will do anything? I doubt it; some people's zealousness for herbal or natural medicine blinds them to the truth: **Cancer kills.**

SUMMARY

The above case histories are true. Consider **Figure 28-2,** which is a letter I received in March 2001. The woman had a mastectomy of her right

3.15.01

Hello,

I was given your address by Second Opinion Pub. Co.. I am interested after reading "Into the Light" by W.C. Douglas M.D. in the photoluminescent therapy. I read and saw a video on the practices of oxygenation therapies in Russia. They have had wonderful results for years now.

I had a mastectomy of the right breast two years ago. I did this after my soul search and deep-long studies of all my alternatives. I let them take only 2 lymphnodes, because I felt one was involved in my right armpit, and it was. Now I have a swollen armpit lymphnode in the left side. (Approx 2 mos.) I am on a herbal regime - Essiac that I make myself, CELLFORTE, and other herbs, foods and teas, too many to mention here, that help my immunity and are especially good for healing cancer and strengthen the liver etc. If I feel I need to "step-it-up" I would like to do the photoluminescent / oxygenation route. Could you help me? What exactly do you do? Are your charges for this reasonable?

I do appreciate your time and attention to this matter.

Sincerely,
K.B.

Wisconsin

Figure 28-2: Letter from an Actual Prospective Patient Sent to Caring Medical
This person is playing Russian roulette by not having a physician follow-up for her breast cancer.

vitamins and minerals, and intramuscular nutrients instead of surgery. Do I cure everyone? No. But even those that I do not cure are happy that I tried. For the more than 90% who are helped or cured, they are abundantly grateful.

CASE OF VANESSA DOWNEY BASHAM (BREAST CANCER SURVIVOR): A SMART ZEALOT

Her letter (See **page 250.**) speaks for itself—Vanessa did not start treating her cancer on her own. She did some research and finally came to a physician whom she trusted. Though her doctors recommended chemotherapy, she decided to do alternative medicine but under the guidance of a **natural medicine specialist who treats a lot of cancer patients.** She underwent extensive cancer marker testing, as well as tests for cancer physiology. She had a lot of cancer physiology still in her system, which has been corrected with natural medicine. She continues to be tested every six months. After three years of her cancer markers being normal and cancer physiology being reversed, she will go from being tested every six months to yearly testing. Just because a person is tumor free does not mean that he or she is free from cancer marker and cancer physiology testing.

CASE OF SUZANNE SOMERS, ACTRESS

"SOME MAY WANT TO KNOW WHAT YOU THINK OF ACTRESS SUZANNE SOMERS TAKING AN EXTRACT OF MISTLETOE, INSTEAD OF CHEMOTHERAPY, FOR HER BREAST CANCER."

-David B. Biebel, D.Min., Editor, Today's Christian Doctor

When I read that Suzanne Somers (actress in *Three's Company*) was treating her

• March 1, 2001 • Re: Vanessa Downey Basham • To Whom It May Concern:

On May 13th, 1999 I underwent surgery (lumpectomy with axillary node dissection along with sent node procedure) for Grade 2 infiltrating ductal carcinoma of the left breast with metastasis to the lymph nodes. My particular type of breast cancer was very aggressive with my S-phase faction by flow cytometry showing a potential doubling time of 19 days. Dr. Krajcovic, Head Surgeon, of the Breast Care Center at St. Luke's Hospital, Chesterfield, MO. advised me at that time to seek chemotherapy, radiation therapy and the drug therapy, Tamoxifen. He then referred me to Dr. Albert L. Van Amburg, oncologist at St. Lukes. Dr. Van Amburg advised me to take eight treatments of CMF, followed up by radiation therapy. Also, he advised me to take the drug Tamoxifen for five years. If I followed his recommendations, he gave me an 85% chance of recovery. After consideration of the pros and cons of said treatments, I chose to look into alternative treatments.

On 8/7/99, I had my first visit with Dr. Ross A. Hauser at his office in Oak Park, IL. My symptoms included: general wasting away, severe fatigue, insomnia, night sweats, mouth ulcers, abnormal bowel function, fibrous tissue disease of the breasts, and abnormal menses with dysmenorrhea, menorrhagia, and PMS. Dr. Hauser ran the following tests on me to determine my condition:

He ran an AMAS-Initial-Lab to determine if cancer cells were still present in my body. The results indicated the cancer was present and that my system was very pro-cancer.

He ran a Comprehensive Digestive Stool Analysis. This was to determine digestion, absorption and colonic environment. Results indicated that my digestion of protein was inadequate within my small intestine, in which, Dr. Hauser corrected with digestive enzymes and diet. It also indicated sufficient amounts of E-coli in my stool with inadequate amounts of lactobacilli and bifidobacteria. Klebsiella infection was also present, as well as, an overgrowth of yeast. Stool pH was elevated, while butyrate was depressed. Overall Bacterial Dysbiosis Index was severely elevated, suggesting extreme alteration in bacterial gut ecology. Dr. Hauser corrected these conditions by giving me Fluconazole (an anti-fungal medication) and by adding a Small Intestine Support Formula to aid the body's assimilation and utilization of nutrients and to help rebuild the good flora in my intestines. Supplementation and diet were also utilized.

He ran a Comprehensive Hormone Profile, which also indicated my system was still pro-cancer. Because the cancer had been 90% estrogen and Progesterone receptive, Dr. Hauser was checking for abnormalities in my estrogen levels. My overall estrogen quotient was low and my bad estrogen, estradiol was high. Also, my DHEA level was low. Dr. Hauser corrected this by having me take 25mg of DHEA daily, which also helped correct the estrogen imbalance. He added tofu to my diet to increase the amount of phytoestrogens and phytoprogestins in my diet, which helped increase my overall estrogen quotient.

He ran a Thyroid-Panel-Lab and a CBC. Results of the Thyroid Panel indicated hypothyroidism, which Dr. Hauser corrected by prescribing Armour Thyroid 30mg daily, plus modifications to my diet. Results of CBC indicated a depressed immune system, which Dr. Hauser corrected with diet, supplementation, and natural chemotherapeutic agents. He did metabolic typing on me to indicate what medication to prescribe and what type diet and nutrients I needed. The following variables were analyzed: Oxidative Rate, Blood, Urine and Saliva pH, Autonomic Nervous System Dominance, Blood Type, Body Type, and testing for Candida Infection. He ran a modified glucose tolerance test to determine oxidative rate. These were within normal ranges. He also ran a Reams Test to check blood sugar, pH, saline, albumin, and urea. My urine was very acidic indicating digestive disorders. My saliva pH was elevated indicating a sluggish liver. I was put on a diet that supported my acidic state, blood type, and medical condition. In addition, because of the effects of the autonomic nervous system on my already depressed immune system he advised me to avoid any type of environment that would cause me stress, this included work. He advised me to omit from my life anyone or anything that might cause stress. He advised me not to even watch the news on television if that upset me. In addition he used supplementation and diet to help rebuild my immune system in order to fight off and destroy remaining cancer cells. He prescribed two natural chemotherapeutic agents; one was Poly-MVA, an oral anti-cancer agent. The other was Ukrain, a drug widely used in Europe. Both these agents kill cancer cells and help to fortify the immune system. Because these agents fortify and build the immune system to help the body's natural defenses against cancer, anemia and low white blood count (common with conventional chemotherapy) are not seen.

In addition, Dr. Hauser prescribed supplements to detoxify the body and to work as an astringent to vital organs. He advised me to consume lots of clean water, at least eight eight-ounce glasses daily. Lastly, he advised me to remove amalgam fillings from my mouth and have them replaced with non-metal substitutes. Mercury has been found in accumulative amounts in malignant breast tissue and is also known to suppress the immune system. I was then advised to follow up with mercury detoxification.

From all indications of follow up studies done on May 16, 2000 and July 3, 2000, I am now cancer-free. I continue to improve daily. I am still presently taking supplementation to correct metabolic imbalances. Dr. Hauser still has me on a modified diet and lots of clean water. All signs of wasting away have stopped and I have gained back twenty pounds. My immune system is strong and fatigue is at a minimum. I am no longer bothered by insomnia and my menses have improved greatly, as well as, breast tenderness. Bowel function has also improved with less constipation and plotting. My system is still somewhat acidic which I hope will also be corrected over time. I returned to work as of August 21, 2000 and continue to hold my position.

I will always be appreciative of Dr. Hauser for all he did to save my life. I know that I was led to him by a divine God.

Appreciatively, *Vanessa Basham*

breast cancer with natural remedies (e.g., mistletoe), part of me wanted to jump for joy, but another part of me wanted to cringe. I have used in my practice many natural remedies from around the world. Mistletoe, in my opinion, is not one of the stronger agents; if Suzanne Somers has a high tumor load, mistletoe will keep it in check for awhile, but then it will grow. If she succumbs to the cancer, the media will have a field day, and mistletoe will be relegated to the "quack" remedy file. I hope and pray she has a natural medicine specialist who knows about IPT. IPT and mistletoe together would be a much more potent combination in my opinion.

A few weeks after I wrote the above paragraph, Suzanne Somers was the lead article in the April 30, 2001, *People* magazine. She explained that she had a lumpectomy followed by radiation treatments but chose to forgo the high-dose chemotherapy treatments in lieu of receiving Iscador, an extract of mistletoe. This is what I expected. Suzanne Somers is *not* treating her cancer with mistletoe as reported in the media. She had the overwhelming majority of her cancer (probably all of it) removed surgically and then was zapped with radiation. **What she really did was to choose not to receive high-dose chemotherapy.** As one can imagine, her whole body has been wracked by these treatments, and what she feels she needs is an immune stimulant. Sounds great to me. I do know that Iscador is a compound that one would have to be familiar with in order to use it, so I am confident she is under the care of a natural medicine specialist. Good for her!

Another danger with her story is that people will think that Suzanne Somers is treating her breast cancer with mistletoe. A woman may have a breast lump, not get it checked out, take some mistletoe because she read that Suzanne was doing it, and not see a physician. I know I have harped on this point so many times, but it is too dangerous to wait and monkey around when you have cancer. The next time you hear something in the news or read it in the paper or on the Internet about cancer or a cancer treatment, please talk to a natural medicine physician about it.

CANCER AND IMMUNITY

When the immune system responds to the presence of a foreign substance, or antigen, it does so in two possible ways. In the humoral

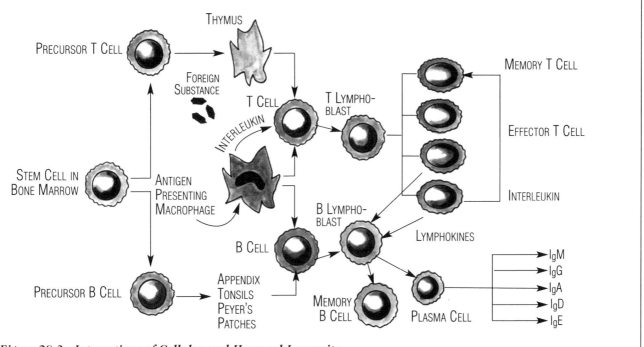

Figure 28-3: Interactions of Cellular and Humoral Immunity
Cytokines such as interleukins play a primary role in immune regulation.

FIGURE 28-4: BASIC FUNCTIONS OF THE COMMON CYTOKINES

INFLAMMATORY:	Tumor necrosis factor α (TNFα) Interleukin-1 (IL-1) Interleukin-6 (IL-6)
ANTIVIRAL:	Interferons (IFNα, B and γ)
LYMPHOPOIETIC/ HEMATOPOIETIC:	Interleukins (IL-2), (IL-4) and (IL-12), Granulocyte-monocyte colony-stimulating factor (GM-CSF)

response, B lymphocytes recognize and attach to the antigen. Plasma cells are then formed to produce antibodies against the antigen. In the cell-mediated response, T lymphocytes (T helper cells or cytotoxic T lymphocytes) recognize the foreign substance and either directly kill the invader or elicit the production of antibodies from plasma cells. Regulation of T lymphocyte proliferation and activity is largely mediated by cytokines such as interleukin-1 (IL-1), interleukin-2 (IL-2), and tumor necrosis factor (See **Figure 28-3**).

Cytokines are molecules that mediate communication between cells of the immune system. Most cytokines are made by cells of the immune system as part of an immune response. They are soluble proteins produced by mononuclear cells of the immune system (usually lymphocytes or monocytes) that have regulatory actions on other cells of the immune system or target cells involved in immune reactions. Cells expressing receptors for a particular cytokine can be positively or negatively stimulated by that cytokine, leading to an alteration of cellular functions. These functions may include enhanced cytotoxic activity (cell-killing ability), secretion of antibody, or secretion of additional cytokines. Some of the more basic functions of the common cytokines are seen in **Figure 28-4.** Cytokine release can recruit and activate additional immune cells. Thus, cytokines play a critical role in immunity. Some cytokines are being used in primary cancer therapy.

For the person who is concerned about a weakened immune system, it is now possible to directly test various cytokine levels (See **Figure 28-5**). Most people who do cancer work believe that it is important to keep a person's immune system strong while undergoing cancer therapy. For this reason, we often give people interferon-alfa during their IPT treatments. We have also used IL-2. As can be seen in **Figure 28-6,** both of these agents have a wide range of immunostimulatory functions.

The concept known as natural immunity or immune surveillance implies that the immune system is capable of recognizing all tumor cells as foreign. Natural killer (NK) cells (another type of lymphocyte) and macrophages confer this type of immunity. However, views are divided on the concept of immune surveillance because not all human tumors elicit an immune response or are not particularly sensitive to the effects of NK cells.

IMMUNE STIMULATION MAY LEAD TO CANCER GROWTH

According to R.T. Prehn of the Institute for Cancer Research in Philadelphia, much data suggest that immunosurveillance is actually a weak and inefficient defense mechanism.

Mistletoe is one of many treatments used by alternative medicine physicians to treat cancer. It acts primarily as an immune stimulant. The problem is that cancer is not an immunodeficiency disease. Most cancer patients whom we see who have not had chemotherapy or radiation therapy have excellent immune function. A good summary of the immune function in the process of cancer formation is from the *American Journal of Pathology:*[1]

> Most and perhaps all neoplasms arouse an immune response in their hosts. Unfortunately, this response is seldom effective in

```
NOTE: PLEASE REFER TO #100431996 FOR TEST RESULTS.

Results reported from: Specialty Laboratories, Inc.
                       2211 Michigan Ave
                       Santa Monica, CA 90404

     Interleukin-2                 0                < 31 pg/mL

     **PLEASE NOTE UPDATED REFERENCE RANGE 05/02/00**    For Research
     use only
```

Figure 28-5: An Interleukin-2 Blood Test

Cytokine blood levels are one of the tests that are available that relate to immune function.

FIGURE 28-6: IMMUNE FUNCTIONS OF INTERLEUKIN-2 AND INTERFERON-ALFA

Both of these agents can be used with IPT to stimulate a cancer patient's immune system.

CYTOKINE	BIOLOGIC ORIGIN
IL-2	Costimulates T cells; activates cytotoxic responses in T cells; stimulates monocytes to become tumoricidal; chemotactic for T cells; cofactor for growth and differentiation of B cells; induction/release of cytokines; induces non-MHC-restricted CTL killing; costimulates proliferation and differentiation of B cells.
IFN-α	Antiproliferative to certain tumor cells; promotes partial reversal of the malignant phenotype; enhances the expression of surface molecules, including b2-microglobulin, Fc receptors, tumor-associated antigens, and MHC class I antigens; augments NK activity; modulates B cell function; inhibits suppressor T cell activity; activities monocytes/macrophages; exerts antiviral activity; interacts (enhance, inhibit) with growth factors, oncogenes and other cytokines; activates CTL.

limiting tumor growth. Immunologic surveillance, as originally conceived, probably does not exist. The early weak response to nascent tumors stimulates rather than inhibits their growth. A truly tumor-limiting reaction occurs only in exceptional tumor systems, and then it is relatively late and ineffective. Immunity may be of great importance in limiting the activity of oncogenic viruses, but is probably seldom the determiner of whether or not an already transformed cell gives rise to a lethal cancer.[1]

In 1959, Lewis Thomas proposed the concept that immune surveillance was an active process controlling the emergence of malignant clones from somatic cells that undergo precancerous mutations during the lifetime of a normal, immune-competent individual.[2] This hypothesis would have predicted that individuals affected with genetically determined immune deficiencies should experience much higher rates of all types of cancers than seen in the general population. However, surveys of patients with primary and acquired immune deficiencies have not revealed an increased risk of all cancer types.[3]

The above paragraph is from one of the most up-to-date cancer books in the country, *Clinical Oncology*, second edition, published in 2000. It is about 3,000 pages long. It has hundreds of pages on the immune system, as it should. The immune system is important in regard to cancer, but realize this, it is the cancer therapy that causes a person's immune system to decline, not the cancer itself. The person who is taking an herb to strengthen the immune system is delusional to think that this will be strong enough to shrink a tumorous mass. Thus the title of this chapter: **Warning: Herbs are no substitute for an IPT physician.**

For the sake of the natural medicine zealot who does not believe me on this point, I will refer to some good papers on the immune system and cancer and give the references. Consider the following:

"In a series of papers I made the prediction, based on a survey of the literature, that a weak and/or incipient immune reaction would be directly stimulatory, rather than inhibitory, to target tumor cells.[4,5] This prediction has been substantiated, both in my laboratory and by others.[6,8] In essence, the experimental findings are that specific immune lymphoid cells (in some cases probably of the T cell variety or their precursors), in sufficiently low dilution, stimulate the growth of target tumor cells both in vitro and in vivo. Lymphoid cells harvested a very short time after immunization are more stimulatory than are those harvested at somewhat longer intervals, the latter tending to be inhibitory."[1,9]

"Although we have cited a considerable amount of evidence in this review, this evidence is suggestive only; the immunostimulation hypothesis is obviously far from established. However, the hypothesis seems particularly attractive because it might offer an elegant explanation of the reason why most and perhaps all neoplasms are endowed with tumor regression antigens. It may be that a weak immune reaction is actually necessary to enable a nascent neoplasm to overcome the known nonimmunologic homeostatic devices, such as inhibition by surrounding normal cells."[10]

"Although such data support immune surveillance, the original hypothesis had several major problems or limitations:

1. The majority of human tumors associated with immunodepression have been leukemias and lymphoproliferative diseases, rather than a complete array of the common types of malignancy.

2. There has not been a consistent association between immunodepression and tumors.

These hypotheses have led to the suggestion that immune surveillance may be operative only against tumors induced by oncogenic viruses, which have strong transplantation antigens and for which immune T cells have been shown to be important in resistance." [11,12]

"More recent attempts at immunotherapy, while based on more complete understanding of immune mechanisms, have often been disadvantaged by involving preterminal patients with disseminated tumors in whom already impaired immune mechanisms had little chance of producing demonstrable improvement. However, the possibility exists of *enhancing* tumor growth in patients who have favorable prognoses if managed with other forms of therapy.[13]

For the avid researcher, the above is interesting reading. It should be a wake-up call to natural medicine providers, herbalists, and especially cancer patients that using immune stimulation herbs to treat cancer could be making the cancer grow. The cancer patient needs specific agents that kill cancer. Cancer therapy needs to be done by a physician who has experience in treating cancer patients and preferably one who utilizes IPT. Immune-stimulating herbs are no substitute for IPT.

IMMUNODEFICIENCY CAUSES

What role does the immune system play in comprehensive cancer therapy? It is well known that the heterogeneous nature of neoplasms with regard to their antigenicity and immunogenicity makes them susceptible to antibody-dependent cellular cytotoxicity and to natural killer (NK) cells, T cells, cytokine-activated NK cells, tumor-infiltrating lymphocytes, and cytotoxic T lymphocytes.[14] In other words, the heterogeneity of neoplasms generally causes an immune reaction in the host to recognize and destroy some of the cancer cells. But remember that the tumors are heterogeneous in that the antigenicity differs between primary tumors and their metastases and among different metastatic lesions.[15,16] So a tumor mass can be made of many different cell populations, any of which can metastasize. (This concept was also discussed in **Chapter 29**.) It is up to the immune system to mount a full-blown immune reaction against all the cells of the cancer, but this seldom happens. It is for this reason that we strongly suggest that cancer patients do not rely on immune stimulation as their sole cancer treatment.

Most assuredly, one of the main reasons for a bad outcome in cancer therapy is infection. It is imperative that a cancer patient keep his or her immune system strong while undergoing cancer therapy, whether it is IPT or high-dose chemotherapy. Nothing can set a cancer patient back more, or kill the patient quicker, than a serious infection.

Immune system testing is part of the comprehensive cancer program at Caring Medical. It is best for the cancer patient to have various immune system tests prior to, during, and after therapy is completed. Various tests are available, but some of the more common ones that we use are a complete blood count, albumin, total protein levels, and NK cell counts and activity levels.

A long-time patient of Caring Medical is A.L. She had a history of breast cancer and a mastectomy but refused chemotherapy. She was followed by several doctors, including us. It was alarming when her NK activity level came back severely depressed in early 2001 (See **Figures 28-7A** and **B**). Shortly thereafter, her cancer recurred. So we have seen the effects of immune depression, but it is imperative for the cancer patient

Figure 28-7A and B: Blood Tests for Immune Functions

These results show depressed natural killer cell (NK) activity levels, indicative of low immune system function.

Figure 28-7A

*** NK CELL COUNT ***			
%NATURAL KILLER CELLS	13.0	5.5-20%	mm3
% IMMUNOCOMPETENT -NKHT3+	4.0	1.5-5%	mm3
% NKHT3 NEGATIVE	12.0	4-15%	mm3
% T3 POSITIVE CELLS	65.0	53-79%	mm3

Figure 28-7B: Natural Killer Cell Activity

*** NK CELL ACTIVITY ***			
NK CELL ACTIVITY	8.40 LOW	20-50	LUs

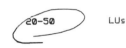

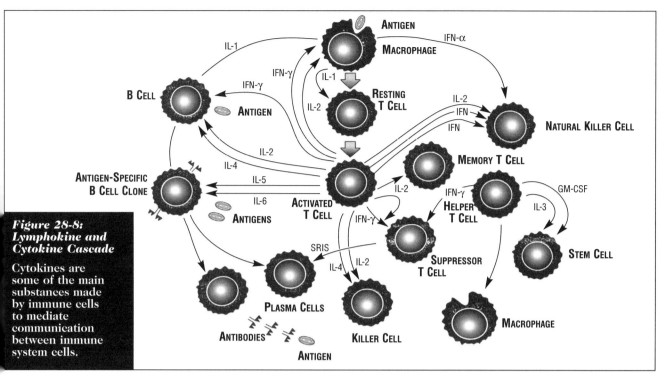

Figure 28-8: Lymphokine and Cytokine Cascade

Cytokines are some of the main substances made by immune cells to mediate communication between immune system cells.

not to use immune stimulation as his or her sole form of cancer therapy.

NK cells are a subpopulation of lymphocytes that differ from mature T or B cells or macrophages in that they bind to and directly destroy certain tumor populations. They kill directly without prior sensitization and have a selectivity for malignant cells. Some research suggests that NK cells may be part of the first line of defense against cancer by destroying tumor cells before T cells and macrophages can be mobilized. NK cells can be readily activated by exposure to IL-2, a cytokine released by T helper cells. In vitro or in vivo exposure to IL-2 causes activation and proliferation of NK cells. These IL-2-activated NK cells mediate in vitro destruction against a broad range of tumor cell lines and freshly isolated tumor cells.

As can be seen in **Figure 28-8,** the interactions between cytokines and cells of the immune system are quite complex. Cytokines as a whole are molecules that mediate communication between cells of the immune system. Most cytokines are made by cells of the immune system as part of an immune reaction. The two main classes of cytokines are the interleukins and the interferons. These biological response modifiers, as they are called, have many functions:[17]

➢ Enhance cytotoxic activity of NK cells
➢ Differentiate T and B cells
➢ Activate additional immune cells
➢ Stimulate leukocyte proliferation
➢ Enhance tumor-associated antigen expression
➢ Suppress angiogenesis
➢ Direct anti-tumor activity

Cytokines are important in the management of cancer because they can also be deficient and a cause of immunosuppression in the cancer patient. When immunodeficiency is found in a cancer patient, it is important to correct the cause as soon as possible so an infection does not develop. As we have discussed many times before, most people assume that a person gets the cancer because of a suppressed immune system; however, when tested, this is rarely found. When cancer patients are found to be immunodeficient, it is almost always because of the traditional medical treatments they have received. This is another reason people with cancer should receive a powerful and effective treatment such as IPT, which has much less risk of causing immune suppression than traditional chemotherapy or radiation therapy.

Most cancer patients understand the immunosuppressive effects of high-dose chemotherapy. Most of them to varying degrees cause suppression of the immune system when used in typical dosages. This is because the chemotherapeutics decrease the bone marrow's ability to produce blood cells. The white blood cells help to protect the body against infection. This is why anyone receiving chemotherapy, either high-dose or IPT, needs to receive regular checks of their blood counts.

Unfortunately, according to modern allopathic medicine, the recovery of the immune system after high-dose chemotherapy has not been well defined.[17] What natural medicine practitioners have known for years is that many people are not the same after high-dose chemotherapy. If high-dose chemotherapy fails, then it is doubtful anything else is going to work because of the ravaging effects it has on the person's immune system. It is common after one or two sessions of high-dose chemotherapy that the person's white and red blood cell counts are so low that Neupogen to raise white blood counts and Epogen (or Procrit) to raise red blood counts must be given. These medications are sometimes given with IPT but in much less frequency than in high-dose chemotherapy.

Immunosuppression can also have other causes, including malnutrition. Insufficient calories, protein, or essential nutrients, such as vitamins, minerals, and fatty acids, can all lead to deficits of immune function. This is another reason that periodic blood tests and body weight be monitored to ensure adequate nutrition is being supplied by the person's diet. If dehydration or malnutrition is found, then intravenous nutrients are given. It is common in our office to give intravenous nutrients on days when IPT is not given if the cancer patient is having a difficult time eating or drinking. On rare occasions, a feeding tube is put in for proper nutrition.

A lesser known cause of immunosuppression in the cancer patient is narcotic medications. Considerable data are available that opioids (narcotics) suppress immune function. Like high-dose chemotherapy, narcotics are damaging to the immune system and hurt cancer

Nothing will send a cancer patient to the grave quicker than narcotics.

recovery prognosis. This is why we say, "Nuke the narcotics!"

NUKE THE NARCOTICS!

Cancer patients are put on narcotics as fast as flies go to cr-p. We are sorry, but it is true. The second a cancer patient starts hurting, on goes the Duragesic patch. Nothing will send a cancer patient quicker to the grave than narcotics.

Narcotics are horribly immunosuppressive. Hopefully after reading this section, you will see why we are adamant about getting cancer patients off narcotics. If all a cancer patient needs is pain control, then use anti-inflammatories. It should be noted that one of the wonderful effects of IPT is that it gets rid of pain, as do many of the alternative medicine therapies, such as high-dose vitamin C, Neural Therapy, or Prolotherapy. In case you don't believe us, references will be given about the immunosuppressive effects of narcotics.

THE KNOWN EFFECTS OF NARCOTICS ON THE IMMUNE SYSTEM

- Suppression of the cytotoxic activity of NK cells[18]
- Enhanced growth of implanted tumors[18]
- Depressed T lymphocyte responsiveness to stimulation[19]
- Ablate delayed hypersensitive skin response[20]
- Spleen atrophy[21]
- Thymus atrophy[21,22]
- Decreased T lymphocyte numbers[22]
- Decreased T cell function[23]
- Inhibited antibody production[24]
- Inhibited B cell activity[25]
- Decreased levels of interferon[26]
- Increased incidence of infections[27]
- **Depressed function of all cells in the immune system**[27]

If the last statement is true, then is it any wonder that chronic pain or cancer patients never get off narcotics once they start on them? Once a person is on regular dosages of narcotics for more than two months, it is doubtful he or she will ever get off. This is a sad but true statement. We probably should rephrase this: The patients will get off narcotics the day they die. **Narcotics have the same depressive effects on the immune system as high-dose chemotherapy!** If you do not believe us, then listen to what the premier neuroimmunology journal in the world says. The *Journal of Neuroimmunology* in an article by Toby K. Eisenstein and Mary E. Hilburger from the department of microbiology and immunology at Temple University School of Medicine stated it plainly.[27] The article is a review on the information known to date about what narcotics do to the immune system. The authors conclude that, **"In aggregate, the literature supports the existence of an in vivo neural-immune circuit through which morphine acts to depress the function of *all cells* of the immune system."** In other words, taking the medical literature as a whole, narcotics suppress *every* cell of the immune system. The body needs an intact immune system to heal. It does not matter if it is after an accident, sports injury, or cancer, the body heals by an immune reaction. The person who is on narcotics needs to nuke the narcotics if healing is to take place.

WHAT ARE NARCOTICS?

The term *narcotic* is derived from the Greek word for "stupor" and at one time applied to any drug that induced sleep, but most refer to drugs that have morphine-like, strong analgesic properties.[28] Narcotics are medications that are morphine-like, analogous to nonsteroidal anti-inflammatory drugs (NSAIDs) that are aspirin-like. There are numerous NSAIDs because each touts to be safer and more efficacious than another. So it is with the various narcotics. Each tries to become an even stronger pain reliever with fewer side effects. By definition, narcotics that act in a manner similar to morphine are immunosuppressive. This goes for Vicodin, Darvocet-N, Duragesic, morphine, OxyContin, codeine, Percodan, and any other such addictive substance.

At Caring Medical, this information is explained to the patient on the first visit if he or she is narcotic dependent. It is not necessary to be off narcotics in order to begin IPT, although this is preferred, but there must be a willingness to get off them. For the person unable to do so, there is little hope of a cure. Typically, a person's dose of narcotics is gradually weaned by 5 to 10 mg/week until he or she is completely off the narcotics. Some peo-

ple, when told about the immunosuppressive effects of narcotics, are able to get themselves off narcotics in a few days. Ideally, this should be done under doctor supervision.

REVERSING IMMUNDEFICIENCY

It is important for a cancer patient to have a strong immune system. This may not help slow cancer growth or cause a decrease in tumor load, but it will help decrease secondary infections from forming. The cancer patient is especially at risk for developing serious lung, bladder, and blood infections. A comprehensive natural medicine program for immune strengthening typically involves eight steps:

1. Insulin Potentiation Therapy to reduce tumor load
2. Adequate and proper nutrition
3. Stopping narcotic medications
4. Using anti-inflammatory medications for pain control
5. Giving biological response modifier prescription medications
6. Taking immunostimulator nutraceutical agents
7. Maintaining a positive outlook
8. Prayer and deepened faith in God

INSULIN POTENTIATION THERAPY

"It should be said that in reality the attempts at using the immunological system in the treatment of malignant tumors in man has not shown very effective results, but when Donatian Therapy (IPT) is used, then a more effective stimulation of the immunological system is obtained."[29]

For the person with cancer, the best way the immune system can be stimulated is to get rid of the cancer. Generally, when a person with cancer has a symptom, whether it be pain, nausea, anorexia, weight loss, or a weak immune system, it is from the cancer. So by definition, an aggressive cancer treatment is needed to correct *the cause* of the symptom. The treatment that we recommend for most cancers is IPT.

The key points of IPT have been discussed many times in this book but are important to repeat. Insulin is a hormone that pushes substances into cells. When a person's body does not have insulin, the blood sugar rises, and diabetes results. **Insulin can potentiate the effects of many different remedies because it has the unique ability to increase a cell's permeability to certain substances.** Since cancer cells have many more insulin receptors on their cells than normal cells, insulin can be used to push medications or herbal remedies into the cancer cells to destroy them. Specifically, the technique involves giving a person intravenous insulin to induce a hypoglycemic state. Once this state is reached, low-dose chemotherapy is given to destroy the tumor cells without harming the normal cells.

IPT takes advantage of several characteristics of cancer cells. Research has shown that some solid tumors have more insulin receptors than normal cells. Insulin also causes some cancer cells to go into a proliferative growth phase, during which chemotherapy works better. This is crucial because in many instances, less than 10% of the cells constituting the tumor mass are actively proliferating by the time the tumor is detected; thus the remaining 90% of cells are not susceptible to most chemotherapeutic agents because they are not engaged in DNA synthesis.

What most people with cancer do not realize is a tumor that has reached the size of clinical detectability (1-cm mass) has already undergone approximately 30 doublings to reach 10^9 cells. Only 10 further doubling cycles are required to produce a tumor burden of approximately 1 kg, which is usually lethal.

One can easily surmise that once a tumor mass is detected, the immune system is overloaded. The cancer at this stage is often in accelerated growth. The quickest way for a person to help improve his or her immune system is to quickly reduce the tumor load. The person has only a few options, including surgery, radiation therapy, high-dose chemotherapy, or low-dose chemotherapy with IPT. It is hoped as more people learn about IPT that this will be the chosen option because, unlike high-dose chemotherapy, IPT has a much lesser chance of causing immune system depression. The main reason for this, of course, is that much lower doses of chemotherapy are given, and physicians who use IPT often encourage patients to do the other seven steps that help stimulate the immune system.

ADEQUATE AND APPROPRIATE NUTRITION

This book covers two main topics: Insulin Potentiation Therapy and cancer physiology. Insulin Potentiation Therapy is the method in which insulin can be used to potentiate the effects of chemotherapy to kill cancer cells. It works because cancer cells have more insulin receptors than normal cells. These insulin receptors help the cancer preferentially get food from the body. In other words, the cancer can grow while the body starves.

Research has been provided that shows that cancers, besides having more insulin receptors, can actually secrete insulin. It appears in many of the cancers studied that the higher a person's own insulin levels are in the blood, the higher his or her risk of cancer. A logical conclusion of this would be that to help starve the cancer, a person would need to keep his or her blood insulin levels as low as possible. Since insulin is secreted by the pancreas in response to high blood sugar levels, the diet needed by a cancer patient is one in which the blood sugar is kept as low as possible. In other words, for many cancer patients, this would be a diet that is high in protein and low in carbohydrates.

The concept that the cancer patient needs a high-protein diet rather than a macrobiotic diet is politically incorrect and is sure to get many natural medicine zealots mad. One must realize that we have made these statements after reviewing the science of cancer physiology and after treating patients with the Gerson and/or macrobiotic/juicing method for almost 10 years. We review the insulin/cancer connection/cancer physiology topic in depth in **Chapter 29** and the diet in **Appendix A.** Suffice it to say, the appropriate diet for most cancer patients will still be one high in vegetables but with much more protein than is currently being recommended in natural medicine/herbal circles. It is important that the cancer patient's insulin levels and nutritional markers be monitored during therapy.

STOPPING NARCOTIC MEDICATIONS

There is nothing that kills cancer patients quicker than slapping Duragesic patches on them or getting them on OxyContin. **No ifs, ands, or buts about it . . . narcotics hasten the demise of cancer patients.** Since we are being politically incorrect, why not go all out? Practitioners who treat cancer patients have been told that real compassionate care involves relieving the suffering of the cancer patient. This primarily means getting them on narcotics.

We are all for relieving pain and suffering. This is what we do for a living and have written nine books about, but cancer doctors often do not tell their cancer patients that the narcotic medications being prescribed for them will quicken their death. Narcotics are fine if there is no hope of survival. If we have bony metastases, there is no hope of survival, and it is clear that death is near, then give us a morphine drip. Many of the patients we see are definitely not ready to die; as a matter of fact, they insist that we help them in the fight for life. For the person with cancer who wants to live, the narcotic medications must go.

USING ANTI-INFLAMMATORY MEDICATIONS FOR PAIN CONTROL

No one has written more about the detrimental effects of anti-inflammatory medications than we have. They are much overused for pain management and much underused in regard to cancer care. Anti-inflammatory medications stop the normal healing inflammatory reaction that is needed for the body to repair such structures as cartilage, menisci, ligaments, tendons, and muscles. After injuries to these structures, using anti-inflammatory medications hampers healing and accelerates the degenerative process. (For the person desiring more information on this topic, please see www.benuts.com and order one of the nine books on Prolotherapy that we have written.)

With regard to cancer therapy, however, there are several reasons to use anti-inflammatory medications:

- Control pain
- Reduce swelling
- Don't suppress the immune system
- Help prevent cancer formation

Anti-inflammatory medications, such as ibuprofen, Advil, Celebrex, Voltaren, and tramadol, help control pain and swelling by inhibiting prostaglandin synthesis. Unlike narcotic medications, though, they have been found not to suppress T lymphocyte and NK cell function.[30] NSAIDs have also been shown to decrease the risk of colon cancer.[31,32] These compounds exert their antiproliferative effects on colonic cells by inhibiting prostaglandin synthesis by reversibly binding to the enzyme cyclooxygenase. NSAIDs are currently being studied for numerous other cancers to see if they also show a preventive effect. It is for these reasons that it is common for patients to receive NSAIDs during their IPT treatments.

USING BIOLOGICAL RESPONSE MODIFIERS IN CANCER THERAPY

Interleukin-2, interferons, colony stimulating factors, tumor necrosis factor, and other interleukins belong to a group of humoral factors known as biological response modifiers. As discussed already, biological response modifiers are substances that are secreted by immune cells to modify the biological response of the immune system, typically stimulating it.

Interferons have been the most extensively studied cytokines in cancer treatment. Three types of interferons have been identified: interferon-alfa, produced by leukocytes; interferon-beta, produced by fibroblasts; and interferon-gamma, produced by T lymphocytes. Interferon-alfa is perhaps the one that has been studied the most and has been approved for use in several types of cancers. At low doses, it can be used in a comprehensive cancer program (along with IPT) for direct immune stimulation effects on T cells, NK cells, and macrophages.

Hematopoietic growth factors are glycoproteins that bind to specific cell surface receptors and stimulate the proliferation, differentiation, and activation of blood cells from different lineages. They can be used to increase red blood cell counts (erythropoietin; Epogen or Procrit), white blood cell counts (colony stimulating factor; Neupogen), or platelets (oprelvekin; Neumega).

NUTRICEUTICALS THAT STIMULATE THE IMMUNE SYSTEM

There are numerous books and studies on nutrients and nutriceuticals that help cancer patients and those that specifically stimulate the immune system. We refer the reader to *Beating Cancer with Nutrition*[33] and *Herbal Medicine: Healing and Cancer*[34] to get a more detailed analysis on this topic. In regard to the nutriceutical supplements that we use in our practice, the main ones are listed in Appendix B. Some of the more common nutriceuticals that stimulate the immune system are shown in **Figure 28-9.** For many of the herbal

FIGURE 28-9: NUTRICEUTRICALS THAT STIMULATE THE IMMUNE SYSTEM

Aloe Vera	Germanium	Schizandra
Ashwagandha	Glutamine	Selenium
Astragalus	Glutathione	Shark Liver Oil
Bee Pollen	Green Tea	Shiitake Mushrooms
Beta Glucan	Inositol	
Boswella	Hexaphosphate	Soy Protein
Burdock	Lactobacillus	Thuja
Celandine	Licorice	Turmeric
Chinese Skullcap	Milletia	Uno de Gato
Chorella	Mistletoe	Whey Protein
Cod Liver Oil	Panax Ginseng	Zinc...
Colostrum	Quercetin	...& Many Others
Echinacea	Reishi Mushrooms	

substances, the immunostimulatory compounds in them have been isolated (See **Figure 28-10**).

Almost every day in the office we hear from clients about a friend of a friend who took some multilevel marketed herbal product that cured them of his or her cancer. No doubt a few of these stories are true, but the vast majority of them are not. We have never verified one story of an herbal remedy curing a person of metastatic cancer. If you know someone who has been cured of cancer with a herbal remedy, please send us the pathology, CT scan, and doctor's reports to our office, as well as the phone number of the person because we would like to talk to that person. If it is found to be true, then we will gladly recommend that herbal product to our clients. In the meantime, please do not rely on immune stimulatory herbs for cancer care—an IPT physician is much more reliable.

MAINTAINING A POSITIVE OUTLOOK
"WHERE THERE IS LIFE, THERE IS HOPE."

- Steven G. Ayre, M.D.

If one goes to the Web site of Dr. Ayre at www.contemporarymedicine.com, in large print it says, "A champion of patient advocacy and empowerment, Dr. Ayre's patients frequently exclaim, 'At last, I've found a doctor I can work with. Someone who listens to me, and hears what

I say!'" Dr. Ayre is one of the pioneers who brought IPT to the United States. He takes a comprehensive approach to cancer management and is an authority on the mind-body connection. Nothing will get him more excited than talking about this topic. He enjoys listening and talking with his patients. He has noticed, as have others who treat the sick, that the person who has a lot of fight and a tremendously positive outlook on life will have a better prognosis than the person with a more negative outlook.

Science is starting to prove the saying that "A positive thought has a positive effect on the body, and a negative thought has a negative effect." Findings from a number of studies show that there is an association between psychological response factors and disease outcome on follow-up in cancer patients. Greer and colleagues showed a significant association between psychological response to early breast cancer and 10-year survival, with "fighting spirit" and optimism associated with longer survival;[35] Reynolds and Kaplan reported elevated risk of both cancer incidence and mortality from hormonally dependent tumors in unhappy and socially isolated women on 18-year follow-up;[36] and Levy and associates found that breast cancer patients who expressed more joy at baseline had a longer disease-free interval.[37]

These results are not surprising, as we all have experienced getting sick when we are stressed and not getting enough sleep or know people who have lost a spouse often get sick or die soon afterward. The more stressors a person experiences, the likelier an illness will occur. This makes sense since psychological stress has a tremendous inhibitory effect on the immune system. Some of these are as follows:[38-42]

- Reduced proliferative response to mitogen stimulation
- Reduced NK cell cytotoxicity
- Decreased B cell, NK cell, and monocyte levels
- Depressed lymphocyte function
- Changes in interleukin levels
- Increased risk of cancer
- Increased risk of infection

Vickie Girard in her book *There's No Place Like Hope* talks of her struggles with cancer and

FIGURE 28-10: IMMUNOSTIMULATORY HERBS

Herb	Compound	Compound Type	Immune Effect
Celandine 　Chelerythrine 　Protopine 　Sanguinarine 　D-Limonene 　Nomilin	Chelidonine	Alkaloid	Anti-tumor, antiviral; increased lymphocytes and natural killer-cells; increases bile flow
Echinacea 　Arabinogalactan 　Echinacin	Echinacoside Polysaccharide Pentacadiene Caffeic acid	Glycoside	Antibacterial, anti-tumor effects, offers nonspecific immune stimulation
Garlic 　Methyl allyl 　trisulphide	Allicin	Allyl sulfide	Anti-tumor effects; kills candida; inhibits cyclo-oxygenase and lipoxygenase; slows tumor growth
Goldenseal 　Hydrastine 　L-canadine	Berberine	Alkaloid	Antibiotic, antiviral, anti-tumor
Pau d'Arco 　Lapachone 　Alpha and beta 　xyloidone	Lapachol Quinone	Naphthoquinone	Provides mild anti-tumor action
Schizandra 　Sesquicarene 　Citral 　Schizandrol 　Sterol stigmasterol	Gomisin A-Q	Lignan	Antihepatotoxin, anti-oxidant, nonmutagenic; protects against chemo and radiation
Turmeric 　other oxidant, 　anticurcuminoids	Curcumin and compounds	Phenolic	Anti-tumor, hepatotoxin; increases lymphocyte production
Uno de Gato 　and other 　alkaloids, 　quinovic acid	Isopteropodin Glycosides Steroids Triterpenes	Alkaloids	Immune system booster, tumor-inhibitor, intestinal antiseptic
Venus' Flytrap (Carnivorous 　Plant)	Plumbagin Drosren Hydroplumbagin	Napthoquinone	Provides gene repair mechanism; immune activator; cytotoxic, antiviral, antibiotic, antifungal

Many of the compounds in herbals that are responsible for their immune stimulating properties have been isolated.

Adapted from Herbal Medicine: Healing and Cancer, D. Yance, Chicago, IL, Keats Publishing, 1999

what it took to beat it. She has many great thoughts in the book, for example,

> I will not tell you that you won't feel helpless at times, for I know far too well that feeling. What I am telling you is that you can climb back out of that dark pit of despair—that hope exists for all of us. . . Remember always, cancer is only a small part of who and what you are—never the sum total. . . Above all, know this: Cancer is a beatable, treatable, and survivable disease.[43]

One of Winston Churchill's famous lines during World War II was, "We will never, never, never, never give up." If this is the attitude of the cancer patient and his or her family, the likelihood of success is greatly enhanced.

The practical steps that we emphasize to our cancer patients are as follows:

- Try not to be negative.
- Try to not be around negative people.
- Be positive.
- Be around positive people.
- Have family unity in the treatment course decided.
- Once a treatment course is decided, do it with all the strength, hope, optimism, and prayer you and your friends can muster.

The practical side of this is that if there is a dispute between family members on what treatment course is to be done, it is important that unity be achieved before the cancer patient undergoes the first treatment. Nothing will hurt a cancer patient's chances of survival quicker than an unsupportive spouse or child. This completely discourages the patient when survival demands a massive amount of encouragement from family and friends.

Get rid of stress. Many people's stress is from their jobs. If your job is causing you a lot of stress and you have cancer, then immediately quit your job. It may be killing you.

We recommend that the person with cancer not watch the news or pick up a newspaper. These are too depressing. It is best to listen to uplifting music, read uplifting books, and most of all—be around uplifting people. If you can find something uplifting on television, then go for it, but it won't be easy to find.

Do activities that you love. If you love to exercise, then keep it up. If you love your dog, spend lots of time with your dog. If you enjoy the country, then rent a cabin out in the woods for an extended period of time.

Laugh hard and laugh often. See the funniest movies. Read the funniest books. Be around the funniest people. Laugh 'til your belly hurts.

Have positive thoughts. Positive thoughts have a positive effect on the body. Be an encourager, even in the midst of your cancer diagnosis. A good example of this is our friend Steve Meyer. He was diagnosed with a very rare form of cancer, mantle cell lymphoma. It has a poor prognosis. Instead of being doom and gloom, he used his circumstance to encourage others. (See **Figure 28-11**.)

Steve underwent a successful bone marrow transplant. As is evident by his compassion, he used his cancer diagnosis as a means to help others. He put his trust in God and his doctors.

When his doctors said he was cancer free, he tried to go back to work but just couldn't. Instead, he has decided to continue his cancer ministry and other volunteer work. This includes being cochair with his wife Robin on the Hospitality Team at Calvary Memorial Church in Oak Park (the church we attend) and helping us as one of the volunteers at Beulah Land Natural Medicine Clinic, a Christian missionary clinic, along with being very active in the community and politics. He is a good example of a person who makes his life count—cancer or not.

PRAYER AND DEEPENED FAITH IN GOD

"I KNOW GOD WON'T GIVE ME ANYTHING I CAN'T HANDLE. I JUST WISH HE DIDN'T TRUST ME SO MUCH."
- Mother Teresa

Nothing should be able to perk up people better than knowing that the God of the universe loves them. I once told a cancer patient this, and she smirked back, "I hate God." A few short months later, she was dead.

Nothing can help heal a person more than strong faith in God. Reading the Bible, praying, and having your friends and family pray for you is putting faith into action. Doctors can be great, IPT can be great, but God is great. He has already put in print many of the points that we have been discussing. Consider these verses from the Bible (*New International Version*):

- **Proverbs 15:30:** A cheerful look brings joy to the heart, and good news gives health to the bones.

- **Proverbs 16:9:** In his heart a man plans his course, but the Lord determines his steps.

- **Proverbs 17:22:** A cheerful heart is good medicine, but a crushed spirit dries up the bones.

- **Proverbs 19:21:** Many are the plans in a man's heart, but it is the Lord's purpose that prevails.

- **Matthew 9:22:** Jesus turned and saw her. "Take heart, daughter," he said, "your faith

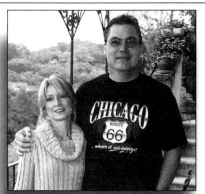

Figure 28-11: Steve and Robin Meyer stand under the veranda of a bed and breakfast in Venasque, France.

MANTLE CELL: QUALITY OF LIFE

Steve participates in an email listserv for Mantle Cell patients. One new victim of this disease posted a question to the group about what could be expected as a "quality of life" with this disease. Here is Steve's reply...

Dear Sir (or Ma'am).

I am not happy to have this disease, nor is anyone who has it. Chemotherapy is not a refreshment. Bone Marrow Transplants are less fun than going to the lake in the summer. And having ones life ripped apart by a disease that has historically killed all its victims is not my first choice.

On the other hand when you are surrounded by people who love you, people who pray for you, people who bring you meals, send you cards, rake your leaves, cry with you, laugh with you, do your chores for you, shovel your snow all winter, cut your grass all summer, come over on Sunday to watch football with you, call you on the phone, pick up your medicine for you, drive you places when you can't, offer you their homes, offer support to your healthy parents, offer support to your brothers and sisters, come over to keep you company, take you out to dinner, bring you books, CDs, tapes, loan you their laptop, offer their friendship and love...When your kids tell you they love you, again and again and again and cry at the thought of losing you...When your wife or husband tells you they love you even when you act like an idiot and they cry themselves to sleep at the thought of losing you...

When you see your parents eyes at the thought of losing a child to this disease and they say, "I wish it were me" and they mean it...When people you've never met pray for you, send you mail, encourage you, meet you for dinner...when the Doctor weeps for you because he wishes he could do more...When the pain gets so bad it takes your breath, or you get so sick you think you're gonna die.

I'll tell you what I do.

I thank God for my life just the way it is! I have had a good life, and I intend to live for many years to come. I plan on seeing my Becky grow up. Today she was the happiest little girl in the third grade, and so proud to read her grades one by one to her dad, who she has no doubt loves her with all of his heart. I plan to see my twelve year-old son's penmanship improve even if it takes forever and someday he will beat me in chess. I plan to see my sophomore daughter in college someday grow up the rest of the way and get married and give me grandkids. I plan to see my parents finish their lives with their son alive, and I'll bury them when they die. I plan to see my beautiful wife grow old, get gray hair, and sag, so I can love her more than I do now, and we can retire to Florida.

Did we all get a bad break? Yes. Do we have the right to complain? A little. Would I change my life if I could? Never!

I'm glad you asked the question. And I pray that you and everyone else with this disease gets cured, and those who have died from this disease, I plan to see them again. The quality of my life has never been better!!! May God bless all those with MCL and the loving caregivers and families.

Steve Meyer, Oak Park, Illinois *(11 days to Bone Marrow Transplant)*

Below is one response of many published at Steve's web site:

Again, I read with amazement—thank you Steve for your loving input. It couldn't have been better said. I wanted to post, then I wanted to just sign off the attack list. But all input is good, even if it is to vent frustration and disappointment. ANY treatment greatly depends on how the person feels who is getting it and making the decisions. If you love your doctor that helps greatly too. If I were to believe one hospital and one hospital alone would be the answer then I guess Tim would be gone now. So much new stuff going on in MANY Hospitals. Most of the successful ones work on grants, common sense tells you that if they have success they have more money pouring into the program. Tim picked his treatment, not I. He likes and trusted his previous doctors, Even after changing one of them. His odds were not good, he has already lost a kidney to cancer. Not MCL, only later was he diagnosed with MCL. He would not have been a candidate for a stem-cell transplant anywhere if he did not meet the criteria..."thank you god for answering" I thank this list for what our kind founder said to me when we were searching for an answer. "The most important factor in your treatment is how you feel about it." I agree, and I agree that you also need a good hospital and one that does transplants.

Tim did not have his transplant at any hospital mentioned here, and he at times wonders if it was the correct choice. Scary, that we can put doubts in the very minds that are searching. Everyone can't go to NY, TX, WA etc., but we fight, we live and we love. Anger defeats it all, does it not? I will hang on to my father's words..."Sis, there are no signposts along the road of life. If you take a wrong turn, do your best to get back on the path. Trust you will be guided." And so it goes...Bless you Steve, I needed your input; we are fighting too.

Much love to the group and blessings,

Tammy

has healed you." And the woman was healed from that moment.

- **Luke 17:5-6:** The apostles said to the Lord, "Increase our faith!" He replied, "If you have faith as small as a mustard seed, you can say to this mulberry tree, 'Be uprooted and planted in the sea,' and it will obey you."

- **John 3:16-17:** For God so loved the world that he gave his one and only Son, that whoever believes in him shall not perish but have eternal life. For God did not send his Son into the world to condemn the world, but to save the world through him.

- **Ephesians 4:29-32:** Do not let any unwholesome talk come out of your mouths, but only what is helpful for building others up according to their needs, that it may benefit those who listen. And do not grieve the Holy Spirit of God, with whom you were sealed for the day of redemption. Get rid of all bitterness, rage and anger, brawling and slander, along with every form of malice. Be kind and compassionate to one another, forgiving each other, just as in Christ God forgave you.

- **Galatians 5:22-23a:** But the fruit of the Spirit is love, joy, peace, patience, kindness, goodness, faithfulness, gentleness and self control.

- **John 6:28-29:** Then they asked him, "What must we do to do the works God requires?" Jesus answered, "The work of God is this: to believe in the one he has sent."

- **Philippians 4:6-7:** Do not be anxious about anything, but in everything, by prayer and petition, with thanksgiving, present your requests to God. And the peace of God, which transcends all understanding, will guard your hearts and your minds in Christ Jesus.

- **Philippians 4:8:** Finally, brothers, whatever is true, whatever is noble, whatever is right, whatever is pure, whatever is lovely, whatever is admirable—if anything is excellent or praiseworthy—think about such things.

- **James 5:13:** Is any one of you in trouble? He should pray. Is anyone happy? Let him sing songs of praise.

These verses are only a small fraction of the wisdom and encouragement found in the Bible. Yes, that big book on your shelf. Yes, it is okay to pick it up. Yes, it is even okay to open it up and read it. Please read it; it may be in there that you find the healing for which you have been looking.

As with a positive attitude, modern medicine is realizing the power of prayer and faith in healing. In other words, they are finally catching on to what the Bible says. Our lives have been transformed through the reading of the Bible and applying its principles. For the cancer patient looking for hope, it is there on every page. We have found nothing stronger to help heal a person both physically and spiritually than putting complete trust in God.

As the Bible says in Psalm 46:1: "God is our refuge and strength, an ever-present help in trouble." Pastor Peter preached on this passage on December 18, 1994. I (Ross) know this because it is marked in my Bible. His main point was that fear and faith are at polar extremes; the one repels the other. You cannot have both faith and fear. Pastor Peter was a man of great faith, yet he still died of his cancer.

Faith is not a guarantee that a person with cancer will be healed physically, but it will heal the person spiritually. As in the case of Pastor Peter, as he was being "cleansed" spiritually, he brought his family and friends with him. He never cursed God because of his ailment; he just showed us all what true faith looks like. To this day, his courage during his battle inspires us. Our natural medicine charity work in southern Illinois is an outgrowth of his great faith and the God that he served.

Perhaps the above can be summed up in the poem following.

SUMMARY

Many people with cancer have died because they have used herbal remedies on the recommendation of a friend and did not see a qualified

> ## Cancer is limited...
>
> It cannot cripple love;
>
> It cannot cripple faith;
>
> It cannot eat away peace;
>
> It cannot destroy confidence;
>
> It cannot kill friendship;
>
> It cannot shut out memories;
>
> It cannot silence courage;
>
> It cannot invade the soul;
>
> It cannot reduce eternal life;
>
> It cannot quench the Spirit;
>
> It cannot lessen the power of the Resurrection!
>
> *(Author Unknown)*
>
> ### Praise the Lord for His omnipotence!

physician to get care for their condition. Warning: herbs are no substitute for an IPT physician.

Most herbal remedies that are recommended for cancer stimulate the immune system. Since cancer is not an immunodeficiency disease, these herbal remedies do not bring about cancer remission.

Most newly-diagnosed cancer patients, when tested, are shown to have a normal immune system. When immunodeficiency exists, it is generally because of the treatments the cancer patient has undergone, including high-dose chemotherapy and radiation therapy. Another treatment that suppresses the immune system is narcotic medications. It is best for cancer patients not to use narcotics, and to use anti-inflammatory medications for pain relief.

When immunodeficiency does exist, there are many steps a cancer patient can take to reverse this state. The first step is to reduce the tumor load with Insulin Potentiation Therapy. Proper nutrition, stopping narcotic medications, using anti-inflammatory medications for pain control, giving biological response modifiers such as cytokines, nutriceutical stimulation, maintaining a positive outlook, plus prayer and deepened faith in God are also important.

Clinical experience has demonstrated that patients with a strong faith and a "fighter" attitude, who have strong family support, have better outcomes. As such, it is important for the cancer patient to laugh often with people whom they love. Love is the best medicine, and God is the best doctor. ∎

CHAPTER 29

Learn to Starve Tumors—Because Cancers Crave Sugar!

"IN THE PRESENCE OF MALIGNANCY, CARBOHYDRATE TOLERANCE IS DEFINITELY DECREASED, THE DEGREE OF DECREASE VARYING DIRECTLY WITH THE DEGREE OF MALIGNANCY OF THE TUMOR." [1]
-D. Jackson, M.D., 1934

Between 1910 and 1940, research on cancer patients clearly focused on cancer physiology. The main question to answer was, "How did the biochemistry of the blood and tissues in a person with cancer compare to somehow who was healthy?" This research clearly demonstrated that there were differences (**Figure 29-1**).

FIGURE 29-1: NORMAL PHYSIOLOGY VERSUS CANCER PHYSIOLOGY

BIOCHEMICAL PARAMETER	PHYSIOLOGY		
	CANCER	NORMAL	SOURCE
BLOOD pH	ALKALOSIS	NORMAL	STURROCK/1913[2]
GLYCOLYSIS	HIGH	NORMAL	CORI/1925[3]
LACTIC ACIDOSIS	PRESENT	ABSENT	WARBURG/1926[4]
CELL pH	ACID	NORMAL	HARDE/1927[5]
ENERGY PRODUCTION	ANAEROBIC	AEROBIC	WARBURG/1930[6]
CARBOHYDRATES FEED TUMORS?	YES	NO	GOLDFEDER/1933[7]
CARBOHYDRATE TOLERANCE	DECREASED	INCREASED	JACKSON/1934[1]
CELL pH DECREASED WITH GLUCOSE?	YES	NO	KAHLER/1943[8]

As in other fields of medicine, when nitrogen mustards were found to have tumoricidal effects in the 1940s, cancer research shifted from the physiological basis for the disease toward patentable medications—chemotherapy drugs. This has continued to this day as pharmaceutical companies race to find the magic bullet cancer drug.

POSITRON EMISSION TOMOGRAPHY— MODERN DAY PROOF THAT CANCER LIVES OFF SUGAR

Positron emission tomography (PET) is an imaging technique that allows the visualization of the whole body at once; it shows body metabolism and other functions rather than simply the gross anatomy and structure that is revealed by conventional x-rays, CT (computer tomography) scans, and magnetic resonance imaging (MRI) scans. No other imaging modality has comparable potential because PET has the unique ability to image functional processes, such as tumor metabolic activity, in vivo. The basic principles of PET are based on the detection of photons emitted from the patient after the intravenous injection of a short-lived radiopharmaceutical fluorodeoxyglucose (FDG). Because tumors utilize more glucose than normal tissues, they are seen on the PET scan as dark nodules as they pick up the radioactive glucose (See **Figure 29-2**). PET scanning has demonstrated great clinical utility in imaging a variety of cancers, including lung, head and neck, breast, bladder, and brain, as well as lymphomas and colon cancer. It is currently the most accurate modality available in detecting the spread of lung and colon cancer.[9,10]

PET scanning is a more sensitive modality for showing early cancers than MRI or CT scans

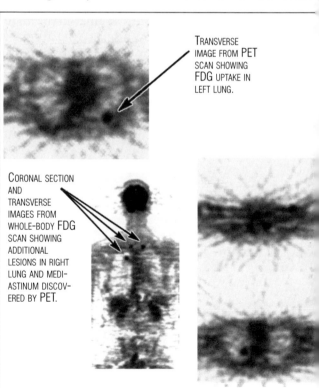

TRANSVERSE IMAGE FROM PET SCAN SHOWING FDG UPTAKE IN LEFT LUNG.

CORONAL SECTION AND TRANSVERSE IMAGES FROM WHOLE-BODY FDG SCAN SHOWING ADDITIONAL LESIONS IN RIGHT LUNG AND MEDIASTINUM DISCOVERED BY PET.

Figure 29-2: Positron Emission Tomography (PET) of Lung Cancer

PET scanning uses radioactive glucose to pick up cancers—proving that cancers do indeed crave sugar.

because it involves cancer physiology. When cells start using more glucose than normal cells, PET scanning picks up the abnormality—this is one of the earliest signs of cancer physiology. MRI and CT scans are typically not abnormal until a 1-cm mass forms. For the cancer patient desiring to know whether he or she has cancer left after treatment or if the cancer is shrinking with treatment, PET scanning can prove invaluable. So why are not more PET scans done on cancer patients? Because most often they are not covered by insurance.

You see even today the simple fact that cancer craves and feeds off sugar is being ignored by modern allopathic medicine. Cancer patients, who bear the consequences by being fed sugar in their tube feedings and intravenous drips in the hospital, are told by their oncologists to "eat whatever you want," and are refused a test by their insurance companies that could help save their lives. We hope this chapter will help reverse these trends. We hope that you will learn that you must starve your tumor because it craves sugar.

THE RESEARCH OF CORI, CORI, AND WARBURG

The concept that cancer craves sugar is based on the research of C. Cori, G. Cori, and Otto Warburg in the 1920s. Cori and Cori observed that blood passing through a sarcoma growing in a chicken wing contained 23 mg % less sugar and 16.2 mg % more lactate than blood that passed through the opposite normal wing. This finding was confirmed by other researchers for tumors of different species.[12,13] Cori and Cori discovered that the initial breakdown of glucose to yield energy (a process known as glycolyis) was markedly increased in cancer cells.[3] Science rewarded them by naming the process by which lactate is recycled in the body as the Cori cycle (also known as the lactic acid cycle).

Otto Warburg in the 1920s did much of the early work in tumor oxygenation. He calculated oxygen consumption rates for many types of tumors as assessed in tissue biopsy. He also discovered aberrant metabolic states present in tumors. Some of his research findings are as follows:[4,6]

- Perfused tumors with arterial blood extracted 57% of the sugar from it, whereas in normal tissues the sugar lost from the blood ranged between 2% and 18%.
- As long as adequate oxygen was supplied to normal tissues, none of the sugar was utilized for production of lactic acid, but tumors produced from 46 to 49 mg of this acid for each 100 mL of blood.
- When the sugar concentration is reduced by insulin shock, the formation of lactic acid is also reduced (See **Figure 29-3**).
- Rat tumor cells possessed a high rate of anaerobic and aerobic glycolysis compared to normal cells.
- In rapidly growing, undifferentiated tumors, aerobic glycolysis was increased, and respiration was decreased.
- Neoplastic change occurred when cellular respiration was damaged (caused by damage to oxidative metabolism), and the cell, in response, increased its glycolytic rate.
- Cells failing to adapt in this fashion died, but the cells able to increase the glycolytic rate high enough to produce a normal ATP (adenosine triphosphate) concentration became cancer cells.

FIGURE 29-3: THE LACTIC ACID PRODUCTION IN NORMAL GLUCOSE AND IN INSULIN SHOCK SERUM

Experiment Number	Lactic Acid Production in Normal Glucose Serum (mg)	Glucose Levels	Lactic Acid Production in Insulin Shock Serum (mg)	Glucose Levels (mg)
1	.036	140	.023	35
2	.036	155	.101	26
3	.025	144	.018	33
4	.042	136	.017	44
5	.021	122	.014	32
AVERAGE:	.032	139	.016	30

Figure 29-3 Insulin injections, by lowering blood glucose levels, decrease lactic acid production in tumor tissues.

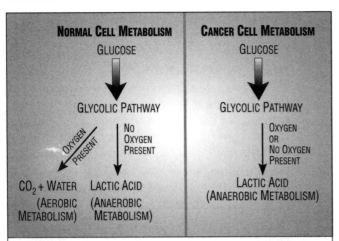

Figure 29-4: Normal Cell Metabolism Versus Cancer Cell Metabolism
Cancer cell metabolism proceeds at a high rate of glycolysis regardless of the presence of oxygen. Normal cells switch from anaerobic to aerobic metabolism in the presence of oxygen. This is known as the Pasteur effect.

colysis) (See **Figure 29-4**). This observation prompted Warburg to postulate that the respiratory processes of malignant cells are impaired and that normal cells become malignant after they suffer such impairment. The basic findings of Warburg have survived some eight decades of experimentation. Some research has, of course, shown that the Warburg hypothesis does not apply to every cancer, but many of the principles he set forth apply to most cancerous conditions. Otto Warburg was rewarded for his research by winning the Nobel Prize in Medicine in 1930.

Cori, Cori, and Warburg discovered in the 1920s that tumor cells consumed more sugar than normal cells and converted it to lactic acid. They found the tumor cell was able to metabolize glucose (glycolysis) with the production of lactic acid. With one molecule of oxygen, malignant tissue produces from three to four times as much lactic acid as did benign tissue. The tumor cell is a facultative anaerobe and aerobe.

CANCERS CRAVE SUGAR

Glucose net uptake and lactate release by malignancies exceed the peripheral exchange rates *30- and 43-fold,* respectively.[13]

Otto Warbug discovered that there was a quantitative difference in the way cancer cells extract and utilize energy. The normal cell desires to extract the maximum amount of energy per molecule of glu-

The Warburg hypothesis implied that every cancer cell had decreased respiration, increased glycolysis, and normal ATP production. He made two fundamental generalizations: (**1**) Cancer is caused by damage to oxidative metabolism, and (**2**) the decrease in oxidative metabolism and increase in fermentative metabolism (anaerobic) explain the nature of all cancers. Warburg postulated that cancer cells originate from normal cells in two phases: an irreversible injury to respiration, followed by a long intracellular struggle in replacing lost respiration energy with fermentation energy and conversion of the cells into undifferentiated cells. This second stage involves selection and requires many consecutive generations of cells, accounting for the long latency of carcinogenesis.

Warburg developed his theory based on the differential behavior of glucose metabolism between normal and malignant cells. When normal tissues were switched from anaerobic to aerobic conditions, the lactate formation from glucose (glycolysis) was virtually ceased (Pasteur effect), while beyond the high glycolytic rate observed in malignant tissues, glycolysis persisted even after exposure to an aerobic environment (aerobic gly-

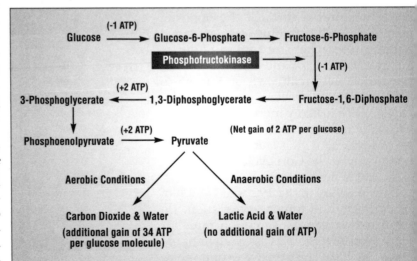

Figure 29-5: The Breakdown of Glucose for Energy
Aerobic metabolism produces much more energy per glucose molecule (36 ATPs) compared to anaerobic metabolism (2 ATPs). Aerobic metabolism is thus a more efficient method of energy extraction than anaerobic metabolism.

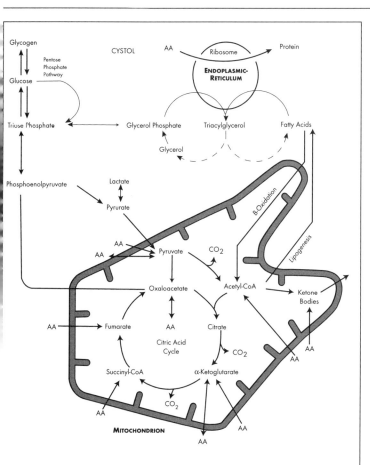

Figure 29-6: Normal Aerobic Metabolism:
Aerobic metabolism proceeds through the citric acid cycle
(Krebs Cycle) in the mitochondria of the cell.

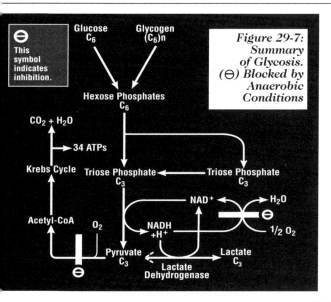

cose that it absorbs. The method in which glucose is broken down to the energy source ATP is called glycolysis. At the last stage of glycolysis, pyruvate is formed plus 2 ATP molecules per glucose molecule. Glycosis occurs in the cytoplasm of cells. The most efficient way to metabolize pyruvate is by aerobic metabolism. As long as oxygen is present, aerobic metabolism will break down the pyruvate to carbon dioxide (CO_2) and water (H_2O) and form an additional 34 ATP molecules per glucose molecule metabolized. When sufficient oxygen is not present, pyruvate is shunted down a different pathway to form lactic acid and water with no additional gain of ATP molecules. This is anaerobic metabolism (See **Figure 29-5**).

Aerobic metabolism proceeds through the Krebs cycle (also known as the citric acid cycle) as pyruvate diffuses from the cytoplasm into the mitochondria of cells (See **Figure 29-6**). What happens in fast-growing cancer cells is that glycolysis proceeds at a much higher rate than is required by the citric acid cycle. Thus, more pyruvate is produced than can be metabolized. This in turn results in excessive production of lactate, which favors a relatively acid local environment in the tumor.[14]

Glycolysis can function under anaerobic conditions and is similar to the process of fermentation in yeast. When oxygen is excluded, glycogen (the storage form of glucose) disappears, and lactate appears as the principal end product. When oxygen is available, aerobic recovery takes place: glycogen reappears, while lactate disappears. The reactions in glycolysis are the same in the presence of oxygen as in its absence, except in extent and end products.

Under aerobic conditions, pyruvate is taken up into the mitochondria. After conversion to acetyl coenzyme A, it is oxidized to carbon dioxide by the Krebs cycle to produce an additional 34 ATP molecules per glucose molecule. In anaerobic conditions, pyruvate is reduced by NADH (nicotinamide adenine dinucleotide) to lactate, with the reaction being catalyzed by lactate dehydrogenase (See **Figure 29-7**). Inhibition of this enzyme is key to reversing cancer's anaerobic physiology.

The overall equation for glycolysis from glucose to lactate is as follows:

$$Glucose + 2ADP + 2\,Pi \rightarrow 2\text{-Lactate} + 2ATP + 2H_2O$$

Under anaerobic conditions, the lactate formed is transported to the liver and kidneys where it reforms glucose, which again becomes available via the circulation for oxidation in the tissues. This process is known as the Cori cycle or lactic acid cycle (See **Figure 29-8**). The glucose that is formed from the Cori cycle can then be reused. Thus, under aerobic conditions, there is a net gain of 36 ATP molecules formed per molecule of glucose used, whereas under anaerobic conditions only 2 ATP molecules are formed per molecule of glucose. It is obvious that oxidative phosphorylation via aerobic metabolism is a much more efficient way to extract energy.

Cancer cells primarily use glucose for fuel, with lactic acid as an anaerobic end product. This inefficient pathway for energy metabolism yields only 5% of the ATP energy available in food and is one of the main reasons why 40% of cancer patients die from malnutrition or cachexia.

The scientific literature on in vivo studies of tumor metabolism offers overwhelming evidence that glucose is the primary energy source for malignancies.[15-19] The consumption of glucose in cancer cells is often many times that of normal cells. According to one study, "cancer cells demonstrate a 3- to 5-fold increase in glucose uptake compared to healthy cells."[20] In another study done on 17 patients with colon carcinoma, glucose net uptake by the carcinomas exceeded peripheral glucose retention by a factor of 30 and was related to tumor blood flow. Lactate output from the tumors was about 43 times greater than the peripheral release. With regard to both the glucose and lactate balance, the carcinomas differed from the periphery at $p < 0.001$ statistical significance.[13] (See **Figure 29-9**).

It should now be obvious that cancer truly does crave sugar. As it turns out, the more aggressive a tumor, the more it craves sugar. Several investigators have shown that the glucose consumption of individual tumors correlated with their grade, growth, and recurrence rates.[17,21,22] For instance, a study of 100 patients revealed an average glucose uptake rate in grade I and II astrocytomas (brain cancer) of 0.21 micro-moles/gram/minute compared to 0.3 in cases in grade III and 0.41 micromoles/gram/minute in verified cases of grade IV astrocytomas.[17]

As discussed previously, Warburg, Cori, and Cori established that the rate of glycolysis is high in cancers. It was apparent from their data that a considerable part of the energy supply of tumors is obtained through this glycolysis and that tumors are capable, unlike other tissues, of survival under anaerobic conditions by means of energy derived from glycolysis. Warburg actually cut out the center portions of rat tumors and analyzed them for lactic

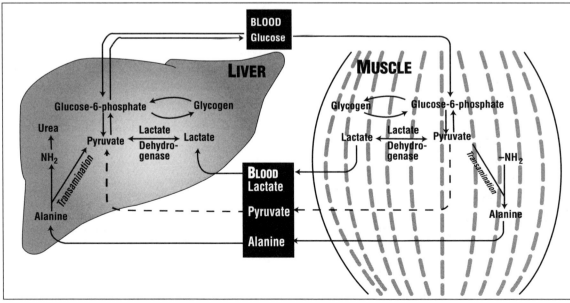

Figure 29-8: The Lactic Acid (Cori) cycle and Glucose-Alanine Cycle

The Cori cycle allows lactate from muscles or cancer cells to form glucose. This anaerobic metabolism is very inefficient compared to aerobic metabolism.

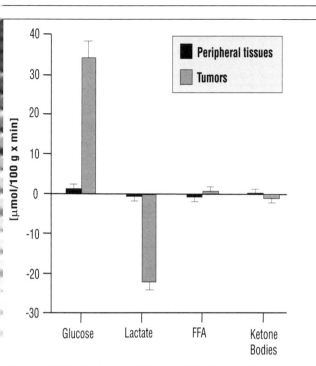

Figure 29-9: Balance of Energy-Yielding Substrates Across Both Peripheral Tissues and the Colonic Tumors

As one can see, glucose consumption and subsequent lactate production from the tumors was significantly greater than from peripheral tissues.

FIGURE 29-10: LACTIC ACID LEVELS OF VARIOUS TISSUES (MICROMOLES PER 100 GRAMS)

Lactic acid production is much greater in cancerous tissues than normal ones.

NORMAL TISSUES

BRAIN	141
MUSCLE	188
LIVER	230
KIDNEY	155
HEART	578

CANCEROUS TISSUES

PRIMARY MOUSE CARCINOMA	832
PRIMARY RAT LIVER CARCINOMA	590
HUMAN BREAST CARCINOMA	1,450

acid in the fluid collecting there.[4,6] Cori and Cori analyzed for lactic acid in the ingoing and outgoing blood supply of tumors.[3]

Most researchers have found that the lactic acid level in tumor tissue is consistently three to four times that found in resting differentiated tissues. This is easily seen in a study that looked at lactic acid levels in various tissues, animal cancers, and human breast cancer[23] (See **Figure 29-10**). Various researchers have confirmed that lactic acid levels in the blood can be markedly elevated in patients with cancer.[24-26] With regard to circulating levels of lactate, Holroyde found elevated fasting plasma lactate levels of 1.76 mM in patients with metastatic solid tumors and progressive weight loss.[27] Russell found mean blood lactate levels of 1.12 mM in 31 untreated patients with small cell lung cancer and 0.62 mM in 20 healthy volunteers.[28] Lactic acid and various other metabolites of aerobic and anaerobic metabolism can easily be measured in the blood. They should be part of a cancer physiology study (**Figure 29-11**).

As a general rule, the amount of lactate released by tumor cells is linearly related to the amount of glucose they consume (See **Figure 29-12**). Assuming steady state conditions and glucose as the only substrate source of lactate, the glycolytic rate can be determined as the ratio of lactate release to glucose uptake (lactate release rate:glucose uptake rate). With this assumption, most human cancer cell lines investigated show a 40-85% glycolytic rate.[29-32] In other words, for cancer cells, about one half to three fourths of the glucose that is delivered to them is converted to lactate. This is in vast contrast to normal cells in which the glycolytic rate is negligible.

In 1960, H. Busch at the University of Illinois College of Medicine found in an animal tumor line for a period of one to eight minutes following injection of the labeled glucose that lactate in the tumor contained 70-90% of the isotope of utilized glucose.[33] He concluded that "these data have a bearing on the possibility of approaching cancer chemotherapy by inhibition of glycolysis." The author showed that doing this revealed some cancer inhibiting effects.[34,35]

If helping to shut down the tumor supply would have the effect of decreasing tumor growth, then the reverse must also be true. If the glucose supply to a tumor is increased, tumor growth will be enhanced. A good example of both of these principles was done by Pietro Gullino at the Laboratory of Biochemistry at the National Cancer Institute, with the results published in 1967.[16] In this experiments, the in vivo relationships among glucose availability, utilization, and glycolysis were studied in three types of animal

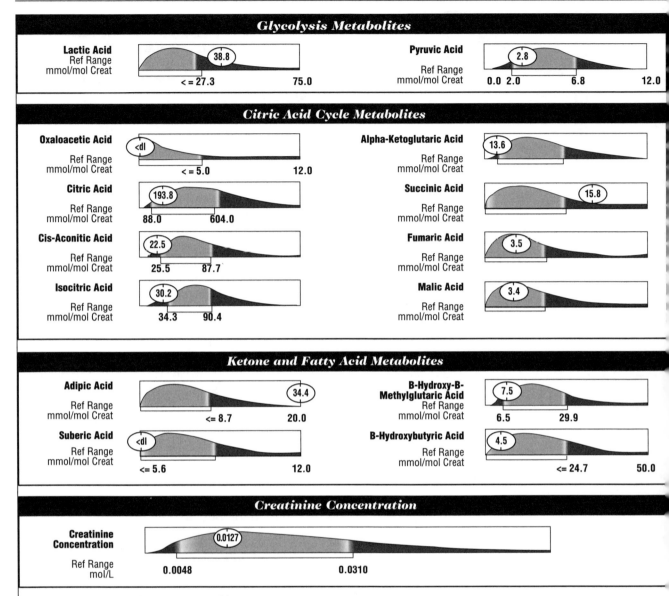

Figure 29-11: Cellular Energy Profile

This is one of the tests done at Caring Medical to detect cancer physiology. In the test above, notice the elevated blood lactic acid levels, indicative of some anaerobic metabolism.

Adapted from Great Smokies Diagnostic Laboratory, Asheville, NC.

tumors. The study found that about 35% of the glucose consumed was eliminated as lactate regardless of the tumor type. In normoglycemia (blood sugars maintained within the normal range), the amount of glucose consumed and glycolyzed was directly related to the glucose available, which decreased per unit weight as the tumor size increased (See **Figure 29-13**). During hyperglycemia, produced either by dextrose injections or diabetes, the tumors increased

glucose utilization from 3- to 10-fold as compared with normoglycemia. **When the animals were given an insulin shot that caused hypoglycemia all three of the tumor lines tested (carcinomas, hepatomas, and fibrosarcomas) had decreased glucose uptake in proportion to the amount of glucose available (the glucose level in the blood).** This study showed that glucose consumption of tumors in vivo is directly related to glycemia (blood level of glucose). Other research has also

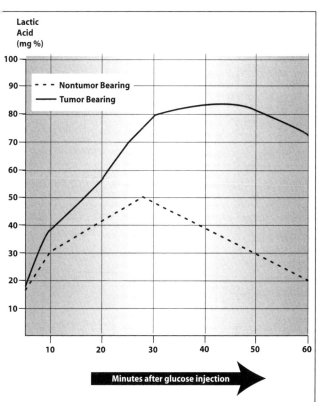

Figure 29-12: Lactic Acid Production after Glucose Injection

Tumor cells consume more glucose and produce more lactate than normal cells.

Adapted from The blood lactic acid of tumor-bearing and tumor-free mice, by T. Norman, Cancer Research, 1955, 5:1027-1030.

shown that when sugar concentration is reduced by insulin shock, the formation of lactic acid is also reduced by about 50%.[36]

Tumor energy production is directly correlated to the amount of glucose the tumor consumes because cancer craves sugar. Research done in the early 1990s by researchers at Carnegie Mellon University in Pittsburgh, Massachusetts General Hospital, and Harvard Medical School helped prove this.[37] The research sought to determine in vivo whether tumor energy production depends on oxygen or glucose delivery to the tumor. As can be seen in **Figure 29-14**, tumor energy status markedly dropped with a drop in blood flow. The question to the researchers was, "What contributed to the drop in tumor energy supply: oxygen deprivation, glucose deprivation, or a combination of both?" The researchers answered this question by cutting off the oxygen supply to the tumors for 60 to 90 minutes and then in a similar fashion ran a glucose-free medium through the tumors. The energy supply of the cancer was measured as the ratio of nucleoside triphosphate to inorganic phosphate (NTP/Pi). One can see in **Figure 29-15** that the hypoxia had no effect on energy production, whereas reducing the glucose concentration to the tumor had a dramatic effect. The authors stated, "In conclusion, the energy status of the isolated ex vivo-perfused mammary adenocarcinoma is similar to that in

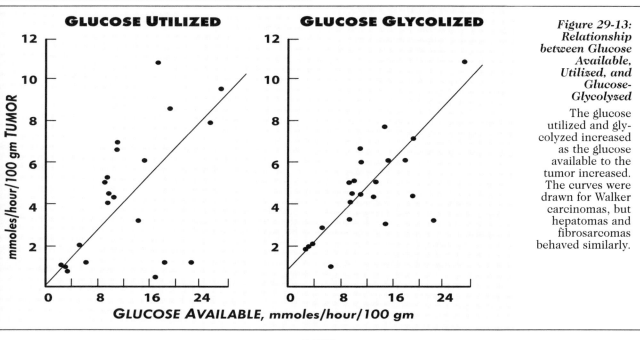

Figure 29-13: Relationship between Glucose Available, Utilized, and Glucose-Glycolyzed

The glucose utilized and glycolyzed increased as the glucose available to the tumor increased. The curves were drawn for Walker carcinomas, but hepatomas and fibrosarcomas behaved similarly.

273

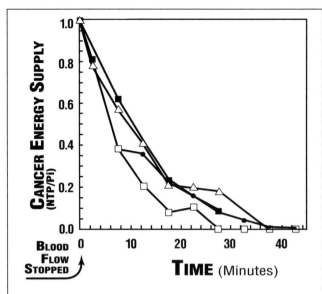

Figure 29-14: Response of the in Vitro Status of Several Tumor Lines to Ischemia

As can be seen, ischemia caused a dramatic drop in the cancers' ability to extract energy from the blood.

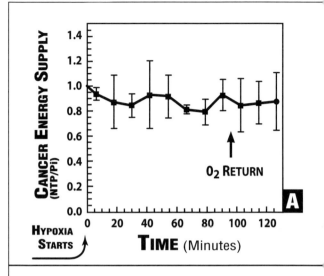

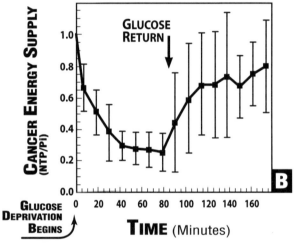

Figure 29-15: Average Response of the NTP/Pi Ratio to Acute Hypoxia (A) and Acute Glucose Deprivation (B)

At zero minutes in A, the gas in the gas exchanger was switched to 95% N_2/5% CO_2. At zero minutes in B, the glucose content of the medium was decreased to zero. The arrows mark the return of the 95% O_2/5% CO_2, or glucose, respectively. Error bars represent standard deviation. Decreasing oxygen in the blood had no effect whereas depriving the cancer of glucose had a dramatic effect or decreasing the cancers energy supply. This proves that cancers do indeed crave sugar.

vivo. The perfused tumor is dependent on glucose for maintenance of NTP levels."

GLUCOSE INTOLERANCE AND CANCER INCIDENCE

From this overview of cancer physiology, it should be clear that cancer craves sugar. Thus, it makes sense that people who consume a lot of sugar end up with more cancers than those who do not. Likewise, people who have blood sugar-related medical conditions such as diabetes would likewise have a higher risk of cancer.

> Glucose intolerance is one of the earliest metabolic abnormalities described in cancer populations. In our experience, the rate of glucose intolerance in cancer is high. In a recent study, we found that more than 60% of neoplastic patients undergoing a glucose loading test showed an intolerant or overtly diabetic response.[38,39]

These authors also state that "reversing abnormal carbohydrate metabolism may represent a possible point for therapeutic intervention in patients with cancer." Exactly! Unfortunately, the average oncologist does not think like this.

Believe it or not, the first time abnormally high blood glucose levels in response to a carbohydrate load (glucose intolerance) were found in cancer patients was in 1885! In that year, Freund reported glucose intolerance in 62 of 70 tumor patients![40] Over the years, many others have found glucose intolerance common in cancer patients. Glicksman found 35% of 557 consecutive cancer patients exceeded 200 mg/dL on glucose tolerance tests.[41] Glicksman cited an eight times higher inci-

TABLE I: THYROID DISEASE IN FEMALES

INCIDENCE	AGE GROUP	RATE	PERCENT
†Expected	20-64	10.9-14.2/1000	1.09-1.42
Breast Cancer	18-75	120/1000	12

† Data from Metropolitan Life Insurance Co.

TABLE II: DIABETES IN FEMALES

INCIDENCE	AGE GROUP	RATE	PERCENT
*Expected	15-84	6.77/1000	.67
Breast Cancer	18-75	49.1/1000	4.9

* Courtesy of American Cancer Society.

Figure 29-16: Thyroid Disease and Diabetes in Females
The incidence of thyroid disease was ten times and the incidence of diabetes eight times greater in women with breast carcinoma than in women of comparable ages in the general population.

dence of diabetes in breast cancer but emphasized that the diabetes encountered in malignancy is usually mild. What we want to know is this, "How mild can it be if it contributed to the person's cancer?" R. Repert, M.D., followed 306 cases of breast carcinoma entering Butterworth Hospital between 1939 and 1949, with special regard to clinical endocrinologic factors.[42] His findings are shown in **Figure 29-16.** He found that the incidence of thyroid disease was 10 times and the incidence of diabetes mellitus eight times greater in women with breast carcinoma than in women of comparable ages in the general population. In addition to the above findings, other evidence suggestive of hormonal imbalance was found. Fifty-seven (25%) of 306 females had had pelvic operations. Sixteen patients had menorrhagia; 27 had metrorrhagia; and six had oligomenorrhea or amenorrhea. The incidence of sterility was 10%. Do you see what happened when the hormonal problems of these women were not corrected? Most likely because of estradiol excess, they subsequently developed breast cancer. Dr. Repert concluded that a general hormonal imbalance accompanies breast carcinoma.

Many researchers have looked at the relationship between diabetes mellitus and cancer risk. Significantly elevated relative risks (RR) among subjects with diabetes have been observed for cancers of the liver (RR = 2.8), pancreas (RR = 2.1), and endometrium (RR = 3.4). Other cancers

shown to be elevated in diabetics include thyroid, larynx, rectum, and colon cancers.[43]

Thus far, the discussion has primarily focused on diabetes and cancer risk. Diabetes is the end-stage result of glucose intolerance. Glucose intolerance begins with a person developing elevated blood sugars in response to carbohydrate loads, but not so elevated as to meet the criteria for diabetes. Some people with "early" glucose intolerance develop overt diabetes, but many do not. The most widely accepted test for glucose intolerance and diabetes is the glucose tolerance test. In this test, varying amounts of glucose via a sugary drink are given to the person (generally 100 g), and glucose levels are checked every 30 minutes to one hour for three to six hours. The person starts the test after an overnight fast. Glucose intolerance is generally diagnosed if the maximum blood sugar level during the test is greater than 160 mg/dL, and diabetes is diagnosed if it is greater than 190 mg/dL. Natural medicine doctors who do glucose tolerance tests generally have stricter criteria: Glucose intolerance is present if, during the test, the following are observed:*

- Fasting glucose levels are greater than 120 mg/dL.
- Fasting glucose levels are below 70 mg/dL.
- Glucose levels rise more than 50%.
- Glucose levels rise above 140 mg/dL.
- Glucose levels drop below 70 mg/dL.
- Glucose levels fail to rise 20%.
- The person becomes symptomatic.

In one study from Universitats-Frauenklinik in Germany, 837 women with breast cancer, benign tumors, and other breast conditions requiring excision or mammography were given a glucose tolerance test by oral ingestion with 100 grams of glucose or intravenous injection of 0.33 grams glucose/kg body weight.[44] The results in 327 women with breast cancer were compared with those in 510 women with benign breast affections. The criteria used to interpret the test are listed on the top of page 276.

In this prospective study the researchers found a diabetes incidence of about 22% in the breast cancer patients but only 3% in those patients with benign tumors (See **Figure 29-17**). Another 6.7%

* Depending on clinical experience, physicians do use various criteria.

GLUCOSE TOLERANCE TEST CRITERIA

	NORMAL (mg/100ml)	ABNORMAL (mg/100ml)	PATHOLOGICAL (mg/100ml)
1. 2-hour Value	120	121-140	140
2. Maximal Value	160	161-180	180

These were the criteria used in this study comparing the incidence of glucose intolerance in women with breast cancer versus benign breast lesions.

Adapted from Stoffwechselkrankheiten, *by H. Mehnert, H. Förster, p. 216, Thieme, Struttgart, 1970,*

of breast cancer patients and 2.5% of benign lesion patients presented with glucose intolerance (subclinical diabetes). Of interest was the fact that 46% of the breast cancer patients were overweight, compared to 26% of those with benign lesions. The authors noted, "The significantly increased coincidence of breast cancer, diabetes mellitus, and being overweight suggests that dietetic factors may be important." Unfortunately for the cancer patient (especially breast cancer patients), this obesity factor has been translated to eat less fat. Almost universally, "low-fat" foods are laced with tremendous amounts of carbohydrates. It is evident by the various studies discussed in this book that cancers crave carbohydrates—not fat. The driving force is insulin. It should be noted that B. Muck and associates performed other studies on glucose intolerance and female cancers and found overall glucose intolerance in 50% of the women with endometrial cancer, suggesting that similar somatic, clinical, and metabolic characteristics exist in breast cancer patients as well as in women

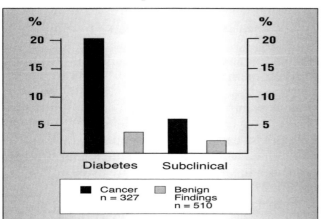

Figure 29-17: Incidence of Diabetes in Women with Benign and Malignant Breast Diseases

As one can see, diabetes is much more common in malignant breast diseases, than in nonmalignant conditions.

with endometrial cancer.[45] This concept is consistent with the research discussed in this book.

In 2001, the American Cancer Society published a mammoth textbook on cancer and cancer therapies entitled *Clinical Oncology.*[46] We would now like to show you in totality what they wrote about carbohydrate metabolism:

> In cancer patients, the changes seen in carbohydrate metabolism are an increase in glucose production and development of insulin resistance. Combined, they tend toward a state of glucose intolerance. Tumor cells may act as a glucose drain; they are able to metabolize glucose at high rates and are critically dependent on glycolytic pathways for more than 50% of their energy requirements. Particularly important in this process is the mitochondria-based hexokinase type II enzyme, which has been shown to be expressed in higher levels in tumor cells versus normal cells. Other significant pathways for glucose production are an increase in Cori cycle activity and an increase in hepatic glucose production, mediated by lipid-mobilizing factor, which acts to stimulate adenylate cyclase in a guanosine triphosphate-dependent manner.[46]

The American Cancer Society knows about glucose intolerance in cancer patients, and the glucose metabolism abnormalities in cancer. They state that tumor cells may act as a glucose drain...in other words, cancer craves sugar. Unfortunately for cancer patients across America, the American Cancer Society does not tell them how to reverse this physiology.

SUGAR INCREASES CANCER GROWTH THROUGH INSULIN

Endocrinology 101 says that if you eat sugar or a lot of carbohydrates, your blood sugar goes up. To normalize the blood sugar, your pancreas secretes insulin. The higher the blood sugar, the more insulin that is secreted (See **Figure 29-18**). If a person continues to eat too many carbohydrates over a long period of time, the cells of the body become resistant to the glucose-lowering effects of insulin. This medical condition is called insulin resistance. If the person doesn't change his or her diet and lifestyle, the condition can progress into overt diabetes or syndrome X. Syndrome X is a term used to describe a constellation of risk factors for heart disease, including insulin resistance, high cholesterol and triglyc-

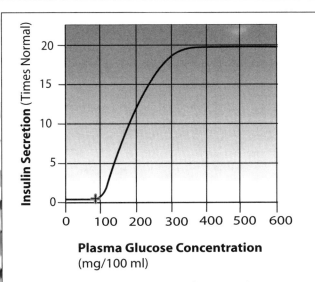

Figure 29-18: Approximate Insulin Secretion at Different Plasma Glucose Levels
The higher the blood sugar, the more insulin is secreted.

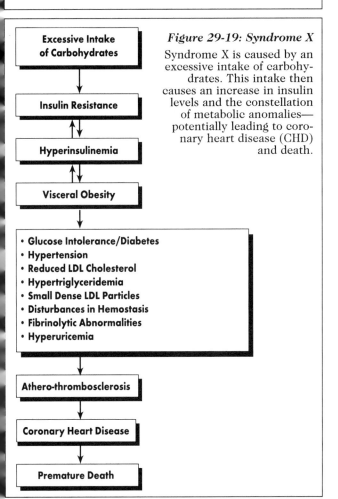

Figure 29-19: Syndrome X
Syndrome X is caused by an excessive intake of carbohydrates. This intake then causes an increase in insulin levels and the constellation of metabolic anomalies—potentially leading to coronary heart disease (CHD) and death.

eride levels, high blood pressure, and obesity (See **Figure 29-19**). The underlying metabolic denominator in syndrome X is elevated insulin levels. There is little doubt about what contributes to these elevations—an elevated intake of refined carbohydrates.

The relationship between glucose intolerance and insulin and its relation to cancer can be easily seen in a study done by A. Carter at the State University of New York Department of Medicine.[47] In this study of glucose tolerance, insulin and Growth Hormone levels were compared between breast cancer patients and healthy women. Both groups of women were given a standard six-hour, 100-g glucose tolerance test. During this time, glucose, insulin, and Growth Hormone levels were checked. The results can be seen in **Figure 29-20**. The study found that the mean glucose tolerance was impaired in women with breast cancer; mean plasma glucose at one hour was 190 mg/dL; at two hours, it was 165 mg/dL. Insulin secretion was delayed and prolonged in cancer patients. The peak plasma insulin value was 11 times the baseline value. The mean baseline level of Growth Hormone in cancer patients was 1.8 mg/mL, which was significantly greater than the mean in healthy subjects of 0.74. Carter noted that the results were not attributed to age, obesity, inanition, or stress. "These metabolic abnormalities may characterize host susceptibility to breast cancer or be effects of the tumor."

Insulin levels increase because of the high carbohydrate diet that many people eat. Research has shown that countries with the highest consumption of sugar also have the highest breast cancer mortality[48] (See **Figure 29-21**). Associations are, of course, not causations, and even high correlations provide no proof that sugar causes breast cancer. However, this association should be taken seriously because of the connecting link between sugar and insulin. Insulin is an absolute requirement for the proliferation of normal mammary tissue, and 70% of experimental mammary tumors regress after destruction of the insulin-secreting capacity of the pancreas.[49,50]

In regard to animal studies, it is clear that animals fed high carbohydrate diets have increased tumor growth.[51,52] Comments such as "I concluded that the addition of large amounts of carbohydrates to the food intake stimulated the growth and size of the tumor" call attention to the fact

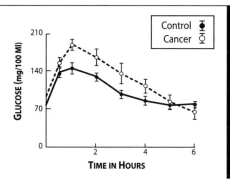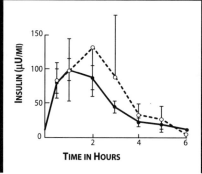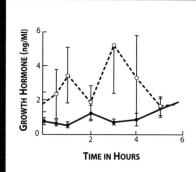

Figure 29-20: *Comparison of Breast Cancer Patients and Healthy Patients*

Mean plasma glucose, insulin, Growth Hormone levels, in 10 patients with metastatic breast cancer and 11 healthy, women given 100 gm of oral glucose. The vertical lines represent ± 1 standard error of the mean (SE). In this study, women with breast cancer had significantly higher insulin, glucose, and Growth Hormone levels than healthy women.

FIGURE 29-21: SUGAR CONSUMPTION AND BREAST CANCER MORTALITY

COUNTRY	YEAR MORTAL STATITISTICS	MORTALITY PER 100,000 IN AGE GROUPS				AVERAGE CONSUMPTION G/DAY 1965-1969		
		35-44	45-54	55-64	65-74	SUGAR	GLUCOSE	TOTAL
UK	1979	23.0	64.7	96.9	122.2	131.8	13.5	145.3
Ireland	1977	19.3	69.0	72.2	112.5	126.8	11.3	138.1
Canada	1977	18.9	50.6	90.4	104.9	137.1	—	137.1
US	1978	16.9	51.0	83.0	98.9	133.7	—	133.7
France	1977	13.4	39.5	64.1	85.6	92.2	4.1	96.3
Japan	1979	6.8	14.6	18.2	17.0	57.4	—	57.4

Figure 29-21: Based on the epidemiological findings, there appears to be a correlation between sugar intake and cancer.

that animals given a rich carbohydrate diet and inoculated with tumors died much more quickly than did the control animals. The animals injected with glucose showed an earlier development of the tumor, and the tumor reached a larger size than it did in the control animals, which is evidence that the tumor can be influenced by local measures."[53] These results are expected because cancers crave sugar. Sugar provides the energy source for cancers and stimulates insulin and Growth Hormone secretion, which further stimulates cancer growth.

The above study shows that breast cancer patients have higher glucose, insulin, and Growth Hormone levels than women who are healthy. As we have already discussed, all three of these substances cause cancer growth if a cancer is present. The higher the person's glucose level in the blood, the higher the insulin and Growth Hormone levels. Since some cancer cells have an excessive number of insulin and Growth

Hormone receptors (and/or IGF-1 [insulin-like growth factor] receptors), elevated insulin and Growth Hormone levels should be avoided by the cancer patient.

SUGAR POISONS THE BODY

A poison, as defined by *Stedman's Medical Dictionary,* is any substance, either taken internally or applied externally that is injurious to health or dangerous to life.[53] Surely sugar meets this definition as its effects on the human body over time can lead to the following conditions:

WHAT HAPPENS WHEN SUGAR POISONS THE BODY...

- Cancer
- Candidiasis
- Cataracts
- Cavities
- Chronic Fatigue
- Diabetes
- Glucose Intolerance
- Heart Disease
- High Blood Pressure
- Infections
- Low Immunity
- Obesity
- Poor Circulation
- Poor Healing
- Premature Aging
- ...Many Other Degenerative Disorders.

Poorly controlled blood sugar poisons the body (See **Figure 29-22**). When the blood sugar becomes too high, metabolism is altered, and disease processes begin. In regard to cancer, this means cancer physiology. High blood sugars have the following effects that aid cancer physiology:

- Increase amount of energy source for cancer cells
- Increase insulin levels that stimulate cancer growth
- Elevate lactic acid levels that lower tumor pH
- Encourage anaerobic metabolism
- Increase protein kinase C, which increases cancer risk
- Increase prostaglandin E-2 levels, increasing platelet stickiness
- Lower immunity

High blood sugars occur because a person is eating too many carbohydrates for his or her metabolism. Carbohydrates are food components that are composed of carbon, oxygen, and hydrogen. One or more basic sugar molecules bind together to form all carbohydrates. All sugars are reduced to the simple sugar, glucose, through digestion or conversion in the liver. Starch and glycogen are complex sugars that contain numerous glucose molecules. Carbohydrates such as wheat, bread,

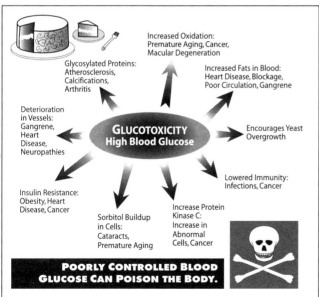

Figure 29-22: Poorly Controlled Blood Glucose Poisons the Body

Poor blood glucose control can set the stage for cancer physiology.

Adapted from Advances in Care of Diabetes, *Vol. 15, No. 2, p. 255, May 1999.*

and pasta are polysaccharides because they contain three or more chains of sugar molecules (See **Figure 29-23**). They are broken down by enzymes in the small intestine and are absorbed into the bloodstream as monosaccharides, which are individual sugar molecules, or disaccharides, which are pairs of sugar molecules.

The rate of glucose transport, as well as the transport of other monosaccharides into the cells, is greatly increased by insulin. When large amounts of insulin are secreted by the pancreas, the rate of glucose transport into most cells increases to 10 or more times the rate of transport when no insulin is secreted.[54] After absorption into the cells, glucose can either be used immediately for release of energy to the cells or stored in the form of glycogen, which is a large polymer of glucose.

Insulin is secreted in response to elevated blood sugars (See **Figure 29-24**). Glucagon, which is also made in the pancreas, is released when the blood sugar becomes too low. Insulin and glucagon have opposite roles in the body (See **Figure 29-25**). The larger the carbohydrate content of the diet, the higher the fasting insulin/glucagon ratio that is secreted into the bloodstream from the pancreas (See **Figures 29-26A** and **B**).

One of the amazing facts that most people do not realize is that the body has no essential need to consume carbohydrates. **There is not one single carbohydrate that is essential for the human body,** yet there are many amino acids and fatty acids that are essential.

When people are told to lower the carbohydrate content of their diets, they are shocked at just how many carbohydrates are in everyday foods (See **Figure 29-27**). A single glass of orange juice can have 50 grams of carbohydrates. Most are also surprised at just what is sugar. Most people will be startled when confronted with their sugar addictions. "I don't eat sugar." "I don't have candy bars." Well, sugar has many different names. Glucose is the final product that is formed from the breakdown of all carbohydrates in the blood. So when blood sugar is mentioned, this refers to glucose. Glucose is also a sugar, found usually with other sugars, in fruits and vegetables. Dextrose, also called corn sugar, is derived synthetically from starch. Fructose is fruit sugar. Maltose is malt sugar. Lactose is milk sugar. Sucrose is refined sugar made from sugar cane and sugar beet. As

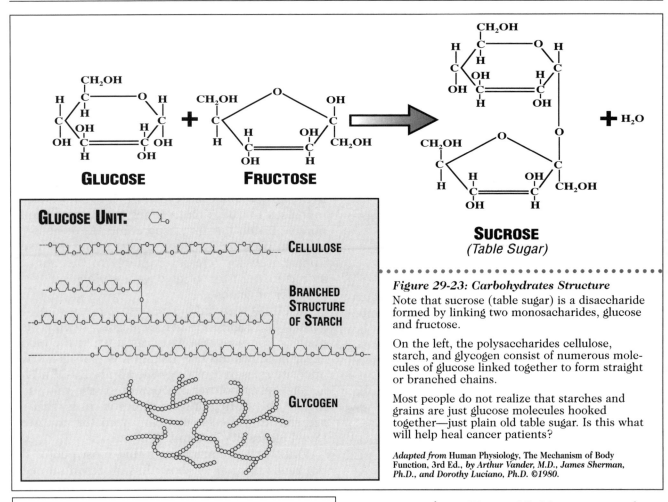

GLUCOSE + **FRUCTOSE** → **SUCROSE** *(Table Sugar)* + H_2O

GLUCOSE UNIT:

CELLULOSE

BRANCHED STRUCTURE OF STARCH

GLYCOGEN

Figure 29-23: Carbohydrates Structure

Note that sucrose (table sugar) is a disaccharide formed by linking two monosaccharides, glucose and fructose.

On the left, the polysaccharides cellulose, starch, and glycogen consist of numerous molecules of glucose linked together to form straight or branched chains.

Most people do not realize that starches and grains are just glucose molecules hooked together—just plain old table sugar. Is this what will help heal cancer patients?

Adapted from Human Physiology, The Mechanism of Body Function, 3rd Ed., *by Arthur Vander, M.D., James Sherman, Ph.D., and Dorothy Luciano, Ph.D. ©1980.*

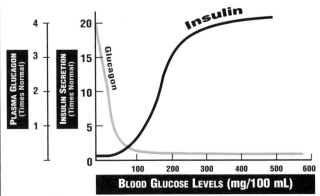

Figure 29-24: Plasma Insulin and Glucagon Concentrations at Different Blood Glucose Levels

Cancer patients are wrongly urged to load up on carbohydrates, when, in reality, this pushes insulin levels up. When insulin goes up, the cancer patient's physiology is modified more in a direction that favors cancer.

Adapted from A. Guyton, Textbook of Medical Physiology, *9th ed., W.B. Saunders, Philadelphia, PA, p. 1022.*

one can see from **Figure 29-28,** sugar can have many different names, but they are all sugar.

"Come on, doc, what is the big deal about sugar?" Haven't you been paying attention to this book? Cancer craves sugar! Just keep eating sugar and see what happens! Even the American Cancer Society believes that 70% of cancers are caused by lifestyle factors[46] (See **Figure 29-29).** People are doing a great job of eating their sugar as evidenced by the fact that the average person in America consumes some 150 pounds of sugar per year (See **Figure 29-30).**

So what are the consequences of all this sugar that people are consuming? The most obvious effect is obesity. The Centers for Disease Control and Prevention report that 61% of Americans are now overweight and that 26% are obese (at least 20% over ideal body weight). Just 10 years ago, only 56 percent of us were overweight and 23 percent were obese.[55] There is also an epidemic of child-

FIGURE 29-25: THE ROLES OF INSULIN AND GLUCAGON *Adapted from Protein Power by Michael Eades, Bantam Books ©1996.*

INSULIN
- Lowers elevated blood sugar
- Shifts metabolism into storage mode
- Converts glucose and protein to fat
- Converts dietary fat to storage
- Removes fat from blood and transports it into cells
- Increases the body's production of cholesterol
- Makes the kidneys retain excess fluid
- Stimulates the growth of arterial smooth muscle cells
- Stimulates the use of glucose for energy

GLUCAGON
- Raises low blood sugar
- Shifts metabolism into burning mode
- Converts protein and fat to glucose
- Converts dietary fat to ketones and sends them to the tissues for energy
- Releases fat from fat cells into the blood for use by tissues as energy
- Decreases the body's production of cholesterol
- Makes the kidneys release excess fluid
- Stimulates the regression of arterial smooth muscle cells
- Stimulates the use of fat for energy

DIET	FASTING INSULIN/ GLUCAGON PERCENT RATIO
STARVATION	0.4
LOW-CARBOHYDRATE DIET	1.8
BALANCED DIET	3.8
HIGH CARBOHYDRATE DIET	16.0

Figure 29-26A: Fasting Insulin to Glucagon Ratios in Response to Diet

A high-protein low-carbohydrate diet causes much more glucagon and less insulin to be produced by the body compared to a high-carbohydrate diet. This helps the cancer patient reverse cancer physiology.

Adapted from W. Muller, The Influence of the Antecedent Diet Upon Glucagon and Insulin Secretion, 1971, 285:450-1454.

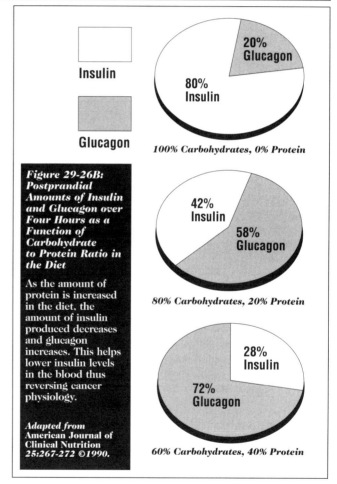

Figure 29-26B: Postprandial Amounts of Insulin and Glucagon over Four Hours as a Function of Carbohydrate to Protein Ratio in the Diet

As the amount of protein is increased in the diet, the amount of insulin produced decreases and glucagon increases. This helps lower insulin levels in the blood thus reversing cancer physiology.

Adapted from American Journal of Clinical Nutrition 25:267-272 ©1990.

hood "globesity." The Centers for Disease Control and Prevention report that 25% of children ages two to 20 years are, or are at risk of becoming, overweight or obese—twice the rate of obesity seen just a decade ago.[56] This obesity is extremely dangerous, as adipose tissue (fat) undergoes constant renewal, and lipogenesis (fat accumulation) requires insulin; therefore, obesity is an obligatory hyperinsulinemic state. An obese person may secrete five to eight times more insulin than a person of normal weight[57] (See **Figure 29-31**).

It might be helpful to review again exactly why this massive amount of blood insulin is dangerous to people. We will use breast cancer as the example. Scientific research has confirmed the following in regard to breast cancer patients, breast cancer tumors, and breast cancer cells:[58-66]

➢ Countries with the highest intake of sugar have the highest breast cancer mortality.

➢ Diabetics have an increased risk of breast cancer.

➢ Glucose intolerance is higher in breast cancer patients.

➢ Breast cancer patients have increased insulin levels.

➢ Insulin stimulates breast cancer tumor growth.

➢ Breast cancer cells have six times more insulin receptors than normal cells.

➢ Insulin receptors on breast cancer cells do not down-regulate (decrease) as much as normal cell insulin receptors to high insulin levels in the blood.

➢ The insulin receptor content of breast tumors correlates positively with tumor size, histological grade, and the estrogen receptor content.

CARBOHYDRATE CONTENT OF FOOD

Source	Amount	Carbohydrate (g)
Orange Juice (100% Unsweetened)	8 Ounces	30
Soft Drink	8 Ounces	26
Low-Fat Milk	8 Ounces	12
Cereal	1 Cup	30
Rice	1 Cup	51
Potato	1 Medium	20
Bread	2 Slices	30
Pizza	1 Slice	30
Cookie	1 Medium	30
Pasta	1 Cup	36
Rice Cake	1 Cake	15

Figure 29-27: Carbohydrates Are Everywhere
Most people have no idea just how prevalent carbohydrates are in their diets.

FIGURE 29-28: VARIOUS NAMES OF SUGARS

Sugars often appear on food labels and ingredient lists under different names. Be aware when you see these kinds of terms:

- Barley Malt
- Cane Juice
- Dextrose
- Fruit Juice
- Glucose
- Honey
- Maltose
- Molasses
- Sucrose
- Brown rice syrup
- Corn Syrup
- Fructose
- Fruit Juice Concentrate
- High-Fructose Corn Syrup
- Lactose
- Milk Sugar
- Naturally Sweetened

➤ Most (90%) of breast cancer cells demonstrate significant binding of insulin.

➤ High insulin levels are linked to deaths from breast cancer.

In visual form, these facts look like **Figure 29-32**. The cancer cell loves insulin because insulin helps push glucose into the cancer cell. The person who eats an excessive amount of carbohydrates produces an excessive amount of insulin. This insulin then sets off a cascade that enables the cancer cell to feed indefinitely on the person. The end result for many is cancer and cancer cachexia (See **Figure 29-33**). If a person with cancer does not change his or her diet to lower insulin levels, the end result is a greater risk of death.[65]

Consider the following study. Researchers from the University of Toronto Mount Sinai Hospital led by Pamela Goodwin, M.D., followed 535 women with breast cancer for 10 years and studied the

FIGURE 29-29: CAUSES OF CANCER IN THE UNITED STATES*

RISK FACTOR	PERCENTAGE
Tobacco	30
Adult Diet and Obesity	30
Sedentary Lifestyle	5
Occupational Factors	5
Family History of Cancer	5
Viruses and Other Biological Agents	5
Perinatal Factors and Growth	5
Reproductive Factors	3
Alcohol	3
Socioeconomic Status	3
Environmental Pollution	2
Ionizing and Ultraviolet Irradiation	2
Prescription Drugs and Medical Procedures	1
Salt and Other Food Additives or Contaminants	1

Over 70% of the causes of cancer relate to reversible lifestyle factors. Notice the most significant factors relate to the things people put in their mouths: cigarettes and carbs—the two evil "Cs."

American Cancer Society

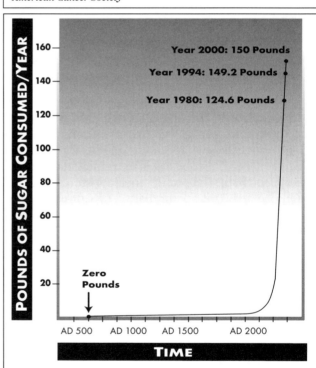

Figure 29-30: Total Refined Sugar Consumption per Person per Year in the U.S.A.
Be clear on this: not only do cancers crave sugar—so do Americans.

relationship between breast cancer grade and stage and insulin concentration. Fasting insulin concentrations were measured to avoid postpran-

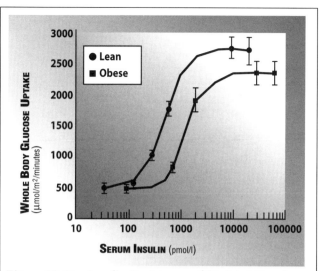

Figure 29-31: Insulin Resistance of Skeletal Muscle Glucose Uptake in Obesity

In obesity, insulin levels increase to get the same amount of glucose uptake from the cells.

Adapted from Decreased effect of insulin to stimulate skeletal muscle blood flow in obese men: A novel mechanism for insulin resistance, by M. Laasko, S.V. Edelman, G. Brechtel, and A.D. Baron. Journal of Clinical Investigation, 1990, 85: 1844-1852.

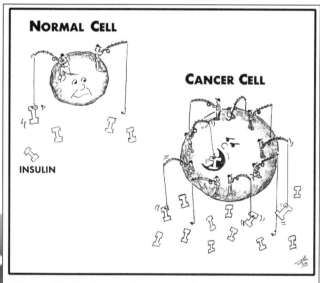

Figure 29-32: Insulin Receptor Concentrations on Normal and Cancer Cells

Cancer cells have many more insulin receptors to "catch" the insulin. This is needed to satisfy the cancer cells' ferocious appetite for sugar.

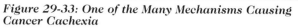

Figure 29-33: One of the Many Mechanisms Causing Cancer Cachexia

In many respects, cancer cachexia (muscle-wasting syndrome) is insulin driven.

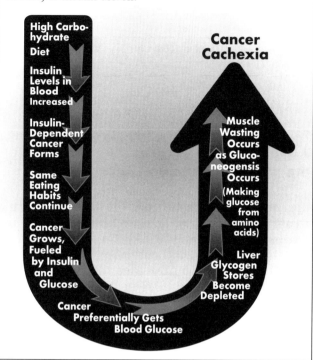

dial fluctuations. Patients enrolled in the study received standard accepted treatments of surgery with chemotherapy, hormonal therapy, and radiotherapy if indicated. **The researchers found that women with the highest insulin levels were eight times more likely to die during the study than women with the lowest insulin levels,** with 70% of such patients being alive after seven years compared with 95% of those with normal insulin levels. Women of normal weight in the study who also had high insulin levels showed the same increase in death rate as the obese women.

When a cancer patient has high insulin levels, the cancer can go on an eating frenzy, somewhat like a school of piranhas that finds an elephant trapped in the water. Tumors just keep eating and eating. As long as the person's diet keeps blood glucose levels elevated, the person's weight will stay the same, and the cancer will grow. If a person with cancer loses his or her appetite, be assured—the cancer does not. It will then extract glucose from the person's glycogen stores in the body. Consider an animal study in which lactate levels and liver glycogen stores were measured before and after a tumor was implanted in 30 rats. The results are dramatic (See **Figure 29-34**).[67] For the person desiring to prevent cancer or survive once the diagnosis is made, it is critical to keep insulin levels as low as possible.

FIGURE 29-34: BEFORE AND AFTER RESULTS ON LACTATE LEVEL AND LIVER GLYCOGEN LEVELS

In this animal study, once implanted with a tumor, blood lactate levels increased dramatically as liver glycogen levels plummeted. Literally, the cancer was sucking the sugar right out of its host!

CONDITION	TOTAL GLYCOGEN IN LIVER (MG)	PLASMA LACTATE (MG/100 ML)
CONTROL	147	32
LEUKEMIA	8	92

TOO MANY CARBS IN THE STANDARD AMERICAN DIET AND THE MACROBIOTIC-JUICING DIET

"For once, the experts on health are nearly unanimous. Most agree that the food we eat for breakfast, lunch, and dinner and for those in-between snacks should be low in fat and high in carbohydrates."[67] This statement is taken from *The Glucose Revolution*, one of thousands of books that promote the high-carbohydrate diet.

We wholeheartedly agree that the health care experts on both sides of the fence, allopathic and alternative, agree that a high-carbohydrate diet is needed to maintain health. Even the U.S. Department of Agriculture and U.S. Department of Health and Human Services have gone so far as to develop the food guide pyramid, which says that a person is to eat up to 11 servings of bread, cereal, rice, and pasta per day (See **Figure 29-35**). The government is doing a great job because Americans are listening and gorging those carbs. **Figure 29-36** shows the top 20 sources of carbohydrates in the American diet.

In 1981, a team of scientists led by David Jenkins, M.D., a professor of nutrition at the University of Toronto, Ontario, Canada, developed a method of comparing foods to find out which ones would be good for people with diabetes. The system developed became known as the glycemic index. The glycemic index of foods is simply a ranking of foods based on their immediate effect on blood sugar levels. To make a fair comparison, all foods are compared with a reference food such as pure glucose and are tested in equivalent carbohydrate amounts. The higher the glycemic index, the higher a person's blood sugar will go after eating the food.

Research has confirmed the validity of the glycemic index. One such study determined the plasma glucose and insulin responses of various

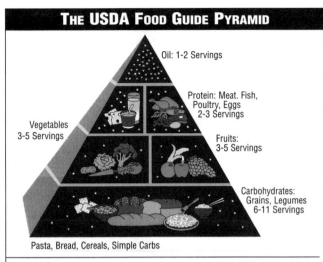

THE USDA FOOD GUIDE PYRAMID

Oil: 1-2 Servings

Protein: Meat. Fish, Poultry, Eggs 2-3 Servings

Vegetables 3-5 Servings

Fruits: 3-5 Servings

Carbohydrates: Grains, Legumes 6-11 Servings

Pasta, Bread, Cereals, Simple Carbs

Figure 29-35: The USDA Food Guide Pyramid
The food guide pyramid was released in 1988 by the U.S. Department of Agriculture to encourage people to eat more grains and carbohydrates. As a result, Americans have become sicker and fatter, and cancer rates continue to climb.

TOP 20 SOURCES OF CARBOHYDRATE IN THE AMERICAN DIET*

1. Potatoes (mashed or baked)	8. Pizza	15. Pancake
2. White Bread	9. Pasta	16. Table sugar
3. Cold Breakfast Cereal	10. Muffins	17. Jam
4. Dark Bread	11. Fruit Punch	18. Cranberry Juice
5. Orange Juice	12. Coca-Cola	19. French Fries
6. Banana	13. Apple	20. Candy
7. White Rice	14. Skim Milk	

Figure 29-36

* *Adapted from Dr. Simon Liu, Harvard University School of Public Health, Data represents the findings of the Harvard Morses Health Study.*

doses of glucose, sucrose, fructose, and white bread in normal human subjects.[68] As can be seen in **Figure 29-37**, they all had similar responses. The authors stated:

> It is concluded that, in normal subjects, as carbohydrate intake is increased from 0 to 100 grams, plasma insulin responses increase at a greater rate than plasma glucose responses. The insulinaemic responses elicited by glucose, sucrose or fructose are similar to those that would be expected from a starchy food with the same glycaemic index.[69]

It is common practice in natural medicine circles to tell patients to eat a high-carbohydrate, macrobiotic diet. Even more popular is for them to juice. This type of diet is very high in carbohy-

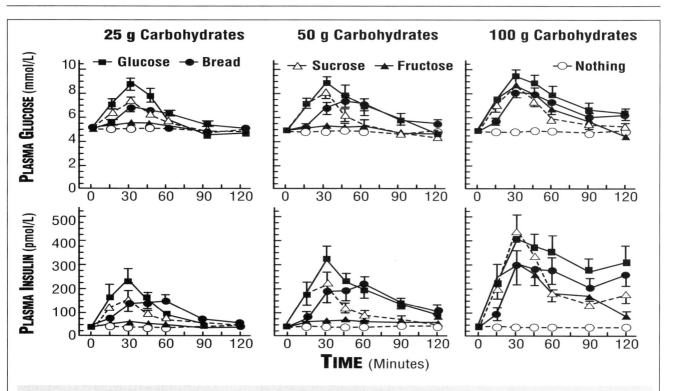

Figure 29-37: *Plasma Glucose (top row) and Insulin (bottom) Responses after Consuming 25 grams (left), 50 grams (center) and 100 grams (right) of Carbohydrate from Glucose, Sucrose, Fructose, or White Bread*

The results for 0 grams of carbohydrate are shown on each panel also (**O**). Statistically, they all raised blood glucose and insulin levels the same. This is one of the many studies that proved that is the quantity—not the quality of the carbohydrates consumed—that determines the postprandial (after meal) glucose and insulin levels.

FIGURE 29-38: GLYCEMIC INDEX OF FOODS

HIGH		MODERATE	
Glucose	100	Brown Rice	55
Maltose	105	Oatmeal	55
White Bread	95	Yams	50
Baked Potato	95	Grapes	50
Rice Cakes	80	Barley Grain	45
French Fries	80	**LOW**	
Corn	75	Apples	40
Graham Crackers	75	Oranges	40
Honey	75	Black-Eyed Peas	40
Puffed Wheat	75	Pinto Beans	40
Cream of Wheat	70	Lima Beans	30
Watermelon	70	Grapefruit	25
Pineapple	65	Soybeans	15
Grape Nuts	65	**ZERO**	
Ice Cream, Premium	60	Chicken	0
		Turkey	0
		Fish	0
		Tofu	0

drates. High-fiber vegetables, fruits, and grains have a lesser effect on elevating the blood sugar as does sugar, as can be seen in **Figure 29-38**. Grains and vegetables have a much lower glycemic index than fruit (because of the fructose) and substantially lower than high-sugar foods such as ice cream, honey, and beer (maltose). What most glycemic index charts do not show is the glycemic index for high-protein foods. The reason is that the glycemic index for these foods is close to 0. This principle can be seen in **Figure 29-39**. If a person eats protein as his or her main calorie source and eats to the beginning sensation of fullness, blood sugar stays stable. In other words, a high-protein diet causes both glucose and insulin levels to stay low. This helps starve the cancer. This is in stark contrast to the macrobiotic-juicing diet that so many cancer patients are following (See **Figure 29-40**).

GRAINS AND FRUIT ARE THE CULPRITS

The problem with most macrobiotic diets as they pertain to cancer is that they include too

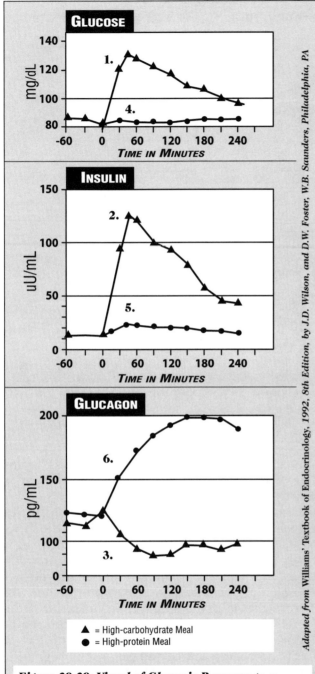

Adapted from Williams' Textbook of Endocrinology, 1992, 8th Edition, by J.D. Wilson, and D.W. Foster, W.B. Saunders, Philadelphia, PA

▲ = High-carbohydrate Meal
● = High-protein Meal

Figure 29-39: Visual of Glycemic Response to a High-Carbohydrate Meal versus a High-Protein Meal

Following a high-carbohydrate meal, glucose levels rise rapidly (**1**) stimulating the release of insulin (**2**), which promotes utilization of glucose, but also signals the body to store fat. Glucagon secretion is suppressed by the high glucose level (**3**). A high protein meal, however, causes only an imperceptible rise in blood glucose (**4**) and, consequently, a very small rise in insulin (**5**), but a significant increase in the glucagon level (**6**).

many grains and fruit. These carbohydrate sources cause very high elevations of blood sugar levels after eating. While many studies have shown a positive effect by eating a diet rich in vegetables and fruits, it is our contention that the significance of these studies is from the vegetables. It is clear that the fructose from fruit has many detrimental effects, including the following:[70]

➤ Elevates total cholesterol.
➤ Increases risk factors for heart disease.
➤ Increases blood lactic acid levels.
➤ Elevates blood insulin levels, especially for women using oral contraceptives.
➤ Reduces the affinity of insulin for its receptor.
➤ Increases risk for hyperinsulinemia.

It is our contention that if researchers look at the effects of fruit and grain consumption and eliminate vegetables as a variable, these foods will not be protective against cancer but will indeed increase some cancer risks. In one large meta-analysis from 1982 to 1997 involving 23,038 breast cancer patients, it was shown that vegetables did indeed decrease cancer risk, but once vegetables were eliminated as an independent variable, fruits no longer showed a protective effect.[71]

The idea of the glycemic index is a good one, but it does not cut the mustard when one studies it in clinical practice. When carbohydrate-rich foods are tested individually, a specific difference in the plasma glucose response is noted. However, when these foods are tested as a group, it is the **total** amount of carbohydrates eaten that determines blood glucose and insulin levels, **not** the type of carbohydrates. As can be seen in **Figure 29-41**, when normal subjects and those with Type 2 diabetes are fed meals of equal carbohydrate amounts but with varying glycemic potentials, the blood sugar elevations are the same after the meal.[72] In a similar study using high, intermediate, and low glycemic index meals, blood glucose and insulin levels were not significantly different[73] (See **Figure 29-42**). Even when the sucrose intake of a high-carbohydrate diet is increased from 1% to 16%, the blood glucose and insulin levels are not changed[74] (See **Figure 29-43 A and B**). What if the percentage of simple versus complex carbohydrates was changed in the diet? Same result: **As long as the total amount of car-**

HAUSER DIET VS. MACROBIOTIC DIET

	HAUSER DIET	MACROBIOTIC DIET
Carbohydrate Content	Low	High
Protein Amount	High	Low
Vegetables	High	High
Fruit	Low	High
Glucose Levels	Low	High
Insulin Levels	Low	High
Lactate Levels	Low	High

Figure 29-40: For actually *reversing* cancer physiology, the Hauser High Protein Diet makes a lot more sense than the macrobiotic diet.

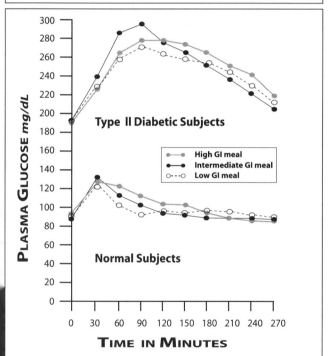

Figure 29-41: Plasma Response to Meals with Varying Glycemic Potential

When carbohydrate-rich foods are tested individually, a difference in the plasma glucose response is noted. The plasma glucose response to a given food has been named "the glycemic index (GI)." However, when mixed with meals planned to contain foods with a high (●), interm ediate (●), or low (○) GI level, either consumed by normal glycemic patients or those with Type 2 diabetes, there is no difference in the plasma glucose response to the meals. This proves that it is the quantity, and not the quality of the carbohydrates consumed, that determines blood glucose elevations.

Adapted from Comparison of predictive capabilities of diabetic exchange lists and glycemic index of foods. Diabetes Care, by D.C. Laine, and W. Thomas, M.D. Levitt, and J.P. Bantle. 1987, 10:387-394.

bohydrates stayed the same, the elevation in blood glucose and insulin remained constant.[75] Even when the amount of fiber was increased in the diet, the elevated blood glucose and insulin levels were unchanged[76] (See **Figure 29-44**). The reason? It is the carbohydrate content of the diet that affects these levels, <u>not</u> the type of carbohydrates eaten. Ever hear of the saying "it is quality not quantity?" Well, when it comes to blood sugar and insulin levels, it is the *quantity* of the carbohydrates that makes all the difference.

If you still are not convinced that complex carbohydrates raise blood sugar levels, consider **Figure 29-45,** which shows, if anything, the more complex carbohydrates in the diet, the higher the postprandial (after meal) glucose levels. Clearly, they are not depressed.

CUTTING OFF THE TUMOR ENERGY SUPPLY BY CUTTING OUT THE CARBS

For most of the people with cancer who come to Caring Medical, testing reveals metabolic dysglycemia or glucose intolerance. The question of what is an abnormal glucose tolerance test is determined primarily by how much glucose is given initially during the test. One of the most comprehensive studies on the subject was done by Joseph Kraft, M.D., in 1975, when he reported on 3,650 glucose/insulin tolerance tests.[75] In this study, people were given 100 grams glucose, and their blood sugar and insulin levels were checked during the fasting state and then at a half, one, two, and three hours after the glucose meal. He found that 95% of the people tested had a mean fasting insulin level of 13.37 microunits. Under normal circumstances, insulin peaks within the first hour and then levels start to decline. The criteria that he used for an abnormal test can be seen in **Figures 29-46A** and **B**. One has to realize that he used for a normal fasting insulin level, a number that is three standard deviations from the mean (30 microunits is approximately three standard deviations from 13.37).

There are many types of abnormal patterns in glucose/insulin tolerance tests. One can see some of the patterns in **Figures 29-47A** and **B**. As can be seen, in mild states of glucose intolerance, hyperinsulinemia frequently exists, whereas in individuals with mild diabetes (glucose intolerance), insulin levels are generally in the normal range; in more severe cases of non-

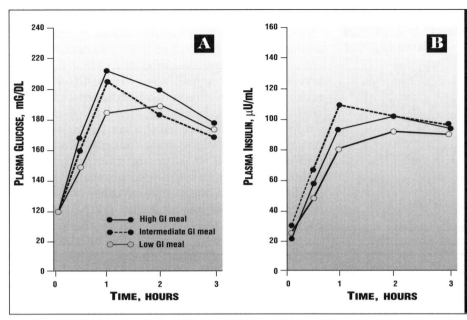

FIGURE 29-42: PLASMA RESPONSE TO MEALS WITH VARYING GLYCEMIC POTENTIAL

Plasma glucose (A) and insulin (B) response to meals with varying gycemic potential. In a study similar to that by Laine (see Figure 29-41), plasma glucose and corresponding insulin responses did not vary in single meals provided with predicted differing glycemic potential when consumed by patients with Type 2 diabetes. These meals contained 45% carbohydrates with 60% starch, 30% fruit, and 10% vegetables for the carbohydrate-rich foods.

Adapted from Effect of source of diabetic carbohydrate on plasma glucose and insulin responses to mixed meals in subjects with NIDDM. Diabetes Care, by A.M. Coulston, C.B. Hollenback, A.L.M. Swislocki, and G.M. Reaven 1987, 10:395-400.

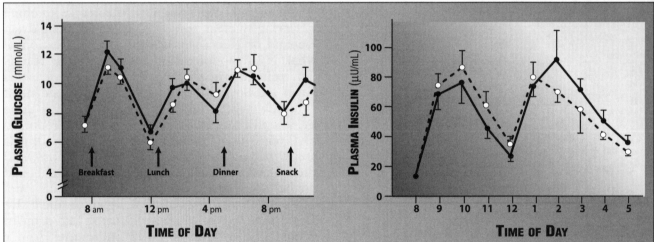

Figure 29-43A: Impact of Types of Carbohydrates on Plasma Glucose Concentration
Using a crossover design, patients with Type 2 diabetes were randomly assigned to diets that contained 55% carbohydrates for one month. In one period, 3% of the calories were from sucrose (O), and in the other period, 19% were from sucrose (●). The total amount of carbohydrates eaten did not vary. There was no difference in the day-long plasma glucose concentration, whether the diet contained 3% or 19% sucrose.

Figure 29-43B Impact of Type of Carbohydrate on Plasma Insulin Concentration
Using a crossover design, patients with type 2 diabetes were randomly assigned to diets that contained 50% carbohydrate for 15 days. In one period, 1% of the calories were from sucrose (O), and in the other period, 16% were from sucrose (●). The total amount of carbohydrates eaten did not vary. There was no difference in the daylong plasma insulin concentration whether the diet contained 1% or 16% sucrose when total carbohydrates remained the same at 55%.

Adapted from Metabolic effects of added dietary sucrose in individuals with non-insulin-dependent diabetes mellitus (NIDDM). Metabolism 1985, 34:962–966.

insulin-dependent diabetes mellitus (NIDDM), insulin levels are low.

There are many different glucose/insulin tests that can be done to document hyperinsulinemia and glucose intolerance. One that is commonly done by natural medicine doctors is seen in **Figure 29-48** after a person receives a 75-g glucose load. One must realize that labs are required by CLIA (governing body for labs) to set normal ranges that, in our opinion, are inaccurate because the "nor-

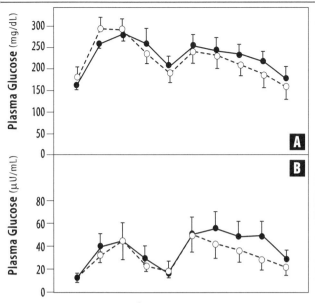

Figure 29-44: Impact of Dietary Fiber on Plasma Glucose (A) and Insulin (B)

Using a crossover design, patients with Type 2 diabetes consumed diets that contained 11 g/1000 kcal of dietary fiber (high-carbohydrate, normal-fiber diet) (●) or 27 g/1000 kcal of mixed dietary fiber (high-carbohydrate, high-fiber diet) (○) for one month. There was no change in the fasting or postprandial plasma glucose or insulin levels. Again, showing that it is the total amount of carbohydrates that determines a person's blood glucose and insulin levels.

Adapted from American Journal Clinical Nutrition, 1986, 43:16-24.

mals" are determined on many abnormal people. There are very few people who have optimal health, so we like to use the term *optimal range* when treating our patients.

In our office, when giving a glucose/insulin tolerance test, we desire our patients to have an *optimal* test result, so much stricter "norms" are used. Dr. Kraft found the mean fasting insulin level to be 13.37, so we try to keep our cancer patients under 10. In regard to glucose levels, as much as possible under 100 in the fasting state is optimal, and under 120 after meals. For the cancer patient, it is helpful to get a glucose/insulin tolerance test before and during treatment.

In addition to the glucose/insulin tolerance test, another good test for the cancer patient to have before and during treatment is a cellular energy profile. (See **Figure 29-11** on page 264.) This test is used to check the levels of substrates that are involved in aerobic and anaerobic metabolism. *High levels of lactic acid* would indicate the person has some anaerobic metabolic physiology. Once this is found, a natural medicine program can be started, with the response easily documented by a repeat test.

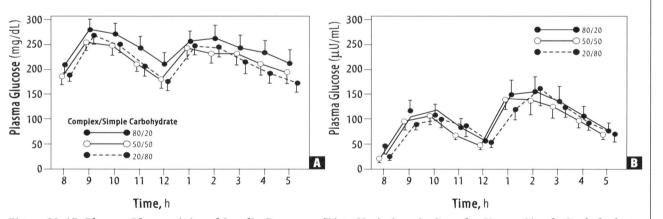

Figure 29-45: Plasma-Glucose (A) and Insulin Response (B) to Variations in Complex Versus Simple Carbohydrates

Patients with Type 2 diabetes consumed one-day test diets of a constant (50%) carbohydrate content in a randomized, crossover design (all participants received all diets). Breakfast and lunch meals were planned to contain 80% complex and 20% simple carbohydrates, 50% of each, or 80% simple and 20% complex carbohydrates. Although there was some variation in the plasma-glucose and insulin concentrations in the three diets, there was no significant or clinical impact of the variation in the type of dietary carbohydrate on plasma-glucose or insulin concentration. If anything, the more complex carbohydrates in the diet, the **higher** the postprandial plasma concentration was of glucose and insulin

Adapted from The effects of variations in percent of naturally occurring complex and simple carbohydrates on plasma glucose and insulin response in individuals with non-insulin dependent diabetes mellitus. Diabetes by C.B. Hollenbeck, A.M. Coulston, and C.C. Donner, et al. 1985, 34:151-155.

FIGURE 26-46A: CRITERIA FOR ABNORMAL GLUCOSE LEVELS
(Plasma Glucose Table)

TIME	mg per 100 mL	WILKERSON POINTS*
Fasting	130 or more	1
1 hour	195 or more	$1/2$
2 hours	140 or more	$1/2$
3 hours	130 or more	1

*Wilkerson point system. Two or more points are judged diagnostic of diabetes.

FIGURE 29-46B: TABLE OF INSULIN PATTERNS

PATTERN I: NORMAL
1. $1/2$ or 1 Hour Peak Value
2. 2nd Hour Less than 50 microunits
3. 3rd Hour Less than 2nd Hour
4. 2nd Hour plus 3rd Hour Value less than 60 microunits
5. Subsequent Hour Values at Fasting Range (0-30 microunits)

PATTERN II: NORMAL PEAK, DELAYED RETURN
1. 2-3 Hour Total > 60 and < 100 = Borderline Value Range
2. 2-3 Hour Total > 100 = Abnormal Value

PATTERN IIIa:
1. Second Hour Delay Peak

PATTERN IIIb:
1. Third Hour Delay Peak

PATTERN IV:
1. High Fasting > 50 microunits

PATTERN V:
1. Low Insulin Response
2. (High Value < 30 microunits)

STARVING CANCER BY THE HAUSER DIET

A tumor must be fed, or it will not grow. The growth of tumor cells generally involves the same nutrients required for the growth of normal tissue. The diet is the distal source of all tumor nutrients, but the proximal source of nourishment for the cancer cell is the body fluids of its host. In regard to glucose, it is the blood glucose level of the person that will determine whether it will be feast or famine for the cancer.

It is evident that cancer cells prefer glucose as their primary energy source. To ensure an adequate supply of glucose for food, cancer cells have more insulin receptors than normal cells. It is clear in many different human and animal models that many of the cancers tested are insulin dependent (See **Figure 29-49**). For the person to starve the cancer, it would be prudent to keep both insulin and glucose levels as low as possible.

TYPES OF PATTERNS FROM THE GLUCOSE/INSULIN TOLERANCE TEST

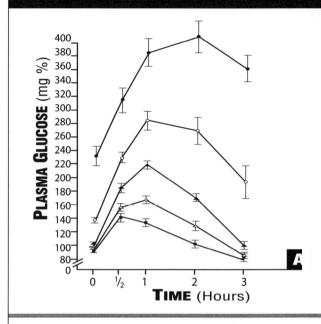

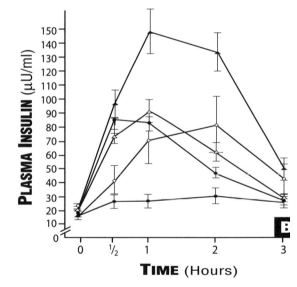

Figure 29-47A & B: The mean (**A**) (± SE) is plasma glucose reponse to oral glucose in the five patient groups. A ■ is normal, △ is borderline tolerance, ▲ is impaired glucose tolerance, ○ is fasting hyperglycemia (110 to 150 mg/dl), ● = fasting hyperglycemia (>150 mg/dl). **B**: mean (±SEM) plasma insulin response to oral glucose in the five patient groups. The symbols are the same as for **A**.

The criteria we use is to keep fasting insulin levels below 10 and at one hour after meals below 20. Glucose levels should not go over 120 after meals.

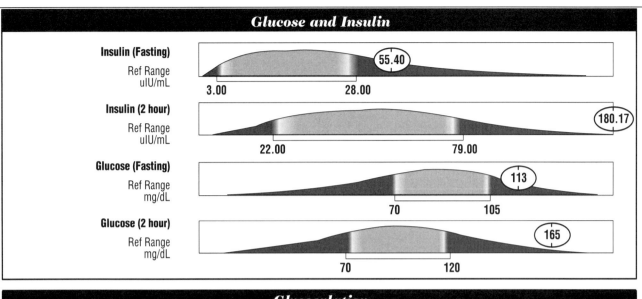

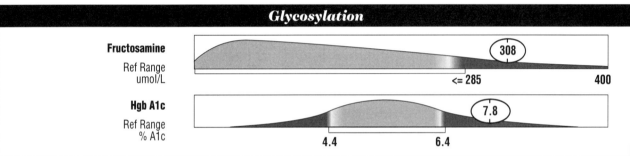

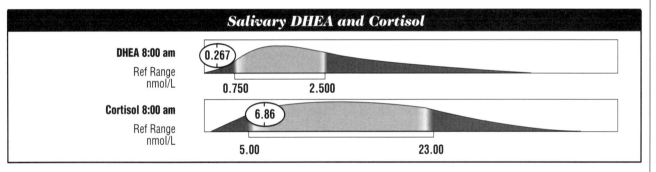

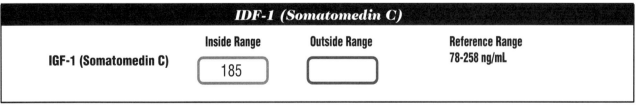

Figure 29-48: Metabolic Dysglycemia Profile

This is one of the panels natural medicine doctors use to show glucose intolerance in cancer patients. Notice the high glucose and insulin levels found on this exam, indicative of cancer physiology.

Adapted from Great Smokies Diagnostic Laboratory, Asheville, NC.

FIGURE 29-49: CANCER/INSULIN RELATIONSHIPS
Many cancers are dependent on insulin.

HUMANS	EXPERIMENTAL TUMORS
INSULIN-PRODUCING/ SECRETING TUMORS	**INSULIN-PRODUCING/ SECRETING TUMORS**
Insulinoma	Murine Myeloid Leukemia
Intrathoracic Mesothelioma	Murine Aplastic Carcinoma
Cervix Carcinoma	Murine B-16 Melanoma
Corpus Uteri Carcinoma	Murine El 4-Lymphoma
Bronchial Carcinoma	Rat RIN Type Cells m5F
Abdominal or Retroperitoneal Fibrosarcoma	Rat or Hamster Insulinoma
Renal Adenocarcinoma	
Hodgkin's Lymphoma	
Non-Hodgkin's Lymphoma	
Caecum Adenocarcinoma	
INSULIN-DEPENDENT TUMORS	**INSULIN-DEPENDENT TUMORS**
MCF-7 Breast Cancer	Murine Thymoma
T-47 D Mammary Tumor Cells	Murine Ehrlich Tumor
Other Breast Cancers	Murine Ehrlich Ascites Carcinoma
Respiratory Cancers in Diabetic Males	Murine Mammary Adenocarcinoma[b]
	Murine Squamous Cell Carcinoma[c]
Retroperitoneal Mesothelioma	Murine Granuloma
Abdominal Sarcoma	Rat Mammary Adenocarcinoma[c]
	Rat Hepatoma, Azo Dye Induced
	Rat Mammary Carcinoma[b]
	Rat Novikoff Hepatoma
	Rat Walker 256 Carcinosarcoma[b, d]
	INSULIN-INDEPENDENT TUMORS
	Rat Sarcoma (MCA)[e]
	Rat Morris Hepatoma[e]
	INSULIN-SENSITIVE TUMORS
	Rat R 3230 AC Mammary Carcinoma
	Rat Walker 256 Carcinosarcoma[b]
	Murine Cloudman S 91 Melanoma Cells
	Fao Hepatoma Cells in Culture in the Absence of Glucose

Classification based on direct or indirect evidence from scientific reports. [a]Insulin or substances immunologically cross-reactive with insulin. [b]Tumor capable of enhancing host insulin secretion and causing remission of diabetes in host. [c]Tumor growth enhanced by insulin administration. [d]Tentative classification: inconsistent results. [e]Insulin administration benefits host by diminishing the cachexia. Abbreviations: DMBA: 7; 12-Dimethylbenz(a)anthracene. MCA: Methylcholanthrene.

Adapted from Insulin-cancer relationships: Possible dietary implication, by D. Yam, Medical Hypotheses, 1991, 113.

with fasting glucose levels being under 100. The reason for these strict criteria is the fact that only small elevations in blood sugar cause a dramatic increase in insulin secretion (See **Figure 29-50**). As long as the blood sugar does not change much, insulin levels will not either. The only way a person can do this is by eating a high-protein diet. A high-protein diet will help starve cancer cells.

It is helpful to have general guidelines when starting a dietary program, but in this case it is easy to obtain *objective evidence* by cancer patients testing their blood sugars fasting, one hour after meals, and just before the evening meal. This can be done simply by buying a glucometer, a device that measures blood sugar. A blood sugar measuring device is now available that looks like a watch; it can measure blood sugar levels without the person having to prick his or her finger. For the person desiring to reverse cancer physiology, this added monitoring is a very vivid and effective way to help ensure that the goals are being met.

The goals of the ideal cancer diet are as follows:

- To stimulate immunity
- Thin the blood
- Inhibit anaerobic metabolism
- Enhance aerobic metabolism
- Promote detoxification
- Provide cancer-fighting substances
- Optimize hormone milieu
- Eliminate cancer-causing agents
- Help starve the cancer
- Complement other treatments the person is receiving

Unfortunately for the cancer patient, not all of these goals are being met by the various cancer "diets" on the market. The vast majority of books on cancer at chain bookstores say that if you have cancer you should eat 25% fat, 55% complex carbohydrates, and 20% protein. The fat can come from flaxseed and olive oils, perhaps a little poultry or fish; the complex carbohydrates from whole grains, legumes, fruits, and vegetables; and the protein from vegetable sources, including beans, peas, and lentils. The diet advice given out by most registered dietitians, nutritionists, and alternative health care providers is simple: "Cut out sugar and start being a vegetarian."

This "politically correct" cancer diet advice does, in many respects, meet many of the goals of the ideal cancer diet. By eliminating sugar and chemicals in their diet, people will not be putting cancer-causing substances into their systems. By increasing the amount of vegetables in their

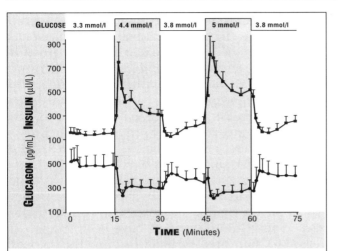

Figure 29-50: The Effect of a Small Change in Glucose Concentration within the Physiological Range upon the Secretion of Insulin and Glucagon

Keeping blood sugar levels low is the key to keeping insulin levels low. This is what is needed for cancer patients to starve their tumors.

Adapted from Diabetes mellitus, by R.H. Unger, D.W. Foster in J.D. Wilson, D.W. Foster, Williams Textbook of Endocrinology, 7th ed., 1985, pp. 1031, W.B. Saunders Company, Philadelphia, PA.

diet, the fiber content increases, as does the number of bowel movements. This will promote detoxification, and, of course, vegetables stimulate immunity, thin the blood, enhance aerobic metabolism, provide cancer-fighting substances, and complement other treatments being received. These diets fall short because they have way too many carbohydrates for the average cancer patient and thus do not inhibit anaerobic metabolism, starve the cancer, and optimize the person's hormone milieu.

The various principles of the Hauser diet as formulated by Marion, a registered dietitian, and Ross, a medical doctor, are as follows:

- Eliminate sugar and sugar substitutes from the diet.
- Use chemical-, hormone-, and preservative-free foods.
- Eat organic foods as much as possible.
- Eat food that is fresh.
- Carbs are the enemy.
- Consume an inordinate amount of soy.
- Remember natural fat is your buddy.
- Protein rules.

The complete Hauser diet is depicted in **Appendix A.** In the first four principles, the Hauser diet is similar to many other cancer diets. Cancer patients need to eat organic and fresh foods and eliminate sugar, sugar substitutes, chemicals, dyes, and preservatives from their diets. It is vastly different, however, in the percentages of components, as the Hauser diet contains 30% fat, 45% protein, and 25% complex carbohydrates. In other words, the Hauser diet has the opposite percentages of protein to complex carbohydrates compared to the "politically correct" cancer diet.

For cancer patients desiring to truly starve their cancer, they must lower the carbohydrate grams in their diet until they keep their blood sugars and insulin levels low. This will be slightly different for each person. In general, cancer patients should first make the change of eliminating sugar from the diet and increasing vegetable sources. Next learn how many carbohydrates are in the foods eaten. They will soon learn that fruits are very high in carbohydrates and must be eliminated from the diet. Vegetable juices are not in the Hauser diet for the same reason. In the strict Hauser diet, only foods that have a carbohydrate content of 6% or less are eaten. The general amount of carbohydrates allowed in a day is typically 60 grams or less, depending on the health of the individual, body weight, and, of course, glucose and insulin levels found during a glucose/insulin tolerance test. For specific servings sizes and more information on carbohydrate/ protein content and The Hauser Diet, please see **Appendix A.**

SOY IS GOOD.

"NO MATTER WHAT OTHERS SAY, SOY IS GOOD."
—Ross A. Hauser, M.D.

The Hauser diet is a high-soy diet. Soy protein typically makes up 25 to 50% of the protein content of the diet. Soy products should be eaten every day and include tempeh, natto, tofu, miso, whole soybeans, soy protein powders, and soy milk. Soy is important to the cancer patient because soy has the following qualities:

- is an excellent protein source
- stabilizes blood sugar and insulin levels
- contains soy isoflavones, including genistein and diadzein, which are phyto-estrogens (cancer-fighting substances)

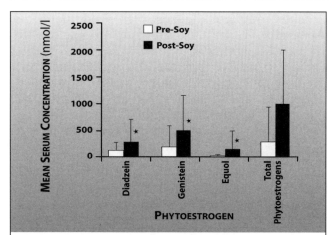

Figure 29-51: Soy Increases Phytoestrogens
Mean serum phytoestrogen concentration in patients before and after 14 days of soy treatment (n = 19).
* Significantly different than pre-soy serum concentration ($P < 0.05$).

- provides precursors to the lignans enterodiol and enterolactone and to phytoestrogens
- decreases circulating estrogens.

Soy is an excellent protein source. One cup of soybeans contains 28g of protein, fiber, zinc, B vitamins, half a day's supply of iron, and lots of highly absorbable calcium.[76] On the basis of their vitamin and mineral content, soy foods are of high therapeutic value, yet the bad press of late has caused many people to question the value of eating soy.

"Doctor, I thought I wasn't suppose to eat soy?" "Won't soy make my breast cancer worse?" "Doesn't soy contain estrogens that would cause my cancer to grow?" The effects of soy are considered to be due to the isoflavones that many soy products contain. Isoflavones are sometimes called phytoestrogens or plant estrogens that act like weak forms of estrogens naturally produced in the body. Genistein and diadzein, both soy isoflavones, are thought to be responsible for the cancer protective effects of soy.

In a study done in 1998, the effects of soy-protein supplementation on epithelial proliferation in the normal human breast were studied. Forty-eight women were randomly assigned to receive their normal diet either alone or with a 60-g soy supplement (containing 45 mg isoflavones) taken daily for 14 days. The phytoestrogens, genistein, diadzein, equol, enterolactone, and enterodiol were measured in serum samples obtained before and after supplementation. As can be seen from **Figure 29-51**, the concentrations of the isoflavones genistein and diadzein increased in the soy group at 14 days. The study also found that the proliferative rate of breast lobular epithelium significantly increased, showing that short-term dietary soy stimulates breast proliferation.[77] This caused an alarm in the media that soy products cause breast cancer to grow, which is the exact opposite of the facts that scientific studies have shown.

If soy increased breast cancer risk, then young women who ate it, especially during development, would have a significant increase in breast cancer risk. When Chinese women have been studied in regard to their breast cancer risk and the amount of soy consumed during adolescence, there is an inverse relationship. In one particular study, the inverse association was observed for each of the soy foods examined and existed for both pre- and postmenopausal women. It was clear in this study that the more soy food that an adolescent ate, the lower the risk of subsequent breast cancer.[78] Other studies have also shown an inverse relationship between soy consumption and breast cancer development.[79, 80]

Researchers have determined that some of the soy protective effects on breast cancer are due to its ability to modulate female hormone production. Soy products have been shown to cause a significant decrease in the amount of ovarian estrogen produced, especially estradiol levels.[81-84] In one study, estradiol levels decreased by 25%, and this decrease was positively associated with urinary isoflavone excretion.[85]

Soy contains substances called isoflavonoids. There have been multiple studies showing that urinary isoflavonoid levels correlate inversely with breast cancer risk. Two of the isoflavonoids, diadzein and genistein, have been studied and are shown to do the following:[86-90]

- inhibit the development of breast cancer cells
- inhibit new blood vessel formation
- decrease cancer cell adhesiveness
- inhibit cell proliferation in estrogen-receptor-positive breast cancer cells (which was reversed by increasing estrogen concentrations)
- block estradiol binding

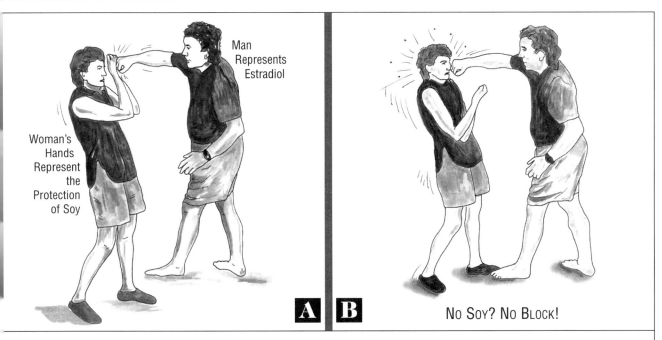

A **B** NO SOY? NO BLOCK!

Figure 29-52A & B: The Protective Effects of Soy
Here is an illustration of the protective effects of the hands to a punch. This is similar to the way that soy blocks the effects of estradiol.

Genistein binds to the estrogen receptor with an affinity approximately 100-fold less than that of estradiol.[91, 92] As has been discussed previously for many female cancers, estradiol is the main culprit in their formation. Genistein, by blocking its binding to female tissue cells, such as the ovary, cervix, and breast, acts as an estrogen blocker, though it itself has some mild estrogen-stimulating effects. A good analogy is blocking a punch. The person who is being hit still feels his or her own arms and hands hit them in the face but not nearly with the same force as when the punch from an opponent goes unblocked (See **Figures 29-52A** and **B**). Because you still feel the punch even though it is blocked does not mean that you should not block it. In the same way, soy should be used by cancer patients (especially those with female cancers) because it helps decrease estradiol concentrations and blocks its binding.

CASES FROM THE ARCHIVES OF CARING MEDICAL

Increasing the soy content along with total protein in a person's diet is an effective way for many patients to start reducing their cancer physiology. One of our clients who has learned this is Mary Lunz. She learned about the high-protein diet for cancer from Doug Kaufmann, a nutritionist, whose show *Health Matters* airs on FamilyNet daily, Monday through Friday (www.FamilyNetTV.com). The diet is discussed in his book *The Fungus Link.* Doug is a friend and colleague and is one of the foremost authorities on the fungal etiology of various diseases, including cancer. Mary, upon hearing Doug, started on an aggressive antifungal program, including herbal remedies, medications, and a drastic diet change. As one can see from her breast cancer markers in **Figure 29-53**, the high-protein diet definitely made a difference.

FIGURE 29-53: CANCER MARKERS AS A RESULT OF A HIGH-PROTEIN DIET

CANCER MARKERS

DATE:	CA 27-29	CA 15-3
8/16/00	120	81
10/16/00	115	81
1/29/01	107	107
HIGH-PROTEIN DIET STARTED		
3/8/01	77.7	77
7/16/01	62.5	56

One may wonder why she was monitored for these particular cancer markers for her breast cancer. Her other cancer markers, including CA 19-9, have been within normal limits. This is another example of why the cancer patient must be monitored closely using *numerous* cancer markers.

The high-soy, high-protein diet helps a cancer patient because it decreases a person's blood sugar, thereby decreasing insulin levels. For the female cancer patient, it is especially helpful because it helps lower body estrogen and estradiol levels. Good examples of this are Karrie Stopka and Annie Geranda.

Karrie is in her late 40s and has taken control of her health. She "allowed" the surgeon to do a lumpectomy, but no one was going to irradiate, chemo, or perform further surgeries on her. She had one surgical margin that was not clear of cancer, a good indication that the cancer will come back if nothing is done. She did not even want the small doses of chemotherapy in IPT, though this was recommended. She decided to just reverse her cancer physiology. She was started on a high-soy, high-protein diet and given nutritional supplements. Her results in **Figure 29-54** show just how quickly some aspects of cancer physiology can be reduced. It is amazing how low one can get the estrogen levels if a proper diet is eaten.

FIGURE 29-54: TOTAL DAILY URINARY LEVELS IN MICROGRAMS/24 HOURS

DATE	TOTAL ESTROGENS	ESTRADIOL	ESTROGEN QUOTIENT	
2/14/00	168.2	143.8	0.05	**BEFORE** HAUSER DIET
5/8/00	58.5	30.6	0.44	**AFTER** HAUSER DIET

Annie came in with a low total estrogen level but most of it was estradiol causing her to have a low estrogen quotient. She had a recurrence of her breast cancer in the "other breast" and decided to see what Caring Medical had to offer. As it turned out, on reviewing the pathology report, it was clear that her second tumor was a completely different population of breast cancer cells; in other words, it was a new cancer that came from her previous cancer. This concept of tumor heterogeneity is discussed later in this chapter. As one can see, the high soy high protein diet had a dramatic effect on her estrogen cancer physiology (See **Figure 29-55**).

Before proceeding, however, it is important to review anaerobic metabolism and how nutritional supplementation can also help starve cancer cells.

FIGURE 29-55: ESTROGEN LEVELS OF A BREAST CANCER PATIENT

DATE	TOTAL ESTROGENS	ESTRADIOL	ESTROGEN QUOTIENT	
6/16/99	58.5	40.0	0.08	**BEFORE** HAUSER DIET
7/15/01	9.9	1.4	0.33	**AFTER** HAUSER DIET

STARVING THE CANCER BY LACTATE INHIBITION

Since Warburg's early demonstration of elevated glycolysis in tumor cells, many investigations have been carried out on the intrinsic respiration and glycolytic activity of neoplasms, both in laboratory animals and humans. There seems little question that anaerobic glycolysis is high in tumor cells and that aerobic glycolysis (lactate production in the presence of oxygen) is characteristic of malignant neoplasms in general.

Normal metabolism of glucose ends with many ATP molecules being formed to give short-term energy to the cell, whereas in tumor metabolism the main end product being formed is lactate (See **Figure 29-56**). Lactate has many purposes for the cancer cell, but its primary purpose is to recover glucose through the Cori cycle so the cancer will have enough glucose. If there is not enough glucose in the cancer patient's blood, glycogenolysis and gluconeogenesis occur. Glycogenolysis involves the breakdown of glycogen in the liver to make glucose, and gluconeogenesis is the formation of glucose from substances such as amino acids. The end result of this is a net energy loss for the cancer patient but energy gain for the cancer as more glucose is formed (See **Figure 29-57**). The cancer grows while the person starves. Natural medicine treatments, including IPT, reverse this trend.

The functional significance of glycolysis in cancer appears to be twofold: as a source of energy production (growth) for the tumor and as a source of lactate in the host that causes a marked stimulation of gluconeogenesis, which causes a significant energy loss for the person with cancer. There are two main mechanisms by which to starve the cancer:

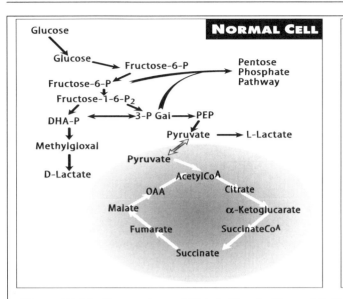

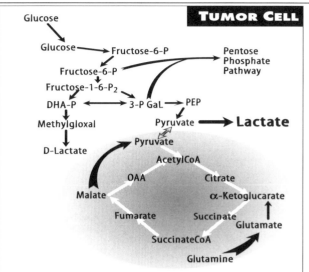

Figure 29-56: Comparison of Metabolism in Normal Cells and Tumor Cells

Abnormal enzymes in tumor cells cause an increase in lactate production in the presence of oxygen. Darker arrows show an increase in lactate formation due to the altered enzymes.

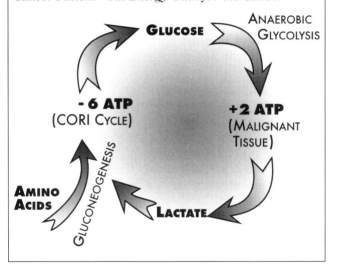

Figure 29-57: Schematic Representation of Systemic Metabolic Circuit Responsible for Energy Loss in the Cancer Patient—but Energy Gain for the Cancer

1. Provide it with no glucose.

2. Do not let the glucose form into lactate (lactic acid).

The end product of glycolysis is pyruvate. During anaerobic metabolism, which occurs during starvation, sprinting, or during cancer metabolism, the pyruvate is shunted away from the Krebs cycle to form lactate through the action of the enzyme lactate dehydrogenase (See **Figure 29-58**). Some consider lactate dehydrogenase to be the most significant enzyme in cancer cell metabolism.[93] Thus, it should be possible to partially starve a cancer through inhibition of lactate dehydrogenase.

I know some of you are still not getting it even though you are on **Chapter 29** of this book. Cancer cells primarily use glucose as their main energy source through glycolysis. The by-product of glycolysis is lactic acid. Lactic acid is a potent glyconeogenic substance. Thus, cancer cells are assured of a continuous supply of glucose for their relentless growth because of this lactic acid. Lactate dehydrogenase is the enzyme that catalyzes the production of lactic acid. Blocking this enzyme should prove very helpful to the cancer patient.

One of the most effective inhibitors of lactate dehydrogenase and lactate transport is quercetin. Quercetin belongs to an extensive class of flavonoid compounds almost ubiquitous in plants and plant food sources (See **Figure 29-59**). Quercetin is the major bioflavonoid in the human diet. The estimated average daily dietary intake of quercetin by an individual in the United States is 25 mg.[94]

The term *bioflavonoid* is used to connote flavonoids that have biological activity in humans. Quercetin has been found to be an inhibitor for certain enzymes. Quercetin has been shown to suppress the high glycolytic rate of tumor cells. It

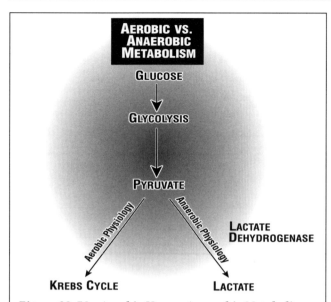

Figure 29-58: Aerobic Versus Anaerobic Metabolism
Anaerobic metabolism starts with lactate being formed through the action of lactate dehydrogenase.

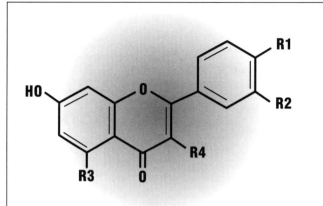

Figure 29-59: Structure of Naturally Occurring Flavonoids Showing Numbering of Ring Atoms
In quercetin, R1, R2, and R3 are all OH.

does so by suppressing lactate transport, especially the excretion of lactate from tumor cells. As the lactate accumulates, intracellular acidification increases, which also acts to decrease the glycolytic rate of tumor cells.

Quercetin has a potent ability to inhibit lactate production in tumor cells. In a study done at Cornell University in 1975, E. Suolinna found that quercetin not only inhibited lactate production but also leukemia cell growth[95] (See **Figures 29-60A** and **B**). Other researchers have also confirmed this finding[96,97] (See **Figure 29-61**). Many in vitro studies have been done and have confirmed that quercetin has potent effects for inhibiting tumor cell growth (See **Figure 29-62**).

Quercetin has also been shown to be a potentiator of chemotherapy. An in vitro study using human ovarian and endometrial cancer cell lines found that the addition of 0.01 to 10 mM quercetin to cisplatin caused a 1.5- to 30-fold potentiation of the cytotoxic effect of cisplatin.[98] The potentiating effects of quercetin and other nutriceutical products are explained further in the next chapter.

Other nutriceutical agents can be used to decrease lactic acid formation. Some of the more common ones that have been studied include alpha lipoic acid, NADH, AMP (adenosine monophosphate), DMG (dimethylglycine), malic acid, and carnitine.[93,99,100] Generally for the patient desiring to reverse cancer physiology, a high-dose of these substances is recommended, with the most important one being quercetin.

WHY ALL OF THE ABOVE PROBABLY WILL NOT WORK—THE CONCEPT OF TUMOR HETEROGENEITY

If nothing else, people will say, "Dr. Hauser's writing is very interesting." It is true that if a person with cancer follows the tenets of this chapter, it will not cure him or her of cancer, but it will work in reversing some aspects of cancer physiology. To become cured of cancer, the person often has to do several modalities, including diet, herbs, lifestyle changes, and some aggressive treatment such as IPT. The main reason, however, that these will sometimes not work in curing the person of cancer is because tumors contain a heterogeneous population of cells that are vastly different.

As I (Ross) alluded to with the case of Annie, when someone has a recurrence of cancer, the pathologic characteristics of the secondary tumor are usually *different* from the primary tumor. The growth rate, S phase fraction, tumor antigens, and amount of differentiation may be entirely different when a tumor recurs. Sure, both tumors are breast cancer, but generally the one that recurs has a much poorer prognosis, not because there is a recurrence, but because it is a much stronger and more aggressive cancer. **In many respects, it is a completely different tumor than the first tumor.** This concept makes sense when one understands tumor heterogeneity.

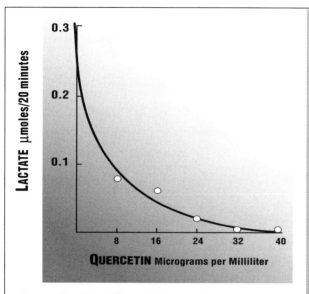

Figure 29-60A: *Effect of Quercetin on Lactate Production in Erlich Ascites Cells*
Quercetin significantly inhibited lactate production.

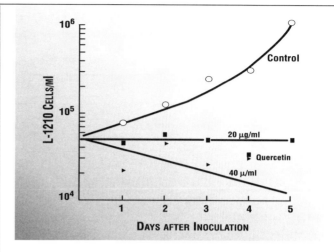

Figure 29-60B: *Effect of Quercetin on the Growth of L 1210 Leukemia Cells in Vitro*
This study found that Quercetin by itself had a chemotherapy effect causing cancer cell death at concentrations of 20 mg/ml or above. Samples were taken for counting at one-day intervals. Arrowheads show when the medium was changed.

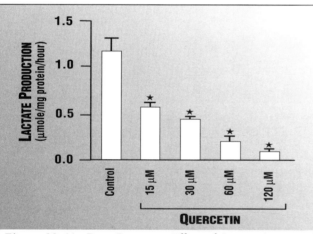

Figure 29-61: *Dose-Response Effect of Quercetin on the Glycolytic Activity of Colon Cancer (HT29) During their Exponentially Growing Phase*
Quercetin significantly decreased the cancer cells' lactate production, signifying that cancer cells were dying.

When a person is diagnosed with a tumor or cancerous mass, it is easy to think of this mass as consisting of one cell type, such as breast cancer. Generally, the pathology reports from the surgery or the biopsy will tell many facts about this cell type, so it is relatively easy for an oncologist to tell a person his or her prognosis. The problem with this concept is that the pathology report describes only one of the many cell types that probably exist in the person's cancer. It may be that the cells that the pathologist tested were on the outside of the tumor; these generally carry a good or better prognosis than the ones inside the tumor mass. This is because the physiology of the tumor is much different inside the mass than outside.

From many studies performed thus far using experimental animal tumors, it is clear that the oxyhemoglobin (how much oxygen is attached to red blood cells) is significantly lower in tumors than in normal host tissues, and oxyhemoglobin values drop as the tumor volume increases[101, 102] (See **Figure 29-63**). In addition, data obtained from biopsies indicate that tissue hypoxia and/or anoxia already exist in smaller tumors and worsens with increasing size. During tumor growth, spatial heterogeneities of the oxygen supply substantially increase due to an increasing nonuniformity and inadequacy of the tumor microcirculation. It appears that the vasculature is better at the tumor periphery; thus, oxygenation at the outer aspect of the tumor is significantly higher than in the tumor center[103,104] (See **Figure 29-64**.)

These factors mean that the center of the tumor will rely more on anaerobic glycolysis for energy and become more acidic. As we will see in the next chapter, the center of the tumor is acidic, but the tissues outside the tumor site, especially

Figure 29-62: **In Vitro Studies of Quercetin on Malignant Growth**

IC50 is the quercetin concentration at which tumor growth was inhibited by 50%. Quercetin has been shown in vitro to significantly inhibit tumor cell growth.

Malignant Cell Line	IC50
Bladder	Not Given
Breast (MDA-MB-435)	55 μM, LC50 = 26 μM
Breast (MDA-MB-468)	21 μM
Breast (MDA-MB-435)	31 μM
Breast (MCF-7)	4.9 μM
Breast (MCF-7)	15 μM
Colon (HT29 and Caco-2)	45-50 μM
Colon (HT29 and Caco-2)	30-40 μM
Gastric (HGC-27, NUGC-2, MKN-7, and MKN-28)	32-55 μM
Head and Neck (HTB43)	Significant Inhibition above 100 μM
Head and Neck (HTB43 and CCL135)	Significant Inhibition above 100 μM
Leukemia (14 AML Lines and Four ALL lines)	2 μM
Leukemia (CML Line K562)	59 μM
Melanoma (MNT1, M10, M14)	7 nM, 20 nM, 1-10 μM
Ovarian (OVCA 433)	10 μM

Adapted from R. Mans, Relationship between size and oxygenation status of malignant tumors. Adv Exp Med Biol. 1983;159:391-398.

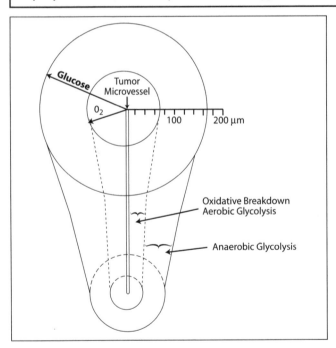

Figure 29-63: Tumor Microvessel

This is a representation of a tissue cone surrounding a tumor microvessel with critical diffusion distances for oxygen (inner cone) and glucose (outer cone). Tumors depend on oxygen and glucose from these microvessels. Experimental data obtained from cryobiopsies are indicative of tissue hypoxia and/or anoxia already existent in smaller tumors that worsen with increasing size. During tumor growth, spatial heterogeneities of oxygen and glucose supply substantially increase due to an increasing nonuniformity and inadequacy of the tumor microcirculation.

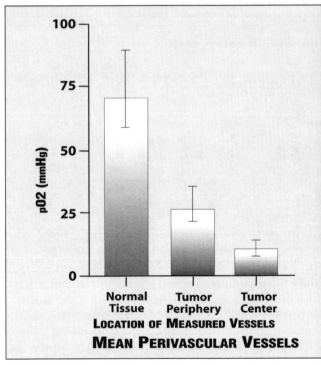

Figure 29-64: Perivascular oxygen tension in tumor window chambers. Mean pO_2 in normal tissue surrounding the tumor is significantly higher than in the tumor (p = 0.002). Also, pO_2 in the tumor periphery is significantly higher than tumor center (p = 0.002). Tumor center oxygen tensions of some functional vessels were found to drop to 0 mmHg at some readings.

Adapted from Dewhirst, et al. Radiation Research 130:171-182, 1992.

the blood pH, are alkaline. The tumor populations on the periphery and in the center are different. They are heterogeneous.

The heterogeneous nature of neoplasms is well recognized in the scientific literature. Populations of human and animal cancers frequently demonstrate a great variation in chromosome number and DNA content. Tumors are known to be heterogeneous with regard to their antigenic properties, immunogenicity, hormone receptors, pigment production, metabolic characteristics, and growth rate, as well as in their susceptibility to a variety of cytotoxic drugs.[105-108] It is not surprising that cells within the same tumor mass can be heterogeneous with regard to invasion and metastasis, that is, they contain a variety of subpopulations of cells with differing metastatic potentials. This last fact means that highly metastatic variants of cells may exist within a primary tumor site. The pathology report from a tumorous mass is only valid for the cells that were tested. So a woman with breast cancer whose cancer has all good prognostic indicators per the biopsy report may have a very anaplastic cell type in the middle of the tumor mass of which she or her oncologist is not yet aware. They will become aware, like Annie did, when the tumor recurs three years later.

Tumor heterogeneity is an important concept to understand because it is another reason for a person diagnosed with cancer to undergo aggressive care such as IPT. Even if the prognosis appears good based on the pathology report, it is generally best to be conservative and do some treatment that is systemic at eliminating *any* cancer cells. **Remember, in the majority of patients with clinical cancer, excluding those with skin tumors, metastasis has already occurred at the time of diagnosis.**[109-111] Therefore, even the most extensive surgical procedures cannot hope to bring about a high "cure" rate. Short of the complete prevention of cancer, the urgent goal of any health care provider caring for cancer patients should be the prevention or the successful treatment of micrometastases. The latter are best treated with IPT.

The heterogeneity of cancer also means that when using various chemotherapy agents, it is likely that the various populations of the cancer will respond differently to treatment. This explains why conventional oncology shrinks the cancer mass but not completely. The chemotherapy was effective against the peripheral tumor cells but not against the more hypoxic fraction. Typically, IPT physicians take the heterogeneity factor out of the loop by incorporating many different chemotherapy medications during a treatment course. IPT physicians will often use three to five cancer-killing medications during a session and, if needed, will change the regime to maximize the effectiveness of IPT against **all** tumor cell populations.

There is one more reason that tumor heterogeneity is important: The central tumor hypoxia may have to be addressed. If the center of a tumor mass is hypoxic (which is likely especially for larger tumor masses), then it is doubtful that the circulation is good enough to bring chemotherapy medications to the site. Tumor hypoxia is a real entity that is an independent risk factor for poor prognosis. In one study from the University of Mainz Medical School in Mainz, Germany, hypoxic tumors were found to exhibit larger tumor extensions and more frequent (occult) metastases compared to well-oxygenated tumors.[112] In other words, the less oxygen a tumor has, the more likely it will be aggressive and metastasize.

To increase the oxygen content of a tumor, heat or substances that increase blood flow, such as pentoxifylline (Trental), can be given. Low-dose hyperthermia and pentoxifylline have been shown to increase tumor oxygenation, which has helped cancers become more sensitive to the killing effects of radiation therapy.[113-115] Whenever significant tumor heating is possible, this is done in our office. For tumors that are relatively superficial, pentoxifylline is given via a subcutaneous injection just before the IPT is given to, at least theoretically, increase the chemotherapy levels at the cancer site.

WHY DOESN'T MY ONCOLOGIST TELL ME THIS STUFF?

Oncologists are *not* known to be nutritional wizards. There is still a notion in oncology that food feeds cancer. We believe this stems from the fact that intravenous feedings given to cancer patients in the hospital have been shown to feed the cancer. Numerous human and animal studies have shown that intravenous feedings, formally known as parenteral nutrition, stimulate cancer growth.[116-118] For many years, Marion was on a nutrition support team at a major medical center. The nutritional support that is given in tube feedings and by intravenous lines is typically approximately 50% dextrose, sucrose, glucose, or some other simple sugar. Sometimes the blood sugars go so high in the patients given these feedings that they need insulin. Is it any wonder when cancer patients receive 50% dextrose straight into the blood with a little insulin added that their cancers grow? Thus the notion from oncologists that food feeds cancer. Food does not feed cancer; carbohydrates especially in the form of sugars, do.

For the person who doubts this, go to the grocery store and look at the ingredients of the most popular tube feeding product of all-time—Ensure. What is the first ingredient? How many carbohydrate calories does the product have? The results may shock you... you'd better be sitting down.

SUMMARY AND ACTION PLAN

The typical American diet is high in carbohydrates. Over time, this type of diet causes high insulin levels to occur in order to keep blood sugar levels within normal ranges. If the person continues to eat a diet

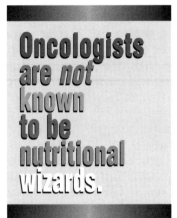

Oncologists are *not* known to be nutritional wizards.

high in carbohydrates, glucose intolerance and diabetes can form. These latter two conditions are much more prevalent in the cancer population versus those without cancer. Because cancers can grow with or without oxygen as long as they have glucose, one can say that cancers crave sugar.

Cancers take the sugar they consume and form lactate, also known as lactic acid. This lactate can then be turned back into more glucose to help feed the cancer. Cancer physiology is thus more anaerobic than aerobic. Because cancer cells have more insulin receptors than a normal cell, the blood glucose is preferentially attracted to those cells instead of the host's normal tissue cells.

The way to starve the tumor is to reduce blood sugar and insulin levels. It is helpful for cancer patients to get these levels checked via a glucose/

insulin tolerance test periodically to make sure they are reversing their cancer physiology. Blood sugar levels can best be lowered by eating a high-protein, low-carbohydrate diet. It is the amount of carbohydrates consumed during a day, not the glycemic index of the foods eaten, that determines the level of glucose or insulin that will be produced from the food.

One of the high protein foods that is recommended in the Hauser Diet for cancer patients is soy. Soy contains Isoflavones, including genistien and diadzein, which have anti-cancer effects. Studies have shown that consuming soy and soy isoflavonoids can lower estradiol levels. These substances also block estradiol binding. It is for these and many other reasons that Ross A. Hauser, M.D. is quoted as saying, "No matter what others say, soy is good."

Cancer cells depend on anaerobic metabolism for energy. One of the main enzymes of anaerobic energy production is lactate dehydrogenase, which converts pyruvate the end product of glycolysis to lactate. Quercetin, a bioflavonoid from plants, has been shown to inhibit this enzyme and help lower the amount of lactate produced by cancer cells.

Tumors are not uniform, as they are made up of a heterogeneous population of cells. The center of a tumor mass generally has less blood circulation and thus is more hypoxic than the periphery. This heterogeneity makes metastases more likely and also increases the risk of tumor resistance to chemotherapy. IPT regimes take this into account they typically consist of many different cancer-killing agents to increase the likelihood of success For these and many other reasons, cancer patients are turning to a high-protein diet to starve the cancer, and receiving IPT to help destroy it. ■

CHAPTER 30

Warning: Adjunctive Therapies Are No Substitute for an IPT Physician!

"IF EVERYTHING WERE ALRIGHT, IT WOULDN'T MATTER, BUT EVERYTHING IS NOT ALRIGHT. EVERY MINUTE AN AMERICAN DIES OF CANCER—10,000 A WEEK, OVER 500,000 A YEAR, EQUAL TO TEN TIMES THE CASUALTIES OF THE VIETNAM WAR—EVERY YEAR."

-Dan Haley, Politics in Healing, Potomac Valley Press, Washington, D.C., © 2000

After Henry's IPT treatments, I (Ross) sent him to see a surgeon, because IPT had shrunk Henry's lung cancer considerably. Henry came to us with a huge neck mass. He had been referred to us because we had helped to cure another cancer patient whom Henry's wife knew. After 10 IPT treatments, Henry's neck mass was gone, and all that was left was a very small lung nodule. At this point, I thought Henry should see if he had other options beside continuing IPT. While Henry was at the surgeon's office, the doctor called me and said, "Ross, keep doing what you are doing. You are his only hope."

You would think after 10 years of treating cancer patients that we would have heard it all, but they still keep coming in:

- "I bought this zapper. Do you think it is going to cure my cancer?"
- "I am coming so you can show me how to give bee venom shots to get rid of my cancer."
- "I am sure Laetrile is going to cure my cancer."
- "I had a spiritual healing. The lump is just scar tissue."
- "This reverend has people take Barley Green and cures a lot of cancer. Should I try it?"

The stories go on and on. Anyone who knows us realizes that we use prayer in the office, recommend Superfood (similar to Barley Green), believe in parasites/fungus and cancer association, and have used as much Laetrile in the office as probably any American doctor. We have a unique perspective because most of the treatments that people propose to us have been used by us to some degree but with limited success. Because these treatments do not cure cancer, we say they are adjunctive. Adjunct means something joined or added to another thing but not essentially a part of it.[1] I love that definition because this is what these therapies are for most cancers—adjuncts to IPT. IPT can stand alone, but in many circumstances, it is better that some of these adjunctive therapies be added to the IPT regime.

The adjunctive therapies discussed in this chapter are ones we use to varying degrees in our practice. We have put them in the order by which they are used, from most used to least used. As every doctor treats cancer patients differently, some or all of these therapies are not done by other IPT doctors. There are also adjunctive therapies that other IPT doctors do with IPT that we do not do in our clinic. This is why we go to conferences together to learn the best therapies for our patients.

Each adjunctive therapy is used to either help the person's quality of life or to hopefully increase the effectiveness of IPT. For the person who is in cancer remission, these adjunctive therapies may be used as part of a comprehensive program to reverse cancer physiology. The adjunctive therapies to be discussed are as follows:

- AMP (Adenosine Monophosphate) Injections
- Anabolic Hormones
- Cesium
- Doug Kaufmann's Antifungal Program
- Germanium
- HCl Injections
- Herbal Potentiators
- Intravenous Therapies
- Laetrile
- Low-Dose Oral Chemotherapy
- Magnetic Therapy
- Naltrexone
- Nutriceuticals for Specific Purposes
- Oral Hypoglycemics

The following will contain a brief overview of these adjunctive therapies. For the inquiring mind, it is recommended that the references in the bibliography be read thoroughly.

HERBAL POTENTIATORS

There are many reasons for the cancer patient to take herbal remedies, including immune stimulation, reversing medication side effects, ensuring adequate nutrition, and assisting in cancer control. But what most people do not know is that simple nutrients and herbal remedies can be used to potentiate the effects of chemotherapy.

Various substances can be used to optimize the cancer-killing effects of chemotherapy, in addition to insulin, dimethyl sulfoxide (DMSO), oxygen therapies, and hyperthermia. Scientific studies have shown that beta carotene, bupleurum, coenzyme Q_{10}, *Coriolus versicolor,* diadzein, genistein, glutamine, glutathione, green tea, melatonin, milk thistle, N-acetylcysteine, quercetin, rabdosia, selenium, vitamin A, vitamin C, vitamin E, and vitamin K have been shown in studies to potentiate the killing effects of chemotherapy.[2-6]

The activities of some of these dietary substances are seen in **Figure 30-1**. Because many of these compounds have some antioxidant activities, they could theoretically interfere with the oxidant-killing effects of chemotherapy. When one reviews the literature, there is resounding evidence that nutrients and herbal remedies

enhance the killing effects of chemotherapy and subsequently reduce its side effects. It is more than overdue that modern oncologists realize this fact and start prescribing some of these nutriceuticals for their patients.

BETA CAROTENE

Beta carotene has been shown to enhance the cytotoxicity of melphalan and BCNU on human squamous carcinoma cells and of cisplatin and dacarbazine on melanoma cells. In mice with transplanted mammary carcinoma, beta carotene enhanced the anti-tumor effect of cyclophosphamide, and in mice transplanted with fibrosarcoma, beta carotene enhanced the anti-tumor effect of melphalan, BCNU, doxorubicin, and etoposide.

VITAMIN C

In vitro studies with several tumor cell lines have shown vitamin C to enhance the cytotoxic activity of doxorubicin, cisplatin, paclitaxel, dacarbazine, 5-fluorouracil, and bleomycin. Vitamin C has also been shown to increase drug accumulation and to partially reverse vincristine resistance of human non-small cell lung cancer cells. Animal studies have shown that vitamin C at 500 mg/kg and 1,000 mg/kg enhances the chemotherapeutic effect of cyclophosphamide, Vinblastine, procarbazine, BCNU, and doxorubicin.

VITAMIN E

Vitamin E, in vitro, has been shown to enhance the cytotoxic effect of several anticancer drugs including 5-fluorouracil, doxorubicin, vincristine, dacarbazine, cisplatin, and tamoxifen. Studies with laboratory animals have shown that parenteral administration of vitamin E enhances the anticancer effect of 5-fluorouracil and cisplatin.

QUERCETIN

Quercetin has been shown to enhance the cytotoxicity of several antineoplastic agents. In multidrug-resistant cancer cells, quercetin markedly enhanced the growth-inhibitory effects of doxorubicin. In drug-sensitive cancer cells, quercetin has been shown to enhance the antiproliferative activity of cisplatin, nitrogen mustard, busulfan, and cytosine arabinoside. Quercetin also enhanced the anti-tumor activity of cisplatin in mice implanted with a human large-cell lung cancer.

FIGURE 30-1: ACTIVITIES OF DIETARY SUPPLEMENTS	
ANTIOXIDANT	**ACTIVITIES**
Vitamin E	Chain-Breaking Lipid-Soluble Antioxidant Inhibitor of Protein Tyrosine Kinases
Vitamin C	Water-Soluble Antioxidant
Coenzyme Q_{10}	Lipid-Soluble Antioxidant, Cofactor for Electron Transport
β-Carotene	Lipid-Soluble Antioxidant
Glutathione	Water-Soluble Antioxidant
N-Acetylcysteine	Water-Soluble Antioxidant, Source of Cysteine for Glutathione Synthesis
Glutamine	Cellular Fuel for Enterocytes and Lymphocytes, Source of Glutamate for Glutathione Synthesis
Selenium	Incorporated into Selenoproteins
Genestein	Antioxidant, Inhibitor of Topoisomerase I and II, Inhibitor of Protein Tyrosine Kinases
Daidzein	Antioxidant
Quercetin	Antioxidant, Inhibitor of Topoisomerase II, Inhibitor of Protein Tyrosine Kinases

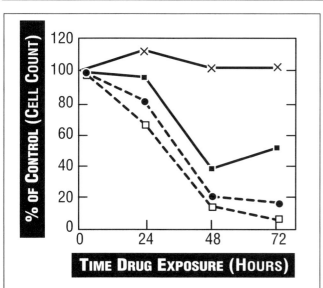

Figure 30-2: Alpha-tocopherol (Vitamin E) significantly enhanced the cancer-killing effects of fluorouracil (5-FU) in this leukemia cell line.

Enhancement of 5-FU cell growth inhibition by α-tocpherol.
×——× = Vitamin E
■——■ = 5-FU
●——● = Vitamine E plus 5-FU

Alpha-tocopherol (Vitamine E) significantly enhanced the cancer-killing effects of 5FU in this Leukemia cell line.

FIGURE 30-3: Some Non-Antioxidant Properties of Common "Antioxidants"

RETINOIC ACID DERIVATIVE
Exhibits anti-angiogenic properties
Induces metalloprotease-1 gene expression
Down-regulates insulin-like growth factor binding proteins
Inhibits IGF-1
Induces TGF beta
Inhibits telemerase
Inhibits thrombomodulin
Increases connexin
Induces osteopondin expression

VITAMINS C AND/OR E
Inhibits androgen induced AP-1 and NF-KB DNA binding sites
Induces apoptosis
Activates calcineurin
Inhibits protein kinase C

CAROTENOIDS
Inhibits or regulates gene expression of connexins
Pro- and anticarcinogenesis
Enhances cell transforming activity
Suppresses RAR-beta and increase activator protein-1
Induces TGF beta
Inhibits carcinogen induced neoplastic transformation

MELATONIN
Induces apoptosis in EAC cells
Regulates sleep-wake cycle
Regulates gluco-corticoid receptor
Blocks activation of estrogen receptor for DNA

RESVERATROL
Induces apoptosis in HL-60 cells

QUERCETIN
Induces apoptosis in colorectal tumor cells

PDTC (PYRROLLIDINE DITHIOCARBAMATE)
Induces apoptosis by raising redox-active copper
Induces apoptosis by cytochrome C dependent mechanism
Affects binding of NF Kappa B to DNA

SILIBININ AND OTHER FLAVONOIDS
Induces G-cell arrest in prostate cancer cells
Induces p53-independent apoptosis

PDTC AND VITAMIN E
Induces apoptosis in CRL cells by induction of p21WAF1/CIP1 inhibition of cell cycle

POLYPHENOLS
Induces G2/M phase cell arrest in PC-3 tumor cells

Adapted from Cancer Therapy Through Modification of Blood Physico-Chemical Constants (Donatian Therapy), by García D, García y Bellón, translated by M. Dillinger, 1978. Available at: www.IPTQ.org.

SUMMARY OF STUDIES

These studies can be reviewed by looking at references two to six in the bibliography. Most of the studies on the potentiating effects of nutrients are based on cell cultures (See **Figure 30-2**).

The take home message for the cancer patient is to make sure you are taking a good multivitamin. Depending on the medications that will be used during IPT, various nutriceutical agents may be added to your regime to potentiate the effects of the chemotherapy.

NUTRICEUTICALS FOR SPECIFIC PURPOSES

There are many reasons to take nutriceutical products. Many of them have intrinsic anticancer effects (See **Figure 30-3**). Typically we give various oral (by mouth) chemotherapy agents to our cancer patients in our office. The most common ones that we use are high-dose vitamin D and vitamin A.*

---

* *These are available by calling 1-877-RX-BEULAH or ordering on-line at www.benuts.com. Be "nuts" for your health—buy your nutritional supplements at Beulah Land Nutritionals! Dr. Hauser serves as a consultant to Beulah Land Nutritionals.*

FIGURE 30-4: CHEMOTHERAPY DRUG TOXICITIES AND NUTRICEUTAL TREATMENTS

CHEMOTHERAPY DRUG	TOXICITY	NATURAL MEDICINE TREATMENT
Bleomycin	Lung	Alpha Lipoic Acid, N-Acetyl-Cysteine
Carmustine	Stomach	Ginger, Probiotic, (Stomach Enyzme)*
Cisplatin/Carboplatin	Kidney	IV Glutathione, Alpha Lipoic Acid, Uve Ursi (Cystatin)*
Doxorubicin	Heart	Coenzyme Q$_{10}$, L-Carnitine, Hawthorne Berry (Cardiomax)*
Gemzar/Mitomycin	Low Blood Counts	Shark Liver Oil, Mushroom Extracts, (Marrow Plus)*
Vinblastine/Vincristive	Nerve	B Vitamins, Microhydrin*

Herbal products available at www.benuts.com or 1-877-RX-BEULAH.

FIGURE 30-5: CHEMOTHERAPY DRUG SIDE EFFECTS AND POSSIBLE TREATMENTS

	ALLOPATHIC TREATMENT	NATURAL MEDICINE TREATMENT
Anxiety	Xanax, Atavan	Valerian, Hops, GABA, Blue Vervain
Anemia	Epogen Shot	Iron, Liver Extract, Beet Juice, Marrow Plus*
Anorexia	Megace, Marinol	IV Nutrients, Enzyme Juicing, Ginger, Peppermint
Nausea	Zofran, Compazine	Ginger, Stomach Enzyme,* Small Intestine Powder*
Diarrhea	Lomotil, Imodium	Psyllium, Enzymes, Papaya, Bromelain
Constipation	Ducolax Suppositories	Super Aloe,* Cascara, Probiotics, Magnesium
Hair Loss	Wig	Vitamin E, Antioxidants, Hauser Hair Formulas,* ProCollagen*
Fatigue	Prozac, Anti-depressants	L-Carnitine, Ginseng, Ashwaghada
Low White Blood Cell Counts	Neupogen	Shark Liver Oil, Astragalus Marrow Plus*
Candida Infections	Nystatin, Diflucan	Probiotics, DE Yeast*
Insomnia	Ambien, Xanax	5-HTP, Valerian Root, Melatonin, Kava Kava
Pain	Narcotics	Bromelain, Prolotherapy, Neural Therapy

Herbal products sold at www.benuts.com or 1-877-RX-BEULAH.

Nutritional products are especially effective at helping reduce the side effects of chemotherapy. Natural herbal products can be used to decrease the specific toxicities of the various chemotherapy drugs (See **Figure 30-4**). For the cancer patient undergoing high-dose chemotherapy, nutriceuticals can be used to better tolerate the treatment (See **Figure 30-5**).

Anorexia and weight loss are major concerns for cancer patients. The gastrointestinal side effects of chemotherapy, cancer physiology, infections, and poor health are among the factors that contribute to their malnutrition (See **Figure 30-6**). Nutrient intravenous infusions with vitamins, protein powders, and herbal supplements are methods to combat malnutrition. Perhaps the greatest weapon, however, against the anorexia of cancer is IPT.

Donato Pérez Garciá, M.D. (Donato 1), and Donato Pérez Garciá y Bellón, M.D. (Donato 2), in their book *Cellular Cancer Therapy,* put it this way, "Cachexia is the most important physiological effect of malignant tumors. In man, one of the most prominent symptoms of cancer is the loss of weight..."[7]

Insulin Potentiation Therapy helps reverse the anorexia, cachexia, and malnutrition of cancer by

- Stopping cancer growth
- Killing cancer cells
- Reversing cancer physiology
- Decreasing lactate levels
- Detoxifying the body
- Stimulating appetite
- Increasing the person's energy
- Providing the person a sense of well-being

IPT is the cancer method of the future because it helps a person regain health while undergoing tumor remission. It does not destroy the person while destroying the cancer.

For the cancer patient in remission, nutrients can be used to *stay* in remission. Many nutrients have definite chemopreventive effects, such as selenium, vitamin C, and vitamin E. As discussed in other parts of this book, nutritionals are sometimes needed to reverse aspects of cancer physiology, such as reducing estradiol levels, to keep female cancers from recurring.

DOUG KAUFMANN'S ANTIFUNGAL PROGRAM

When Pastor Peter was diagnosed with immunoblastic lymphoma, we just assumed that he would get well. He underwent surgery, irradia-

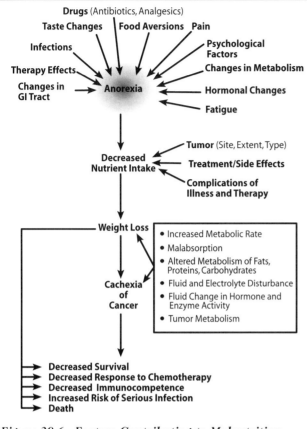

Figure 30-6: Factors Contributing to Malnutrition in the Cancer Patient

Nutriceuticals can alleviate this problem, but the best method is to aggressively treat the cancer with IPT.

Adapted from The Cancer Chemotherapy Handbook, *by David Fischer, M. Tish Knopf, J. Henry Durivage, Page 503, 1997, 5th Edition, Mosby, St. Louis.*

tion, and many rounds of chemotherapy. After about nine months of this, like many of our patients, we realized that there needs to be a better way. We went on a search, and the search led us to Dallas, Texas, and the office of Doug Kaufmann.

Doug has been in the natural health field for over 30 years, having run a comprehensive food allergy testing lab, authored a best-selling book on food allergies in the 1970s, and ending up in private practice in Dallas. He currently is the host of the national cable show *Health Matters* on FamilyNet and is author of the book *The Fungus Link.* His much anticipated book on the fungus etiology of cancer has recently been released. Needless to say, he is a remarkable man.

He is the main proponent of educating people on the fungus link to human disease. Because of the way food is produced, food is contaminated with high levels of mycotoxins. Most of the mycotoxins are in the grains that people eat. He has devised a very effective diet to eliminate fungus and fungus mycotoxins, appropriately termed the *Kaufmann Diet*. As you would expect, the Hauser diet and the Kaufmann diet are very similar; both are based on the premise that cancer physiology may be reversed by the diets.

On his radio and television programs every week across America, Doug tells people about the fungal etiology of disease. Because of the massive use of antibiotics, people lose the protective bacteria in their intestines, which sets up the opportunity for a fungal infection. This fungal infection can cause carbohydrate cravings in the individual. The physiology on which a cancer cell extracts energy is the same process that a fungus cell utilizes, namely anaerobic fermentation, using glucose instead of oxygen as the substrate on which to get energy. Patients with fungal infections such as candida often crave sugar; thus they eat it. One can easily see that if they continue to eat this sugar, cancer could form (See **Figure 30-7**). The Kaufmann program to eliminate fungus and fungus mycotoxins from the diet includes getting on a good probiotic (acidophilus), taking antifungal herbs and medications, and following the Kaufmann Diet. We have seen first-hand that the Kaufmann antifungal program does indeed help clients reverse cancer physiology and become cancer-free.

For many years, Doug had worked with a dermatologist. He would often prescribe antifungal medications because

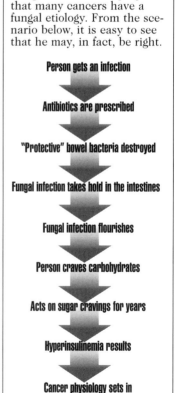

Figure 30-7: The Fungus-Cancer Link

Doug Kaufmann has proposed that many cancers have a fungal etiology. From the scenario below, it is easy to see that he may, in fact, be right.

Person gets an infection

Antibiotics are prescribed

"Protective" bowel bacteria destroyed

Fungal infection takes hold in the intestines

Fungal infection flourishes

Person craves carbohydrates

Acts on sugar cravings for years

Hyperinsulinemia results

Cancer physiology sets in

Cancer forms

> *...the addition of large amounts of carbohydrate to the food intake stimulated the growth and size of the tumor...*

of the fungal rashes people would present. What they noticed was that some of the people's cancers were shrinking. It was at this point that Doug realized the cancer-fungus link. Now he recommends that cancer patients be placed on antifungal medications in addition to eating a low-carbohydrate, high-protein diet. We follow the Kaufmann antifungal program by having cancer patients on antifungal medications throughout their treatment program. This means using medications such as ketoconazole, diflucan, sporonox, and/or nystatin to decrease the body burden of fungus. In the hundreds of cancer patients whom we have tested, we have not found one who did not have evidence of a fungus infection by blood and stool testing.

LOW-DOSE ORAL CHEMOTHERAPY

Once a cancer takes hold in an individual, it can grow exponentially as long as the glucose supply is present. Since most cancer patients eat too many carbohydrates, they have to resort to high-dose chemotherapy to stop the growth. Hopefully this book and the many IPT doctors will help reverse this trend.

For the cancer patient who is going to use IPT, some low-dose chemotherapy by mouth may be needed for a time. It is always possible in between IPT treatments that the cancer could grow, especially if the cancer load is great. It takes time to reverse cancer physiology. Depending on the cancer, it may take four to 12 IPT treatments to start cancer shrinkage; therefore it may be necessary to halt tumor growth with some oral chemotherapy medication. The person typically begins to feel better the day there is more cancer being destroyed than being formed.

In our office, we will use some type of oral chemotherapeutic agent. This could be high-dose vitamin A; vitamin D; or something such as poly-MVA, carnivora, PC SPECS; the latter three are *natural* chemotherapeutic agents. For the person with a big tumor load, it may be necessary to use a typical chemotherapy medication, though it will be prescribed in a low dose.

HCL INJECTIONS

"IRRESPECTIVE OF WHETHER ALKALOSIS IS A LOCAL OR A GENERAL BODY CHANGE, IT SEEMS LOGICAL THAT AN ACIDOTIC THERAPY SHOULD BE USED TO REDUCE THE ALKALINITY IN THE BLOOD CAUSED BY THE TUMOR. IF ONE SUCCEEDS BY ANY MANIPULATION IN SHIFTING THE TUMOR REACTION MORE OR LESS TOWARD THE ACID SIDE, THEN IT SHOULD BE POSSIBLE EITHER TO RETARD CANCER GROWTH OR TO CAUSE THE DISAPPEARANCE OF THE TUMOR." [8]

This quote above is from an article after surveying some recent investigations in cancer research. The author noted:

> In its metabolism the tumor cell resembles the yeast cell. The tumor cell is able to produce glycolysis of glucose with the production of lactic acid. With one molecule of oxygen, malignant tissue produces from three to four times as much lactic acid as does benign tissue. The tumor cell is a facultative anaerobe and aerobe... I concluded that the addition of large amounts of carbohydrate to the food intake stimulated the growth and size of the tumor...The carbohydrates increase the growth energy of the tumor...I believe therefore that for the development and origin of malignant tumors a certain degree of alkalinity and a disturbance of the carbohydrate metabolism is of great importance."[8]

Other researchers in the 1930s found the same thing. Fischer-Wasels found that the alkalosis of the blood stimulated metabolism and that in an alkaline medium, glycolysis, cell division, and growth energy of the tumor were stimulated.[9]

It was actually as early as 1906 that cancer research found that people with cancer had increased alkalinity in their blood.[10,11] The research was confirmed in later years. McDonald reported in 1927 that the blood of untreated or advanced carcinoma patients was more alkaline than normal, except in cases of skin or superficial cancers, in which it was found to be normal.[12] McDonald noted:

> People cursed with acidosis are practically immune from cancer. Their blood may reach the figure of 7.2 on the biochemist's scale of acidity. A victim of cancer, on the other hand, would show a record of about 7.45.[12]

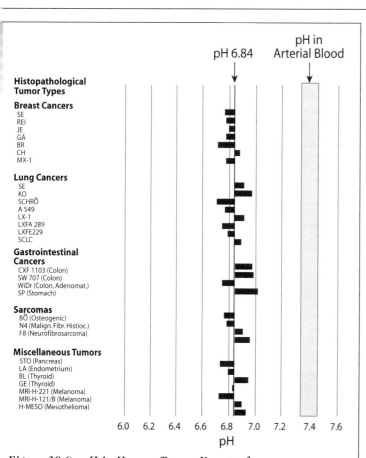

Figure 30-8: pH in Human Tumor Xenografts

The vertical line at pH 6.84 indicates the average value of all the single-point measurements recorded in a total of 68 xenografts. Black bars indicate the difference between the former value and the mean pH of individual tumor xenografts. Of each tumor line, 5-12 individual xenografts were analyzed. Grey area: physiological range of pH values in arterial blood of tumor-bearing rats.

that the rise in pH was not due to the cancer. He was the first that I know of to prove that there is cancer physiology; even if one takes out the cancer, it is still there. Perhaps this explains the 50% of cancer recurrences after surgery.

The state of the blood in cancer is of great importance because cancer becomes a systemic disease, and cancer cells receive their nourishment from and give off their waste products to the blood. Therefore it is to be expected that the blood of cancer patients should differ from normal blood.[14]

It was clear to researchers in the early part of the 20th century that the secret to curing cancer was in the blood, yet cancer patients some 100 years later have only one cancer marker drawn every year and are given a clean bill of health when it is okay. Modern oncology is not looking at cancer physiology, to the detriment of the cancer patient.

Research done at the cancer research laboratories at the University of Pennsylvania and Philadelphia General Hospital found the following:

- The average pH of 26 untreated cancer patients is 7.44, or considerably more alkaline than normal.

- The average of 8 untreated superficial cases is 7.38; that of 18 untreated internal cancer cases was 7.47.

- The degree of alkalinity is closely related to the prognosis of the disease.[14]

The higher a cancer patient's pH, the worse the prognosis. In other words, the worse the cancer physiology, the more likely the cancer will either be large and/or metastatic.

While the blood in cancer patients is alkaline, the actual malignant tissues are acidic (See **Figure 30-8**). Many researchers have confirmed this both in animal and human studies.[15-17] This would make sense because cancer cells produce lactic acid, which would make these cells and their surroundings acidic. *Perhaps this is why we always hear in alternative medicine circles about cancer patients being so acidic, when in reality they are too alkaline.*

In 1928, Reding reported that (a) the blood of untreated cancer patients exhibits a high pH; (b) the pH in cases of benign precancerous tumors is elevated but not to the same degree as in malignant cases; (c) about 50% of the relatives of cancer patients show a pH slightly above normal, thus indicating a familial predisposition to cancer; and (d) the increased blood alkalinity or rise in pH habitually persists after removal of the tumor.[13] Reding came to the conclusion that "cancer is always associated with alkalosis."

Wow! Isn't this exciting? Research like this excites me! I (Ross) collect old medical books. Most of the answers modern medicine is searching for can be found in these old books. Reding found that the rise in pH preceded the appearance of malignancy and continued after surgery, meaning

When carbohydrates are given to a person or animal, or are injected into them, the cancer sites become more acidic,[18-20] which is indicative of the cancer growing and producing more lactic acid. One study showed that cancer patients given glucose by mouth produced the same decrease in tumor extracellular pH as did intravenous glucose.[19] This shows again that the amount of carbohydrates that a cancer patient intakes will determine the amount of growth of the cancer. This is sad because many of the feedings in the hospital for sick cancer patients are intravenous glucose, or their tube feedings are full of glucose. The cancer patient needs the opposite—a high-protein, low-carbohydrate diet.

Reversing the blood alkalinity of cancer physiology may be one of the keys to curing a cancer patient because it would help decrease the cancer's ability to make lactic acid. In regard to lactic acid production, the following is clear:

- The concentration of lactic acid in the blood rises when the alkalinity of the blood is increased. A decrease in the alkalinity is followed by a reduction of the lactic acid.

- These changes are determined by the pH of the blood. Below a pH of about 7.4, the rate of removal of lactic acid is greater than the rate of its accumulation. Above this value, the opposite takes place.

- It appears that the concentration of lactic acid in the blood is not determined by the oxygen tension, but by the pH of the blood.[21]

To quote the late Willy Meyer, M.D.: "We may find alkalosis without cancer, but no cancer without alkalosis."[22] He made this statement in the early 1930s, and he and handful of doctors started treating cancer with dilute hydrochloric acid (HCl) injections. Some of their results are found in the book *Three Years of HCl Therapy*. When we first heard about this, we researched to find the best pH monitor possible. We have been doing blood, urine, and saliva testing on cancer patients for about 10 years and have found Dr. Meyer's statement correct in every person we have tested except one. A lady with a very advanced case of cancer came in and was found to have an acid pH at 7.31. She died within two weeks. Apparently all of her alkaline reserves were used up.

The history of intravenous HCl injections is very interesting, and we recommend the above book for a thorough explanation. What some innovative doctors found was that HCl could be injected at a dilution of 1:500 without any evidence of toxic effect—yet with uniformly good results clinically.[22] Typically, a person with alkalinity is given 10 cc in an intravenous bag. We use HCl, not only to reverse cancer physiology, but other aberrant physiology that occurs with many chronic and disabling diseases.

HCl injections have been shown to:
- help resolve infections
- increase white blood cell counts
- enhance phagocytosis
- increase oxygen content of red blood cells
- decrease blood pH
- decrease blood lactate levels
- reverse some aspects of cancer physiology

Alkalosis is easily tested by checking the pH in blood, urine, and saliva. If alkalosis is found, HCl injections can be given. We tested the effect 25 grams of vitamin C would have on the blood pH in 1998 on one of our patients before and after infusion and found that it decreased by 0.1. Since vitamin C is ascorbic acid, it makes sense that it lowers the blood pH, which might help explain some of its beneficial effects in cancer. So in regard to IPT, HCl and/or Vitamin C is given in an IV bag after the chemotherapy is given to aid in the reversal of cancer physiology.

INTRAVENOUS NUTRIENT INJECTIONS

Part of the usual regime with IPT is intravenous vitamins. The vitamins are given to help decrease anorexia, provide nutrition, increase the efficacy of IPT, and reverse cancer physiology. If a person is experiencing weight loss or is malnourished, it is helpful to give some vitamins and fluids in the vein intravenously. Besides helping quality of life, it may in fact help preserve life. The nutritional status of the person needs to be maintained for immune function to be optimal. Once the blood protein level (albumin) drops below 3.5, immunodeficiency starts to set in, which increases the cancer patient's risk of infection. By giving intravenous vitamins and minerals, the bad taste in the person's mouth and nausea can often be relieved, and he or she starts eating again.

At the Caring Cancer and Interventional Natural Medicine Center (CCINMC), we use over

310

20 different intravenous nutritional formulations. Besides the normal vitamins and minerals, we also have available to the cancer patient herbals such as licorice root, trace minerals such as germanium, glutathione, hydrochloric acid, and various amino acids such as taurine.

Some IPT doctors will give their patients high doses of vitamin C intravenously. In some individuals, giving 50 to 100 grams of vitamin C over a two to three hour period has a chemotherapeutic effect in decreasing cancer markers and causing some tumor shrinkage. I have personally seen this, though I would caution that I have not seen this cure a person of cancer. It is a useful adjunctive therapy along with IPT. Remember the chapter title: **Warning: Adjunctive Therapies Are No Substitute for an IPT Physician!**

ANABOLIC HORMONES

The most common reason that some cancer patients look so lousy is because they feel lousy. Nothing can help the cancer patient feel better than anabolic hormones. Anabolic means to build up. Anabolic hormones, such as Growth Hormone, insulin, testosterone, DHEA, and pregnenolone help make the body stronger, specifically by building up muscles. Insulin is given, of course, in the IPT regime, but we also often give additional anabolic hormones such as Growth Hormone and testosterone, especially if the person is weak and losing weight. It has been shown that Growth Hormone and insulin can reduce whole-body and skeletal muscle protein loss in patients with cancer.[21] Furthermore, the infusion of insulin can ameliorate net protein breakdown during catabolic metabolism.[23]

Sometimes patients are asked to use testosterone, DHEA, or progesterone at home. These are given in pill form or creams that are rubbed onto the skin. These hormones would be expected to increase appetite and help with weight gain. When a cancer patient starts eating more and gaining weight, it is a good sign that the cancer's catabolic (breakdown) physiology is starting to reverse.

MAGNETIC THERAPY

"IN EACH PHASE WE FIND THAT WHEN MAGNETIC ENERGY OF THE NEGATIVE (N) POLE IS APPLIED TO THE CANCER SITE, A REMARKABLE REDUCTION IN THE CONDITION AND ALSO A MARKED ARREST IN FURTHER DEVELOPMENT OF THE CANCER CONDITION TAKES PLACE."[24,25]

WHEN A NEGATIVE MAGNETIC FIELD IS APPLIED TO THE BODY, IT HAS THE ABILITY TO REMOVE THE CANCER-DEVELOPING CONDITION OF ACID-HYPOXIA AND REPLACES IT WITH AN ALKALINE AND OXYGENATED ENVIRONMENT. THEREFORE, A NEGATIVE MAGNETIC FIELD EXPOSURE CAN BE USED TO TREAT AS WELL AS PREVENT CANCER."[26]
- William Philpott, M.D., in his book Magnet Therapy

Magnets are becoming mainstream in medicine. They provide the discrete detail of a magnetic resonance imaging (MRI) scan, and physical therapists use them to help ease pain and speed the healing of broken bones.

A magnet has two poles, as does the earth. The poles of a magnet can be determined with a magnetometer. This instrument is composed of a compass that registers the presence of positive and negative electromagnetic poles. The magnet's north pole (south seeking) is the one that has negative electromagnetic energy, whereas the south pole has positive energy. Generally, the magnet's south pole is marked in red and the north pole in green.

In 1974, physicist Albert Roy Davis noted that positive and negative polarities have different effects on biologic systems. He found that magnets could be used to kill cancer cells in animals and could also be used in the treatment of arthritis, infertility, and chronic diseases related to aging. He concluded that negative magnetic fields have a beneficial effect on living organisms, whereas positive magnetic fields are detrimental.[24,25]

In his book *Magnetic Therapy,* William H. Philpott, M.D., describes the reasons why negative magnetic fields help heal the body.

According to him, acid-hypoxia (high acidity and low oxygen) is a central condition in both degenerative diseases and acute symptoms from maladaptive reactions. In contrast, alkaline-hyperoxia (low acidity and high oxygen) is the biologically normal state needed for energy production, oxidoreductase enzyme function, defense against infection, detoxification, and overall healing. Exposing the body to a negative magnetic field produces a biological response of alkaline-hyperoxia, helping to reverse undesirable symptoms and degenerative diseases.[26]

Figure 30-9 summarizes the different effects between positive and negative magnetic energy.

I (Ross) can personally attest to the knowledge of Dr. Philpott, as he has consulted on many of my cancer patients. I am also on his board as he is currently conducting clinical research on the effi-

NEGATIVE MAGNETIC FIELDS	POSITIVE MAGNETIC FIELDS
pH Normalizing	Acid producing
Oxygenating	Oxygen Deficit Producing
Resolves Cellular Edema	Evokes Cellular Edema
Usually Reduces Symptoms	Often Exacerbates Existing Symptoms
Inhibits Microorganism Replication	Accelerates Microorganism Replica
Slows Down Infections	Speeds up infections
Biologically Normalizing	Biologically Disorganizing
Reduces Pain and Inflammation	Increases Pain and Inflammation
Governs Rest, Relaxation, and Sleep	Governs Wakefulness and Action
Evokes Anabolic Hormone Production—Melatonin and Growth Hormone	Evokes Catabolic Hormone Production
Clears Metabolically Produced Toxins from of the Body	Produces Toxic By-products of Metabolism
Eliminates Free Radicals	Produces Free Radicals
Slows Down Electrical Activity of the Brain	Speeds up Electrical Activity of the Brain

Figure 30-9: The Physiological Effects of Negative and Positive Magnetic Fields
Negative magnetic fields help the body heal. They help reverse localized cancer physiology.

cacy of magnets on the treatment of cancer. When he talks to a cancer patient of mine, he will send me a report of exactly what the patient needs (See **Figure 30-10**). He also tells the patient and me the exact strength of the magnet needed (in gauss). He continually emphasizes that a cancer patient needs to always use the negative (south-seeking) magnetic field. This side of the magnet is placed on the skin.

Magnetic therapy can be used as adjunctive treatment with IPT. According to Dr. Philpott, a negative magnetic field helps treat cancer and specifically the cancer site by

- Creating an alkaline environment
- Activating aerobic metabolism
- Aiding detoxification[26]

This creates bodily conditions (especially at the cancer site) in which cancer cannot exist. This oxygen-rich and highly alkaline environment inhibits the energy-making functions of cancer cells. Because of this fact, a negative magnetic

CARCINOMA OF THE BREAST WITH METASTASIS TO THE AXILLA

ORIENTATION:

This magnetic research protocol is for a 38-year-old woman recently diagnosed by lumpectomy of a carcinoma of the left breast with one node in the left axilla. The node in the breast was 2.5 × 2.4 cm.

MAGNETIC THERAPY:

MAXIMUM THERAPY:
- One-hundred and forty 4" × 6" × 1" magnets.

MINIMAL THERAPY:

- Two 4" × 6" × ½" ceramic block magnets with Velcro on both the positive and negative pole sides.
- Two 5" × 12" double magnet, multimagnet flexible mats.
- A magnetic mattress pad composed of mini-block magnets that are 1⅞" × ⅞" × ⅞". These are placed one and a half inches apart throughout the bed pad.
- Four 4" × 6" × 1" magnets placed ¾" apart in a wooden carrier that holds them up against the headboard. These can be raised or lowered depending on the height of the pillow. They come shipped at the top of the carrier and need to be lowered so the wooden dowel they are resting on is level with the back of the head when the head is on the pillow.

Place across the left side of the chest and across the front of the armpit a 5" × 12" double magnet, multimagnet flexible mat. Place on top of this, directly over the left breast, a 4" × 6" × ⅞" magnet and place on top of this over the front of the armpit, with the magnet being 6" lengthwise, a 4" × 6" × ½" magnet. This is awkward because it somewhat restricts the use of the left arm. Yet, this is necessary. There is no way to put the magnet directly under the armpit, so for this reason, it is being treated from the front of the armpit. This is held in place with the 4" × 52" body wrap. It may be necessary to have two of these body wraps—one to hold the flexible mat in place, and the second one to hold the block magnets in place. The block magnets will have Velcro on both the positive and negative pole sides.

Figure 30-10: Magnetic Prescription for Breast Cancer
Adapted from Carcinoma of the Breast with Metastasis to the Axilla, Magnetic Research Protocol, Feb., 2000, William H. Philpot, Publisher, Choctaw, OK. This protocol was prescribed by Dr. Philpot for one of Dr. Hauser's patients.

field of sufficient strength and duration can cause the death of cancer cells.

When we went to a medical conference in Dusseldorf, Germany, in 1998, we were astounded at just how much more advanced other parts of the world are compared to the United States in regard to various methodologies for treating disease. There are now centers in Europe and Asia using huge magnets to treat cancer patients. For the doubting Thomas' out there, we have included a few of the possibly hundreds of references that confirm that magnetic therapy can kill cancer cells.[24-33] One of the references is a review of research in Europe by the former director of the National Institute of Public Health in the Czech Republic, Jiri Jerabek, M.D. In his book *Magnetic Therapy in Eastern Europe,* he describes research on the use of magnets for many diseases, including cancer, and how magnetic therapy can also be used as a potentiator of chemotherapy.

ORAL HYPOGLYCEMICS

Why are cancers more prevalent with age? Is it because our diets are that much worse when we get older? Partly. It is because many of us have continued to eat too many carbohydrates, and as we age, our glucose tolerance becomes impaired (See **Figure 30-11**). The result is that our insulin levels after eating dramatically increase with age (See **Figure 30-12**).

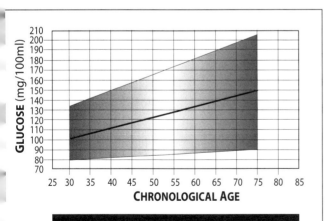

CHANGE IN GLUCOSE TOLERANCE WITH AGE
(Oral glucose tolerance test at one hour.)

Figure 30-11: Changes in Glucose Tolerance with Age
Above can be seen age-related changes in glucose tolerance one hour after eating.

Adapted from The Neuroendocrine Therapy of Aging, *by V. Dillman and W. Dean, The Center for Bio-Gerontology, 1992*

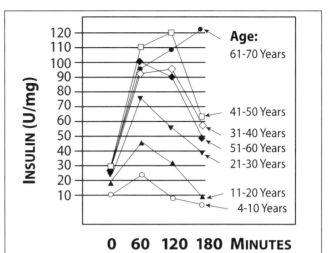

Figure 30-12: Age-Related Change in Blood Insulin Levels Two Hours after Eating
Note that insulin levels increase dramatically after age 20. This can only be interpreted to mean that nearly everyone over age 20 suffers from "prediabetes." This may explain the dramatic increase in cancer with aging.

Adapted from The Neuroendocrine Therapy of Aging, *by V. Dillman and W. Dean, The Center for Bio-Gerontology, 1992*

In their book, *The Neuroendocrine Theory of Aging,* Dilman and Dean discuss how nearly everyone over age 40 is "subclinical diabetic" because of their decreased glucose tolerance and high insulin levels.[34] This causes the tissues not to respond to insulin normally. The remedy they recommend is an oral hypoglycemic agent called metformin (Glucophage). This medication helps tissues respond more normally to insulin. According to them, it helps lower glucose and insulin levels to much younger levels.

Dilman and Dean depict several experiments using metformin on animals with cancer in which it showed some anticancer effects. Because of their enthusiasm, some antiaging societies and natural medicine doctors are recommending this medication for healthy aging because of its many positive effects (See **Figure 30-13**).

There are many oral hypoglycemic drugs such as Glyburide, Diabinase, and Micronase. First we test someone's glucose tolerance and insulin levels. If they are high, we generally start with diet, but if they are really high (fasting glucose over 200 or insulin over 30), then an oral hypoglycemic agent is probably warranted. Remember, the best way to lower glucose and insulin levels is via the Hauser diet, one that is high in protein and low in carbohydrates.

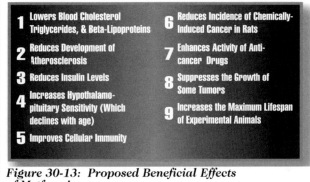

Figure 30-13: Proposed Beneficial Effects of Metformin

Adapted from Parsons P. Differential effects of NAD, nicotinamide, and related compounds upon growth and nucleoside incorporation in human cells, by P. Parsons Biochem Pharmacol. 1983;32:871-876.

About seven years ago, a patient of ours went to a Mexican clinic and was prescribed the Warburg therapy. Part of this treatment involved the administration of insulin shots under the skin, much like a diabetic would receive. The theory was that this would lower the blood sugar and have a positive effect on the cancer. It did have a positive effect, but not the one that he was hoping for; it caused the cancer to grow. The theory behind lowering blood sugar is a good one with the Warburg therapy, it just should not be done with insulin. Cancer patients already have high insulin levels, so more insulin is not needed. To help cure the person of cancer, the insulin levels must be lowered, whether it be by diet or medications. If a tumor is present, therapies that are stronger than these will be needed, so Insulin Potentiation Therapy is prescribed. In this case, insulin is given just before chemotherapy to drive the medications into the cancer cell. This is the only method in which insulin should be used for a cancer patient. Insulin given by itself runs the risk of increasing cancer growth. However, when combined with chemotherapy medications, insulin is a powerful weapon against cancer.

NALTREXONE

There are many little-known cancer therapies used by natural medicine doctors. They remain little known because the doctor who discovered it does not have enough cases to publish a scientific paper or the doctor is not a writer or publicist. This does not mean that the therapy is not valid or that the doctor has not tried to get it accepted. One of the cancer therapies that fits in this category is low-dose naltrexone.

Naltrexone is a medication used to block the effects of synthetic opioids, as when someone overdoses on heroine. Naltrexone can save a person's life. From a biochemical point of view, naltrexone has been shown to increase the body's production of beta- and metenkephalin endorphins. Blood tests done by Bernard Bihari, M.D., a physician in New York City, have shown that naltrexone can double or even triple the activity of natural killer cells, presumably by increasing the body's own natural production of endorphins.

Beta-endorphins and metenkephelin have numerous immune-stimulating properties (See **Figure 30-14**). Dr. Bihari found that with many serious illnesses, such as AIDS and cancer, the body's endorphin levels are low. He also notes that certain types of cancers are dense with opiate receptors in their cell walls. Dr. Bihari and his colleagues have found that malignancies that arise from human tissues that are dense with opiate receptor sites are the ones that either have responded positively to treatment with naltrex-

FIGURE 30-14: IMMUNOREGULATORY EFFECTS OF NEUROPEPTIDES

HORMONE/NEUROPEPTIDE	EFFECT
β-Endorphin	Enhancement of Ig and IFN-γ synthesis Modulation of T cell proliferation Enhancement of generation of T_C cells Enhancement of NK cell activity Chemotactic for monocytes and neutrophils
Leu- or metenkephalin	Suppression of Ig synthesis Enhancement of IFN-γ synthesis Enhancement of NK cell activity Chemotactic for monocytes

*Ig, immunoglobulin; IFN-γ, interferon-γ; NK cells; natural killer T cells; T_C cells, cytotoxic T cells.

Adapted from Endocrinology, Vol. 3, Third Edition, Leslie J. DeGroot, Editor, 1995, W.B. Saunders, Philadelphia

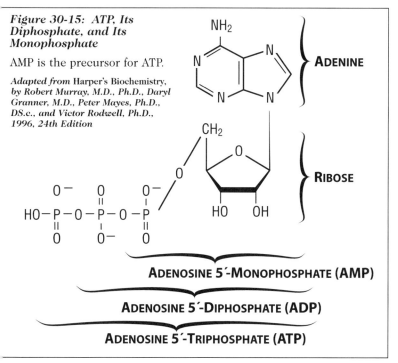

Figure 30-15: ATP, Its Diphosphate, and Its Monophosphate

AMP is the precursor for ATP.

Adapted from Harper's Biochemistry, *by Robert Murray, M.D., Ph.D., Daryl Granner, M.D., Peter Mayes, Ph.D., DS.c., and Victor Rodwell, Ph.D., 1996, 24th Edition*

normal biochemical processes. It is one of the nucleotides involved in protein synthesis, an intermediate in the Krebs cycle, and a precursor to the energy carrier molecule (ATP). It is also a key component in certain enzyme reactions necessary for proper fat and carbohydrate metabolism.

Research shows that AMP is a precursor or building block for ATP (See **Figure 30-15**). As already discussed, ATP is the principal energy carrier in all living cells because energy is stored in its "high energy" phosphate bonds. For example, when a living cell breaks down (oxidizes) a compound such as glucose, some of the energy released is caught and packaged into ATP. This stored energy can be subsequently released to meet metabolic demands. Aerobic metabolism produces a lot more ATP molecules per unit energy than does anaerobic metabolism.

Many essential coenzymes and related compounds are derivatives of AMP (See **Figure 30-16**). Many of these natural adenosine derivatives, such as NADH, NAD, as well as ATP and AMP, have been shown to inhibit cell proliferation in a variety of tumor cells in vitro.[35-38] In one particular study on a breast cancer cell line, it was found that AMP caused a significant decline in glycolysis and cell proliferation. The cancer cells were studied without any AMP, and the amount of lactate they produced was found to be proportional to the amount of glucose they were fed (See **Figure 30-17**). When the cancer cells were subjected to AMP, lactate production declined dramatically, and many metabolites in the glycolytic pathway were also reduced. AMP was found to inhibit several enzymes in the glycolytic pathway, including lactate dehydrogenase[39] (See **Figure 30-18**).

We give AMP by an intramuscular injection. AMP injections cause ATP levels to rise for 24 to 48 hours.[39] Because of its many functions, including the stimulation of aerobic metabolism and the inhibition of anaerobic metabolism (at least in some studies), it makes sense to us to

one or are ones that Dr. Bihari expects would respond. These cancers include the following:

- Cancer of the Pancreas
- Colon Cancer
- Cancer of the Small Intestine
- Rectal Cancer
- Malignant Melanoma
- Prostate Cancer
- Multiple Myeloma
- Lymphoma (Hodgkin's and non-Hodgkin's)
- Lymphocytic Leukemia
- Cancer of Some Endocrine Glands
- Neuroblastoma

We were notified about naltrexone through the research of Christina White at the Brewer Science Library in Richland Center, Wisconsin. She has a newsletter called *New Horizons*, which often depicts the best in natural medicine.* Christina loves helping cancer patients improve their health, and naltrexone is one of the methods of which she has written.

AMP Injections

Adenosine monophosphate (AMP) is a natural cellular metabolite. It's directly involved in many

* *The Brewer Science Library is located at 325 North Central Ave., Richland Center, WI 53581; phone: 1-608-647-6513; fax: 1-608-647-6797; E-mail: drbrewer@mwt.net; web site: www.mwt.net/~drbrewer.*

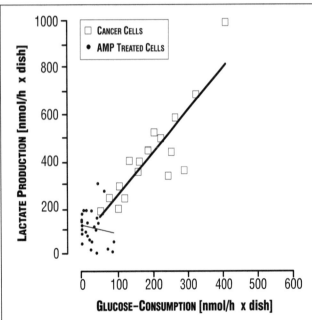

COENZYME	R	R'	R''
Active Methionine	Methionine*	H	H
Amino Acid Adenylates	Amino Acid	H	H
Active Sulfate	SO_3^{2-}	H	PO_3^{2-}
3', 5'-Cyclic AMP	H	H	PO_3^{2-}
NAD*	†	H	H
NADP*	†	PO_3^{2-}	H
FAD	†	H	H
CoA-SH	†	H	PO_3^{2-}

* *Replaces Phosphate*
† *R is a B-vitamin Derivative.*

Figure 30-16: Many coenzymes and related compounds are derivatives of adenosine monophosphate.

Adapted from Harper's Biochemistry, *by Robert Murray, M.D., Ph.D., Daryl Granner, M.D., Peter Mayes, Ph.D., DS.c., and Victor Rodwell, Ph.D., 1996, 24th Edition*

Figure 30-17: Relationship between Lactate Production and Glucose Consumption

This is another study confirming that cancer cells love glucose. Notice how AMP caused a drastic decline in lactate production.

use AMP for our cancer patients. It should be noted that we started using AMP because it seemed to give the patients added energy—the rest of this is just gravy.

GERMANIUM, LAETRILE, AND CESIUM

Germanium, Laetrile, and cesium have been grouped together because they have all had their share of lumps. The cancer research on all of them is excellent in animal studies, but unfortunately no researcher is doing more definitive studies on human beings with cancer. Thus, they are considered old relics that showed some promise, but because no one uses them, they must not work.

We have and do use all of these natural substances but only as adjunctive therapies. We do not believe it is in the cancer patient's best interest to use any of these as the primary cancer therapy. Yes, we have used all of the above, including Laetrile. When a tumor load is large, we can guarantee you that Laetrile, by itself, is like a BB gun to a charging grizzly bear; it won't do much.

Germanium showed promise as an anticancer agent through the research of Hiroshi Oikawa, D.Sc., and Kazuhiko Asai, Ph.D., both of Japan. In the book *Miracle Cure: Organic Germanium,* Dr Asai describes the many beneficial effects of germanium sesquioxide. In regard to cancer therapy, these beneficial effects include:

- increased oxygen supply
- nontoxicity
- depriving cancer cells of electrons
- killing pain
- increased natural killer cell activity

Figure 30-18: Comparison of the Intracellular Metabolite Concentrations[1]

METABOLITE CONCENTRATIONS [nmol/mg protein]

METABOLITES	CONTROL-CELLS	AMP-CELLS	TEST OF SIGNIFICANCE
Glucose-6-phosphate	0.41	0.30	n.s.
Fructose-1, 6-biphosphate	1.23	2.17	$p \leq 0.01$
Pyruvate	0.84	1.61	$p \leq 0.01$
Lactate	43.63	13.86	$p \leq 0.001$
NAD	3.03	1.21	$p \leq 0.001$
Free Phosphate	3.31	2.15	n.s.

[1] All metabolites were measured at an average cell density of 4×10^6 cells/dish; n = 5; n.s. = not significant.

AMP inhibits several enzymes in the glycolytic pathway, including lactate dehydrogenase.

Figure 30-19: Cancer Therapy and pH
The Brewer high pH therapy alkalizes the cancer cell environment, causing cancer cell death.

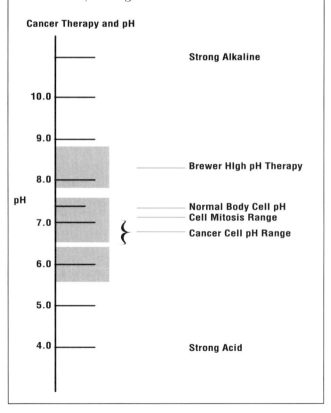

- enhanced interferon production
- prevention of metastases
- reduced blood viscosity[40]

Germanium is given to our patients in capsule form, as well as intravenously.

Cesium, like germanium, is a trace mineral. Cesium was studied as an anticancer agent by a physicist, Keith Brewer, for whom the Brewer Science Library in Richland Center, Wisconsin, is named. The writings of Dr. Brewer are fascinating. He hypothesized that cancer cell death could take place by alkalinizing cancer cells to a high pH (around eight) with cesium[41] (See **Figure 30-19**). Research showed that cancer incidence is lower in areas such as Vilcabamba, Ecuador, and the Hunza Valley of northern Pakistan, which have soils rich in potassium, rubidium, and cesium.[42] He did some animal research that showed that high pH therapy was very effective at causing tumor regression.[43] Unfortunately, he died before definitive human studies could be done.

Laetrile is perhaps the best known and most widely publicized of the alternative cancer therapies. Laetrile is a concentrated extract of amygdaline prepared from apricot kernels specifically for cancer therapy. Substantial amounts of amygdaline are found in apricots, peaches, cherries, berries, buckwheat, millet, alfalfa, and some strains of beans and peas.[44]

When Laetrile (or amygdaline) is acted on by the enzyme beta-glucosidase, it breaks down into two molecules of glucose, one molecule of benzaldehyde (an analgesic) and one molecule of hydrocyanic acid (also known as hydrogen cyanide, a poison). Thus, as beta-glucosidase breaks down amygdaline into its component parts, toxic cyanide is released. Studies on animal cancers have shown that various types of cancer cells contain from 100 to 3,600 times more of this enzyme than noncancerous cells, so much greater amounts of cyanide are released where there are active cancer cells present.[45, 46]

Although most cancer cells have high levels of beta-glucosidase, they are deficient in some other enzymes, especially rhodanese. Rhodanese detoxifies hydrocyanic acid into nontoxic thiocyanate. Ultimately, the cyanide ion becomes part of the vitamin B_{12} (cyanocobalamin) molecule. Since cancer cells have difficulty metabolizing cyanide, it is selectively toxic to cancer cells when released from Laetrile (See **Figure 30-20**).

Do these substances work? It is our opinion that the answer is yes. We believe part of the problem is in the "potency" of the supplement taken. If one looks at the doses of germanium that Dr. Asai describes in his book, it is up to 200 g/day, though most are given 3-4 g/day. When people take this supplement, they are generally taking two 150-mg capsules. This dose is about one-tenth of what is needed. We generally prescribe 3,000 mg/day, so a person takes six 500-mg capsules.* An added dose is given intravenously during the IPT treatment.

Cesium may work, but it takes 6 to 9 grams just to get a therapeutic amount of cesium into a person. This amount of cesium has not been well tolerated in our experience. The person often devel-

ops abdominal cramping and diarrhea, so he or she stops taking it. Unfortunately, there is no way to measure cell pH in the office, so it is difficult to assess the physiological changes with cesium.

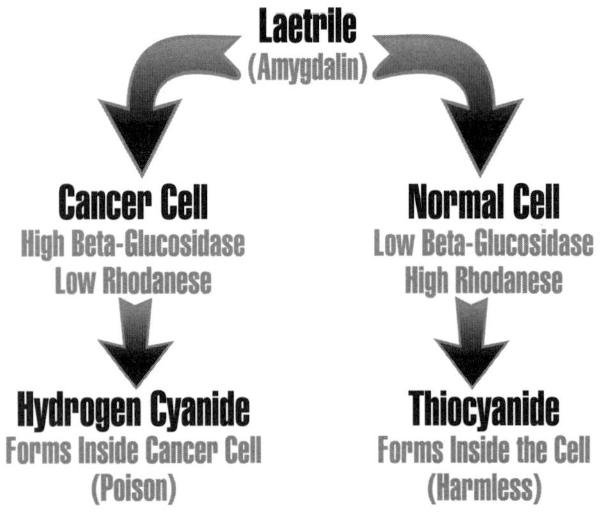

In regard to Laetrile, it is important for the person to monitor thiocyanate levels closely. We like to keep people between 2 and 3 mg/dL (See **Figure 30-21**). This minimizes toxicity and ensures that the Laetrile the person is taking contains amygdaline. We have found some patients' levels of thiocyanable to be zero, even though they were taking Laetrile. The only explanation is that the "Laetrile" they are taking has no amygdaline in it, at all. When they switch to a different company, then the thiocyanate level registers.

There are many alternative medicine treatments that could be used as adjunctive cancer therapies. We have not discussed 714X, Ukraine, and a whole host of other therapies we have used. We have book references for the reader if further information on this subject is desired.[46,47]

SUMMARY

The cancer patient has many options. Comprehensive natural medicine centers, such as Caring Medical in Oak Park, Illinois, have used many of these therapies on cancer patients. Generally, they have proven to be helpful at increasing a cancer patient's quality of life but not in obtaining tumor remission. As such, we recommend that these therapies be adjuncts to the primary cancer therapy the person is undergoing.

Insulin Potentiation Therapy is effective not only because of its cancer-killing effects but also in reversing cancer physiology. This is the primary cancer therapy that a cancer patient should con-

Figure 30-20: Different Metabolism of Laetrile in Cancer and Normal Cells
Cancer cells have high levels of beta-glucosidase, which causes a poison called hydrocyanide to form when the cell is exposed to Laetrile.

TESTS	RESULT	FLAG	UNITS	REFERENCE INTERVAL	LAB
THIOCYANATE, SERUM:					
THIOCYANATE	2.7		MG/DL		
PERFORMED AT:					
MEDTOX LABORATORIES, NEW BRIGHTON, MN CLIA# 24-D0665278					
TOXIC THIOCYANATE CONCENTRATIONS: GREATER THAN 10 MG/DL					

Figure 30-21: Thiocyanate Blood Levels
This test ensures that the Laetrile supplement the person is using contains some amygdalin in it.

---

* *These are available by calling 1-877-RX-BEULAH or ordering on-line at www.benuts.com. Be "nuts" for your health—buy your nutritional supplements at Beulah Land Nutritionals!*

sider. This potent cancer therapy can be combined with other adjunctive treatments to produce a comprehensive approach in cancer management.

In our clinic, we often combine IPT with other treatments, such as Doug Kaufmann's antifungal program, low-dose oral chemotherapy, HCl injections, intravenous therapies, anabolic hormones, magnetic therapy, oral hypoglycemics, low-dose naltrexone, AMP injections, germanium, Laetrile, and cesium. Each of these therapies can help certain aspects of cancer therapy and must be decided on a case-by-case basis. ■

CHAPTER 31

Cancer as a Chronic Disease

"IN THIS FORM, WHEN CORRECTLY APPLIED, BIOLOGICALLY GUIDED THERAPY CAN, IN MANY CASES, BRING UNDER CONTROL EVEN FAR-ADVANCED MALIGNANCIES."

-Emanuel Revici, M.D., in his book, Research in Physiology as Basis of Guided Chemotherapy with Special Applications to Cancer

"THE TRUTH IS, IF YOU ASKED ME TO CHOOSE BETWEEN WINNING THE TOUR DE FRANCE AND CANCER, I WOULD CHOOSE CANCER. ODD AS IT SOUNDS, I WOULD RATHER HAVE THE TITLE OF CANCER SURVIVOR THAN WINNER OF THE TOUR, BECAUSE OF WHAT IT HAS DONE FOR ME AS A HUMAN BEING, A MAN, A HUSBAND, A SON, AND A FATHER."

-Lance Armstrong, testicular cancer survivor, from his book, It's Not About the Bike.

Cancer is a systemic disease. Even if all the tests show that a person has a localized tumor, it is still a systemic disease. IPT and a comprehensive natural medicine program can reverse the "cancer milieu." If one thinks about cancer care, there are only three possible outcomes: remission, control, or death. That is it. The treatment the person receives will either cause the cancer physiology—and the cancer itself—to be gone (remission), or the disease process to stay the same (control), or be unsuccessful and lead to ultimate death.

The term *cure* is not used by oncologists because they seldom cure people. There is a very high cancer recurrence rate even when the tests show the cancer is gone because it is not really gone. The cancer milieu in the blood and tissues is still there. Surgery, radiation therapy, and high-dose chemotherapy make the cancer physiology worse, not better. They sometimes help cancer patients get better, but they do so in spite of themselves. The best approach for the cancer patient is to look at *all* cancer diagnoses as a systemic disease that needs comprehensive treatment.

Honestly, we do not like the word *cure* as it relates to cancer because it gives the person a sense of eternal security that is not true. If the person returns to his or her previous lifestyle, including dietary, emotional, spiritual, and psychological habits, the cancer physiology will return with the cancer.

It is the hope of every cancer patient and the doctors and health care providers who care for them that the therapy given will indeed cure them. We believe that this is often possible with a comprehensive natural medicine approach, with the power and effectiveness of IPT. We believe that the long-term effectiveness of IPT will be found to be far better than traditional high-dose chemotherapy.

IPT, as with other therapies, can be used to help a cancer patient control his or her disease. This was the goal of Bruce Kaye when he came to Caring Medical for IPT. He had been recently diagnosed with chronic lymphocytic leukemia with a white blood cell count of 588,000 (normal is under 10,000). He did not want immunosuppressive chemotherapy but desired IPT. I (Ross) discussed with him that aggressive treatment was recommended because any white blood cell count over 100,000 is dangerous and blood clotting can be affected. He received a total of 12 IPT treatments over a two-month period. He had no side effects from the treatment. As can be seen from **Figure 31-1**, his white blood cell count came down gradually over this period. We last spoke with him in June 2001, and he was under the care of his oncologist who has him taking an oral chemotherapy drug. He continues to take supplements to reverse his cancer physiology.

IPT did not cure Bruce Kaye of his cancer, but it did give him a treatment option to control his cancer. Once his cancer was under control, based on the recommendation of his oncologist, he decided to take some traditional oral chemotherapy. We are supportive of his decision and are happy that his disease is controlled.

There are many people who live full, productive lives with cancer. As we explain to new patients, everyone has something wrong with them. Many of us are not aware exactly what "it" is. The first step to regain health is to find out what a person can do to get the cancer under control. When as many cancer cells are being destroyed as are forming, the disease is said to be controlled. We do not like the term *arrested* because this signifies that the disease is stopped or inactive. Cancer is rarely inactive; it can be controlled or killed. These are better terms.

FIGURE 31-1: WHITE BLOOD COUNT OF BRUCE KAYE: BEFORE, DURING, AND AFTER IPT

PRIOR TO IPT:

DATES (NORMAL LEVELS):	7/21/00
WBC	588
RBC	3.21
HGB	10.1
HCT	30.8
PLT CT	165

Figure 31-1:
As shown, IPT treatments caused a dramatic decline in the cancer cell blood counts.

DURING IPT:

DATES:	8/28/01	8/30/00	9/6/00	9/18/00	9/25/00
WBC	479	427	386	267	201
RBC	3.25	2.79	2.66	2.83	3.00
HGB	10.9	8.3	8.8	8.6	9.0
HCT	31.3	26.5	24.8	26.8	27.3
PLT CT	105	136	109	136	147

DATES:	10|02|00	10/09/00	10/16/00	10/23/00
WBC	168	165	102	65.50
RBC	3.97	2.93	3.05	3.14
HGB	8.9	8.7	9.0	9.3
HCT	27.2	26.9	28.0	28.3
PLT CT	106	108	90	87

NATURAL MEDICINE TO CONTROL CANCER

Ruth Hanson had been in good health her whole life until she was diagnosed with colon cancer at age 70. She had a colon resection on November 30, 2000, and, unfortunately, two out of two lymph nodes were positive for moderately differentiated, infiltrating adenocarcinoma. She was recommended to undergo radiation therapy and chemotherapy. She refused and sought the help of various natural medicine practitioners, including us. As can be seen by some of her lab work, she had some nutrient deficiencies. Specifically, her antioxidant assay and many of her lipid-soluble antioxidant levels were low. Her insulin sensitivity screening result was normal but not optimal. (See **Figures 31-2A, B, and C**) She was placed on a glucose/insulin lowering diet, as well as supplements to not only correct her low antioxidant status but also help reverse other cancer physiology. She is followed every three to six months, and thus far her cancer markers are all negative. Is she cured of her cancer? Probably, but we take no chances. Continue to take your supplements, Ruth; we will talk again after you have your cancer markers drawn in a few months. Ruth's greatest chance at curing her disease is, of course, now! Her tumor load is either zero or very low. Now is the time to eat right. Do unto others as you would have them do unto you, pray, and receive close medical follow-up. If she does have an elevation of her cancer markers, then she knows where to turn—IPT.

LJILJANA VUKOSAVLJEVIC CASE STUDY

On September 11, 2000 Ljiljana came to see me (Ross) with her family. At the time, she was 60 years old. She had a left modified mastectomy on June 5, 1998 because of a cancerous lump.

The pathology on the mass showed infiltrating ductal carcinoma (5.1 cm) with three of nine axillary lymph nodes containing metastatic carcinoma. She had eight high-dose chemotherapy treatments and 29 radiation treatments. She was

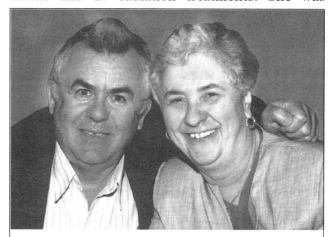

Ljiljana and Mike Vukosauvljevic
Married 42 years—and because of IPT—they plan to be married for many more years...

APPROVED FOR RELEASE		SIGNATURE		DATE
TEST	**NORMAL RANGE**	**RESULT**	**UNITS**	**FLAG**
AOA (PRE TX)	0.95 - 1.6	**0.42**	mmole / L	LOW

AOA = Antioxidant Assay

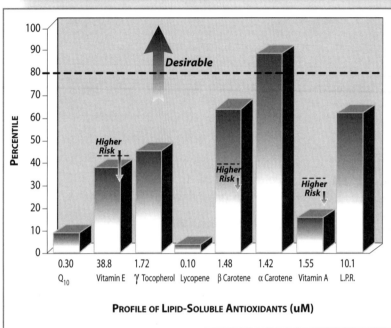

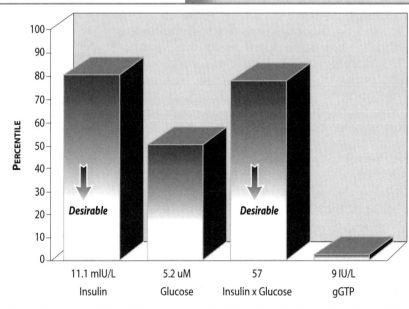

Figures 31-2A, B, C: Nutrient Lab Results of Ruth Hanson

Ruth was found to have a significant antioxidant deficiency and a sub-optimal glucose tolerance.

admitted to the hospital in the winter of 1999 because of pneumonia. A CT scan of the chest at that time showed that her cancer had come back in the lungs and bones including the left 9th and 12th ribs, thoracic and lumbar vertebrae and right femoral neck. She then had 16 chemotherapy treatments. Her last chemotherapy treatment before the visit to CMRS was 8/18/00.

She was taking codeine cough syrup at the time of her first visit. She was also on narcotic pain medication because of severe pain in the chest and upper back. Because of her previous chemotherapy, she was left with tingling and numbness in her fingers and toes. Her review of systems showed that she was currently suffering from chronic fatigue, shortness of breath, sinus congestion, recurrent infections, stomach upset, chronic pain, and a myriad of other symptoms. Her latest chest CT scan prior to the first visit to CMRS showed multiple pulmonary metastatic nodules with the largest one being in her right middle lobe, measuring 2 x 2 cm. This test showed a worsening of her mediastinal adenopathy. Thus, her cancer was continuing to grow— despite all of the high-dose chemotherapy she had

Wow—what a handful! This is a typical patient case coming to an IPT physician. It is hoped that after this book, this will *not* be the case. **Please see an IPT physician before your body is wrecked by high-dose chemotherapy and the cancer continues to grow.** Ljiljana was being followed at one of the top five hospitals in the country. Every year, this hospital is rated one of the best in the country. Yet, even with all of its big guns and mass knowledge, it is completely missing the boat in regard to cancer. Specifically in Ljiljana's case, once her cancer recurred after the initial chemotherapy and radiation therapy, one could easily surmise that clearly traditional therapy was not reversing the reason her body was allowing the cancer to grow.

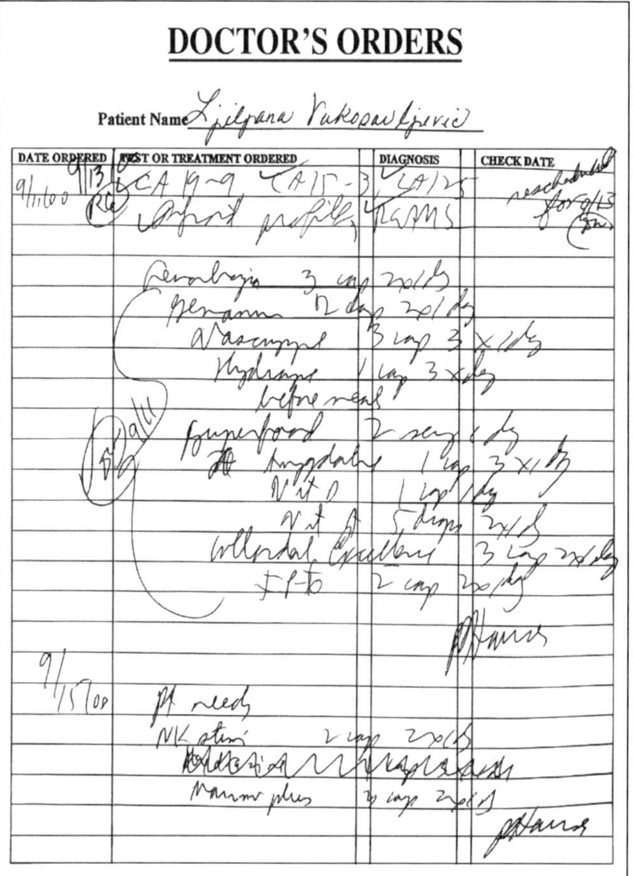

Ljiljana's natural medicine regime consisted of many natural supplements that we have discussed in this book (See **Figure 31-3**). In addition, she was prescribed Lamasil to decrease fungal load, Glucophage to keep her blood glucose levels down, Femara (later switched to Arimidex) to lower her estrogen levels, Coumadin to thin her blood, low-dose Naltrexone to stimulate her immunity (prescribed after she was off of narcot-

Figure 31-3: Initial Medicine Orders for Ljiliana

ic medications), and low-dose Cytoxan, an oral chemotherapy medication.

It was noted on initial testing that her fasting blood sugar was 133. Therefore she was placed on a high protein low carbohydrate diet. She was clearly eating the opposite prior to this. Her initial breast cancer markers in the blood were all negative, so her response to therapy would have to be based on CT scan findings.

Because she was physically going down hill fast, it was agreed that she should start Insulin Potentiation Therapy right away. She received a total of 18 treatment sessions from 9/26/00 to 1/23/01. Her first CT of the chest since starting IPT indicated an obvious shrinking of her metastases—or in the words of the radiologist, "clearly decreased in bulkiness from previous." It should be noted that after her second IPT treatment, she was not having any more chronic pain so her narcotic medications could at that time be discontinued. Her second CT scan of the chest after start-

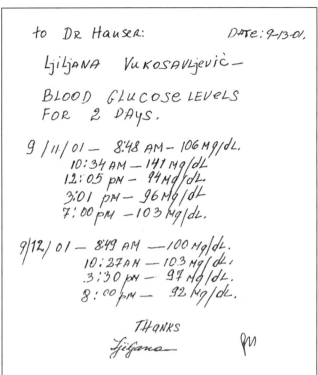

to DR HAUSER: DATE: 9-13-01.

LjiljanA VukosAvljevic—

BLOOD GLUCOSE LEVELS
FOR 2 DAYS.

9/11/01 — 8:48 AM — 106 Mg/dL.
   10:34 AM — 141 Mg/dL
   12:05 pM — 94 Mg/dL
   3:01 pM — 96 Mg/dL
   7:00 pM — 103 Mg/dL.

9/12/01 — 8:49 AM — 100 Mg/dL.
   10:27 AM — 10.3 Mg/dL.
   3:30 pM — 97 Mg/dL.
   8:00 pM — 92 Mg/dL.

THANKS
Ljiljana

Figure 31-4: Blood Glucose levels of Ljilana Vukosauljevic

Ideally, these should all be under 100. These are vastly improved because of the high-protein diet she is eating now.

ing IPT was done on 2/11/01. This showed continued overall improvement in her lung metastases. There was no definite evidence of pathologic adenopathy. So, clearly, the natural medicine program including IPT was working. I desired Ljiljana to continue with IPT, but she and her family wanted to treat her with just the diet and nutritional supplements, as well as the few medications I had prescribed. I agreed to this, as long as she received close follow-up. She agreed and has been an ideal patient.

BLOOD CHEMISTRY-TUMOR MARKERS				
CA 15-3	24.9		U/mL	[< 31.3]
CA 125	24.8		U/mL	[0.0-34.9]
CA 19-9 @	8.4	f	U/mL	[0.0-33.0]
CEA	2.5	f	ng/mL	[0.0-5.0]
HCG TUMOR @	<1	f	IU/L	[0-5]

CA 19-9 (08/28/01 -- Current)

Figure 31-5: Blood Cancer Markers

As can be seen, these are all negative for Ljilana, so her x-ray studies are a better monitor for her in regard to her response to treatment.

Periodically, I have Ljiljana check her blood sugars at home, and for the most part, she does a good job at keeping them at 100 or less. (See **Figure 31-4**.) Her latest fasting Insulin level was 12. I would like it less than 10. She also sets periodic testing for her Coumadin dose (PT/INR test). Every three to four months she gets a chest CT scan. As of January, 2002 she still has some small nodules in the lungs and in a few of the bones, but with each test they keep getting smaller. Her blood breast cancer markers continue to be negative. (See **Figure 31-5**.) She continues to have the vibrant life she has had after her second IPT treatment.

AUNT KAREN
"YOUR LIFE IS GOD'S GIFT TO YOU. WHAT YOU DO WITH THAT LIFE IS YOUR GIFT TO GOD."

Two days ago, Marion and I visited Aunt Karen. We dropped in "unexpectedly." Marion doesn't like to do that, but I sure do. As usual, Aunt Karen greeted us with enthusiasm and a big smile. "I just got out of the hospital for another week of chemotherapy." "How do you like my new doll?" Displayed on her dresser in a lovely glass container was one of the Gene Marshall collection of dolls. This one was entitled "Simply Gene." She was made up like an elegant Hollywood starlet. She showed us her many different outfits.

She did indeed look beautiful. Aunt Karen was in the middle of making the doll some earrings and other accessories. She then took out one of the red, white, and blue rosaries that she was making for the patients at the local hospital where she receives chemotherapy. "The chaplain gives these to patients. They just love them." She then proceeded to put on a special headgear and I said "Karen you look like a jeweler." "Yeah, I am. I have all of the instruments." She proceeded to clean our rings and give Marion one of her many artistic-designed rings.

Though Karen has lost a kidney and had a year's worth of chemotherapy, lives alone, and still has some colon cancer metastases in her lungs you wouldn't know it. As she puts it, "I am not ready to give up. There is just too much to do. There are many others in our family who have the real problems." Aunt Karen is busy advising her nieces and nephews about life.

You see, Aunt Karen is confident in her God. As she describes it, "God is my buoy!" We left her presence that day inspired. As a side note, on her television was the *I Love Lucy* show. As I told Marion later that day, "Karen was doing the perfect activities for a cancer patient. She was going to watch an *I Love Lucy* marathon while doing an activity that she loves (making jewelry). She was also going to give part of her work (rosary beads) to charity." Perhaps these are some of the reasons that Karen is doing so well. She still has cancer—but you wouldn't know it. Cancer patients around the world would be wise to follow Karen's example. Make your life count, whether you have cancer or not.

SUMMARY

Cancer is a chronic disease. It is best if a cancer patient realizes that once the diagnosis is made, life will not be the same. It does not mean that a person can never have pizza, for example; it will just turn into a rare treat instead of an everyday occurrence. A proper diet is necessary for life as well as a wholesome lifestyle.

IPT can be used not only to get cancers into remission but also for cancer control. Sometimes all that can be obtained by a cancer treatment is to hold the cancer in check. In such an instance, it is necessary to understand that it does not mean that the tumor is inactive; it just signifies that the rate of cancer cells being destroyed is equal to the rate of those forming. For some people, cancer needs to be thought of as a chronic condition. Since we all have some condition, though many of us do not know what "it" is, a person can live a full and active life with the diagnosis of cancer. ∎

CHAPTER 32

What would I do if I got cancer? Great question...

Cancer runs in my (Ross') family. My mother had breast cancer; my grandmother died of colon cancer; my aunt is struggling for her life because of colon cancer; a great aunt had breast cancer; my great uncle had kidney cancer—and who knows about numerous cousins and other relatives. Cancer is a very present risk for me.

GET ON A CANCER PREVENTION PROGRAM

Besides having a high family history of cancer, I have type A blood and a cancer personality, as I suppress my more intense or upsetting feelings. Left to my own devices, I can be very melancholy. This is my temperament. Cancer is a real risk for me so, I need a cancer prevention program.

Unfortunately, the average person waits until he or she is diagnosed with cancer before starting to think about the disease. Currently one in three women and one in two men will die of cancer. With these types of statistics, everyone needs a cancer prevention program.

A cancer prevention program first starts by visiting a conservative cancer doctor. So my first step would be to get under the care of a natural medicine physician. I see Jenifer Van De Pol, M.S., P.A.-C, at Caring Medical in Oak Park, Illinois. I have been screened, and my CEA (carcinoembryonic antigen) level (for colon cancer) is within normal limits. My blood sugar and insulin levels are low. My risk factors for heart disease are also low (cholesterol is in the 140s). I exercise almost every day.

Jenifer has talked to me about eating more green vegetables. I struggle with constipation, which I believe makes me a greater risk for colon cancer. My non-love for vegetables also puts me at risk. I love to look at vegetables...all those colors...green, yellow, orange, red—I just wish I did not have to put them into my mouth. As such, I think about taking a vegetable powder drink (Superfood) daily, as well as a fiber drink (a pow-

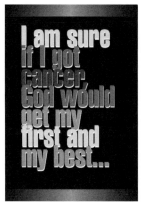

I am sure if I got cancer, God would get my first and my best...

der containing essential fatty acids). I just wish I was more successful at getting these drinks down my throat. I eat a high-protein, high-soy diet. Fortunately for me, there is a Thai restaurant only three doors down from the office. My favorite meal there? Thai Tofu Satay with peanut sauce. Yum. So I do eat tofu every week.

Because of my risk for colon cancer, I take butyrate capsules. I also take a probiotic (SMI powder*) and periodically cleanse the colon, along with an antifungal program that may include medications such as nystatin. Of course, I take a "reasonable" amount of supplements such as a multivitamin (Supervits*), quercetin (Natural D-Hist*), enzymes for soft tissue healing (MSCLR enzyme*), and various antioxidants (Unique E*). I get so many samples of free vitamins that when I feel up to it, I pop a few of them. My favorite supplement: pure, unadulterated Dale Alexander's cod liver oil.* (I take a big swallow or two of the orange-flavored stuff daily.) My second favorite is Aloe Vera 10x, a concentrated aloe vera drink.

DO PERIODIC LABORATORY TESTING

About twice a year, I get some laboratory tests done. This may include pH levels, insulin, glucose, blood thickness, routine chemistries, and cancer markers. Each individual case determines which tests need to be run and how often.

TEST CHEMOTHERAPY DRUGS ON MY SPECIFIC TUMOR

Oncologists, as well as IPT physicians, have general guidelines as to which types of tumors are sensitive to certain chemotherapy drugs. The real question is whether my specific tumor is sensitive to a particular drug. It is now possible to test the sensitivity of cancer cells to chemotherapy drugs via a cytotoxicity assay used to measure drug-induced cell death following drug exposure. (See **Figure 32-1**.) The test can be done on a persons

---

* All the supplements discussed in this chapter are available by calling 1-877-RX-BEULAH or ordering on-line at www.benuts.com.

TREATING CANCER WITH INSULIN POTENTIATION THERAPY

What would I do if I got cancer? Great question...

RATIONAL THERAPEUTICS

Cancer Evaluation Center

750 East 29th Street
Long Beach, CA 90806
Tel 562.989.6455 Fax 562.989.6454
web site http://www.rationaltherapeutics.com

DRUG SENSITIVITY REPORT

Patient:	
Dx:	Breast
Prior Rx:	Yes
Physician:	Dr. Ross Hauser
Assay Date:	11/4/00
Report Date:	11/13/00
Assay Quality:	Good
Specimen Number:	

SINGLE DRUG DOSE EFFECT ANALYSIS

Drug	IC50	Units	Interpretation
Nitrogen Mustard*	1.4	ug/ml	*Sensitive*
Taxol	7.5	ug/ml	*Sensitive*
Docetaxel	16	ug/ml	Intermediate
Doxorubicin	0.3	ug/ml	Intermediate
Topotecan (2)	0.2	ug/ml	Intermediate
5-Fluorouracil	46	ug/ml	Resistant
Cisplatin	2.6	ug/ml	Resistant
Gemcitabine (1)	201	ug/ml	Resistant
Mitomycin-C	1.2	ug/ml	Resistant
Navelbine	>10	ug/ml	Resistant
Trimetrexate #	39	ug/ml	Resistant
Vincristine	>0.6	ug/ml	Resistant

MULTIPLE DRUG DOSE EFFECT ANALYSIS

Drug	Ratio	IC50	Units	Interpretation	Synergy
Doxorubicin & Taxol	1.2:50	6.4	ug/ml	Intermediate	No Synergy
Cisplatin & Gemcitabine (1)	6.6:263	17	ug/ml	Intermediate	*Synergy*
5-Fluorouracil & Nit. Mustard	100:5.4	15	ug/ml	Intermediate	*Partial Synergy*
5-Fluorouracil & Trimetrexate	100:50	21	ug/ml	Intermediate	*Partial Synergy*
Gemcitabine (1) & Nit. Mustard	263:5.4	32	ug/ml	Resistant	*Partial Synergy*
Mitomycin-C & Navelbine	2.4:10	3.1	ug/ml	Resistant	*Partial Synergy*
Navelbine & Taxol	10:50	5.3	ug/ml	*Sensitive*	*Partial Synergy*
Cisplatin & 5-Fluorouracil	6.6:100	27	ug/ml	Intermediate	Mixed Synergy
Cisplatin & Topotecan (2)	6.6:0.92	1.1	ug/ml	Intermediate	Antagonism

INTERPRETATION:

Laboratory results represent only one part of the overall determination of therapy for patients and do not guarantee outcomes nor indicate the specific drugs that should be used in a particular patient.

The drug referenced is the index agent for the described class of drugs. Prior in vitro analyses have provided data indicating relative equivalence of activity.

Ex Vivo best regimen (EVBR®) would be Cytoxan plus Taxol (Taxotere); or Navelbine plus Taxol (Taxotere).

Robert A. Nagourney, MD
Laboratory and Medical Director
Rational Therapeutics

The performance characteristics of these assays have not been established and the results are provided for investigational use only.

Figure 32-1: Chemotherapy Drug Sensitivity Report on Breast Cancer Tissue

For this particular patient, the cytoxic regime recommended is Cyclophosphamide and/or Navelbine and Taxol/Taxotere.

own cancer cells if tumor tissue is available. So this type of test would be a definite if I ever got cancer.

GET AN IPT DOCTOR

If I were actually diagnosed with cancer, I would immediately see an IPT doctor and receive treatment. I would do all of the things I need to do to reverse cancer physiology. Hopefully, if I do them now, this will never happen. I do slip occasionally, okay more than occasionally, on my diet. I did not mention my coffee habit which I am trying to quit. I cannot get into this...too personal.

I would probably go to one of the IPT doctors mentioned in **Appendix E**. These are doctors whom I personally know and trust.

Would I go to an oncologist? Probably, just to see what he or she has to offer. I am sure it would convince me even more to have IPT.

Would I have surgery? I would definitely consider it, depending on where the tumor was located. If I had colon cancer, I definitely would have it removed. I would then start IPT. Even if the margins were clear, I would still do IPT. I would get 10 treatments, once per week and then close follow-up with cancer marker testing.

I WOULD TAKE MY SUPPLEMENTS

If I got cancer, I would down that green drink, fiber drink, and every other awful-tasting slushy, drink, capsule or tablet the IPT doctor told me to take. I would also do it with joy. I would ask him or her what else they would want me to take and then—I would take that with gusto. Cancer is a tremendous motivator.

WORK LESS

I work too much. I wrote this book just after finishing a grueling 900-page sports book entitled *Prolo Your Sports Injuries Away!* I am writing this chapter on Labor Day (2001) evening, after running a half marathon this morning. My thighs and legs are very sore. I should be getting a massage, but instead I am finishing this book. Like you, I work too much. I know it, but I love it.

PLAY MORE

I enjoy running. I love playing golf. I like spending time with Marion. I need to do more of all three, not necessarily in that order. Marion has picked up running. She is doing great. We are running in our first race together in two weeks. She is my best friend; I need to do more fun things with her.

I would also try to laugh more—see funny movies, read funny books, buy a clown outfit and wear it around the house. Perhaps then I would not take myself and life as seriously as I do now. Enjoy the moment more.

BE MORE CHARITABLE

Marion and I and a group of friends in the Oak Park area started a "free" clinic in rural Illinois. It is now a not-for-profit called Beulah Land Ministries. We still don't have a full-time facility out of which to run the clinic. Currently, I am "too busy" to help raise the funds for this project. The cost for the land, supplies, and building would be about two million dollars. Something tells me that if I got diagnosed with cancer—I would become "unbusy" and this missionary clinic would take a top priority in my life.

TELL MORE PEOPLE I LOVE THEM

There are just not enough hugs in the world. We don't complement each other enough. If I got cancer, I would surely let those around me know that I loved them. In case I forget to tell you—"I love you."

BE MORE SERIOUS ABOUT MY FAITH

Honestly, I have turned into one of those once-a-week Christians. I go to church but do not give God my best. I used to, but now I work. I am sure if I got cancer, God would get my first and my best. I hope that writing this publicly will help me get my priorities right again. God deserves all of our best—our best time, energy, thoughts, and works.

SUMMARY

If I were diagnosed with cancer, I would definitely do IPT with the best IPT doctor I could find. I would, of course, try to prevent cancer in the first place by eating lots of protein, soy, and vegetables, as well as take a "reasonable" amount of supplements. If surgery would help the prognosis for the disease, I would consider it. Periodically, I would undergo laboratory testing to see if the cancer physiology was being reversed. I would work less and play more. God would have my attention and get my best. Why I don't do that now is beyond me. If you figure out the reason, will you let me know? ■

The Hauser Diet

We devised the Hauser diet in response to the many questions we receive every day from cancer patients, as well as from people who just want to prevent cancer. Everyone wants to know how to eat. We are bombarded every day with E-mails, phone calls, and consultations with patients and families asking us how to eat. (See **Figure A-1.**) It is no wonder that people are confused. Many different diets, supplements, and quick-fix remedies are available; it is hard to know what to do.

FROM: F. Moulton
Sent: Thursday, October 25, 2001 10:47 PM
To: lptcancernews@aol.com
SUBJECT: Write a book *please*

Thank you for your most recent newsletter. My husband is in his last days of cancer and is at a point where he absolutely cannot survive.

My question is...do you have a book or suggestions on a proper diet for someone who is trying to avoid cancer and also persons who are attempting to beat the disease? If you have done research on this, a book would be wonderful. We have been so terribly confused after reading *many* books on the subject. Some say eat meat, others say eat strictly vegan. Some say eat only raw fruits and veggies, others say fruits convert to sugar too rapidly and avoid them. Some diets say to avoid *all* dairy products and to get your system into an alkaline state where another book says to get into an acidic state. Too confusing for someone without a degree in medicine and nutrition... *Help!!!*

Sincerely, Susan Moulton

Figure A-1: A Common E-mail Question
The Hauser Diet was devised to help patients reverse their cancer physiology.

We hear questions such as these:
- "Should I juice?"
- "What do you think about the macrobiotic diet?"
- "Does soy cause cancer?"
- "Do you want me to become a vegetarian?"
- "Can I put apple juice in with the green drink?"
- "Can I eat meat?"
- "Have you heard of the grapefruit diet?"
- "Do you recommend the Gerson diet?"
- "Can't I get all my nutrients from food?"

These are all very good questions. We have done a lot of research in developing what we call the Hauser diet. This diet represents general recommendations that may be modified slightly to adjust to individual metabolic differences. We want to remind you that there is no one perfect diet for everyone. **Our clinic is known as an interventional natural medicine clinic that practices science-based interventional natural medicine.** You have learned in this book that the strict macrobiotic, vegetarian-type diet is often not in the best interest of most cancer patients. This diet may be excellent at reversing some aspects of cancer physiology, but with respect to insulin, this diet may lead to hyperinsulinemia in many people, which, in fact, actually enhances cancer physiology.

The diet should ultimately be a source of strength to the body, not a regime that is a source of strife. Diet is more than just food. Food is involved in many aspects of people's lives. It is used to provide comfort, to entertain, to show gratitude, and to keep you alive. First and foremost, it is important to select foods that are of the highest quality. We recommend foods that are fresh, unprocessed, organically grown, nonirradiated, and free of chemical additives. A balanced, healthy metabolism capable of inhibiting cancer requires a nutritionally adequate diet. Unfortunately, in today's society, fast food makes up about 40% of food intake and is nearly completely devoid of fresh vegetables and fruits. The fresh foods that are readily available to us in the regular grocery store are usually picked before they are ripe and contain pesticides or other chemical additives. Enzymatic action has been halted in order to preserve shelf life. Processing foods disrupts the natural makeup of the food and adds chemicals and other artificial substances that add toxicity to the food itself.

The goals for the ultimate "anticancer" diet are as follows:

1. Stimulate Immunity
2. Thin the Blood
3. Inhibit Anaerobic Metabolism
4. Enhance Aerobic metabolism
5. Promote Detoxification

6. Provide Cancer-Fighting Substances
7. Optimize Hormone Milieu
8. Eliminate Cancer-Causing Agents
9. Help Starve the Cancer
10. Complement Other Concurrent Treatments

STIMULATE IMMUNITY

We are sure that you, the reader now realize that a weakened immune system is not the primary cause of cancer. This is the reason that many immune-stimulating natural medicine protocols may not cause the cancer to go into remission. A strong immune system is important during and throughout therapy because any type of infection can overwhelm the immune system and allow the cancer to grow. This is especially true for the cancer patient receiving traditional high-dose chemotherapy. Every person undergoing IPT or any form of cancer treatment needs to keep a strong immune system in order to help ensure that the body has maximum cancer-fighting abilities.

Optimum activity in B and T cell immunity is key to achieving an excellent immune response against cancer. Foods that accomplish this will perform one or more of the following activities:

- Stimulate macrophage phagocytosis
- Increase interferon and interleukin production.
- Improve immune cell numbers
- Enhance the cytotoxic activity of immune cells against cancer cells
- Stimulate T lymphocyte and B lymphocyte activity

Numerous substances previously discussed in **Chapter 25 and 31** have these abilities, often accomplishing it via the intake of various food substances. Many nutrients can provide pharmacological changes in immune function. Protein, arginine, glutamine, omega-6 and omega-3 fatty acids, iron, zinc, B vitamins, vitamin E, vitamin C, and vitamin A have all been proven to modulate immune functions.[1]

FOODS THAT ENHANCE IMMUNITY

VEGETABLES:
- Asparagus
- Beets
- Broccoli
- Brussels Sprouts
- Cabbage
- Carrots
- Cauliflower
- Green Leafy Vegetables
- Onions
- Peppers
- Pumpkin
- Tomatoes
- Yams

LEGUMES:
- Black-eyed Peas
- Garbanzo Beans
- Kidney Beans
- Lentils
- Navy Beans
- Pinto beans
- Split peas
- Soybeans

FISH:
- Bass
- Cod
- Haddock
- Halibut
- Salmon
- Sardines
- Sole
- Trout
- Tuna

WHOLE GRAINS:*
- Amaranth
- Barley
- Buckwheat
- Ezekiel bread
- Flax
- Millet
- Oats
- Rice
- Rye
- Spelt Wheat

OILS *(Cold-Pressed and Unrefined "Extra-Virgin"):*
- Borage Oil
- Fish Oils
- Flax Seed Oil
- Hemp Oil
- Olive Oil
- Primrose Oil
- Sesame Oil

FRUITS:*
- Apples
- Apricots
- Berries
- Cantaloupe
- Cherries
- Figs
- Kiwi
- Oranges
- Pears
- Red Grapefruit

OTHER:
- Bee Pollen
- Brewer's Yeast
- Cayenne
- Cinnamon
- Curry
- Garlic
- Ginger
- Green Tea
- Kelp
- Mustard
- Salsa
- Spirulina
- Stevia
- Vinegar
- Wheat Germ

---

* *Whole grains and fruits, as one will see, are only a minor part of the Hauser Diet, because of their glucose and insulin-raising effects.*

Obviously, we recommend that you incorporate many of these foods into your diet every day. Stop going to fast-food places and drive over to the nearest Whole Foods™ grocery store. Start shopping in the produce section. You might find some new and exciting things there!

THINNING OF THE BLOOD WITH FOODS

Research shows that in order for many cancers to start and continue growing in the body, they must cause a thickening of the blood or increased clotting of the blood. The scientific term for this "thickening" is called coagulopathy. Obviously, we want to avoid things that accelerate coagulopathy and encourage things that promote a natural thinning of the blood. Many different natural substances cause the blood to become thinner. These substances and their food sources will reduce coagulopathy and thus contribute to reversing this aspect of cancer physiology and especially helping prevent metastasis of the cancer to other parts of the body. Foods in this category are vegetables, and foods high in omega-3 fatty acids.

Some medical treatments actually worsen coagulopathy, such as high-dose chemotherapy and radiation therapy. Patients receiving these treatments are especially prone to coagulopathy problems. These patients, in particular, need to eat foods that help naturally thin the blood. Likewise, it is important for cancer patients to avoid foods that further thicken the blood. The most common substances that cause thickening of the blood and enhance clotting are polyunsaturated fatty acids and hydrogenated oils. Most cancer patients need to reduce overall fat intake because they are eating the wrong kinds of fats. Foods should be baked, broiled, steamed, or grilled, rather than fried; avoid high-fat meats and gravies.

FOODS THAT ENCOURAGE NATURAL BLOOD THINNING VEGETABLES:

- Avocados
- Broccoli
- Brussels Sprouts
- Cabbage
- Cauliflower
- Garlic
- Kale
- Kelp
- Onions

FATS:

- Cold Water Ocean Fish
- Fish Oils
- Flax Seed Oil
- Walnut Oil

FOODS THAT CONTRIBUTE TO BLOOD THICKENING

Any food that contains hydrogenated fats or oils will contribute to the thickening of the blood. Therefore it is best to avoid these types of foods:

- Deli foods
- Fried foods: french fries, fried vegetables, fried chicken, chips
- Ice creams and frozen desserts
- Margarine
- Mayonnaise
- Packaged products: cookies, crackers, snack items
- Any food labeled "partially hydrogenated"
- Vegetable oils such as corn oil, safflower oil, and "vegetable oil"

OMEGA-3 FATTY ACIDS... MIGHTY CANCER WEAPONS

Dietary fats are generally divided into two series: omega-6 and omega-3. The current American diet contains between fifteen and twenty times the amount of omega-6 fatty acids compared to omega-3.[2,3] Omega-6 fatty acids come from most cooking oils including safflower, cottonseed, sunflower, peanut, and corn oil. These fatty acids are converted in the body to inflammatory prostaglandins that cause platelets to get sticky. When the blood of cancer patients is tested it generally shows a coagulopathy. Their blood is too sticky because of the platelets. The easiest method for a cancer patient to reverse this coagulopathy is by taking an anticoagulant or blood thinner. Medicines such as aspirin, nonsteroidal anti-inflammatory medications (Celebrex, Dolobid, Motrin), heparin and coumadin all fall into this category. The other effective method to reverse this aspect of cancer physiology is for the cancer patient to stop eating foods (oils) that are high in omega-6 fatty acids and start consuming omega-3 fatty acids.

A healthy ratio of omega-6/omega-3 fatty acids in the diet is closer to 1:1.[2,3] Omega-3 fatty acids can be found in high quantities in cold water ocean fish, sardines, salmon, mackerel, cod, halibut, herring, trout, and tuna. This is why cod liver oil is one of our favorite anti-cancer supplements. Smaller amounts of omega-3 fatty acids are in linseed, flax seed and walnut oil. Omega-3 fatty acids are converted in the body to prostaglandins that have potent anti-clotting abilities. Thus, they help reverse cancer physiology. The take-home point is that **fish is an extremely good food for the cancer patient to consume. Likewise, cod liver oil should be in the tummy of every person trying to prevent cancer or who has cancer.**

What about the beef? Grain-fed beef has an omega-6/omega-3 ratio of over 20:1, whereas grass fed beef has an omega 6/omega-3 ratio of 3:1. Grass-fed beef is also high in conjugated linoleic acid, a type of fatty acid with a lot of anti-cancer properties. Animals that graze on pasture have from 300 to 400% more conjugated linoleic acid than animals fattened on grain in a feedlot. So what about the beef? It is fine to eat—just make sure it is organic and grass-fed.

I thought—fat causes cancer? Too many omega-6 fatty acids cause cancer, omega-3 fatty acids reduce one's cancer risk. Yes, even for colon and breast cancer, the two main cancers supposedly increased by fat consumption. The greater the omega-3 fatty acid consumption, the lower the cancer risk.[4]

INHIBIT ANAEROBIC METABOLISM

Cancer cells extract more of their energy from anaerobic metabolism than normal cells. Anaerobic metabolism causes the by-product lactic acid to form. This can cause metabolism to become too acidic, which is the main theory behind the macrobiotic diet. Vegetables are promoted very highly in the Hauser diet, but a strict vegetarian diet, especially one that emphasizes a lot of juicing, may cause elevated insulin levels in some people. Since it is easy to test anaerobic metabolism, insulin levels, and blood pH, these levels should be checked regularly to see if the patient's diet is contributing to this aspect of cancer physiology. The Hauser diet emphasizes substances and foods that inhibit anaerobic metabolism, which would theoretically help decrease the energy supply of cancer cells.

Bioflavonoids, especially quercetin, inhibit anaerobic metabolism. Current studies estimate that over 20,000 different bioflavonoid compounds exist in nature.[5] Bioflavonoids are basically accessory factors used by plants to assist in photosynthesis and reduce the damaging effects from the sun.

SOURCES OF BIOFLAVONOIDS
- Citrus Fruits, especially the white rind
- Bee pollen
- Berries
- Green Tea
- Legumes
- Onions
- Parsley

ENHANCE AEROBIC METABOLISM

Normal healthy cells obtain their energy via the process of aerobic metabolism. Aerobic metabolism uses oxygen as a fuel, whereas anaerobic metabolism primarily uses glucose or sugar. Humans are aerobic organisms with cells that thrive when there is proper tissue oxygenation. One of the primary differences between healthy cells and cancer cells is that cancer cells are anaerobic. They ferment rather than metabolize food and live in the presence of oxygen. Professor Otto Warburg received two Nobel Prizes, in 1930 and 1944, for his work on cell bioenergetics or the process of how the cell extracts energy from food. In 1966, Professor Warburg spoke to a group of Nobel laureates regarding his work on cancer cells:

> ...the prime cause of cancer is the replacement of the respiration of oxygen in normal body cells by a fermentation of sugar.[6]

Cancer slowly destroys the body by using up fuel, causing the body tissues to waste. Cancer patients will begin to convert protein to energy (sugar) in order to maintain a certain level of sugar in the blood. Cancer also hides in the body's oxygen deficient areas. The denser and more anaerobic the tumor mass, the more resistant the tumor is to radiation.[6] So you can see that oxygen is bad for cancer cells and good for the body. Substances that enhance aerobic metabolism will increase the health of the cells of the body to fight the cancer. The mitochondria are the cells where fuel is burned. If the membranes on the mitochondria remain fluid and permeable, oxygen can flow in, carbon dioxide can flow out, and the cell remains in an aerobic state. A high-fat diet (as described previously), especially one high in saturated fat, will contribute to the rigidity and decreased permeability of the mitochondrial membrane, thereby decreasing oxygenation.

FOODS THAT ENHANCE AEROBIC METABOLISM

Foods or specific vitamins/herbs containing B vitamins, including thiamin, riboflavin, biotin, and niacin; coenzyme Q_{10}; ginkgo biloba; and ginseng can all enhance aerobic metabolism. Food sources for B vitamins include green leafy vegetables, wheat germ, liver, pork, whole grains, dried beans, dairy products, fish, poultry, organ meats, broccoli, millet, pine nuts, potatoes, rice, spinach, avocados, oats, raspberries, bananas, oysters, quinoa, barley, artichoke, wild game, tuna, almonds, brussels sprouts, corn, eggs, mushrooms, pepper, licorice root, celery, flax seed, wheat, mung beans, molasses, okra, and pumpkin seeds.[7,8]

Junk foods deplete oxygen stores. They use up more oxygen than they give off. Processed sugar, white flour, hamburgers, french fries, and pizza are major oxygen users. So we recommend that you avoid these foods if at all possible. Incidentally, both emotional and physical stress also create very high oxygen loss. So do not sweat the small stuff!

PROMOTE DETOXIFICATION

It is highly probable that many people with cancer developed the cancer as the end result of having a toxic waste dump in their bodies. This is not too hard to believe for the person who excessively drinks alcohol and smokes cigarettes. Over time, the toxicity from these substances will overwhelm the detoxification capacities of the body, and a cancer will form.

Detoxification is a process whereby we increase the body's ability to eliminate waste materials. Detoxification is an area of extreme importance to our health and is often overlooked by traditional medicine and oncologists taking care of cancer patients.

Here are some basic principles to follow:

- *Get Rid of the Garbage:* Bring in the right nutrients and take out the wrong ones. We are constantly exposed to toxins and are constantly eliminating them via urine, feces, exhaled air, sweat, and tears.

- *Drink Enough Water:* Increase water consumption (filtered water only, please!) so that you can increase urinary output and cause dilution of urine by drinking more clean, purified water.

- *Have Regular Bowel Movements Every Day:* Improve fiber intake until feces are soft in consistency and regular in frequency. This does not mean having a bowel movement every other day or every third day. It is ideal to have a bowel movement a few hours after **every** meal.

- *Fix Digestive Problems,* thus the need for digestive enzymes or hydrochloric acid to help with assimilation of food. The typical American diet is low in fiber, loaded with poisons, and devoid of natural enzymes.

- *Colon Cleansing,* through a variety of methods, is a good idea for whole body detoxification.

- *Exercise to the Best of Your Ability:* Your skin is an organ by which you excrete toxins. Sweating during physical exercise helps remove toxins and has other health benefits as well.

What many people do not realize is that our bodies are being exposed to many toxic substances every day, including the following:

- Mercury and other heavy metals from dental fillings
- Chlorine and other harmful substances in the water supply
- Dyes and chemicals in foods and even vitamin supplements
- Pollutants in the air
- Electromagnetic fields from cellular phones, computers, and high-voltage power lines

MERCURY AND HEAVY METALS

Did you know that more than 90% of the American population has at least a couple of mercury fillings in their teeth? Mercury is a deadly poison and putting it into the mouth to erode over the years and eventually be swallowed does not seem to be a smart thing to do. Some people are very sensitive to the presence of mercury in their bodies, while others appear to tolerate it better. Removing mercury from the mouth has helped some people feel much better and decrease the toxic load on their bodies.

WATER

Two thirds of the human body is composed of water. Water is the medium of life on this planet. Water helps the body to cleanse and dilute impurities, balance pH, and provide a healthy flow of nutrients into cells and toxins out of cells. Tap water is filled with impurities and chemicals that should be avoided, not only by the cancer patient but by anyone who wants to remain healthy. We recommend that you purchase a good water filtration system for your home and start drinking the water! Most of us are walking around dehydrated. We need water! Drink up!

DYES AND CHEMICALS

Have you ever looked at the label on a food package and been unable to pronounce anything that was on the label? Foods, and even vitamins, are loaded with chemicals, dyes, and other unnatural substances. Be careful what you put into your mouth. Read before you eat.

Some of the most common food additives to avoid are the following:

* *Aspartame:* chemical sweetener used in NutraSweet and Equal

* *Bromated Vegetable Oil:* emulsifier in foods and clouding agent in soft drinks

* *Citrus Red Dye No. 2:* used to color orange skins

* *Monosodium Glutamate:* flavor enhancer used in fast, processed, or packaged foods

* *Nitrites:* used as preservatives in cured meats to prevent spoilage

* *Sulfur Dioxide, Sodium Bisulfite, Sulfites:* preserves dried fruits, shrimp, frozen potatoes; commonly used on salad bar foods

* *Tertiary Butylhydroquinone:* used to spray the inside of cereal and cheese packages

* *Yellow Dye No. 6:* used in candy and carbonated beverages as a coloring[9]

AIR

It is clear that the water, air, and food supply is polluted with harmful substances. Many of these things have already been found to cause cancer in animals, and we are sure a substantial proportion of the others will be put on the carcinogenic list in the future.

Fifty million Americans breathe air that is dangerous for their health. Known carcinogens are produced annually and legally from paper mills, petrochemical refineries, burning of medical waste, crop dusting, diesel fumes, leaded exhaust, and so on.[7] This is obviously not something over which we have much control. Therefore, we have to do other things to try to get rid of all the other "garbage."

ELECTROMAGNETIC FIELDS

We are constantly being exposed to electromagnetic fields and radiation. High-energy radiation or ionizing radiation creates many more free radicals. Avoid unnecessary x-rays; avoid excessive exposure to the sun; and reduce exposure to electronic equipment, computers, and cellular devices.

FOODS THAT PROMOTE DETOXIFICATION

The process by which the body removes these harmful substances from the body is called detoxification. It generally involves the removal of the chemical substances via the bowels and urine. The primary organs used for detoxification are the liver, kidney, and skin. Foods and liquids that promote good defecation and urinary excretion are emphasized in the Hauser Diet.

* High fiber foods, especially fresh vegetables*

* Whole grains and fruits to a lesser extent*

* Water: purified, not tap water

* Teas such as catechin, barberry, yarrow flower, milk thistle

* Yogurt with live cultures (if able to tolerate dairy foods)

* Onions

* Lecithin-containing foods such as soybeans and egg yolks

VEGETABLES: NATURE'S DETOXIFIERS

The scientific community continues to recognize and validate the considerable relationship between vegetable intake and cancer.[10,11] Deeply pigmented plants contain important anti-inflammatory and antioxidant properties from various substances in them including anthocyanidins. These are a type of complex flavonoid that produce blue, purple or red colors. Orange, yellow and red-orange foods are rich in carotenoids such as beta-carotene, lutein and lycopene. More than

---

*   The amount of fruits and whole grains allowed or a particular patient depends on their results of the Glucose Insulin Tolerance Test.*

600 carotenoids occur naturally, but carotenes are the most widely known. Carotenes, which destroy free radicals in lipids, enhance immune response and protect cells against UV radiation.

Green plants contain particularly large amounts of chlorophyll, which is a detoxifier. Foods rich in chlorophyll include chlorella and other blue-green algae, beet greens, bok choy, collards, dandelion greens, kale, mustard greens and nettles. Another class of vegetables with potent detoxifying abilities are those of the cruciferous family which includes broccoli, bok choy, Brussels sprouts, cabbage, cauliflower, mustard greens, radishes and turnips. These functional foods cause a coordinated metabolic induction of many of the Phase II liver detoxification enzymes that detoxify carcinogenic (cancer-causing) compounds from the body, thus reducing the susceptibility of cells to these substances.

Though there is some debate as to which substance(s) and mechanism(s) are the reason vegetables protect against cancer, it is clear that they do. (See **Figure A-2.**) For this reason they are major part of the Hauser Diet.

PROVIDE CANCER-FIGHTING SUBSTANCES

Most people not only need to optimize their immune function, but fight the cancer directly. One of the primary purposes of this book is to show the reader that cancer-fighting substances are essential for survival from most cancers. The process of IPT involves the use of insulin to increase the uptake of cancer-fighting chemotherapy drugs into the cancer cells in order to kill them.

Cancer-fighting substances in certain foods may also need to be ingested in the form of supplements in order to achieve an appropriate dosage necessary to have a cancer-fighting effect. Eating foods containing these substances is obviously encouraged (See **Figure A-3**).

FOODS WITH CANCER-FIGHTING SUBSTANCES

- *Vegetables:* Vegetables are rich in antioxidants and anticancer nutrients, have a preferred lower glycemic index, and are rich in cleansing fiber. These foods contain high amounts of carotenoids.
- *Colorful Food:* Beets, spinach, carrots, tomatoes, and squash are good examples of colorful foods with good cancer-fighting phytochemicals.
- *Cabbage Family (Cruciferous):* Cabbage, broccoli, brussels sprouts, and cauliflower.
- *Allium Family Foods:* Onions and garlic contain bioflavonoids, such as quercetin, that can actually revert some cancer cells back to healthy cells.
- *Cold-water Fish:* Salmon, haddock, halibut, bass, cod, mackerel, sardines, tuna, and other fish from deep ocean waters. These fish are loaded with anticancer fats, including EPA and DHA, which slow down the spread of cancer, stimulate immune function, and contain trace minerals from the sea that are not commonly found in our mineral-depleted soils.
- *Legumes:* Soybeans, garbanzo beans, kidney beans, pinto beans, and many other beans contain high amounts of protease inhibitors for cancer fighting, and other substances that help shut down the blood

FIGURE A-2 REVIEW OF EPIDEMIOLOGICAL STUDIES DEMONSTRATING THE RELATIONSHIP BETWEEN VEGETABLE CONSUMPTION AND CANCER PROTECTION

CANCER SITE	RELATIVE PERCENTAGE OF STUDIES DEMONSTRATING CANCER PROTECTION WITH HIGH VEGETABLE INTAKE	RELATIVE MEDIAN RISK: LOW VS. HIGH CONSUMPTION OF VEGETABLES
HORMONE-RELATED		
Breast	57%	1.3
Ovary/endometrium	75%	1.8
Prostate	100%	1.3
EPITHELIAL		
Oral	100%	2.0
Lung	96%	2.2
Larynx	100%	2.3
Esophagus	93%	2.0
Stomach	89%	2.5
Pancreas	82%	2.8
Cervix	88%	2.0
Bladder	60%	2.1
Colorectal	57%	1.9
Miscellaneous	75%	—
Total	75%	

Figure A-2: Eating vegetables decreases one's cancer risk.

FIGURE A-3: PHYTOCHEMICALS IN FOOD

PHYTOCHEMICAL	FOOD IS WHICH NATURALLY FOUND	ACTION IN BODY
Limonene and nomilin	Citrus fruit	Stimulates detoxification enzymes that break down carcinogens.
Citrus pectin	Plant fiber of citrus fruit	Shown to inhibit metastasis in prostate cancer by competing with tumor cell surface galectins which are essential for successful establishment of secondary tumor cell colonies.
Sulfur-containing compounds, sulforphane	Cruciferous vegetables (broccoli cauliflower, kale, brussels sprouts, and other members of the cabbage family), onions	Protects against cancer.
Allyl sulfides	Garlic, onions leeks chives	Increase the production of glutathione S-transferase and other enzymes that enhance carcinogen excretion.
S-allylmercaptocysteine (SAMC)	Aged garlic	Detoxifies hormones and carcinogens.
Dithiolethiones	Broccoli	Trigger the formation of glutathione S-transferase, which may prevent carcinogens from damaging a cell's DNA.
Ellagic Acid	Grapes, strawberries, raspberries, pomegranates	A polyphenol scavenger of carcinogens; prevents alteration in the DNA of cells. Also inhibits lung tumorigenesis induced by nicotine-derived nitrosamines.
Caffeic Acid	Fruit	Enhances production of enzymes that make carcinogens more water-soluable.
Ferulic acid	Fruit	Binds to nitrates in stomach; prevents production of carcinogenic niaosamines.
Phytic acid	Grains	Binds to iron and reduces free radical Iron effects of too much iron.
Indoles	Cruciferous vegetables	Helps detoxify estrogen.
Isothiocyanates	Cruciferous vegetables	Enhances glutathione S-transferase, which helps in carcinogen excretion.
Chlorophyll	Green vegetables	Antigenotoxin that inhibits the mutagenic activity of certain chemicals
Quercetin	Onions, broccoli, eucalyptus, blue-green algae, propolis	Inhibits the tumor-promoting PGE-2 series by blocking proflammatory reactionings in the body. Helps induce apoptosis.

The following four classes of phytochemicals have demonstrated anti-cancer activity.

1. Protease inhibitors	Soybeans, chickpeas, other legumes	Reduces certain enzymes in cancer cells
2. Phytosterols	Soybeans	Slow down the reproduction of cells in the large intestine, which may reduce risk of colon cancer.
3. Glycosides, saponins, and isoflavonoids	Soybeans	Interfere with the process by which cell DNA cells reproduce, which can prevent proliferation of cancer.
4. Genistein and daidzin (isoflavones)	Soybeans Onions, broccoli, eucalyptus, blue-green algae, propolis	Block the entry of estrogen into the cell, thus causing cancer cells to lose their functioning ability. Possibly helps convert cancer cells back to normal cells.

Adapted from **Herbal Medicine, Healing and Cancer, by Donald R. Yance, Jr., C.N., M.H., A.H.G., 1999, Keats Publishing, Lincolnwood, IL, Table 3.2**

vessels from tumors. Legumes also contribute to the detoxification process.

* *Kelp:* Dulse, nori, wakame, and others help provide a special soluble fiber that carries harmful fats and pro-oxidants from the gut, as well as provide a good source of many trace minerals.

* *Colorful Berries:* Raspberries, boysenberries, strawberries, dark cherries, blueberries, and blackberries contain ellagic acid, which can cause cancer cells to self-destruct (apoptosis).

* *Yogurt:* Yogurt can help fortify the body's defenses against infections and cancer by helping to nourish the gastrointestinal tract.

* *Green Tea:* Green tea contains catechins and other phytochemicals that provide cancer-fighting agents.

* *Healthy Seasonings:* Mustard, curry, hot peppers, salsa, cinnamon, garlic, onions, ginger, sage, rosemary, thyme, and other seasonings replace the typical unhealthy American fat, salt, and sugar approach to flavoring foods.

* Water, Clean and Pure: Water helps the body cleanse and dilute impurities, stabilize pH, nourish cells, and remove toxins.

OPTIMIZE YOUR HORMONAL MILIEU

Some scientists are calling for estrogen to be placed on the carcinogenic list. It is our belief that one of the most potent cancer-causing substances is estradiol. Optimizing your hormone milieu means lowering your estradiol levels and estrogen-binding capacity. This produces the effect of decreasing estradiol levels and increasing the estrogen quotient and, thus, decreases your cancer risk. The Hauser diet encourages the eating of foods that accomplish this and omitting foods that enhance estradiol production.

SOY

Soy products appear to have many benefits in the treatment of cancer. One of the things that soy does is to decrease estrogen levels. Soy blocks the cancer-promoting action of natural estrogens. One serving per day of soy may decrease the risk of developing a number of cancers by nearly 40%. Soy also has a cholesterol-lowering effect.

Soybeans contain phytoestrogens, which help protect against heart disease and are effective against skin cancer. Soy contains saponins, which are antioxidants and play a role in cancer prevention. High levels of estrogens are linked to increased risk of breast cancer and other hormone-related cancers. Isoflavones are antiestrogens and act as protectors against elevated estrogen cancers.[13]

A high dietary intake of soy products, as in countries such as Japan and Singapore, has been associated with a reduction in the incidence of breast cancer in premenopausal women. Genistein, an isoflavone found in soy products, has been found to be protective against leukemia and cancer of the colon, breast, lung, prostate, and skin. Genistein is a potent inhibitor of certain enzymes that allow cancer to progress.[14]

Phytoestrogens present in soybeans inhibit human breast cancer proliferation in vitro and breast cancer development in animal models. A study presented in the American Journal of Clinical Nutrition in 1998 showed that serum levels of the isoflavones genistein and diadzein increased in the soy supplemented group after 14 days.[15]

GOOD SOURCES OF SOY

Soy milk is an easy way to get soy into your diet. You can use it on cereal, in cooking, to make smoothies, and in hot beverages. But—please look at soy milk labels. Pure, organic, unsweetened soy milk contains *more* protein than carbohydrates. If the soy milk you are drinking contains more carbohydrate than protein grams in it, then cane sugar has been added. *Always check labels!* Tofu is another wonderful source of soy. You can use tofu in stir-fried meals; to make soy burgers; on salads; and even to make shakes, puddings, sauces, and soups. You can also take the actual soybeans and make wonderful dishes with them as well. Tempeh and miso are alternate sources of soy that may take a little getting used to but are very good all the same.

ESTROGEN AND PROSTATE CANCER

Researchers at the Fred Hutchinson Cancer Research Center reported in 2000 that three healthy portions of vegetables daily cut the risk of prostate cancer by 48%.[12] More importantly, they also found that three half-cup servings per week of cabbage, cauliflower, brussels sprouts, or broccoli decreases the risk of prostate cancer by 41%.[12] These vegetables are all members of the Bassica family, also termed cruciferous vegetables, and all contain, among other things, a phytochemical called indole-3-carbinol, as well as a much more powerful phytochemical termed diindolylmethane, which is actually just two indole-3-carbinol molecules chemically attached to each other.

These substances, as well as vegetables containing them, have all been shown to reduce cancer risk by balancing your estrogen metabolism in a very specific way. These vegetables reduce the amount of a particularly carcinogenic estrogen (16α-hydroxyestrone) that is normally in your body, while increasing a neutral-to-favorable estrogen (2-hydroxyestrone).[16]

The theory of how estrogen metabolism affects prostate cancer is related to the testosterone-to-estrogen cancer hypothesis. This theory states that once testosterone is transformed into estradiol, whether a little or a lot, then some of that estradiol may be converted to 16α-hydroxyestrone. At this point, this form of estrogen will exert the same negative influence in the prostate as it does in the breast and other tissues in women. The worst case result is prostate cancer.[14] If the risk of prostate cancer can be significantly reduced just by eating some cabbage or broccoli, then start eating it!

FLAX SEED'S EFFECT ON ESTROGEN

Flax seed has been shown to be beneficial for lowering the cancer-associated forms of serum estrogens. In a 1999 study, 28 postmenopausal women were asked to add 0, 5, or 10 grams of ground flax seed to their usual diets. The report states, "Flax seed supplementation significantly increased urinary 2-hydroxyestrone secretion and the urinary 2/16α ratio in a linear, dose response fashion."[13] In other words, the more flax seed consumed, the more estradiol is converted to its 2α-hydroxy metabolite (See **Figure A-4**). While this was not a direct study of breast or other estrogen-related cancer prevention, it is a very suggestive piece of evidence.[18] This is a very simple thing to do in your diet. Go to a health food store and purchase some flax seeds. Grind them up and put them on salads, in yogurt, into vegetable dishes, or anywhere you like.

FIBER AND HORMONES

We are told to increase the fiber in our diets because it can help prevent a myriad of diseases, including cancer. Insoluble fiber, such as cellulose, hemicellulose, and lignins found in fruit and vegetable pulp, skin, stems, and leaves, and the outer covering of nuts, seeds, and grains, is the type of fiber that has been associated with decreased cancer risk. In a 1985 study, 62 premenopausal participants ages 20 to 50 years with regular menstrual cycles were given fiber supplementation to a minimum of 30 g/day in the form of muffins and cereals from wheat, corn, and oat bran. Significant reductions in serum estrogen concentrations were found in the wheat bran supplemented group. The changes in serum estrone and estradiol took place without any reduction in dietary fat consumption, which, in itself, can result in decreased serum estrogen concentrations. The mechanism by which the estrogen levels are lowered is most likely from enhanced enterohepatic circulation.[19]

ELIMINATE CANCER-CAUSING AGENTS

Many people who study cancer physiology believe cancer starts by an initiating agent. Such substances cause a change in the DNA of a cell to promote cancer formation. Cancer seems to be caused by a collection of lifestyle and environmental factors that accumulate over the years. We are bombarded by toxic chemicals every day. Because of "modern" technology, our water, food, and air are polluted. People no longer live in the country with their own wells and no longer grow their own food. They depend on government municipalities to purify their water. Because of the amount of chemicals spilling into the water supply from factories and chemical plants, strong oxidants, such as chlorine, are put into the water. People who drink municipal water and who bathe or shower in it are thus getting oxidant exposure in the form of chemicals in the water. This oxidant exposure is also coming in the form of air pollution, as well as chemicals in the food supply. Each year, America sprays 1.2 billion pounds of pesticides on our food crops, dumps 90 billion pounds of toxic waste in our 55,000 toxic waste sites, feeds nine million pounds of antibiotics to our farm animals to help them gain weight faster, and generally bombards the landscape with questionable amounts of electromagnetic radiation.[20]

FIGURE A-4: ESTROGEN METABOLISM

Flax seed and other substances promote the 2-hydroxylation of estradiol, decreasing a person's risk of cancer.

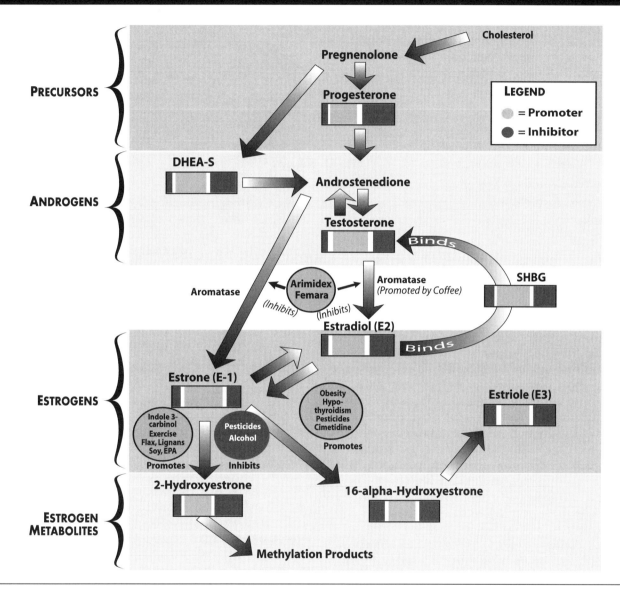

The human body is built from, repaired by, and fueled by substances found in the diet. We definitely are what we eat. Therefore, we recommend that you consume food in its purest and freshest form, without chemicals or artificial ingredients added. You need to find a good organic grocery store where you can be confident of the products sold. Buy fresh organic produce and meats. Avoid packaged foods.

Fast food is also something that certainly needs to be avoided. Much of the reason for this is that most of this type of food is fried at very high temperatures with oils that have become rancid. The chemical structure of the fats has become changed to that of a bad fat. Foods that increase coagulation should be avoided.

It is important for the person with cancer to eliminate as many cancer-causing agents in his or her food, water, and air supply as possible. The Hauser diet makes the person aware of foods and beverages that have cancer-causing agents in them.

Help Starve the Cancer

Cancers love sugar, and, unfortunately, many people who develop cancer also love sugar. The average American consumes between 140 and 150 pounds of sugar per year. This excessive sugar intake has many harmful effects, including the following:

- Lowers immunity
- Feeds cancer cells
- Increases anaerobic metabolism
- Decreases aerobic metabolism
- Increases body toxicity
- Thickens the blood
- Raises insulin levels

Sugar is one of the main promoters of cancer physiology. You can only shudder when you see a three-year-old drinking a sugar-laden cola or "fruit drink." It is evident from the habits of the next generation that we will see the incidence of cancer dramatically increase in the upcoming years. By consuming sugar throughout the day, whether soda pop or the elegant coffee-sugar-ice cream combinations at the local coffee cafe, people are pushing their physiology more and more toward cancer. The excessive sugar consumption causes excess insulin production. The more insulin that is around, the greater the ability of the cancer cells to live and thrive. Insulin pushes glucose into the cancer cell to drive its anaerobic metabolism. If you keep eating those donuts for breakfast, drinking coffee with sugar throughout the day, and eating ice cream desserts, your potential cancer cells are just waiting to grow and live.

Sugar causes cancer physiology to survive. A study was performed where animals were injected with an aggressive strain of breast cancer and then fed diets that would provide either hypoglycemia, normoglycemia, or hyperglycemia. A dose-dependent response in which the lower the blood glucose, the greater the survival percentage at 70 days.[21]

For the person who wants to reverse cancer physiology, the cancer must be starved by keeping sugar levels low. The only way to do this is to avoid foods that are rapidly metabolized into glu-

cose. The following is a list of the top 20 sources of carbohydrates consumed in the American diet.[22] These data were gathered from the Harvard Nurses Health Study. These foods represent things that can rapidly raise your blood sugar and, consequently, your insulin levels. These types of foods just enhance cancer physiology.

1. Potatoes	11. Fruit Punch
2. White Bread	12. Coca-Cola
3. Cold Breakfast Cereal	13. Apples
4. Dark Bread	14. Skim Milk
5. Orange Juice	15. Pancakes
6. Bananas	16. Table Sugar
7. White Rice	17. Jam
8. Pizza	18. Cranberry Juice
9. Pasta	19. French Fries
10. Muffins	20. Candy

Refined simple carbohydrates need to be seriously limited in the diet. If you do enjoy sweet foods, consider sugar substitutes. Choose Stevia, glycine, Sucanat, or fresh colorful fruit over anything with "sugar" on the label.

It is imperative for cancer patients to know the amount of carbohydrates that are in the foods they are eating. As can be seen in **Figure A-5**, chicken, turkey, ham, veal, beef, lamb, pork, and fish have no carbohydrates, whereas just one piece of watermelon has 41g. We are sure that cancer patients are consuming a lot more watermelon than high-protein foods, thinking they are doing themselves a favor.

The amount of carbohydrate grams allowed to each cancer patient to keep glucose and insulin levels low will depend on each individual case. To determine this, it is best to receive a glucose/insulin tolerance test. If a person truly needs a low-carbohydrate diet, then as little as 40grams of carbohydrates may be consumed each day. If this is the case, then basically all fruits and grains cannot be eaten. It is still possible to have vegetables, but the carbohydrate content of each food must be closely watched.

Beware of hidden carbohydrates! Throughout this book, the benefits of soy have been espoused. Many of the soy milk drinks, however, contain as one of the main ingredients organic evaporated cane juice, which in layman's terms is sugar. A true, organic soy milk has 9 grams of protein for every 5 grams of carbohydrates. If the soy milk you are drinking has more carbohydrate calories than protein ones, you are just sucking in the sugar. Bon appétit! Please read the labels.

FIGURE A-5: LOW CARBOHYDRATE DIET

There is only one thing you must do while on this diet—and that is to restrict your carbohydrate intake to less than 60 grams per day.* This can be done by calculating the grams of carbohydrate in each food you eat by using the simple list of values below, making certain that you do not exceed the absolute limit of 60 grams. You will notice that some foods are high in carbohydrate and therefore should be avoided. You will also notice that you may eat all the meat, pure fat, and moderate amounts of most vegetables, cheeses, and eggs that you wish. This means you can eat satisfying meals and need not be hungry while starving the cancer.

FOOD		HOUSEHOLD MEASURE	GRAMS
MILK:	Whole Milk	8 oz.	11.8
	Ice Cream	½ pt. servings	14.8
CHEESE:	Cheese	1 oz. servings	.50
	Cottage cheese	1 rounded tablespoon	1.30
FATS:	Bacon	3 strips	.00
	Butter	1 tablespoon	.00
	French Dressing	1 tablespoon	1.90
	Salad Oil	1 tablespoon	.00
	Mayonnaise	1 tablespoon	.20
EGGS:	1 egg	—	.73
MEATS:	Bologna	2 slices	1.0
	Frankfurter	1 serving	1.9
	Hash	1 serving	7.0
	Chicken, Turkey,	5 oz.	1.0
	Ham, Veal, Beef,	4 oz.	1.0
	Lamb, Pork, Fish	5 oz.	.00
NUTS:	Mixed	10-15	3.0
FISH:	Oysters	4-6	1.2
	Shrimp	5-6	.5
VEGETABLES			
(FRESH)	Asparagus	6 sticks	2.0
	Beans, Green	½ cup	2.0
	Beans, Lima	½ cup	23.5
	Beet Greens	½ cup	5.6
	Beets	2 medium	9.7
	Broccoli	½ cup	5.6
	Brussels Sprouts	6	6.2
	Cabbage	⅔ cup cooked	5.3
	Carrots	1 large	9.3
	Cauliflower	4 tablespoons	3.4
	Celery	2 stalks	1.9
	Corn	1 ear	20.5
	Cucumber	½	1.4
	Eggplant	½ cup cooked	5.5
	Kale	½ cup cooked	7.2
	Lettuce	5 leaves	.9
	Okra	6 pods	19.0
	Onions	⅔ small	10.3
	Green Peas	½ cup	17.7
	Green peppers	1	5.7
	Potatoes	1 small	19.1
	Spinach	½ cup cooked	3.2
	Squash	½ cup	3.9
	Tomatoes	1 medium	.4
	Turnips	½ cup cooked	7.1
	Catsup	1 tablespoon	4.8
	Tomato Juice	1 cup	4.3
FRUIT:	Apples	1 large	22.4
	Apricots	2-3	12.9
	Avocado	medium	5.1
	Banana	1 small	23.0
	Strawberries	10 large	8.1
	Other Berries	⅔ cup	15.1
	Cantaloupe	½ melon	6.9
	Grapefruit	½ small	10.1

FOOD		HOUSEHOLD MEASURE	GRAMS
FRUIT:	Grapes	22	16.70
(CONT.):	Lemons	1 mediuum	8.70
	Oranges	1 small	11.20
	Orange Juice	½ cup	12.90
	Peaches	1 medium	12.00
	Pear	1 medium	25.00
	Pineapple	½ cup	13.70
	Plums	3 medium	12.90
	Rhubarb	1 cup	3.80
	Watermelon	1 slice (6" dia. x 1 ½")	31.60
CANNED			
FRUIT:	Cherries	½ cup	20.00
	Cranberry Sauce	1 tablespoon	10.20
	Pineapple	1 slice	21.10
DRIED:	Apricots	4-6	20.00
FRUIT:	Prunes	2-3	21.30
FLOUR:	Corn Meal	½ cup	15.00
MEAL:	Cornstarch	1 tablespoon	9.00
BREAD:	Whole Grain	1 Slice	13.00
	White	1 Slice	16.00
	Honey Wheat	1 Slice	18.00
	Graham Cracker	1	13.00
	Wheat Rolls	1	16.00
CEREALS:	Cornflakes	¾ cup	27.00
	Oatmeal	½ cup cooked	24.00
	Puffed Rice	¾ cup	14.80
	Shreaded Wheat	1 biscuit	14.10
MACARONI	Spaghetti	½ cup cooked	15.80
	Noodles	1 cup	39.00
	Rice	1 cup	48.00
	Tapioca	1 level tablespoon	14.20
SUGARS:	Honey	1 tablespoon	17.00
	Jam	1 tablespoon	14.80
MISCEL-			
LANEOUS:	Bouillon Cubes	2	4.70
	Gelatin Dessert	1 tablespoon	5.30

*The actual amount of carbohydrates allowed will vary with each person predicated on blood sugar readings.

COMPLEMENT OTHER THERAPIES RECEIVED

Not everyone who has cancer is going to receive IPT. We hope this book will help patients who are diagnosed with cancer seek an IPT physician to determine if they are appropriate candidates for the therapy.

No matter what therapy you receive, it is important that your diet and supplement program complement the other treatments you receive. Cancer, as well as many of the conventional therapies you may receive, may cause a lot of unpleasant symptoms, including nausea, vomiting, anorexia, malnutrition, diarrhea, maldigestion, constipation, gas, anemia, leukopenia, hair loss, fatigue, mouth sores, fungus infections, depression, anxiety, insomnia, and pain.[23]

Many people are coming to natural medicine doctors because they practice holistic care. All aspects of the disease and symptomatology are addressed, preferably from a nutritional approach. Natural medicine physicians understand conventional medicine because they also use these medicines. As it pertains to cancer therapy, these medicines are used in IPT but in much lower doses. Even so, the IPT physician knows the organs and the side effects of the medications, as well as emphasizes diet, herbal supplements, and other medications to reduce these side effects.

The Hauser Diet addresses the most common symptoms and side effects potentially experienced with cancer and cancer treatments and works to reverse them. Specific foods are emphasized that not only help reverse cancer physiology but also cancer symptomatology.

WHEN FIRST DIAGNOSED

The healthiest diet is a whole foods-based diet that keeps blood sugar and insulin levels low. using vegetables; fish; oils; organic, low-fat meats and some fruits and whole grains. Processed and refined foods should be avoided as much as possible. Purchasing organic products will reduce your exposure to chemicals and pesticides. You need a wide variety of nutrients to help build healthy new cells and to fight the cancer.

UNDERWEIGHT

Some people are just naturally thin and have high metabolisms. Other times, low weight is the result of malabsorption or other disorders. You should not be on a severely calorie-restricted diet during your cancer treatment. You will not get enough nutrients. However, this is not license to eat whatever you want. Some tips for sensibly gaining weight are as follows:

- Eat five to six small meals rather than three large ones.
- Try juicing some of your vegetables so that you can sip on it throughout the day.
- Prepare meals that are appealing to sight and smell.
- Snack on high-protein foods, such as nuts and seeds, organic nut-butters, soy cheeses, soy milk, and so on.
- Half an hour before meals, drink a half glass of water with a teaspoon of lemon juice to stimulate the appetite.
- Avoid consumption of liquids with the meal.
- Make meal time pleasant.
- Add oil (flax seed oil, fish oils, and those listed earlier in the chapter) to foods: one to two tablespoons to potatoes, vegetables, salads, smoothies, beverages, and so on.
- Add protein powders to foods or use them to make high-protein drinks.

DURING CHEMOTHERAPY OR IPT

During chemotherapy, the body is under stress. Chemotherapy agents circulate throughout your body, killing cancer cells and knocking off some good cells along the way. Many of the drugs used in chemotherapy interfere with cell division because cancer cells divide faster than most normal tissue cells. When a drug interferes with cell division, the rapidly dividing cells are affected the most. This includes not only cancer cells but also good cells located in the epithelial tissues that line the mouth, throat, and intestines. Chemotherapy can cause mouth sores, tender or bleeding gums, sore throat, swallowing difficulty, changes in menstruation, lower resistance to infections, anemia, kidney and/or liver toxicity, and even more cancer. It may also cause nausea and/or diarrhea. The severity of these side effects is largely related to the drug used, the dosage, the length of treatment, and your individual response. Although most of these side effects are temporary and will gradually go away once treatment ceases, some of them can be permanent.

Herbal and nutritional therapies can make chemotherapy more effective for the particular cancer being treated, as well as protect against side effects. Bromelain and quercetin, for example, are especially compatible with most chemotherapeutics used in cases of breast, ovarian, and colon cancers, as well as leukemia and most melanomas. Reishi, coriolus, astragalus, and Siberian ginseng work well with all chemotherapeutics and can be eaten to reduce many of their side effects. Natural medicine physicians can assist cancer patients, decrease chemotherapy side effects by utilizing various nutritional products.

NAUSEA

We all know what it feels like to be nauseated, and we all hate that feeling. Chemotherapy can sometimes cause the patient to experience this feeling for a prolonged period of time. Nausea may be triggered by certain smells or disturbing sights. In general, a nauseated person does not want to eat. Here are some tips for combating the nausea of chemotherapy:

- Eat smaller, more frequent meals.
- Avoid foods with strong odors.
- Sip clear liquids slowly or suck on popsicles or ice cubes made from your favorite healthy liquid.
- Loosen your clothing and get fresh air.
- Suck on some very strong peppermints, drink peppermint tea, or take peppermint capsules.
- Suck on some ginger lozenges, drink ginger tea, or take ginger capsules.
- Try acupressure wrist bands or acupuncture.

DIARRHEA

Here are some tips for combating diarrhea resulting from chemotherapy:

- Use the tips for nausea.
- Take a good probiotic supplement. (We like *SMI Powder* or *GI Biotic* available at www.benuts.com* or take yogurt with live cultures (avoiding a yogurt that contains a lot of sugar).

- Activated charcoal* may be needed to bind any gastrointestinal irritants.
- Take fiber to bind excessive fluid in the gut. (We use *EFA Powder* or *IVD Enzyme* from www.benuts.com, which also contains enzymes for maximum absorption).

MOUTH SORES

Mouth sores are often caused by chemotherapy or radiation and can be very painful. Because of the severe discomfort they cause, eating can be difficult.

A mouth sore formula[24] is as follows:

- ALOE LEAF EXTRACT: 30mL
- GLYCERIN: 30 mL
- LICORICE: 15 mL
- PROPOLIS: 15 mL
- ESSENTIAL OIL OF CLOVE: 5-10 DROPS
- COLLINSONIA: 10 mL
- ECHINACEA: 10 mL
- CHAMOMILE: 5 mL
- THUJA: 5 mL

Dose: Use 60 drops of this formula (about half teaspoon) per tablespoon or two of warm salt water and rinse mouth every two hours while awake.

Other suggestions:

- *Take a Probiotic internally* and also rinse mouth with ½ to 1 teaspoon or 1 ounce of acidophilus in warm water.
- *L-glutamine Powder:* Take 2-3 teaspoons daily, directly in the mouth. Wash down with water.
- *Natural Vitamin E:* Take 400-1,600 IU of natural vitamin E (mixed tocopherols) prior to starting chemotherapy. Continue during treatments. Natural vitamin E can also be applied topically to the skin three times per day.

HAIR LOSS

Everyone has seen a cancer patient who has lost his or her hair due to the treatments received. You can only imagine what that feels like. Using nutritional means and less toxic treatments such as IPT, patients may actually grow hair during treatments. If you experience hair loss, you can try the following:

- Start 1,200-1,600 IU of natural vitamin E per day, two weeks prior to treatment.
- We use the supplement Pro-Collagen* or Hauser Hair Spray Formula* that contains an herbal combination that helps stimulate hair growth.

---

* *Available from Beulah Land Nutritionals at 1-877-RX-BEULAH or www.benuts.com.*

ANEMIA

When chemotherapy or other treatments produce anemia, the patient's blood counts may drop lower than normal. During this time, it is very important that the patient maintain adequate nutrition.

- Consume heme iron-containing foods: red meat, organ meat.
- Consume nonheme iron-containing foods: spinach, kale, raisins, beets, and beet juice.
- Drink liquid liver extract.
- Ensure adequate B vitamin intake with green leafy vegetables, especially B$_{12}$ and folate supplementation (either orally or via intramuscular injections).
- Supplement with shark liver oil (Immunofin is the product we use*) or a Chinese herbal formula called Marrow Plus.*

LEUKOPENIA

During cancer treatment, levels of white blood cells, which are the immune cells of the body, can drop dangerously low. At this time, the body is put in a state of alert because it is unable to fight off infections, even the common cold. Some ways to help this condition are as follows:

- Avoid being around sick people.
- Avoid consumption of sugar and sugar-containing products.
- Do not consume raw meats or food that has not been refrigerated.
- Wash all fresh foods thoroughly.
- Avoid eating in restaurants.
- Take supplements that help stimulate the immune system, such as Stimmune,* Colostrum, Licorice Root, Garlic, Carnivora* and Astragalus.

FUNGUS INFECTIONS

Fungus feeds on sugar and foods that are rapidly converted to sugar. This means carbohydrates! If you have a problem with fungus, you definitely want to avoid these types of foods. We like to add various herbal remedies to help fight the fungal infection, such as *D-Yeast** and *SMI powder** (available at www.benuts.com). If need-ed, an anti-fungal medication such as Diflucan, Sporonox, or Ketoconazole will be prescribed.

ANSWERING YOUR QUESTIONS ABOUT THE HAUSER DIET

There are many questions people will continue to have about what diet to eat even after reading this chapter or this book. For instance, "How many calories should I consume?" "What if I loose weight on The Hauser Diet?" "Are some protein foods better than others?" "Can I use a little fruit juice to get my pills down?" "How do I know if I am eating the right diet?" So we don't get inundated with emails about The Hauser Diet, we will do our best to answer the most basic questions that we get.

"HOW MANY CALORIES SHOULD I CONSUME?"

A cancer patient must realize that eating too many calories will raise insulin levels. We encourage people to eat a diet that keeps their fasting blood sugars below 80 and their insulin levels below 10. They must eat enough protein to keep their blood albumin counts above 4.0. If on initial assessment their albumin counts are below 4.0, then soy protein powders are given. They are also given some of our secret recipes for Protein Power drinks. (See Figure A-6.)

For example to make a Dreamsickle Tofu Power Drink, one would add 4 ounces of crumbled tofu and one quarter teaspoon of orange extract to the Protein Power Basic Formula. To make a Coconut Almond Power Drink: 15 almonds, a quarter teaspoon almond extract, a third of a teaspoon organic coconut and a packet of stevia are added.

"WHAT IF I LOOSE WEIGHT ON THE HAUSER DIET?"

What if you do—so what? Scientific studies on animals with cancer conclude that calorie restriction aids in cancer survival. Some cancer patients gain weight, while others loose weight while on The Hauser Diet. The most important factor is whether or not the blood cancer markers are going down and the x-rays show the cancer going into remission.

---

* *Available from Beulah Land Nutritionals at 1-877-RX-BEULAH or www.benuts.com.*

FIGURE A-6 CARING MEDICAL PROTEIN POWER DRINK BASIC FORMULA

- 6 OUNCES OF WATER
- 1 Tablespoon of Superfood*
- 4 Ounces of coconut milk
- 1 Cup crushed ice
- 1 Tablespoon of Pro EFA Fiber*
- 1 Tablespoon of Genista*
- 1 Scoop of All in One Powder*
- Additional ingredients to taste

"ARE SOME PROTEIN FOODS BETTER THAN OTHERS?"

If one has to choose between a carbohydrate and a protein, then obviously the protein is a better choice, for the majority of cancer patients. We believe in the healing power of soy versus other protein sources, but overall the most important factor is to eat a diet that keeps blood sugar and insulin levels low so as to not feed the cancer.

"CAN I USE A LITTLE FRUIT JUICE TO GET MY PILLS DOWN?"

Absolutely. (But please keep the juice consumption to 8 ounces a day.)

"HOW DO I KNOW IF I AM EATING THE RIGHT DIET?"

Eat your normal diet. Then check your fasting blood sugar and insulin levels. Keep your fasting glucose level below 80 and your insulin below 10. Then check your blood sugar and insulin levels one and two hours after eating. Try and keep your blood sugar level below 120 and your insulin levels below 25. If they are above these numbers you are either eating too many carbohydrates or just plain eating too much food. The latter is called "gluttony."

THE HAUSER DIET FOOD PYRAMID

To answer the question "What are your general guidelines concerning the relative amounts of protein that should be consumed in relation to carbohydrates and fat?" The typical cancer patient is prescribed a macrobiotic diet by most alternative medicine practitioners. This diet has about 70% of its calories as carbohydrate, 20% as fat, and 10% as protein. The Hauser Diet has 45% of its calories as protein, 35% as carbohydrate, and 20% as fat. **(See Figure A-7.)** In other words, The Hauser Diet has half the amount of carbohydrates as the typical Macrobiotic diet.

"DID YOU JUST MAKE THE DIET UP—OR IS IT BASED IN SCIENCE?"

We appreciate honesty. The Hauser Diet was formulated after Caring Medical started doing Insulin Potentiation Therapy. IPT is based on the concept that most cancers are insulin dependent. If this is true then it would make sense for the cancer patient to keep their insulin levels as low as possible at all times except when they are getting chemotherapy. Imagine, for example, a woman who has breast cancer that is rapidly growing because of insulin. She then consults a doctor who does IPT and she gets on The Hauser Diet. Prior to her getting the actual IPT treatment, her cancer would be starving because their would be no insulin or blood glucose around to feed it because of the diet. Then on the day of the IPT

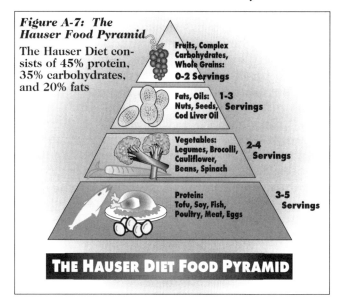

Figure A-7: The Hauser Food Pyramid

The Hauser Diet consists of 45% protein, 35% carbohydrates, and 20% fats

Fruits, Complex Carbohydrates, Whole Grains: 0-2 Servings

Fats, Oils: Nuts, Seeds, Cod Liver Oil — 1-3 Servings

Vegetables: Legumes, Brocolli, Cauliflower, Beans, Spinach — 2-4 Servings

Protein: Tofu, Soy, Fish, Poultry, Meat, Eggs — 3-5 Servings

THE HAUSER DIET FOOD PYRAMID

---

* These nutritional products are available from Beulah Land Nutritionals at 1-877-RX-BEULAH or www.benuts.com. Pro EFA Fiber is high in flax seed and other organic seeds and nuts. Superfood is an organic vegetable powder. Phytocarrots, an organic carrot powder can be substituted for the Superfood. Genista is a high concentrated soy protein powder. For a more creamier taste, some days Sports Doc Meal Replacement (in multiple flavors) can be used. All in One Powder is a hypoallergenic rice based multivitamin powder. Additional ingredients can be added to taste including fruit, stevia, vanilla, cinnamon, coffee extract, and almonds for example. As one can surmise, for the cancer patient, this highly concentrated nutritional drink can do wonders.

treatment, the person gets an insulin shot, which just turns on this ravenous, starving cancer. The cancer thinks the insulin signals that blood glucose levels are going high because the person just sucked down a triple chocolate malted shake. Instead of sucking up sugar, the cancer is confronted with three to five chemotherapy drugs. It has no choice but to let them in because the insulin given had unlocked the "door" to the cell. The IPT-targeted chemotherapy then starts bulldozing the cancer cells. Now do you get it? Makes perfect sense—at least to us.

The actual percentages of protein:carbs:fat in The Hauser Diet come from a study done at The Rockefeller University Hospital and Columbia University College of Physicians and Surgeons in New York City, New York.[25] As has been discussed in this book, the main factor that we see that is implicated in female cancers is estradiol and its metabolism. In regard to the main hormonally driven cancer in males, prostate cancer, the same analogy can be given. The breakdown product of the primary male hormone, testosterone is dihydrotestosterone. This is formed by the action of the enzyme, 5α-reductase, on testosterone to form dihydrotestosterone. In the study noted above, the volunteers were fed a high-protein diet for two weeks and then a high-carbohydrate diet for a second two-week period; there was an interval of three weeks between the study periods during which they consumed their usual home diets. The high-protein diet consisted of 44% of total calories as protein, 35% as carbohydrate, and 21% as fat; the high-carbohydrate diet consisted of 10% of total calories as protein, 70% as carbohydrate, and 20% as fat. Before and after the various diets the metabolism of testosterone and estradiol were measured. As one can see from **Figure A-8**, their were substantial changes in the metabolic breakdown of testosterone and estradiol by the two diets. The mean 5α/5B testosterone ratio decreased approximately 50% when the subjects

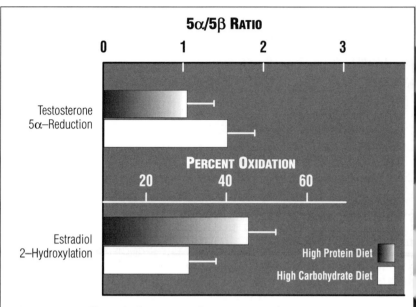

Figure A-8: Effect of Changes in the Amounts of Dietary Protein and Carbohydrate on Testosterone

This study shows that a high-protein diet significantly lowered 5-α reduction of testosterone and increased the 2-hydroxylation of estradiol. Both of these effects are needed to reverse the hormonal aspects of cancer physiology.

Adapted from Nutrition-endocrine interactions: Induction of reciprocal changes in the 5α-reduction of testosterone and the cytochrome P-450-dependent oxidation of estradiol by dietary macronutrients in man, by A. Kappas, and K. Anderson Proceedings of the National Academy of Sciences. 1983; 80: 7646-7649.

were changed from a high-carbohydrate to a high-protein diet (P<0.025). Likewise, the 2-hydroxylation of estradiol increased by approximately 50% when the subjects were changed from a high-carbohydrate to a high-protein diet (P<0.02). Thus, in regard to hormonal milieu, the high-protein diet, helps reverse both male *and* female cancer physiology.

It is clear that the high-protein diet keeps blood glucose and insulin levels much lower than the high-carbohydrate diet. This would be reason enough to recommend this type of diet for the cancer patient. When the hormonal make-up of individuals are compared on the high-carbohydrate versus the high-protein diet, it is quite clear from scientific studies that the diet the patient with cancer needs is the one that is highest in protein.

"SO WHAT WOULD A TYPICAL DAY LOOK LIKE ON THE HAUSER DIET?"

8:00am: Eggs or Protein Power Drink, yum, yum

10:00am: Snack of nuts/seeds

12:00 noon: Big Salad with chicken breast

2:30pm: Protein Power Drink, yum, yum

5:00pm: Piece of Fish with vegetables or Stir fry with Tofu

For drinks, good ol' fashion filtered water. Other liquids consumed would be cod liver oil, fish oils, and/or flax seed oil. Yes it is possible to live without bread and pasta.

SUMMARY OF THE HAUSER DIET

Nutrition can play a vital role in helping you get through your cancer treatment protocol. As always, report any side effects to your physician immediately. Use these recommendations to help you maximize your nutrition and healing while you are undergoing therapy.

We have repeated some themes. These are the basic principles of the Hauser Diet:

- Avoid sugar and sugar-containing foods.

- Avoid junk food; processed food; food chemicals; pesticides; dyes; artificial colors, flavors, and sweeteners; and any other toxic food substances.

- Choose whole, fresh, and organic fruits, vegetables, and meats.

- Increase consumption of vegetables, especially those from the cruciferous family.

- Increase consumption of bioflavonoid-containing foods.

- Increase consumption of soy and soy-containing products.

- Drink water: purified, clean water.

- Reduce fat intake, especially hydrogenated and saturated fats. Consume good fats such as olive and flax oils.

- Increase consumption of cold-water fish.

The Hauser Diet Food Pyramid has the cancer patient eating a diet of 45 percent protein, 30 percent carbohydrates, 25 percent fats and oils, and 0-2 servings of fruits and whole grains.

The diet will be monitored by periodical tests of glucose-insulin intolerance and its parameters, including blood cancer markers. Remember—the most important variable isn't what you are eating—rather it's if your cancer is going into remission.

These principles will not only help you fight cancer but will help you prevent getting cancer in the first place.

CANCER LOVES SUGAR
DIETARY GUIDELINES FOR CANCER PATIENTS

The following dietary guidelines may negate everything that you have learned about anti-cancer nutrition, so brace yourself for some recommendations that may seem a bit against the grain (literally!). These guidelines are supported in the cancer literature.

AVOID EXCESSIVE CARBOHYDRATES.

This is the main principle for an anti-cancer diet. A carbohydrate is ultimately the some as sugar, once it is broken down in the body. Cancer thrives on carbohydrates (or sugar). Your goal is to starve the cancer of its favorite food. Carbohydrates are found in sweet foods like sugar, cakes, cookies, candy, soda pop, chocolate, ice cream etc. Carbohydrates are also the primary nutrients in fruits and grains, including flours. You can effectively starve your cancer by avoiding foods high in carbohydrates and consume food that contains more protein and fat (the good fats).

WHY DOES CANCER LOVE SUGAR?

You may wonder why cancer loves sugar. The answer lies in a hormone called insulin. Insulin finds sugar in the bloodstream, attaches to the sugar, and carries it to the cells of the body. Cancer cells hoard the sugar, making many windows on the cell surface called "Insulin receptors," allowing the insulin to deposit the sugar on the cancer cell. The extra sugar available for food enables the cancer to grow faster than the other cells of the body. When you eat a high carbohydrate food, the cancer cells in your body are having a party—and you are not invited.

ADD PROTEIN AND FAT TO TRICK THE CANCER.

You can play a "metabolic trick" on the cancer by first limiting high carbohydrate foods, and then adding foods that are high in protein and fat. This diet profile helps maintain lower blood insulin levels. In this state, the cancer is starving for sugar.

When you receive an IPT (Insulin Potentiation Therapy) treatment, we inject insulin into the blood stream, making the cancer go crazy with hunger. Instead of providing large dose of sugar, however, we inject small doses of chemotherapy. This means sudden death for the cancer cells, and party time for you!

ORGANIC FOOD CHOICES:

It is very important to find good, high quality protein sources. Purchase meat from a health food store or organic farmers, if possible. Look for organic hormone-free free-range poultry and meat, grass-fed beef and deep sea fish. Choose organic dairy, eggs, soy products, and fresh produce.

FOOD PREPARATION:

Use olive oil, not buffer for cooking oil. Never use margarine or any sort of hydrogenated oil. Check labels, as they are commonly food additives. Lightly steamed or raw fresh vegetables are preferred to canned or frozen. If juicing, use organic vegetables only, avoiding excessive use of carrots, beets, or fruits.

HOW MUCH IS TOO MUCH CARBOHYDRATE?

Try to keep total carbohydrate count per day to under 75 grams. Under 50 grams is ideal.

WHAT CAN YOU EAT?

- Meat (Organic) All meats, including fish, chicken, turkey, beef, lamb, shellfish, pork, and wild game
- Dairy products: Organic, milk, cheese, yogurt, butter (Full fat is usually preferred.)
- Eggs: Organic, free-range eggs
- Nuts and nut butters: Raw only. Roasted nuts often contain rancid oils
- Soy products: Unsweetened soy milk (fortified with protein and calcium is ideal) tofu, tempeh, edamame (frozen fresh soy beans available in the freezer section), and soy protein shakes (using low carbohydrate ingredients)
- Vegetables: Consume dark, deeply colored fresh vegetables, limiting intake of corn, white potatoes, carrots, and beets to two times per week
- Fruit: Limit fruit intake to the one serving or less per day. One serving equals four ounces or half a cup. Berries such as strawberries, blueberries, and blackberries are best. Limit bananas and oranges to two times per week. Avoid all fruit juices, except for immediately following IPT treatment.

WHAT FOOD TO AVOID:

- Grains: Avoid all grains, including all flours. An occasional serving of millet, brown rice or quinoa is allowed, but no more than once or twice per week. Watch your total daily carbohydrate intake.
- Breads Avoid all breads. Limit intake of sprouted grain bread like Ezekiel bread or Essene bread (available in the frozen section of your local health food store) to once or twice per week. Watch total daily carbohydrate intake.
- Pasta: Avoid all pastas. A high protein lentil pasta is acceptable one to two servings per week. Watch your total daily carbohydrate intake.
- Beans: Limit intake of all beans to two servings per week, excluding soybeans, which can be eaten more regularly. Watch your total daily carbohydrate intake.
- Sweeteners: Avoid all sweeteners, including sugar, honey, maple syrup, molasses, sucanat, raw sugar, fructose, corn syrup, brown rice syrup, and artificial sweeteners. Stevia is permissible.

OTHER RESOURCES:

- *Protein Power,* by Dr. Michael R. Eades and Mary Dan Eades. Available at www.Amazon.com.
- *The Nutribase Complete Book of Food Counts,* by Art Ulene. Available at www.benuts.com.
- *Treating Cancer with Insulin Potentiation Therapy* by Ross and Marion Hauser. Available at www.beulahlandpress.com in June, 2002.
- Visit the following web sites to learn more about IPT and cancer: www.iptcancer.com, www.caringmedical.com www.IPTQ.com ■

SUMMARY OF THE BASICS OF THE HAUSER DIET:

FOOD	INCLUDED	EXCLUDED	FOOD	INCLUDED	EXCLUDED
Artificial sweeteners 1 serving per day	Stevia products	Aspartame, saccharine	Nuts Up to 2 servings per day	Raw, include almonds, cashews, pecans, pumpkin seeds, sunflower seeds, soy nuts, walnuts	All others, including processed
Beverages (other than water) Ad lib	Herbal teas	Soda (Regular/Diet) Fruit drinks Fruit juices Alcohol	Oils (cold pressed Extra Virgin) 2 servings per day,	Borage oil Fish oils Flax seed oil Hemp oil Olive oil Primrose oil Sesame oil	Hydrogenated oils, peanut oil
Dairy products Up to 1-2 servings per day	All organic cow's milk products esp. yogurt, cream, butter, cheeses (if tolerated)	Non-organic products, all margarines, butter substitutes	Soy/Soy products 2 servinigs per day	Any without added sugar Soy milk, soy cheese, soy Spreads, misu, tofu,	All with added sugar
Eggs Up to 1-2 servings per day	Organic, fresh, include yolks	Egg substitute products	Sugar	None	All sugar containing products Including fructose, glucose, Dextrose, maltose, and any other forms of sugar
Fish At least 3 times per per week	Bass Cod Haddock Halibut Salmon Sardine Sole Trout Tuna	All Others	Vegetables (Organic) 4 servings per day	All, especially: Asparagus Beets Broccoli Brussels Sprouts Cabbage Carrots Cauliflower Green leafy vegetables Onions Peppers Pumpkin Sprouts Tomato Yams	None
Fruits* 1 Serving per day	Apples Apricot Berries Cantaloupe Cherries Fig Grapefruit Kiwi Lemon Lime Oranges Pears	All others			
Grains* (whole unprocessed) 1 serving per day	Amaranth Barley Buckwheat Ezekiel bread Flax Millet Oats Rice Rye Spelt wheat	Refined white flour processed and all others	Vinegar/Salad dressings	Low carbohydrate brands Apple cider vinegar, Vinegar and oil	High carbohydrate brands, Sweetened dressings
			Water Ad lib At least 48 ounces per day	Bottle or filtered	Tap water
Legumes* 1 serving per week	Black-eyed peas Garbanzo beans Kidney beans Lentils Navy beans Pinto beans Soybeans Split peas	All others	Miscellaneous Ad lib	Bee pollen Brewer's Yeast Cayenne Cinnamon Curry Garlic Ginger Green Tea Kelp Mustard Salsa Spirulina Wheat germ	
Meats Up to 3 servings per day	Organic, no chemicals added	All others including processed			

> "Every time we eat, we vote. Eat fresh, eat local, eat unprocessed!"
>
> –Valerie Metzger, Pumpkin Hollow Farm, North Manchester, IN

* Amounts consumed per day will depend on the person's glucose tolerance.

Serving sizes: 1 serving of fruits, vegetables, and grains = ½ cup, 1 serving of meat, fish = 4 ounces, 1 serving of oil = 1 tablespoon 1 serving of nuts = 1 ounce

Reversing Cancer Physiology with Nutriceuticals:
Dr. Hauser's Top 25

The most important aspect of care for a cancer patient is to make sure he or she is receiving a treatment that has potent cancer-killing ability. For safety and efficacy, the treatment that makes the most sense is Insulin Potentiation Therapy (IPT). IPT has the potency to cause rapid tumor shrinkage while keeping the person healthy.

To help keep the person healthy while undergoing IPT, some physicians recommend nutriceuticals. These are herbal substances (nutri) that have a standardized potency (-ceutical), thus the term *nutriceutical*. Many of the physicians who utilize IPT in their practices are experienced natural medicine doctors; they utilize a wide variety of herbal remedies and interventional natural medicine techniques for their patients. Every doctor has certain substances or medications that he or she uses. This appendix describes Dr Hauser's top 25.* They are no in particular order, but be assured that no one at Caring Medical gets prescribed *all* 25.

FLAV MAX

Flav Max is a soy isoflavone concentrate. Each capsule has 100 mg of Novasoy Isoflavones and 55 mg of Lignans from flax seeds. For those cancer patients who don't want to eat of lot of soy, this is a good substitute.

DIM

DIM takes a comprehensive approach to reversing the physiology of estrogen-driven cancers. It contains diindolylmethane which is one of the substances that helps the 2-hydroxylation of estradiol. This product is a must for women with a female cancer or those desiring to prevent a female cancer.

ONCOGUARD

It is always best to prevent cancers from recurring or, better yet, not to start in the first place. Onco Guard has substances that do just that, including lycopene, green tea extract (catechins), propolis, resveratrol, modified citrus pectin, and red raspberry extract (ellagic acid).

BROMELAIN MAX

Bromelains are proteolytic enzymes derived from the Hawaiian pineapple, *Ananas comosus*. Bromelains can inhibit edema formation. Bromelains cause depolymerization of fibrin and possibly other proteinaceous material, which can increase permeability and enhance the drainage. Bromelain does not have an effect on normal clotting, because it acts on fibrin and not on fibrinogen. Bromelain Max is used to decrease the cancer clotting coat.

ENTEROSIN

Enterosin contains ingredients that aid in apoptosis or cancer- cell death. These include berberine, inositol hexaphosphate, bupleurum chinese Scutellaria baicalensis, burdock root, and more quercetin and soy isoflavones.

CHEMORX

Chemotherapy can have some brutal side effects. Chemorx helps prevent the side effects. It

---

* *Dr Hauser serves as a medical consultants to Beulah Land Nutritionals, for which he receives a stipend. Because he helped to develop some of the products listed, he receives royalties from these products. To view the actual ingredients and further descriptions of the products, go to www.benuts.com. A catalog of the full line of products available through Beulah Land Nutritionals is available free of charge by calling 1-877-RX-BEULAH.*

does so because of the herbal substances that compose it, including ashwagandha, aloe vera, astragalus, eclipta, rabdosia, alpha lipoic acid, and various mushroom extracts.

ENZYME-MAX

No cancer regime would be complete without a potent enzyme combination. Vasuzyme contains very potent combinations of enzymes that are used to decrease inflammation, decrease platelet stickiness, and hopefully enhance immune system and chemotherapy penetration to cancer cells. This product is also helpful for relieving cancer pain.

SUPERFOOD

Superfood is one of Dr Hauser's favorite products. It contains many different kinds of organic vegetable and herbal substances, including spirulina, blue green algae, chlorella, alfalfa, and many others. This is his preferred green drink. Mix two tablespoons in water. For the cancer patient with problems digesting or swallowing capsules, this is a great alternative.

PRO FIBER E.F.A.

One of the concerns of the cancer patient is constipation and toxicity. Pro Fiber E.F.A. has complete proteins, dietary fibers, essentially fatty acids, and fructo-oligosaccharides from seeds, nuts, grains, and beans. Its contents include Jerusalem artichoke, organic fennel seed, sprouted Quinoa, spelt, ground flax, amaranth, and many others. Like Superfood, two tablespoons are mixed in water. This product helps keep the bowels moving, thus removing toxicity.

ALOE MASTER

Aloe Master is a very concentrated extract of whole leaf aloe vera. It is full of mucopolysaccharides, which have immune-boosting activity. Aloe has anti-inflammatory, anti-tumor, and antiangiogenetic activity and inhibits platelet aggregation.

STIMMUNE

This immune system-stimulating supplement that is offered by Beulah Land Nutritionals contains several potent ingredients, including aloe vera, olive leaf extract, and Arabinogalactin. Keeping your immune system strong is important as a person battles cancer.

COLLOIDAL EXCELLENCE

Colloidal Excellence is soft rock phosphate. It is excellent at relieving cancer bone pain. It also has some alkalinizing properties. It contains over 60 minerals in colloidal form for easy absorbability.

VITAMIN D3

Vitamin D3, because of its potency, needs a doctor's prescription. Each capsule contains 5000 IU of vitamin D. It has numerous activities, including inducing the differentiation of certain tumor cell lines, preventing certain cancers from forming, inducing apoptosis, inhibiting angiogenesis, and specific anti-tumor activity. Because of its high potency, it has to be prescribed and monitored by a doctor.

MELATONIN

Cancer is perhaps the biggest stressor that can hit a person. As such, sleep is affected. One of the best natural sleep agents is the natural hormone that helps people sleep, melatonin. Melatonin also has some immune stimulatory effects, antiestrogen activity, and some specific anticancer effects.

GERMANIUM

Dr. Hauser is perhaps one of the last doctors to use this interesting trace mineral. Germanium sesquioxide at high doses has some direct anti-tumor activity, as shown from research from Japan. It appears to be an enzyme inhibitor for a certain step or steps in the (anaerobic) glycolysis sequence.

MARROW PLUS

Marrow Plus is a great Chinese herbal product with many ingredients, including milletia, which has been shown to increase white blood cell counts and counteract cachexia. The product also contains codonopsis which, in particular, is used in China to treat patients with low white blood cell counts due to radiation or chemotherapy; it is also administered to increase red blood cell counts. There are numerous other immune- and organ-strengthening herbal remedies in this product. It is especially useful for the patient receiving chemotherapy.

EZZEAC PLUS

Ezzeac Plus is a tea composed of burdock root, sheep sorrel, slippery elm bark, cats claw, and many other herbs. The combination has a potent detoxification and immune stimulatory effect.

UNIQUE E

Although hard to believe, high-dose natural vitamin E is one of my favorite natural substances for cancer patients. Unique E is unique in that it is natural vitamin E with alpha, beta, gamma, and delta tocopherols in high dose. It is a wonderful blood thinner, helping reverse the coagulopathy of cancer or chemotherapy. Some studies have shown that vitamin E inhibits neoplastic cell growth and mutagenic activity, stimulates immune system activity, and modulates prostaglandin biosynthesis.

DMSO

Cancer often causes significant swelling and pain. For many, a substantial reduction of these complaints can be achieved by simply rubbing DMSO (dimethyl sulfoxide) liquid on the cancerous area.

STOMACH SUPPORT FORMULA
(STM ENZYME)

STM Enzyme contains papaya leaf, marshmallow root, slippery elm, and other substances that substantially help the stomach. Nausea, vomiting, and stomach pain are some of the possible effects of cancer and cancer therapies. A great method of relieving these symptoms is with this stomach support formula.

SMALL INTESTINE SUPPORT FORMULA
(SMI ENZYME)

Cancer physiology and fungus physiology are very similar. Fungus infection is a real threat to the cancer patient. SMI Enzyme is a concentrated powder of cellulase and various probiotics to keep the bowels clear of fungus infection while the cancer patient is being treated.

POLY-MVA *

Poly-MVA is a man-made molecule that contains palladium, B vitamins, and lipoic acid. The compound is soluble in both water and fat. It can easily and safely travel throughout the body and into every cell, crossing the blood-brain barrier as well. The substance acts as a nucleotide reductase, powerful antioxidant, and an intracellular electron donor. It has some direct "chemotherapeutic" (cancer cell killing) effects.

PHYTO CARROTS

What better combination for the cancer patient than organic carrot juice concentrate, sprouted soybeans, and other organic ingredients. To mix up a tasty drink, combine two tablespoons with water.

FLAX SEED OIL

Flax seed and flax seed oil contain lignans and other substances with strong anti-cancer properties. They have the additional benefit of helping decrease platelet-stickiness (which is another attribute of cancer physiology).

AMYGDALINE *

Also known as Laetrile, this is the most famous of all the alternative medicine products. Amygdaline is a natural product from apricot kernels. It is available from Mexican sources in tablet form. ■

* These products are not available at Beulah Land Nutritionals.

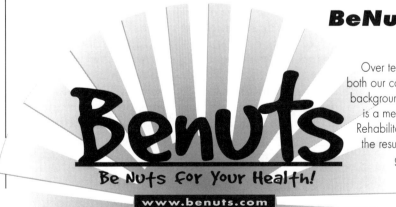

APPENDIX C

Insulin Potentiation Therapy: 25 Case Studies

Insulin Potentiation Therapy (IPT) has been healing people since its first patient, the originator himself, Donato Pérez García, MD, was treated in 1926. Like many natural therapies, large amounts of research dollars have not been put into Insulin Potentiation Therapy, primarily because it uses common medications that are available in generic form. The best evidence that we have that it works is from the patients who have been treated. Consider this e-mail I received from a natural medicine colleague, Dr. Carolyn Bormann. (See **Figure C-1**.) This appendix is a sampling from the archives of the practices of the Garciá family of physicians (Donato 1, 2, and 3) and Ross Hauser, MD. For additional case histories of patients treated successfully with IPT, please see www.IPTQ.org.

IPT CASE HISTORIES FROM DONATO 1, 2, AND 3

1. METASTATIC LUNG CANCER— FAILED PREVIOUS RADIOTHERAPY

A 40-year-old male was seen initially on March 3, 1953, with a history of pulmonary carcinoma in both the right and left lungs and the neck lymph nodes. The patient had been treated previously with radiotherapy. By the time he came for an IPT evaluation, he had severe pain, shortness of breath, cough, poor appetite, and a 50-pound weight loss.

He received a total of 25 sessions of IPT, one per week for six months. On October 15, 1953, he was released as cured.

2. MALIGNANT MELANOMA

A 58-year-old male was seen initially on January 6, 1971, because of a 11- by 7-cm mass on his left side by his pelvis. It had a foul odor, and many secretions were coming from it. It was found to be malignant melanoma.

He received a total of 14 sessions of IPT, one per week. Three and a half months later, the patient was released, totally cured.

3. CERVICAL CANCER—FAILED COBALT THERAPY

A 29-year-old female was first seen for IPT on August 1, 1964. Her cancer had continued to grow

FROM: C.Bormann, N.D.,C.P.
Sent: Saturday, August 18, 2001 10:58 AM
To: Dr. Ross Hauser
Subject: Patients' Experience with IPT

Thanks for you input and support...sounds wonderfully effective...
Carolyn Bormann

Hi Carolyn--I got back from TJ yesterday. It was an interesting treatment.

Afterward, it was like waking up from a fever induced coma. You're all wet and disoriented, and you wander around like you're stoned for three or four hours after. He didn't let us eat anything since supper the night before; then after the treatment all he lets you eat is a fruit bowl and maybe some soup. (Which is ok 'cause you don't feel much like eating anyway.) I crashed about 5 o'clock. The next day I felt fine, no side effects, except not being able to eat any meat. Everyone said that the swelling in my hand looked significant less. It felt a lot softer and was a bit easier to move. My lungs felt better when I took a deep breath, and the tumor under my arm seems to have shrunken about 10 to 15%. There were seven of us receiving treatments.

Everyone had some significant improvement right after. One guy who has Lou Gerig's disease was speaking quite plainly, and everyone could understand him after the treatment.

Another woman that has lung cancer, I noticed that she looked about 70 years old when I first saw her at the airport. After the treatment, she looked like she had put on 10 lbs (that she needed), her skin was pink instead of gray, and she looked healthy. All the while, Donato was preparing formulas and doing the treatments.

Dr. Bergdorf was watching him like a hawk to make sure he wasn't doing anything funny. She questioned everything, and said he held back nothing. He answered every question, gave complete and acceptable explanations for everything he did. Donato is kind of like a stand-up comic who was forced to be a doctor. He made the whole experience fun. I think it was well worth the trip.

I wanted to thank you for your concern about this. It was an interesting experience, traveling with seven women. So Marietta is planning another treatment for all of us in her clinic here in Bountiful, next Friday. I'm curious to see how much she plans to charge, since she doesn't have the connections to get the three different chemo drugs used for the cocktail in these treatments.

Thanks, Klaus

Figure C-1

despite 42 sessions of cobalt therapy. She was noted to have an ulcerated cervix on physical examination.

She received a total of seven sessions of IPT, one per week. On March 12, 1965, she was examined, and her cervix was found to be completely healthy. On March 14, 1965, a pap smear and physical examination done by her previous gynecologist were completely normal.

4. METASTASIS FROM BREAST CANCER— PREVIOUS MASTECTOMY

A 65-year-old female was first evaluated for IPT on February 11, 1970. She had a previous right mastectomy, but her cancer recurred in the lymph nodes on that side, as evidenced by pain and swelling in the axilla.

She underwent eight sessions of IPT, administered one per week. The patient was released as cured from care on July 1, 1970; the tumor, pain, and swelling having disappeared.

5. PROSTATE CANCER

On June 25, 1966, a 77-year-old male was seen for IPT evaluation because of an inability to urinate and blood in the urine. He was found to have a prostate cancer tumor that had grown to the size of a lemon.

He received a total of 22 IPT treatments, one per week. On February 22, 1967, he was released as cured.

6. METASTATIC BREAST CANCER TO THE BONES— FAILED PREVIOUS MASTECTOMY, OVARY REMOVAL, AND RADIATION THERAPY

On February 17, 1963, a very sick 52-year-old female was seen for an IPT evaluation. She had a total mastectomy 20 months earlier. After the operation, she suffered from severe pain in the scapula, thoracolumbar area, and the left half of the pelvis, where breast metastases were found. Her ovaries were then removed, and she was given a total of 10 sessions of radiotherapy. The patient did not improve, and her doctor said nothing more could be done to help her. She was given a prognosis of a few weeks to live. A biopsy at the bony metastases revealed an undifferentiated epidermoid carcinoma. By the time she was seen for IPT, she had lost 40 pounds from her previous average weight (she now weighed 110 pounds). She appeared emaciated.

From February 19 to May 19, 1963, 10 sessions of IPT were given. A series of x-rays was performed after IPT that showed no evidence of osteolytic lesions. She weighed 69 kg or 150 pounds on discharge.

7. TESTICULAR CANCER

On July 16, 1961, a 60-year-old male was seen because of a mass in his testicle the size of an orange. He had excruciating pain and weighed 40 kg (88 pounds), whereas two months prior he weighed 84 kg (190 pounds). He was found to have a seminoma of the left testicle, with metastasis to the corresponding lymph nodes.

He was given seven sessions of IPT. After the second session, there was marked improvement, with substantial reduction in the size of the tumor. On October 23, the patient was released; all signs and symptoms had completely disappeared.

8. CHRONIC LYMPHOCYTIC LYMPHOMA

A 70-year-old female came in for an IPT evaluation on April 23, 1971, because of recurrence of a chronic lymphocytic lymphoma affecting the face. It had previously been treated by surgery. The patient had a tumor the size of a walnut in the region of the left cheek. It was producing a foul smelling, creamy yellow liquid. There were also swollen lymph nodes in the neck.

She received a total of 10 sessions of IPT, one per week. She was released on July 10, 1971. She subsequently had a biopsy of the area after IPT, and the results were negative.

9. THYROID CANCER—RECURRENCE AFTER SURGERY AND RADIATION THERAPY

On April 30, 1962, a 52-year-old female was seen because of severe pain, inability to chew, and difficulty speaking and swallowing because of a thyroid carcinoma. She had lost 22 pounds in the previous three months. The cancer was previously treated with surgery and high-dosage radiation therapy. Despite these therapies, her condition worsened, and she was considered incurable by her doctors.

She received a total of 20 sessions of IPT, from May 1 to July 31, 1963. From the 15th treatment on, the patient complained of no discomfort; the tumor had disappeared. On completion of the treatment, the patient was released, totally cured.

10. STOMACH CANCER

Because of complete anorexia, continuous piercing pain in the epigastrium (stomach area), nausea, and vomiting, a 67-year-old female sought medical care, at which time gastric carcinoma was diagnosed. She decided to use IPT as her primary treatment modality.

The first treatment was given on June 8, 1972. As a result of this treatment, the pain in her stomach and the vomiting disappeared. After the fifth treatment, the patient recovered her appetite. She received a total of 11 sessions of IPT, and radiographic studies of her gastroduodenal area (stomach and part of the small intestine) afterward were normal. She was released on August 30, 1972, totally cured.

11. METASTATIC EWING'S SARCOMA

The mother of a three-year-old reported that her daughter, according to her pediatrician, had a Colles' wrist fracture that did not improve with a cast. The area was biopsied, and she was found to have Ewing's sarcoma. The destruction of the bone was becoming more aggressive, with metastases to the larger bones. The patient had also lost nine pounds and had obvious pain and swelling in her left wrist. The girl was presumed incurable, so she was evaluated on August 18, 1970, for IPT. On examination, it was found that the cancer had spread to many lymph nodes in her neck.

She was given 17 sessions of IPT over a period of several months. The first treatment was given on August 18, 1970. The result of this treatment was that the pain and edema in her hand were diminished. By the fourth treatment, the edema in her forearm was completely gone. After the eighth session, the intense pain in the left wrist had disappeared completely. After the 12th session, the girl showed no problems with her left wrist or forearm. On February 12, 1971, x-rays were taken of the patient's whole skeleton. All bones were normal. She was released as cured. She was followed for eight more years; the case was still totally cured.

12. ADENOCARCINOMA OF THE GALL BLADDER

A 55-year-old female underwent a cholecystectomy (removal of the gallbladder) on April 10, 1964, because of intense nausea and jaundice. The pathology came back as infiltrating adenocarcinoma of the gallbladder and cholelithiasis (gall-stones). After the operation, her whole body jaundice continued. She had intense pain, continuous fever, edema in both legs, nausea, vomiting, and looked cachectic when she was seen for IPT evaluation on June 8, 1964. On physical examination, her liver and spleen were markedly enlarged.

She was given five sessions of IPT, every three days. Twenty-one days after starting, her liver function tests were completely normal, and her jaundice had resolved. She was discharged as cured.

13. CANCER OF THE PANCREAS

A 64-year-old female developed a yellow discoloration in her eyes in September 1986. A CT (computed tomography) scan shortly thereafter revealed a mass in the head of the pancreas that was obstructing one of her bile ducts. She had a Whipple surgical procedure performed, which confirmed adenocarcinoma of the pancreas. In January 1987, she was first evaluated for IPT because of continued nausea, poor appetite, jaundice, and a weight loss of 27 pounds. Physical examination revealed a tender mass palpable in the epigastrium (pancreas).

She had a total of 18 IPT treatments. Throughout the treatment, she began to get her appetite back, eventually regaining all of her weight. Her jaundice completely cleared. Her last treatment was on October 2, 1987. She was in good health until the age of 74 when she died of unrelated causes.

14. SMALL CELL LUNG CANCER

A 46-year-old nonsmoking female developed a pain in her shoulder that radiated down her arm. She had a CT scan on August 22, 1992, which revealed a left upper lobe lung nodule that was 30 mm × 31 mm. A bronchoscopy with biopsy revealed small cell adenocarcinoma of the lung. Her doctor told her that she could extend her life by two years if she underwent surgery to remove half of her lung.

On hearing her various options, the patient decided to use IPT as her primary treatment. Her first treatment was on September 11, 1992, and was effective at getting rid of her pain. The first eight IPT treatments were given once a week. She received a total of 22 treatments of IPT. Regular follow-up visits with x-rays documented progressive improvement in her lung lesion. Her most recent chest x-ray in December, 1998 reported no visible radiologic signs of disease. In the spring of 1999, her CT scan showed no signs of cancer. Her last visit in March 2001 noted that she was surviving with a good state of health.

15. BREAST CANCER WITH METASTASES

In 1996, a 44-year-old female noticed some fatigue and exhaustion. This progressed to some lower back, hip, and upper leg pain. In July 1997, she noticed a sudden change in her breast. She felt a thickening from the breast to her collarbone. A biopsy revealed her worst fear—breast cancer. The tumor mass was 3.9 cm in diameter. She was advised to get a mastectomy with chemotherapy and radiation therapy. If she did not get the treatment, her physicians told her she had "less than a year." She heard about IPT and decided it was the treatment for her.

In September 1997, she started IPT. Even with her first treatment, she felt more energy and strength. She received three treatments within the first week and then two every week thereafter for the next three and a half months. From January through May 1998, she had one treatment per month, resulting in a total of 23 treatments. Follow-up testing with mammography, CT scans, bone scans, and blood tests revealed her to be cancer free. She enjoys good health as of September 2001. She notes, "I never lost any hair. In fact, my hair grew thicker. Thicker than it has been in at least 25 years. I am healthier today than I have been in 25 years, as well."

IPT CASE HISTORIES FROM ROSS A. HAUSER

16. METASTATIC CANCER WITH UNKNOWN ORIGIN

In March 2000, a 49-year-old male came to the office with severe upper back pain. He was desiring Prolotherapy since this helped heal his lower back in the past. Because he had no precipitating event, a chest x-ray was ordered. This showed pulmonary nodules throughout both lung fields. A subsequent CT scan of the thorax and abdomen revealed bilateral lung nodules, as well as multiple ill-defined, low-density lesions in the left lobe of the liver. All signs pointed to metastatic cancer. A bone scan was done and showed metastatic lesions in both femurs. After testing, the patient was given the option of going to an oncologist and possibly having one of the lesions biopsied to find

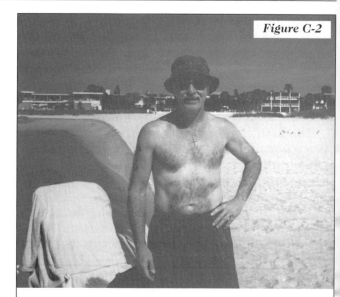

Figure C-2

Dr. Ross Hauser
Caring Medical & Rehabilitation Services, S.C.
715 Lake St. #600
Oak Park, Il. 60301

June 26, 2000

Dear Dr. Hauser,

First, let me state that the name of your facility Caring Medical fits the attitude of your entire staff. Everyone that I've had contact with has been friendly and very helpful.

I have been treated at Caring Medical for for various ailments since about 1995, all successfully. In January of this year I went to Caring Medical for pain in my lower back that. I had this problem for a couple of months. Nothing was discovered so an xray was ordered. After that I had a CT scan. I returned to Caring Medical for the results. I was informed that I had metastatic cancer of the lungs. We discussed and agreed on IPT chemo therapy along with various supplements. After a couple of treatments the results of the CT scan were back. They indicated that I had cancer in the liver and the thigh bone.

In an effort to discover the source of the cancer I went to Midwest Cancer Treatment Center in Zion, Il. This was in mid March. I met with Dr. Sanchez after he reviewed the the xrays, scans, and treatment I had been receiving. He was critcal of the IPT treatment and said that even with high dose chemo my chances for survival were poor. I then went though a battery of tests while there and had a biopsy of the lymph nodes the following week.

Dr. Sanchez called on Good Friday and informed me that I did not have cancer in the lymph nodes or in the liver. He said the bone cancer if any was to small to even biopsy. As far as the lung cancer goes, he could not say that what still showed on the tests was cancer . He concluded by saying that whatever I was doing I should keep it up and call for followup tests in three months. Needless to say it was a joyess Easter .

I concluded the ten weeks of IPT treatment in early June. I then had another series of tests done. I returned to Caring Medical on June 22, 2000 to review the tests. No cancer was showing on the tests. I give praise and thanks to the Lord for my healing. I thank the many people who prayed for me. And finally I thank Dr. Hauser whom God is using in a mighty way. I would urge people to take charge of their own health and to seek alternative healing whenever possible.

Dan Weigand
Oak Lawn, Il.

Metastatic Cancer Survivor, Dan Weigand
Dan Weigand received ten IPT sessions for liver and lung metastases. What does he do now? His picture above speaks for itself.

out exactly what cancer it was. He refused and desired to get IPT since he knew the oncologist would recommend high-dose chemotherapy. (See **Figure C-2.**)

He immediately started receiving weekly IPT treatments. After three treatments, his pain was eliminated. On the fifth visit, he came with his wife who was irate. "How dare you treat my husband. You are not an oncologist, and he doesn't even have a diagnosis of what kind of cancer it is." I (Ross) suggested that because of the wife's insistence that they get an oncology opinion. About a week later he called, "When they reviewed my scans, they said my prognosis was poor. Immediately they wanted to do traditional chemotherapy but weren't optimistic of the outcome. I insisted they rescan me. They came back amazed. The cancer is 90% gone. They said whatever you are doing, keep doing it." He received a total of 10 IPT treatments. He has no evidence of cancer. He enjoys good health to this date. What does his wife think? "Doctor you need to have flashing lights outside your building that says, 'Cure for Cancer Here!'"

17. METASTATIC KIDNEY CANCER

A very sick-looking 56-year-old woman came into Caring Medical in July 2001. She had been diagnosed with a large, left kidney tumor with metastases to the liver and lung. She was losing weight daily and had increasing shortness of breath and fatigue. She was diagnosed with renal cell carcinoma, though a biopsy was never done due to the risk of her bleeding during the procedure. She was born with only one kidney, so surgery was too risky. Her doctors at the university medical center gave her a grim prognosis and said that she should get hospice care at home until the "final days." She had renewed hope when she found out about IPT.

Her first IPT treatment was on July 6. She felt great after the first treatment. Her appetite increased, and her pain decreased. After her third treatment, her back pain was almost all gone, and she was able to go shopping at the mall with her husband. However, after the third treatment, she was admitted to a local hospital because of an infection. A repeat CT scan showed that the kidney tumor had shrunk by 50%. Her oncologist could not believe that the tumor had shrunk, so she was transferred to the university hospital. The oncologist at the teaching hospital told her to stop the "natural" treatment being done and any additional testing and wait and see if the kidney tumor would re-grow. He said that because the

tumor shrunk, it must not be cancerous. Not waiting to find out, she continued IPT for a total of 10 treatments, about one treatment every two weeks. Repeat CT scans are completely negative. She has gained all of her weight back and as of February 2002, she enjoys good health.

18. GASTRIC CANCER

For seven months, a 58-year-old white female complained of stomach discomfort. Despite medications and various treatments, it grew worse. Her appetite started to become poor, and she lost weight. Eventually, she had an endoscopic ultrasound, which revealed a tumor mass in the stomach. She underwent laparoscopy, where a biopsy revealed poorly differentiated adenocarcinoma of the stomach with metastases to the surrounding tissues. Her oncologist recommended surgery, radiation, and high-dose chemotherapy. She sought the advice of a natural medicine doctor in New York, who recommended she come to Caring Medical for IPT.

Her first visit to Caring Medical was on June 27, 2001, where her presenting symptoms were severe nausea, inability to eat solid food, drinking some liquid but only a sip at a time, weakness, and abdominal discomfort. IPT treatment was started the next day. She agreed to do the treatments twice a week. After three IPT treatments, she could drink more liquid without becoming nauseated. On the seventh treatment, her CA 19-9 cancer marker was down from 330 to 78. She was also tolerating solid food by this time and starting to gain weight. Her abdominal discomfort was completely gone. The last of her 12 IPT treatments was on August 28, 2001. She went back to New York and repeat CT scans, endoscopy, and blood markers were better, except a small area in the small intestine. Biopsies of the area were negative, but because the area (according to the endoscopist) did not look normal, six more IPT treatments were done. A PET scan at this time revealed a small area of residual tumor. This was treated with hyperthermia and localized radiation therapy. In March, 2002, she had a PET Scan showing no signs of cancer.

19. METASTATIC LUNG CANCER

In 1999, a 68-year-old retired male was diagnosed with high blood pressure and high cholesterol and was having shortness of breath. He was a two pack per day smoker for 50 years but had quit four years earlier. In March 2001, he noticed a lump on the left side of his neck. The lump continued to grow. He went to an emergency room, where they found his blood sugar to be 319. The chest x-ray identified a rounded 2.5-cm density in the left upper lobe with ill-defined borders. A CT scan showed an irregularly shaped mass measuring 2.0 cm × 3.7 cm in the left upper lobe. The findings were suspicious for a primary lung region and questionably metastasized to the mediastinum. Five days later, he had a bronchoscopy with biopsy. The diagnosis was poorly differentiated adenocarcinoma. He was not a surgical candidate. This patient was not about to get high-dose chemotherapy, so on a friend's recommendation, he came to Caring Medical for cancer therapy.

After examination, he was found to have an extensive mass on the left side of his neck. It was tremendously painful, and he was starting to take hydrocodone. He was experiencing significant shortness of breath on exertion. He began IPT on March 27, 2001. Because of his blood sugars, he was placed on Glucophage (an oral diabetes medication) and a high-protein diet. He was taken off the narcotic because of its immunosuppressive effects. After the third treatment, his neck pain was gone, and there was a noticeable softening of the left neck mass. Visible shrinkage occurred after the fifth treatment. After six IPT treatments, CT scans showed a shrinkage of 50% in tumor size. His lymph node involvement was almost gone. He sought a surgical consultation to decide if he was now a surgical candidate. The surgeon called me (Ross) and said, "You are this guy's only chance. Whatever you are doing, keep doing it." He had six more IPT treatments. A repeat CT scan of the lungs and neck area were clear of tumor. As of December 2001, he enjoys good health.

We wish this was the case history. Unfortunately, this individual did not get the last six IPT treatments. His insurance company would only pay for high-dose chemotherapy, so he elected to switch to that, after his initial great response with IPT. You know the rest of the story . . . High-dose chemotherapy devastated his immune system. The cancer spread and he is not doing well.

20. LARGE PRIMARY BREAST TUMOR

In February 2001, a 58-year-old woman came to Caring Medical because of a large primary breast tumor. The tumor was located in the left breast and measured 10 cm × 8 cm. She refused surgery and an oncology consultation, exclaiming, "Doctor, I am going to trust God and trust you." I (Ross) was hoping she would do it in that order. One of her cancer markers, CA-125, was markedly elevated at 419 (normal is under 37).

She started IPT on March 1, 2001, once per week for 10 weeks. After the fourth treatment, she noted that her breast did not feel as heavy. The tumor, by palpation, appeared to shrink as well. Her CA-125 cancer marker was also down to 185. By the 10th treatment, the mass was no longer palpable. She had a breast MRI (magnetic resonance imaging) scan done at this time, and it showed complete resolution of the mass. Because one of her cancer markers, CA-125, was still elevated at 60, four more IPT treatments were done. After this, the CA-125 went into the normal range. As of follow-up in February 2002, she enjoys good health and is apparently cancer free. (See **Figure C-3**.)

21. RECURRENT BREAST CANCER

A 53-year-old female was diagnosed with breast cancer five years ago (1997). She under-

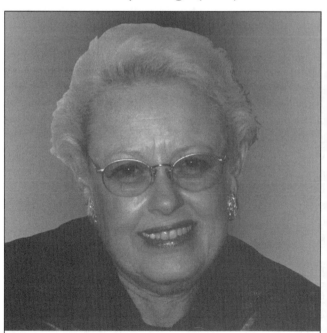

Figure C-3: Betty Jo Davis, February, 2002

Betty Jo decided to take charge of her health, electing to use IPT to treat her large breast tumor (10 cm x 8 cm). IPT helped her save her breast and her life.

Figure C-4

March 29, 2001

Dear Dr. Hauser,

I am writing you let you know of the most recent news with my biopsy. It came back negative. I cannot tell you how happy I am. The physicians thought that I was crazy for wanting to try IPT for treating my cancer but now that they've seen the results they want to know more about it. I couldn't bear to continue with chemotherapy the way I was before I came to Caring Medical. For 2 or 3 days after the chemo I wouldn't feel well, even though they gave me anti-nausea medicine. I would get hemorrhoids and the skin on the soles of my feet began to burn off. I had lost all of my hair, including my eyelashes and had to wear a wig for 6 months and waited another 6 months for my hair to grow back. I really couldn't believe that something that was supposed to save your life could make you so miserable. As you know even after the six months of chemotherapy the cancer still recurred and a masectomy was recommended. I was so happy when I found out about IPT.

All I can say is "it worked." I had NO side effects with IPT physically which definitely made things better for me emotionally. I was very comfortable during the procedure and came out of the hypoglycemic state rapidly. IPT is so much simpler on a patient than chemotherapy. Richard and I have already referred many people to your office for IPT and will continue to support it. After being through both I can say that I wish I would have found IPT first to save my family and me a lot of grief. Thank you for helping save my breast but more importantly my life.

With much gratitude,

Judith Meldahl

Judith Meldahl

22. PROSTATE CANCER, GLEASON SCORE OF EIGHT, PSA 66

In September 2001, a 72 year-old gentleman came to Caring Medical for a second opinion concerning his poorly differentiated adenocarcinoma of the prostate diagnosed via biopsy. His bone scan, CT Scan, and other x-ray studies were normal. He had a PSA of 66.6 and a Gleason Score of eight on the biopsy suggestive of advanced disease beyond the prostate. He had several previous opinions that ranged from aggressive local treatment including radical prostatectomy, radiation therapy, to androgen blockage either with bilateral orchiectomy (removal of both testis) or Lupron therapy. None of these options seemed appealing so he started Insulin Potentiation Therapy once per week.

By the third treatment he noted that his urinary stream was much stronger suggestive of tumor shrinkage. After the sixth treatment his PSA level was down to 15.6. After 12 IPT treatments, his PSA level was 6.2. He received four more treatments after which follow-up PSA levels which were in normal range. His urologist was amazed as he was cancer free and the treatment was essentially side effect free unlike the treatments he had recommended.

As a side note, this particular patient desired to do intravenous Laetrile as one of the chemotherapy agents during the IPT. The Laetrile I.V. bag was given just after the insulin shot. In addition, his dihydrotestosterone levels were high at the start of treatment so hormonal blockade was also given. Dihydrotestosterone feeds prostate cancer, much in the same way estradiol feeds

went high-dose chemotherapy, a lumpectomy, and follow-up radiation. In August 2000, her breast cancer recurred in the same area. She was scheduled for a mastectomy and more high-dose chemotherapy. A friend recommended that she come to Caring Medical for an IPT evaluation.

In September 2000, she started IPT. She received a total of 10 sessions, each given once per week. At the end of that time, an MRI scan of the breast was done, with a subsequent biopsy of a suspicious area on the MRI. The biopsies were negative. Judy explains her feelings best in the following letter (See **Figure C-4.**)

breast cancer. His platelet aggregation study showed a coagulopathy so he was prescribed some natural blood thinners and the medication coumadin. As of March 2002, he appears to be cancer-free and in good health.

23. METASTATIC BREAST CANCER TO THE BONES AND LUNGS: PREVIOUS CHEMOTHERAPY AND RADIATION THERAPY FAILED

On 9/11/00, a 60 year-old female came to see me (Ross) with her family. She had a left modified mastectomy on June 5, 1998 because of a cancerous lump. The pathology on the mass showed infiltrating ductal carcinoma (5.1 cm) with three of nine axillary lymph nodes containing metastatic carcinoma. She had eight high-dose chemotherapy treatments and 29 radiation treatments. She was admitted to the hospital in the winter of 1999 because of pneumonia. A CT scan of the chest at that time showed that her cancer had come back in the lungs and bones including the left 9th and 12th ribs, thoracic and lumbar vertebrae and right femoral neck. She then had 16 chemotherapy treatments. Her last chemotherapy treatment before the visit to CMRS was on August 8, 2000.

She was taking codeine cough syrup at the time of her first visit. She was also on narcotic pain medication because of severe pain in the chest and upper back. Because of her previous chemotherapy she was left with tingling and numbness in her fingers and toes. Her review of systems showed that she was currently suffering from chronic fatigue, shortness of breath, sinus congestion, recurrent infections, stomach upset, chronic pain, and a myriad of other symptoms. Her latest chest CT scan prior to the first visit to CMRS showed multiple pulmonary metastatic nodules with the largest one being in her right middle lobe, measuring 2 x 2 cm. This test showed a worsening of her mediastinal adenopathy. Thus, her cancer was continuing to grow despite all of the high-dose chemotherapy she had.

Her family definitely wanted her to receive IPT, as the traditional chemotherapy was not working. Her natural medicine regime consisted of many natural supplements that we have discussed in this book. In addition she was prescribed Lamasil to decrease fungal load, Glucophage to keep her blood glucose levels

down, Femara (later switched to Arimidex) to lower her estrogen levels, Coumadin to thin her blood, low dose Naltrexone to stimulate her immunity (prescribed after she was off of narcotic medications), and low dose Cytoxan, an oral chemotherapy medication.

It was noted on initial testing that her fasting blood sugar was 133 so she was placed on a high protein low carbohydrate diet. She was clearly eating the opposite prior to this. Her initial breast cancer markers in the blood were all negative, so her response to therapy would have to be based on CT scan findings.

Because physically she was going down hill fast it was agreed that she should start Insulin Potentiation Therapy right away. She received a total of 18 treatment sessions from 9/26/00 to 1/23/01. Her CT of the chest after eight IPT treatments indicated a clear shrinking of her metastases or in the words of the radiologist, "clearly decreased in bulkiness from previous." It should be noted that after her second IPT treatment she was not having any more chronic pain so her narcotic medications could be discontinued. Her second CT scan of the chest on 2/11/01 was done after the 18 IPT treatments and this showed continued overall improvement in her lung metastases. There was now no definite evidence of pathologic adenopathy. So clearly the natural medicine program including IPT was working. I desired her to continue with IPT but she and her family clearly wanted to treat her with just the diet and nutritional supplements, as well as the few medications I had prescribed. I agreed to this as long as she received close follow-up. She agreed and has been an ideal patient.

Periodically I have her check her blood sugars at home and for the most part she does a good job at keeping them at 100 or less. Her latest fasting insulin level was 12, I would like it less than 10. She also gets periodic testing for her Coumadin dose (PT/INR test). Every three to four months she gets a chest CT scan. Her last CT scan of the chest and bone scan done in February of 2002 showed continued improvement. Her latest bone scan also is clear of cancer. Her breast cancer markers continue to be negative.

This patient used IPT to control the disease and shrink it substantially and her natural medicine program was then able to rid the body of the rest of the cancer. She, compared to the case above

Mark appears to have wide-spread metastatic melanoma. At this point now, it appears that we have radiologic evidence of metastasis to lung, bone, adrenal glands and multiple abnormalities in the mesentery and a deposit in the pelvis that may actually be involving small bowel. After 12-13 years, it is unlikely this represents a recurrence. He perhaps has a new amelanotic primary melanoma that indeed may be arising in bowel. I think that involvement of the small bowel is the most likely cause for his anemia and occult GI bleeding.

At this point, the prognosis for cure is limited. We would be happy to take over his care, transfusional support would help him symptomatically. Staging investigations will be completed. He will be placed on long-acting and short-acting morphine for control of his pain. Given the GI bleeding, I would probably choose a nonirritating agent like Vioxx over Motrin for control of his fevers which are probably tumor related.

Figure C-5: Oncology Report on Mark's Condition

(Case #19), continued to have close follow-up at Caring Medical. She was watched like a hawk and with continued documentation with CT scans that her cancer was shrinking, it was clear that her natural medicine program without the IPT was enough to kill her cancer cells. One should state clearly that she was fanatical about taking her supplements and eating foods on the Hauser Diet. She also monitored her blood sugars at home and was seen in the office quite frequently to ensure that the natural program was working.

24. METASTATIC MELANOMA: "YOU'LL BE DEAD IN ONE MONTH."

On 10/15/01 a 45 year-old male came in for consultation because of multiple tumors growing on his neck and face. He was diagnosed with melanoma in 1988 after a lesion was removed from his left thigh. He came with metastatic lesions in the shoulder, pelvis, adrenal gland, lungs, hip, neck, face, and recently the melanoma had started to infiltrate his small intestine and he was having rectal bleeding for six weeks. He was told by the oncologist that if he didn't do something he would be dead in one month. He was also told if he did something most likely he would be dead anyway. The prognosis was grim. (See Figure C-5.)

Of interest in this case was that he was taking morphine, Vioxx, ativan, and/or Tylenol #3 for the pain he was having because of the tumors. He had visible and palpable tumors in his face and neck region. He wasted no time as his first IPT treatment was 10/16/01. When he was seen for his third IPT treatment he had noted that the tumors

were already shrinking. He was feeling much better and was off of all pain medication. He stated, "I came here feeling sick now I feel healthy." After his sixth IPT, his cancer markers were within the normal range. He had repeat CT scans after 12 IPT treatments which showed resolution of his 12 nodules in his right lung and the several nodules in his left lung. He also experienced resolution of his adrenal nodules and 4 x 3 cm lobular mass associated with his small bowel that had eroded away part of his left iliac bone. His facial and neck masses also were gone.

He did an excellent job taking his supplements and keeping his insulin and blood sugar levels down with the Hauser Diet. He, like most cancer patients, tested very glucose intolerant initially with his blood sugars going to 190 and insulin levels to 61 with 100 gram glucose load. On subsequent fasting tests he was able to get his insulin levels to the nondetectable level. Mark sent the office a beautiful Christmas card, as one can see he has much to live for. (See Figure C-6.) As of March 2002, he is back to work for the first time. He has incredible energy and feels great!

25. BREAST CANCER: "MASTECTOMY IS YOUR ONLY OPTION"

On 7/31/01, a 56 year white female came to Caring Medical because she knew that mastectomy was not her only option. Her physicians were pushing for this telling her that, "Mastectomy is your only option." She had been diagnosed with breast cancer on June 22, 2001 via biopsy. She had recommended to her surgery, chemotherapy and radiation. Her breast cancer came back estrogen receptor positive and it was noted on her history that she had started Premarin two years prior. Her initial blood breast cancer markers were negative so her response to therapy would be monitored by PET scans.

She was given 10 IPT treatments once per week. Follow-up PET scan showed complete resolution of the breast mass. (See **Figure C-7.**) You see, some people realize that if you have breast cancer, mastectomy is *not* your only option.

SUMMARY

Today, I (Ross) did a phone consultation with a father whose son is dying of brain cancer. He told me he had researched the traditional medicine options, including radiation and high-dose chemotherapy. The physicians told them that this treatment was palliative, not curative. He was looking for options. The option I (Ross) told him was that his son needed IPT. Only IPT had the ability to get the chemotherapy medications across the blood-brain barrier. Surely IPT was compatible with the oral chemotherapy prescribed by the oncologist and radiation therapy that was being done. (He currently had emergency swelling of the brain, so radiation was required.) In other words, IPT could work with the traditional treatments and most likely potentiate their effects. This father and son are real

Figure C-6

To all the staff at Caring Medical,

God has truly blessed us by leading us to you. You have given us hope and have allowed God to heal miraculously through your dedicated work. We continually rejoice! Words fall short of expressing our thanks.

May God bless you all this Christmas season and abundantly throughout the year.

Mark, Patti, Jeff, Steve and Katie
Thanilla

We Rejoice ~ We Rejoice ~ We Rejoice

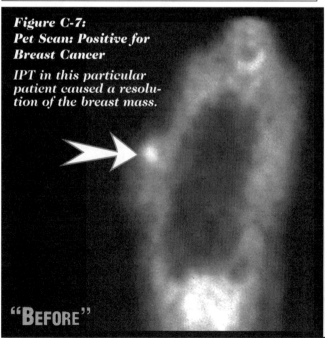

Figure C-7:
Pet Scan: Positive for Breast Cancer

IPT in this particular patient caused a resolution of the breast mass.

"BEFORE"

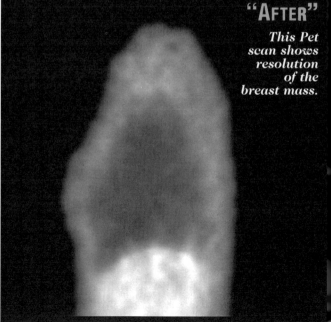

"AFTER"

This Pet scan shows resolution of the breast mass.

people, just like the case studies above. These people have families and are still alive today because of IPT. Just look at them.

Five hundred thousand Americans die each year because of cancer. On September 11, 2001, more than 3,000 Americans died at the hands of terrorist hijackings on three aircraft that toppled several buildings in the World Trade Center and destroyed part of the Pentagon. (A fourth aircraft crashed in a field in Pennsylvania after being hijacked.) Around-the-clock coverage on almost every major network covered the story—as they should. But remember, 150 times that number of casualties occur every year from cancer. The people who died in those aircraft and buildings were real people. Perhaps it has affected us so much because we were able to watch the airplanes explode into the World Trade Center. We saw it over and over again and realized that it could have been us on those aircraft.

On September 10, I (Ross) had flown in three separate airplanes, traveling from Wenatchee, Washington, to Seattle, to Salt Lake City, and finally to Chicago's O'Hare Airport—just one day prior to the hijackings. Yes, it could have been me on one of those planes. So now America sits in fear of terrorism. Well, let me tell you that there is something far more deadly than terrorists that has a 50% chance of taking your life and the lives of your loved ones. You should definitely fear this terrorist, and if it does strike, strike back with IPT. ∎

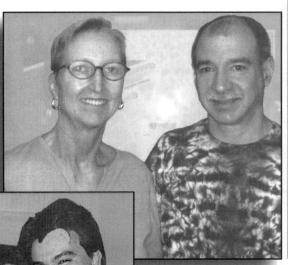

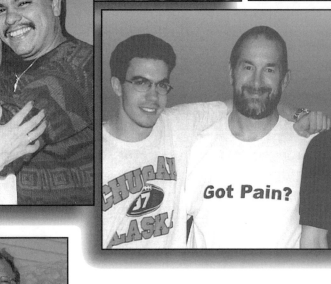

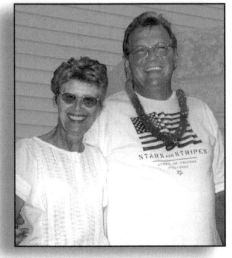

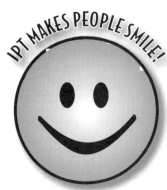

Lives Saved and Changed by IPT:

Left, Brian Guggi poses with his best friend, Michaelene Olson.

Below: Ernie Viano stands with his sons in Alaska, three weeks after treatment.

Middle left, Teresa Miller is gratefully hugged by her son.

Lower left, Betty and Mike Yaun. Betty was told to get her affairs in order. She did just that—heading to get IPT treatments for her kidney cancer. IPT got rid of her cancer.

IPT MAKES PEOPLE SMILE!

IPT and Insurance

In the August 12, 1933, edition of the *Journal of the American Medical Association,* there was an editorial opinion on the use of hydrochloric acid injections, in which the noted beneficial effects of the acid were said to be figments of the imagination. The acid injections were said to hemolyze (burst) red cells and create inflammatory reactions. All reputable physicians were advised under no circumstances to give an injection of a drug so dangerous. The writer offered no evidence of any kind for this adverse opinion. He made no claim to have ever seen an injection of hydrochloric acid given to a single individual. Thus, hydrochloric acid injections never caught on as a medical treatment and are only done by a handful of natural medicine physicians. A similar story could be told about Prolotherapy; Insulin Potentiation Therapy (IPT); and various other safe, remarkable, and powerful therapies.

What does this have to do with insurance? Like the other treatments mentioned, which are not performed by the majority of physicians, there is a good chance that you will not get coverage for Insulin Potentiation Therapy. However, some patients do get coverage (See **Figure D-1**). Probably the number one reason why more people do not get IPT is that insurance companies do not cover it.

Insurance companies are regularly looking for ways to save money. One of those ways is to not cover cancer therapies. Chemotherapy drugs are expensive (See **Figure D-2**). The major expense with IPT is in the drug costs, but if insurance companies would pay for IPT, they would still save a lot of money. It is not uncommon for a cancer patient to have treatment costs of over $100,000; IPT is only a fraction of that cost. The cost comparison of Judy's treatment (case study #21 in **Appendix C**) is

seen in **Figure D-3**. Judy was a recurrent breast cancer patient who had failed previous high-dose chemotherapy. She was recommended for a mastectomy, radiation therapy, and high-dose chemotherapy with nongeneric drugs. Conservative estimates of her health care costs if she had done traditional medical treatment would be $122,000. For $122,000, she would have had a major operation; endured chest radiation; and received high-dose chemotherapy that would have made her blood counts go low, which would have needed hospitalization if she had a fever, or Neupogen or Epogen shots to get the counts back up. She would have vomited, felt terrible for six months, lost a lot of weight, and would have had to buy a wig and a prosthesis that she would have for life. In contrast, she received IPT. Including the cost of supplements, it was approximately $10,000 for the whole course. She did have to eat

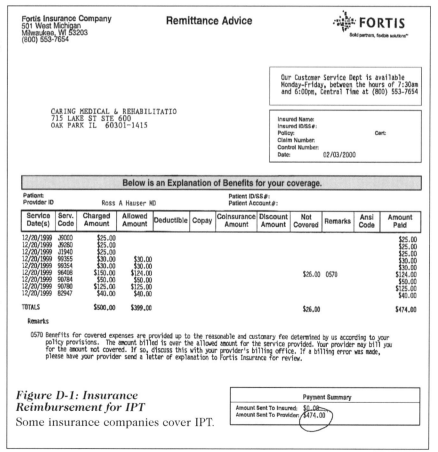

Figure D-1: Insurance Reimbursement for IPT

Some insurance companies cover IPT.

healthy food, but this did not increase her food cost. She had to spend a little more time fixing food, which she was able to do because she felt great. She kept her hair, her breast, and her life. Which sounds better to you?

FIGURE D-2: COSTS OF CHEMOTHERAPY DRUGS

The costs of treatment with particular chemotherapy drugs are listed below. Combination drug therapy is more expensive, since it involves costs for all of the drugs combined.

VERY HIGH COST
(Single drug treatment costs above $10,000)
Interferons, Gemcitabine

HIGH COST
(Single drug treatment costs above $1,000.)
Altretamine, Carboplatin, Carmustine, Cisplatin, Cyclophosphamide, Cytarabine, Dacarbazine, Dactinomycin, Daunorubicin, Doxorubicin, Etoposide, Flutamide, Lurcovorin, Levamisole, Placlitaxel, Streprozocin, Tamoxifen, Vinorelbin, Tartrate

MEDIUM COST
(Single drug treatment costs between $500 and $1,000)
Floxuridine, Fluorouracil, Dydroxyurea, Melphalan, Methotrexate

LOW COST
(Single drug treatment costs from $10 up to $500)
Aminogluthethimide, Bacillus Calmette-Guerin, Bleomycin, Bufilfan, Chlorambucil, Docetaxei, Estradiol, Estramustine, Goserelin, Interleukin-2, Irinotecan, Lomustine, Mechlorethamine, Mercaptopurine, Mesna, Mitomycin, Mitotane, Mitoxantone, Phicamycin, Prednisone, Procarbazine, Testolactone, Thioguanine, Thiotepa, Topotecan, Toremifene, Citrate, Vinblastine, Vincristine

Adapted from Mosby's GenRx: Complete Reference for Brand and Generic Drugs *1998, 1999.*

MEDICALLY NECESSARY

It is unfortunate, but even when IPT is helping a patient, the insurance company can deny his or her claims. The more expensive the claim, the more likely it will be denied. Generally, IPT is approximately $750 to $2,500 per treatment session, depending on the cost of the specific medications used. If generic medications can be used, the cost will be less. If a person has failed a first round of chemotherapy, then most likely a newer type of chemotherapy medication will be needed. This will substantially drive up the cost. Insurance companies generally deny claims with by saying that the tests or services were not "medically necessary."

Carefully review **Figure D-4**, which is an explanation of what an insurance company defines as "medically necessary." It is imperative for the cancer patient to understand this term because it is often the only way to possibly get coverage. Even if IPT cures a person of his or her cancer or shrinks it, insurance still often does not cover the treatment because it is deemed not medically necessary (See **Figure D-5**). It is my (Ross') contention that by calling IPT not medically necessary, the insurance companies themselves are causing the demise of cancer patients. What do you mean, "It is not necessary?" The person has cancer, and cancer kills. You idiots—of course it is necessary; without it, a person with a solid tumor is most likely going to die.

FIGURE D-3: THE DIFFERENCE BETWEEN TRADITIONAL, ALLOPATHIC TREATMENT OF A RECURRENT BREAST CANCER VERSUS IPT

Procedure	Traditional Allopathic in Dollars	IPT Cost in Dollars
Mastectomy	$10,000	$0
Hospitalization	$20,000	$0
Prosthesis	$2,000	$0
Radiation Therapy	$25,000	$0
High-Dose Chemotherapy	$55,000	n/a
Neupogen/Epogen Shots for Low Blood Counts	$10,000	$0
IPT for 10 Weeks	n/a	$10,000
Total Cost:	**$122,000**	**$10,000**

Caring Medical has seen patients get hurt by their insurance companies. This is one of the reasons why this book was written, so patients would have a resource and references with which to fight for the coverage of IPT. One of the books that we recommend to patients is, *Don't Let Your HMO Kill You* by Jason Theodosakis, MD.[1] What impressed us about this book is that Dr. Theodosakis wrote it after his New York Times Number One best-seller, *The Arthritis Cure.* Instead of writing another natural medicine book that most likely would have been a best-seller as well, Dr. Theodosakis, probably, like most natural medicine doctors, has had enough and wrote *Don't Let Your HMO Kill You.* Why do you think he wrote this? Because, like us, he has encountered HMOs

AMERICAN FAMILY INSURANCE GROUP

6000 AMERICAN PKWY • MADISON WI 53783-0001 • PHONE: (608) 249-2111

January 4, 2001

RE: Claim/Policy #:
    Date of service: 07/28/00

Mrs. Francisco,

We have received medical information from Caring Medical. Our Medical Director has reviewed this information and it is of his medical opinion that medical necessity for the above dated lab work is not documented. The lab work does not appear medically necessary, appropriate or acceptable for treatment of your diagnosis.

Your policy excludes coverage of medical services, treatment or supplies which are not medically necessary or which are experimental, even if recommended or ordered by a physician. The policy defines **Medically Necessary** as, "Services or supplies provided by a hospital, physician, or other provider that are required to identify or treat covered conditions and which, as determined by us, are: 1. Appropriate for the symptoms or diagnosis and treatment of your sickness or injury; and 2. Appropriate with regard to standards of acceptable medical practice."

For this reason we are denying the above indicated date of service. If there is any additional medical information supporting the medical necessity of the lab tests please have the physician or medical provider submit that information to: American Family Mutual Insurance Co., Attn: Health Claims, 6000 American Pkwy, Madison, WI 53783-0001.

Kim Landphier, HIA, MHP
Health Claims Specialist
AMERICAN FAMILY MUTUAL INSURANCE COMPANY

cc: Caring Medical

    715 Lake St. Ste 600
    Oak Park, IL 60301

Figure D-4: The"Medically Necessary" Letter
This is how insurance companies deny even cancer patients the very treatments they need.

term "medically necessary" as a way to deny all the care they could get away with. If you look at your explanation of benefits, you are sure to find this phrase. They are only two words, but they have incredible power. Everyone uses the phrase, everyone wants to define it. A debate in Congress continues as this book goes to press between doctors and insurers over who should decide what is medically necessary. Both sides know what is at stake—power over billions of dollars in health services.

Let's take a look at a typical use of the phrase. As one contract puts it, medical services are covered "only if in the judgment of a Plan Physician, they are medically necessary to prevent, diagnose, or treat a medical condition. A service or item is medically necessary only if a Plan Physician determines that its omission would directly affect a Member's health."

Pay attention to how this wording sets you up for denials. The HMO is not asking, "Will this treatment make the patient better?" The contract asks, "Will denying this treatment make the patient worse?"

and other insurance companies that kill people by not paying for their medically necessary treatments. On pages 165-166 of his book, he talks about what is "medically necessary:"

> The strange thing about this term is that no one used it before managed care came along. When indemnity insurance was paying bills, we got all the care that was necessary and quite a bit of care that was unnecessary. No one was asking questions.
>
> When HMOs started taking over and attempted to keep costs down, they invented the

The whole idea is to provide the bare minimum. That's how managed care saves money.

If you keep this in mind, you will already have learned something crucial about how to appeal. Never say that the treatment will make you better. Always emphasize that not getting the treatment will make you worse, perhaps so much worse that you will require more expensive care. Now you are using the HMO's own logic. It may be a strange way to think, but it's the only way to get your point across.

Aug. 28, 2001
Ernie and Donna Viano

Dr. Hauser:

It's almost two and a half years to the date we first came to you for help with Ernie's illness. We had just moved back from Alaska, unemployed with no health insurance coverage.

Ernie' symptoms: severe jaundice, loss of appetite and weight (60 pounds), and nausea. You directed us to the Gerson Therapy and prescribed supplements to support his liver and immune system until a biopsy revealed Lymphoma in the abdomen area.

We knew we did not want to use conventional cancer treatment (chemotherapy) which was pushed at us by both oncologists. We were told, "without it, Ernie had six months." Our thoughts and opinions meant nothing. We were talked to like children—offered one option to his condition. It was insulting and demeaning.

Three weeks later we were in Tijuana and spent 17 days learning the Gerson program a holistic treatment utilizing the body's healing mechanism in the treatment of debilitating illness, thru supplements, juicing, coffee enemas, organic produce, etc. The program was faithfully followed for approximately two years. One year into the program, a CT revealed shrinkage of the tumor by half. We were extremely excited. The next CT, April, 2001, was not so positive. The tumor had started growing.

We had heard of and read about IPT. Our local physician encouraged us to investigate and consider this "other" chemo treatment. The first of 10 treatments was administered on March 20, 2001. Ernie experienced virtually zero side effects; no hair loss, nausea, vomiting, weight loss, or any of the other unpleasant experiences associated with conventional chemotherapy. A CT scan done on June 1, 2001 indicated shrinkage of the tumor. Another CT is scheduled for October 1, 2001 and we anticipate more good results.

IPT has been a positive experience for Ernie. He is a high stress personality. IPT was much easier for him to accept. Insurance is now our present battle. My health insurance carrier has denied payment of his treatments, which I tend to believe is minuscule to the cost of treatments he was to receive during the course of eight four-day confinements in the hospital, per oncologist's orders due to Muga scan results. Denial was stated, based on their opinion, that Ernie could have received conventional therapy by an Oncologist in the Network. My statement to them:

"We believed IPT to be more 'patient friendly,' not to mention the cost-savings. IPT would have been a win-win solution. Their response: "Cost is not an issue here. We are only concerned for the patient's well-being."

I am in the process of appealing my carrier's decision. If my appeal is denied, I am prepared to seek legal counsel. We believe we should have the right to decide the administration of a treatment.

We have been blessed and will overcome. Thanks for your help!

Ernie and Donna Viano

Figure D-5: The IPT Insurance Battle
Even if you show the insurance company that IPT is working, they still claim that it is not "medically necessary."

Read the book; Dr Theodosakis gives a lot of good information that patients need. But sometimes patients need an attorney. If insurance companies will not pay for IPT, then your attorney should write a letter similar to the ones our attorney writes for patients (See **Figure D-6**). The letter in **Figure D-6** was written in response to an insurance company denying coverage for IPT when it was controlling a person's severe lung cancer. The person was "forced" to undergo the treatment the insurance company would pay (more expensive high-dose chemotherapy). One can see the result from an E-mail sent just three months after starting the start high-dose chemotherapy (See **Figure D-7**). We then received a wonderful e-mail from the family summarizing Paul's experience (See **Figure D-8**).

For the cancer patient, it is somewhat discouraging to think that he or she may not get a life-saving treatment because of the politics of medicine. But the simple fact is that it just may happen. The politics of medicine are real. It is for this reason that books such as this need to be written, and patients need to tell everyone they can about natural medicine and therapies such as IPT. People like our attorney, Kirkpatrick Dilling, who have been defending natural medicine therapies, patients, and physicians for 50 years, are an invaluable asset to the cause (See **Figure D-9**).

Caring Medical, like many medical practices that utilize IPT in the care of their patients, requires payment at the time of services because of the unreliability of payment from insurance companies. If a person receives IPT, we do bill the insurance company using the appropriate codes because it does involve traditional chemotherapy agents. If a person needs a letter written, it would say what is found in **Figure D-10**.

A letter from the treating physician is not normally enough to obtain insurance coverage. Data are often what is needed, as well as legal action. We believe this book will help. As we do with Prolotherapy and our other books, we recommend that cancer patients show this book to their family physicians, oncologists, and especially insurers. If possible, obtain many of the articles referenced here to support your claim that IPT is a scientific treatment that is successful and that you need it to save your life. We wish you much success on your quest to do what you think is the best treatment to help save your life. ∎

DILLING & DILLING

ATTORNEYS AT LAW

ESTABLISHED 1917

1120 LEE ROAD
NORTHBROOK, ILLINOIS 60062
(312) 236-8417
TELEFAX NO. (312) 236-8418
EMAIL: dilling1@juno.com

CALIFORNIA LEGAL ASSOCIATE
R. CHANDLER MYERS
PASADENA, 91101

February 20, 2001

Blue Cross/Blue Shield of Illinois
300 East Randolph
Chicago, Illinois 60601-5099

RE: Your member's name: Paul Verest
      Your Identification No.:
      Your Claim Number:

Gentlemen:

We represent Paul Verest, Naperville, Illinois.   Our client is a Cancer victim, with adenocarcinoma and lung and brain metastasis. In desperation last year he sought the services of Dr. Ross Hauser.   Dr. Hauser is an Internationally renowned specialist and medical author, with patients from all over the World seeking treatment from him. At the time Verest retained Dr. Hauser, his only prospect was that of early death with intensive suffering.

Dr. Hauser's treatment for Verest has resulted in a greater quality of life, a less severe cancer progress and undoubtedly extended Verest's survival time. Supporting Dr. Hauser's expert treatment of Paul Verest has been an amplitude of medical research and knowledge.

Dr. Hauser has treated Verest with chemotherapy modified so as to work favorably on cancer conditions but greatly lessen chemotherapy side effects while not impairing treatment effectiveness. Side effects minimized include nausea, vomiting, loss of appetite, diarrhea, anemia, hair loss, fatigue, mouth ulcers, yeast infections, depression, anxiety, insomnia, pain, and death under certain circumstances.

Needless to say, Verest is very satisfied with the treatment he has received.

Paul Verest has been covered by a health insurance policy issued by Blue Cross/Blue Shield of Illinois. However, the insurance has been rendered virtually valueless by your routine denial of any coverage, on the outrageous pretense that the treatments accorded to Verest are "medically unnecessary". Your arbitrary denials are wrong, unjustified and violate his insurance policy, well providing the basis for future awarding of compensatory and punitive damages. Understandably Dr. Hauser believes that it is the proper function of an insurance company to provide coverage for its policyholders, not to dabble in the practice of medicine.

A good illustration of your bad faith is shown by the statement dated January 29, 2001. $1,548.00 had been billed to Blue Cross/Blue Shield for laboratory services, radioisotope tests, injections, drugs, other treatment, and therapy.

The entire $1,548.00 amount was denied as "not covered", no exceptions even being made for any therapy, drugs or injections!

As a result of your bad faith and denial of coverage, Paul Verest has exhausted his meager resources and faces cessation of his vitally needed medical treatment.

Is it your aim to bring about Verest's premature and wrongful death?

It is hereby demanded that the sums you have heretofore wrongfully denied to Paul Verest, as due and owing under his policy of insurance with Blue Cross/Blue Shield of Illinois, shall be paid forthwith and without further delay. Unless we hear favorably that such payment is promptly to be made, we are authorized to institute a suitable lawsuit for damages, attorneys' fees and court costs.

Very truly yours,

DILLING AND DILLING, P.C.

Kirkpatrick W. Dilling

KWD:mem
bc: Paul and Carol Verest

ADELLE DAVIS FOUNDATION
AFFILIATE

NUTRADELLE LABORATORIES, LTD.
AFFILIATE

***Figure D-6:
Attorney Letter
for Insurance
Reimbursement***

Sometimes, patients have to force insurance companies to pay for legitimate health care costs by using the legal system. Perhaps it is through that very legal system that IPT will finally become recognized in a way that the medical community has thus far resisted.

FROM: info@caringmedical.com
SENT: Tuesday, 7/21, 2001 7:42 AM
TO: CARINGMEDICAL; BeNuts
SUBJECT: FW:Paul Verest

All staff—sorry to be passing along sad information, but our former patient, Paul Verest, has passed away. Our thoughts and prayers are with the family.

This email is from his daughter.

----**Original Message**----
FROM: Paul Verest
SENT: Tuesday, 7/21, 2001 7:37 AM
TO: info@caringmedical.com
SUBJECT:

To the staff at Caring Medical, I am sorry to be writing this letter, but my mother and I thought we should inform you that Paul Verest, a former patient of yours, passed away Sunday morning at home with his family. Visitation is scheduled for today, Tuesday and a funeral is scheduled for Wednesday in Naperville. Specifics are available through the Chicago Tribune.

Sincerely, Dawn Verest
(Paul's daughter)

Figure D-7: A Very Sad E-Mail

What treatments insurance companies pay for may not be in the best interest of the patient. Paul Verest, while undergoing IPT, was working full-time, living vibrantly and maintaining his zest for life. Because of Blue Cross/Blue Shield's denial of payment for IPT, Paul was forced to get high-dose chemotherapy. Three months later—he was dead.

September 20, 2001
To Caring Medical

Dawn, Kimberly and I wish to thank you for the beautiful plant and your many expressions of sympathy and support. As you know Paul was a very special person with a warm heart and a gentle nature. Through out this past year Paul never wavered in his resolve to beat the cancer, and he was never bitter or angry over his illness. We knew the medical professions diagnosis and we were determined to beat the odds. Under Dr. Hauser's treatment we had hope and faith in Paul's recovery. Even though the test results showed the cancer was still there, Paul felt great, and functioned completely until four days before he died.

It has been a month since Paul's death and the reality of his no longer being with us is agonizing. Words can not express our grief, but we are consoled in our belief that Paul has earned eternal peace with God. Paul's greatest fear was not dying, but how he would die. He did not want to be a burden to us, and he wanted to have control over his mind and body. God did grant Paul this wish. We found out on August 8th that the cancer had returned to the brain, and they offered no treatment to treat the cancer. When Paul found out the news he knew it would not be long, and I firmly believe he willed his fight to be over. Paul came home on August 15th and died on Sunday morning, August 19th. I was sitting at his side when he took his last breath. He died a peaceful death and he was at home with his daughters and me.

Paul truly enjoyed everyone at Caring Medical, and he always talked about your warmth, compassion and concern. I know we made the right decision in selecting Dr. Hauser's treatment. Although it did not cure Paul, it did give him a quality of life. The events of the past week have been devastating, and my heart aches for all the families and friends who lost love ones. I am thankful that Paul and I had time together. We did not live this past year as if Paul was dying, but we lived it and cherished every day. We appreciate your support and thank you for sharing.

Deepest gratitude, Carol, Dawn & Kimberly

Figure D-8: A Touching Follow-Up

DILLING & DILLING

ATTORNEYS AT LAW
ESTABLISHED 1917

1120 LEE ROAD
NORTHBROOK, ILLINOIS 60062
(312) 236-8417
TELEFAX NO. (312) 236-8418
EMAIL: dilling1@juno.com

CALIFORNIA LEGAL ASSOCIATE
R. CHANDLER MYERS
PASADENA, 91101

February 6, 2001

Dr. Ross Hauser
Caring Medical & Rehabilitation Center
715 Lake St., Suite 600
Oak Park, IL 60301

Dear Doctor:

I continue to be an admirer of the good medical work and writing you are doing. Meanwhile we still have occasional opportunity to publicize what is wrong with so much of the health care system in the United States. This is particularly true of cancer therapies, where due to predominance of harmful orthodoxy thousands are dying needlessly every year.

Several years ago I was able to offer some legal information to Daniel Haley. Since that time Haley has written a monumental book (463 pages) entitled POLITICS IN HEALING, The Suppression and Manipulation of American Medicine.

I find special interest in material concerning Dr. William F. Koch, a great physician we represented in defense of the Koch Treatment. The Koch therapies for cancer were dramatically successful and simple. Basically, Dr. Koch was a homeopath. His Glyoxilide was homeopathic and lead to false claims by the AMA and others that it was only water of no value. Dr. Koch died in 1967 (we visited him in Rio de Janeiro in 1965).

As of this date we know of no one who has knowledge of the Koch treatment. Perhaps you have such knowledge. In any event I am having a copy of the Haley book sent to you. I hope you will read it.

Sincerely yours,

Kirkpatrick W. Dilling

Figure D-9: Kirkpatrick Dilling, a Natural Medicine Crusader...

NUTRADELLE LABORATORIES, LTD.
AFFILIATE

To Whom It May Concern:

Recently your client/insured came to Caring Medical and Rehabilitation Services, S.C., for care for his (her) diagnosis of cancer. He (she) has availed himself (herself) to get advice from his (her) family physician, oncologist, and/or surgeon, and we have discussed with him (her) the possibility of other consultants as needed. After looking at all of the options, and since the cancer diagnosis is a life-threatening illness, he (she) has chosen to take a comprehensive approach to cancer therapy, including a healthy diet, lifestyle changes, and herbal remedies to help keep his (her) nutritional status and immune system strong. In addition, after careful consideration, he (she) has opted to do low-dose, high-frequency chemotherapy (LDHFC).

Because of the Internet, various health-related books, and talking with other patients, the cancer patient understands that there can be significant side effects with the high-dose, low-frequency chemotherapy that is traditionally given. If he (she) receives traditional high-dose chemotherapy, the prognosis for long-term cure is low, even though the medical literature supports such chemotherapy for his (her) particular diagnosis. He (she) has chosen not to receive this type of chemotherapy. He (she) does not want its side effects, which include a high incidence of anorexia, nausea, vomiting, diarrhea, hair loss, malaise, and fatigue.

He (she) does desire to treat the cancer with some chemotherapy—low-dose chemotherapy. He (she) understands that this type of chemotherapy treatment is given weekly as compared to high-dose chemotherapy, which is typically given every three to four weeks. He (she) has been told that in LDHFC, dosages of 10% to 25% of the typical chemotherapy dose are given. He (she) understands that along with the chemotherapy other agents will also be given, such as insulin, glutathione, quercetin, DMSO, selenium, and other potentiating agents to make the low-dose chemotherapy more "potent." These agents are used to increase the killing effect of the chemotherapeutic agents by increasing cell membrane permeability, facilitating the transport of medications across the blood-brain barrier, stimulating tumor cell division (increase in S phase of cell division), and various other mechanisms. The end result for the patient receiving LDHFC is much fewer side effects than traditional high-dose chemotherapy. He (she) understands the risks and benefits of such a treatment plan.

To decrease the risk of drug resistance, multiple chemotherapy medications are used during treatment. I have enclosed the medications to be used in his (her) treatment plan. As you know, these are typically medications that are used in cancer regimes, and, almost universally, insurance plans cover chemotherapy treatments for cancer. Your client/insured is desiring to receive a type of chemotherapy treatment for cancer. Be assured that your insured/client has looked at all the options and has decided for himself (herself) to receive this type of chemotherapy. Please assist him (her) in the fight of his (her) life by covering treatment. Be assured that LDHFC is significantly less expensive than traditional high-dose, low-frequency chemotherapy regimes.

It is my opinion that the LDHFC regime written for your insured/client with the potentiating agents will be successful. If he (she) does not receive the treatment, the cancer is most assuredly going to progress, requiring more expensive treatments. I ask you again to please assist him (her) in the fight of his (her) life by covering this treatment. Together, with the grace of God, we can help him (her) win this fight!

Sincerely with warm regards,

Ross A. Hauser, M.D.
On behalf of the staff of Caring Medical

Figure D-10: A Sample Letter
Above is a good example of a kind of "template" the patient can follow when corresponding with insurance carriers.

IPT Referral List and Physician Training

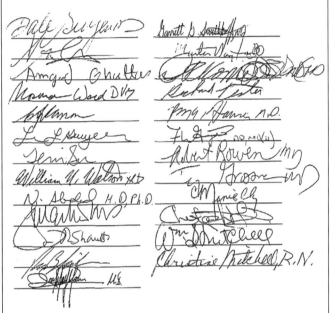

INSULIN POTENTIATION THERAPY COLLABORATIVE GROUP

We the undersigned, jointly affirm Insulin Potentiation Therapy (IPT) as represented in U.S. patent #5155096 and presented at the International Oxidative Medical Association conference, February 21-22, 2001, as well as at major national and international scientific meetings, published in the peer-reviewed medical literature, to be a safe and rational medical therapy, supported with over 60 years of positive clinical outcomes.

Figure E-1: Insulin Potentiation Therapy Collaborative Group
Many physicians are becoming trained in IPT—testifying to its safety and efficacy.

I PT is not taught in medical schools yet. It is also not done in major universities, as such physicians need to receive training in IPT after they have finished their formal training. There are numerous doctors trained in IPT as evidenced by **Figure E-1**. The following is a list of physicians that we personally know, love, and who are mentioned in this book. For a complete list of physicians who have been trained in IPT please see www.IPTQ.org.

IPT DOCTORS MENTIONED IN THIS BOOK:

DONATO PÉREZ GARCÍA, M.D.
Blvd. Agua Caliente #4558-1503A.
Tijuana, B.C. 22420 Mexico
PHONE: 011-52 664-686-5473
FAX: 801-459-9928
www.IPTQ.com
donatopg3@yahoo.com

STEVEN G. AYRE, M.D.
Contemporary Medicine Center
322 Burr Ridge Parkway
Burr Ridge, IL 60521
PHONE: 630-321-9010
www.contemporarymedicine.net
steven303@aol.com

ROSS A. HAUSER, M.D., MARION A. HAUSER, M.S., R.D.
Caring Medical and Rehabilitation Services, S.C.
715 Lake Street, Suite 600
Oak Park, IL 60301
PHONE: 708-848-7789
FAX: 708-848-7763
www.caringmedical.com
www.iptcancer.com
drhauser@caringmedical.com

FRANK W. GEORGE II, M.D.
6748 E. Lone Mountain Road
Cave Creek, AZ 85331
PHONE: 480-595-5508
FAX: 480-575-1570
E-MAIL (OFFICE): home@flashmail.com
E-MAIL (PERSONAL): fwg336@pol.net

FRANK C. NOONAN, D.O.
GAIL GELSINGER, R.N., C.N.N.
The Lincoln Building
1248 West Main Street
Ephrata, PA 17522
PHONE: 717-733-1736
FAX: 717-733-9236
cornerstone@talon.net

ROBERT ROWEN, M.D.
TERRI B. SU, M.D.
Radiant Health Medical Center
95 Montgomery Drive, Suite 220
Santa Rosa, CA 95472
PHONE: 707-571-7560
FAX: 707-571-8929
www.radianthealthmedicalcenter.com
www.doctorrowen.com
www.doctorterrisu.com
E-MAIL drrowen@att.net
E-MAIL terrisu@sonic.net

Garrett Swetlikoff, N.D.
Kelowna Naturopathic Clinic, Inc.
160-1855 Kirschner Road
Kelown, B.C. V1Y4N7, Canada
PHONE: 250-868-2205
FAX: 250-868-2099
gswetlikoff@home.com
gswetlikoff@shaw.ca

For physicians who desire training in IPT, please contact Dr. Steven G. Ayre or Dr. Donato Pérez García above. (See **Figure E-2**.) They are the two physicians who currently train physicians on IPT. Generally, the information on the training courses can also be obtained from www.IPTQ.org. Once a physician is trained in IPT, Dr. Pérez gives the physician access to the physician-only web site, http://groups.yahoo.com/group/IPTdoctors. On this web site the physician will see potential protocols to use as well as case studies that have been successfully treated with IPT.

FOR FURTHER INFORMATION ON IPT

Much information (including the medicine, history and practical application of IPT) can be further researched by accessing the comprehensive web site, www.IPTQ.org. We have included a couple of pertinent books for the reader to investigate:

IPT BOOKS:

■ *Cellular Cancer Therapy Through Modification of Blood Physico-Chemical Constants (Donatian Therapy)*

by Donato Pérez García, M.D. (Donato 1) and Donato Pérez García y Bellón, M.D. (Donato 2) ©1978 *(Translation by Mike Dillinger.)*

(This complete book is published in English on the web site, www.IPTQ.org.)

■ *Medicine of Hope, Insulin-Cellular Therapy* [English Title] *(Médecine de l'Espoir, Thérapie Insulino-Cellulaire)* [French Title]

by Jean-Claude Paquette M.D., ©1995. (This complete book is published on www.IPTQ.org in English, and French.)
Translation by Aimé Ricci. Original book in French.

(The English translation of this book can be purchased at www.benuts.com, or by calling 1-877-RX-BEULAH.)

■ *My Father Is the Best Doctor*
by Donato Pérez García, M.D., © 2002 (This complete book is published on www.IPTQ.org in Spanish and English.) ■

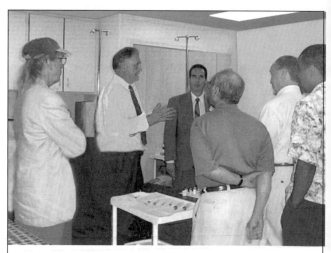

Figure E-2: *Steven G. Ayre, M.D., demonstrates the technique of IPT to a group of physicians at one of the many IPT training seminars that he puts on.*

Certificate

IPTMD06

This is to certify that

Ross A Hauser, M.D.

Attended from February 28 till March 3 of the 2000 year a forty hour Seminar on Basic Clinical principles in the practice of Insulin Potentiation Therapy.

Tijuana. B.C. Mexico a 3 de Marzo del 2000

Dr. Donato Perez Garcia
IPTMD04

Dr. Donato Perez Garcia
Av. Villa Caliente #4558-1503-A
Tijuana, B.C. 22420 MEXICO

Mexico   Tijuana   Oak Park   Buenos Aires

Figure E-3: IPT Training Certificate
Drs. Pérez García and Ayre train physicians in IPT in their respective practices.

FOR MORE INFORMATION!

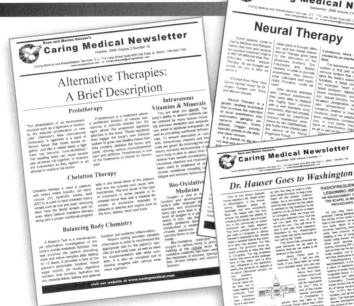

Caring Medical & Rehabilitation Services
Natural Medicine Center

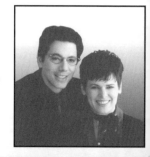

The following is a listing of therapies that are offered at Caring Medical.

- Anti-Aging Regimes
- Biological Aging Measurement
- Bio-oxidative Therapies (Oxygen Therapies)
- Chelation Therapy
- Cryotherapy
- Enzyme Replacement Therapy
- Healing Diseases Naturally
- Herbal Help
- Huneke Neural Therapy
- Infrared Coagulation
- Insulin Potentiation Therapy (IPT)
- Mesotherapy
- Metabolic Typing
- Natural Gynecology
- Natural Hormone Replacement Therapy for Men and Women
- NeuroCranial Restructuring
- Nutritional/Herbal Regimes
- Ozone Therapy
- Photoluminescense
- Prolotherapy
- Radiofrequency
- Therapeutic Skin Care Analysis and Treatment
- *...And Many Others*

The following is a listing of tests and analysis that are offered at Caring Medical.

- 24 Hour Urine for Heavy Metals
- AMAS (Anti Malignin Antibody Serum)
- Babesiosis
- Biological Aging Panel
- Breast Cancer Panel
- Candida Profile
- Food Sensitivity Panel
- Glucose/Insulin Tolerance Test
- Gluten/Casein
- Hair Analysis
- H. Pylori Rapid Test
- Immune Panel
- Metabolic Profile
- Minieral Levels
- Metabolic Typing
- Mycoplasma
- Nova 8
- Nutritional Analysis
- PCR Tests
- pH Testing
- POCKIT HSV 2
- Platelet Aggregation Study
- Quick Strep A ICON
- REAMS Test
- Saliva Hormone Profile (male/female)
- Stool Parasite Analysis
- ...And Many others!

"Where there is Caring, there is Hope."

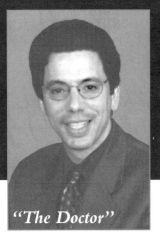
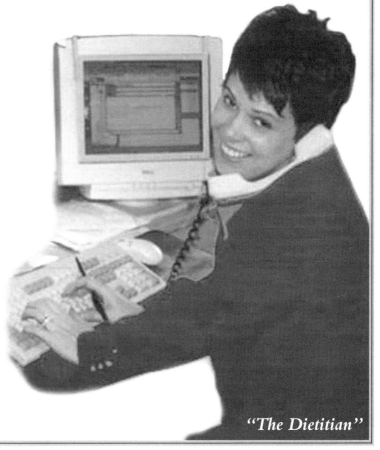
377

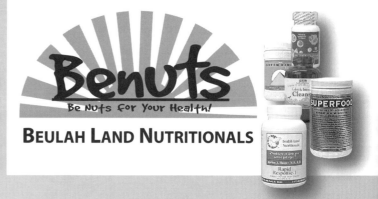

Beulah Land Press

The Doctor: *Ross A. Hauser, M.D.*
The Dietitian: *Marion A. Hauser, M.S., R.D.*

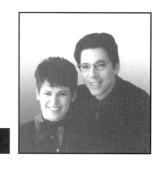

READ FOR YOUR HEALTH! ORDER FROM THE PUBLISHER AT A SUBSTANTIAL DISCOUNT!

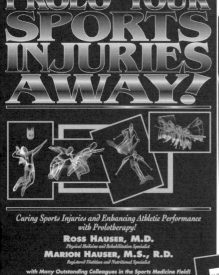

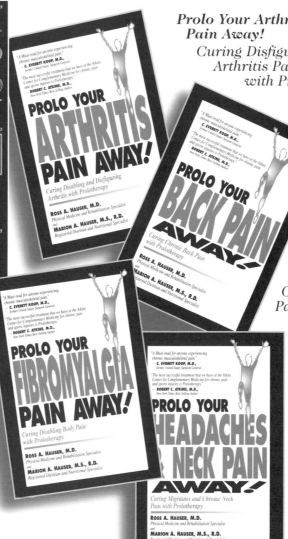

Prolo Your Sports Injuries Away!
Curing Sports Injuries and Enhancing Athletic Performance with Prolotherapy

Prolo Your Arthritis Pain Away!
Curing Disfiguring and Disabling Arthritis Pain with Prolotherapy

Prolo Your Back Pain Away!
Curing Chronic Back Pain with Prolotherapy

Prolo Your Fibromyalgia Pain Away!
Curing Disabling Body Pain with Prolotherapy

Prolo Your Headache and Neck Pain Away!
Curing Migraines and Neck Pain with Prolotherapy.

Prolo Your Pain Away!
Curing Chronic Pain with Prolotherapy

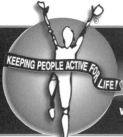
379

CHAPTER 8
NATURAL MEDICINE PRINCIPLES IN CANCER THERAPY

1. Cancer now leading killer of middle-aged. *San Diego Union*. December 26, 1990.
2. Scott J. Cancer watch. *Los Angeles Times*. July 11, 1991.
3. Walters R. *Options: The Alternative Cancer Therapy Book*. Honesdale, Pa: Paragon Press; 1993:1-5.
4. Study finds cancer rate in US children rising. *San Diego Union*. June 26, 1991.
5. Moss R. *Questioning Chemotherapy*. Brooklyn, NY: Equinox Books; 2000.
6. Ries L. SEER cancer statistics review, 1973-1991: Tables and graphs. Bethesda, Md: NCI; 1994.
7. Moss R. *Cancer Therapy*. Brooklyn, NY: Equinox Books; 1996.
8. Pelton R. *Alternatives in Cancer Therapy*. New York, NY: Fireside Book Publishing; 1994.
9. Walters R. *Options: The Alternative Cancer Therapy Book*. Honesdale, Pa: Paragon Press; 1992.

CHAPTER 10
INSULIN POTENTIATION THERAPY: THE HISTORY

1. From www.IPTQ.com, with permission from Chris Duffield, Ph.D.

CHAPTER 11
INSULIN POTENTIATION THERAPY: THE SCIENCE

1. Granner D. Hormones of the pancreas and gastrointestinal tract. In: Murray R, Granner D, Mayes P, Rodwell V, eds. *Harper's Biochemistry*. 24th ed. New York, NY: McGraw-Hill; 1998: 581-596.
2. Santisteban G. *Biochem & Biophys Res Comm*. 1985;132:1174.
3. *Br Med J*. 2000; 320:3.
4. Muck B. Altered carbohydrate metabolism in breast cancer and benign breast affections. *Archiv fur Gynakologie*. 1976;221:83-91.
5. Muck B. Cancer of the breast, diabetes, and pathological glucose tolerance. *Archiv fur Gynakologie*. 1975;220:73-81.
6. Glicksman A. *Cancer*. 1956;9:1127-1131.
7. Repert R. Breast carcinoma study: relation to thyroid disease and diabetes. *JMSMS*. October 1952:1315-1317.
8. Carter A. Metabolic parameters in women with metastatic breast cancer. *JCE & M*. 1975;40:260-264.
9. Vecchia C. A case-control study of diabetes mellitus and cancer risk. *Br J Cancer*. 1994;70:950-953.
10. Pearson O. Serum Growth Hormone and insulin levels in patients with breast cancer. In: *Prognostic Factors in Breast Cancer, Proceedings of 1st Tenovus Symposium, 1968*. Cardiff.
11. Greenwood F. In: *Prognostic Factors in Breast Cancer, Proceedings of 1st Tenovus Symposium, 1968*. Cardiff.
12. Benjamin F, Carter D. *N Eng J Med*. 1969;281:1448.
13. Sanchez A. Role of sugars in human neutrophilic phagocytosis. *Am J Clin Nutr*. 1973;26:1180-1184.
14. Rillema J. Characteristics of the insulin stimulation of DNA, RNA, and protein metabolism in cultured human mammary carcinoma cells. *Biochimica et Biophysica Acta*. 1977;475: 74-80.
15. Cullen J. Insulin-like growth factor receptor expression and function in human breast cancer. *Cancer Res*. 1990;50:48-53.
16. Papa V. Elevated insulin receptor content in human breast cancer. *J Clin Invest*. 1990;86:1503-1510.
17. Holdaway I. Hormone binding by human mammary carcinoma. *Cancer Res*. 1977;37:1946-1952.
18. Mountjoy K. Insulin receptor recognition in cultured human tumor cells. *Cancer Res*. 1983;43:4537-4542.
19. Spring-Mills E. Immunoreactive hormones in human breast tissues. *Surgery*. December 1983:946-950.
20. Zapf J. Insulin-like growth factors/ somatomedins: structure, secretion, biological actions and physiological role. *Hormone Res*. 1986;24:121-130.

21. Furlanetto R. Somatomedin-C receptors and growth effects in human breast cells maintained in long-term tissue culture. *Cancer Res.* 1984;44:2122-2128.

22. Wichert T. Insulin-like growth factor-1 is an autocrine regular of chromogranin A secretion and growth in human neuroendocrine tumor cells. *Cancer Res.* 2000:4573-4581.

23. Pavelic K. Insulin and glucagon secretion by renal adenocarcinoma. *Cancer.* 1981;48:98-100.

24. Pavelic K. Carcinomas of the cervix and corpus uteri in humans: stage-dependent blood levels of substance(s) immunologically cross-reactive with insulin. *J Natl Cancer Inst.* 1982;68:891-894.

25. Pavelic K. Correlation of substances immunologically cross-reactive with insulin, glucose, and Growth Hormone in Hodgkin's lymphoma patients. *Cancer Lett.* 1982;17:81-86.

26. Cullin J. Insulin-like growth factor receptor expression and function in human breast cancer. *Cancer Res.* 1990;50:48-53.

27. McCarty M. Suppression of dolichol synthesis with isoprenoids and statins may potentiate the cancer-retardant efficacy of IGF-1 down-regulation. *Med Hypoth.* 2001;56:12-16.

28. Alabaster O. Metabolic modification by insulin enhances methotrexate cytotoxicity in MCF-7 human breast cancer cells. *Europ J Cancer Oncol.* 1981;17:1223-1228.

29. Schilsky R. Characteristics of membrane transport of methotrexate by cultured human breast cancer cells. *Biochem Pharm.* 1981;30:1537-1542.

30. Hug V. Use of growth-stimulatory hormones to improve the in vitro therapeutic index of doxorubicin for human breast tissue. *Cancer Res.* 1986;46:147-152.

31. Gross G. Pertubation by insulin of human breast cancer cell kinetics. *Cancer Res.* 1984;44:3570-3575.

32. Neufeld O. Insulin therapy in terminal cancer: a preliminary report. *J Am Geriatr Soc.* 1962;10:274-276.

33. Koroljow S. Two cases of malignant tumors with metastases apparently treated successfully with hypoglycemic coma. 261-270.

34. Wyngaarden J, and Smith L, eds. *Cecil Textbook of Medicine,* 18th ed., vol 2. Philadelphia, Pa: W.B. Saunders Company; 1988:2229.

35. Brightman M. Morphology of blood-brain interfaces. *Exp Eye Res.* 1971;25(suppl):1-6.

36. Vander A, Sherman J, Luciano D, eds. *Human Physiology: The Mechanisms of Body Function,* 3rd ed. New York, NY: McGraw-Hill Book Company; 1980:188.

37. Pardridge W. Receptor-mediated peptide transport through the blood-brain barrier. *Endoc Rev.* 1986;7:314-330.

38. Van Houten M, Posner B. Insulin binds to brain blood vessels in vivo. *Nature.* 1979;282:623-628.

39. Frank H, Pardridge W. A direct in vitro demonstration of insulin binding to isolated brain microvessels. *Diabetes.* 1981;30:757-762.

40. Pardridge W. Human blood-brain barrier insulin receptor. *J Neurochem.* 1985;44:1771-1778.

41. Frank H. Enhanced insulin binding to blood-brain barrier in vivo and to brain microvessels in vitro in newborn rabbits. *Diabetes.* 1985;34:728-733.

42. Frank H, Pardridge W. Binding and internalization of insulin and insulin-like growth factors by isolated brain microvessels. *Diabetes.* 1986;35:654-661.

43. Haselbacher G. Insulin-like growth factor II (IGF-II) in human brain: regional distribution of IGF-II and of higher molecular mass forms. *Proc Natl Acad Sci U S A.* 1985;82:2153-2160.

44. Rall D. Experimental studies of the blood-brain barrier. *Cancer Res.* 1965;25:1572-1577.

45. Roth R. *J Biochem.* 1981;256:5350.

46. Yoshimasa Y. *Diabetes.* 1984;33:1051.

47. Ito F. *Endocrinology.* 1984;36:165.

48. Poznansky M. *Science.* 1984;223:223.

49. Pérez García D Sr. La permibldad celular como base en el traitamiento radical de la sifilis: traitamiento de la neuro-sifilis y de la sifilis por la insulina. *Revista Medica Militar.* 1938;2:1-10.

50. Ayre S. New approaches to the delivery of drugs to the brain. *Med Hypoth.* 1989;29:283-291.

51. Ayre S, Skaletski B, Mosnaim A. Blood-brain barrier passage of azidothymidine in rats: effect of insulin. *Res Comm Chem Pathol Pharm.* 1989;63:45-52.

52. Lenka M. Human glioblastoma cell lines: levels of low-density lipoprotein receptor and low-density lipoprotein receptor-related protein. *Cancer Res.* 2000;60:2300-2303.

CHAPTER 12
CHEMOTHERAPY—DON'T LET THE WORD SCARE YOU

1. Fisher D. *The Cancer Chemotherapy Handbook.* St. Louis, Mo: Mosby; 1997:2-3.

CHAPTER 13
WHY I BELIEVE ONCOLOGISTS ARE GOOD, BUT I WOULD GET A SECOND OPINION BEFORE I LET ONE TREAT ME

1. Abel U. Chemotherapy of Advanced Epithelial Cancer: A Critical Survey, Hippokrates, Verlag Stuttgart. 1990.

2. Bjorksten J. *Longevity,* JAB Publishing, Charleston, SC, 1987:22.

CHAPTER 14
BE CAREFUL IN DOING ONLY WHAT YOUR INSURANCE PAYS FOR

1. Wittes R. Accrual to clinical trials. *J Natl Cancer Inst.* 1988;80:884-885.

2. McCabe M. Impact of third-party reimbursement on cancer clinical investigations: a consensus statement of coordinated by the National Cancer Institute. *J Cancer Inst.* 1989;81:1585-1586.

3. Abel U. *Chemotherapy of Advanced Epithelial Cancer: A Critical Survey.* Stuttgart, Germany: Hippokrates Verlag; 1990.

4. Moss R. *Questioning Chemotherapy.* Brooklyn, NY: Equinox Press; 2000:75.

CHAPTER 15
UNDERSTANDING THE PHARMACOKINETICS OF CANCER THERAPY— IT COULD SAVE YOUR LIFE

1. *The Biological Basis of Cancer.* Cambridge, UK: Press Syndicate of the University of Cambridge; 1998.

2. Laszlo J. Oncology introduction. In: *Cecil's Textbook of Medicine.* 18th ed. Philadelphia, Pa: W.B. Saunders Co.; 1988:1082-1089.

CHAPTER 16
CHEMOTHERAPY: THE GOOD, THE BAD, AND THE UGLY

1. Rubin P, ed. *Clinical Oncology.* 3rd ed. Atlanta, Ga: American Cancer Society; 1970.

2. *Cancer Facts & Figures* 2000. Atlanta, Ga: American Cancer Society; 2001.

3. Diamond W, Cowden L. *Cancer Diagnosis: What to Do Next.* Published by Goldberg B, www.alternativemedicine.com; 1998.

4. Murphy G, Lawrence W, Lenhard R, eds. *American Cancer Society Textbook of Clinical Oncology.* 2nd ed. Atlanta, Ga: American Cancer Society; 1995.

5. Steel G. Cell loss as a factor in the growth rate of human tumours. *Europ J Cancer.* 1967;3:381-387.

6. Bingham C. The cell cycle and cancer chemotherapy. *Am J Nurs.* July 1978:1201-1205.

7. McDivitt R. A proposed classification of breast cancer based on kinetic information. *Cancer.* 1986;57:269-276.

8. Gregory W. Chemotherapy of advanced breast cancer: outcome and prognostic factors. *Br J Cancer.* 1993;68:988-995.

9. Hoffman E. *Cancer and the Search for Selective Biochemical Inhibitors.* Boca Raton, Fla: CRC Press; 2000:63.

10. Crewdson J. Cancer-drug treatment: less might prove more. *Chicago Tribune.* April 2, 2000.

11. Evenson B. Discovery could win war on cancer. *National Post.* April 1, 2000.

CHAPTER 20
IPT AS A GENERAL MEDICAL TECHNIQUE

1. *Catalogue of Services.* Beverly Hills, Calif: Immunosciences Lab, Inc. 2001:9-10.

2. Paquette, Jean-Claude. *Medicine of Hope.* Translated from French by Aimé Ricci, 2001.

3. www.IPTQ.org hosted by Chris Duffield, Ph.D.

CHAPTER 21
INSULIN POTENTIATION THERAPY: THE TREATMENT OF THE FUTURE FOR INFECTIONS AND AUTOIMMUNE DISEASES

1. *Catalog of Services,* Beverly Hills, Calif: Immunosciences Lab, Inc.; 2001.

2. Wolfe F. Remission in rheumatoid arthritis. *J Rheumat.* 1985;12:245-249.

3. Kushner I. Changing perspectives in the treatment of rheumatoid arthritis. *J Rheumat.* 1992;19:1831-1834.

4. Harris E. Rheumatoid arthritis: pathophysiology and implications for therapy. *N Engl J Med.* 1990;322:1277-1289.

5. Schartz B. Infectious agents, immunity, and rheumatic diseases. *Arthr Rheumat.* 1990;33:457-465.

6. Tan P. The microbial cause of rheumatoid arthritis: time to dump Koch's postulates. *J Rheumat.* 1992;19:1170-1171.

7. Ford D. The microbiological causes of rheumatoid arthritis. *J Rheumat.* 1991;18:1441-1442.

8. Swift H. Pathogenic pleuropneumonia-like organisms from acute rheumatic exudates and tissues. *Science.* 1939;89:271-272.

9. Clark H. Determination of mycoplasma antibodies in humans. *Bacter Proc.* 1964;64:59.

10. Brown T. Relationship between mycoplasma antibodies and rheumatoid factors. *Arthr Rheumat.* 1970;13:309-310.

11. Rook G. A reappraisal of the evidence that rheumatoid arthritis and several other idiopathic diseases are slow bacterial infections. *Ann Rheumat Dis.* 1993;52:S30-S38.

CHAPTER 22
THE OTHER POTENTIATORS, INCLUDING DMSO, HYPERTHERMIA, ELECTROCHEMOTHERAPY, OXIDATIVE THERAPY, AND NUTRIENTS

1. Jacob S. *The Miracle of MSM.* New York, NY: Berkley Pub Group; 1999:229.

2. Moss R. *Cancer Therapy.* Brooklyn, NY: Equinox Press; 1996:301-305.

3. McGrady P. *The Persecuted Drug: The Story of DMSO.* New York, NY: Charter; 1979.

4. Lasagna L. ed. *Controversies in Therapeutics.* Philadelphia, Pa: W.B. Saunders; 1980:519-528.

5. Jacob S. *Dimethyl Sulfoxide.* Ann Arbor, Mich: Marcel Dekker, Inc.; 1986.

6. Walters R. *Options: The Alternative Cancer Therapy Book.* New York, NY: 1993.

7. Jacob S. *Current Status of Dimethyl Sulfoxide.* Portland: Oregon Health Sciences University; 1994.

8. Denko C. Distribution of dimethyl sulfoxide in the rat. *Ann NY Acad Sci.* 1967;141:77-84.

9. Kolb K. Absorption, distribution, and elimination of labeled dimethyl sulfoxide in man and animals. *Ann NY Acad Sci.* 1967;141:85-95.

10. Pommier R. Synergistic cytotoxicity between dimethyl sulfoxide and antineoplastics against ovarian tumors in vitro. *Surg Forum.* 1987;38:475-477.

11. Pommier R. Cytotoxicity of dimethyl sulfoxide and antineoplastic combinations against human tumors. *Am J Surg.* 1988;155:672-676.

12. Warren J. Potentiation of antineoplastic compounds by oral dimethyl sulfoxide in tumor-bearing rats. *Ann NY Acad Sci.* 1975;243:194-208.

13. Thuning C. Mechanisms of the synergistic effect of oral dimethyl sulfoxide on antineoplastic therapy. *Ann NY Acad Sci.* 1983;411:150-160.

14. Garrido J, Lagos R. Dimethyl sulfoxide therapy as toxicity-reducing agent and potentiator of cyclophosphamide in the treatment of different types of cancer. *Ann NY Acad Sci.* 1975;243:412-420.

15. Diamond W, Cowden W. *Alternative Medicine: Definitive Guide to Cancer.* Tiburon, Calif: Future Medicine Publishing; 1997:879-883.

16. Roberts N. Impact of temperature elevation on immunologic defenses. *Rev Infect Dis.* 1991;13:462.

17. Ngu V. Fever: thermodynamics applied to the leukocyte. *Med Hypoth.* 1990;33:241.

18. Vaupel P. Blood flow, tissue oxygenation, and pH distribution in malignant tumors upon localized hyperthermia. *Strahlentherapie.* 1983;159:73-81.

19. Vaupel P. Pathophysiology of tumors in hyperthermia. In: Issels RD, Wilmanns W, eds. *Application of Hyperthermia in the Treatment of Cancer.* Berlin, Germany: Springer; 1988:65-75.

20. Jain R. Transport of molecules across tumor vasculature. *Cancer Metast Rev.* 1987;6:559-593.

21. Jain R. Tumor blood flow—characterization, modifications, and role in hyperthermia. *IEEE Trans Sonics Ultras.* 1984;SU-31:504-526.

22. Vaulpel P, Kallinowski F. Physiological effects of hyperthermia: recent results. *Cancer Res.* 1987;104:71-109.

23. Elias M. Heat therapy may help against cancer. *USA Today.* March 31, 1986.

24. Hornback N. Radiation and microwave therapy in the treatment of advanced cancer. *Radiology.* 1979;130:459-464.

25. Hornback N. Advanced stage III-B cancer of the cervix: treatment by hyperthermia and radiation. *Gynecol Oncol.* 1986;23:160-167.

26. Scott R. Local hyperthermia in combination with definitive radiotherapy: increased tumor clearance, reduced recurrence rate in extended follow-up. *Intl J Radiat Oncol Biol Phys.* 1984;10:2119-2123.

27. Bicher H, ed. Clinical use of regional hyperthermia. In: *Consensus on Hyperthermia for the 1990s.* New York, NY: Plenum Press; 1990.

28. *American Cancer Society's Guide to Complementary and Alternative Cancer Methods.* Atlanta, Ga: American Cancer Society; 2000:131-132.

29. Suit H. Hyperthermia: potential as an anti-tumor agent. *Cancer.* 1974;34:122-129.

30. Storm F. Magnetic-induction hyperthermia: results of a 5-year multi-institutional national cooperative trial in advanced cancer patients. *Cancer.* 1985;55:2677-2687.

31. Hiraoka M. Site-specific phase I, II trials of hyperthermia at Kyoto University. *Intl J Hypertherm.* 1994;10:403-410.

32. Van der Zee J. Comparison of radiotherapy alone with radiotherapy plus hyperthermia in locally advanced pelvic tumours: a prospective randomised, multicentre trial. *Lancet.* 2000;55:1119-1125.

33. Bicher H, ed. Local hyperthermia for superficial and moderately deep tumors. In: *Consensus on Hyperthermia for the 1990s.* New York, NY: Plenum Press; 1990:353-367.

34. Alberts D. Therapeutic synergisms of hypermia-cis-platinum in a mouse tumor model. *J Natl Cancer Inst.* 1980;65:455-460.

35. Douple E. Therapeutic potentiation of cis-dichlorodiamineplatinum and radiation by interstitial microwave hyperthermia in a mouse tumor. *Nat Cancer Inst Monograph.* 1982;61:259-262.

36. Mella, O. Combined hyperthermia and cis-diaminedichloroplatinum in BD IX rats with transplanted BT4A tumors. *Intl J Hypertherm.* 1985;1:171-183.

37. Los G. Optimisation of intraperitoneal cisplatin therapy with regional hyperthermia in rats. *Europ J Cancer.* 1991;27:472-477.

38. Wiedemann G. Effects of temperature on the therapeutic efficacy and pharmacokinetics of ifosfamide. Neubeuern, Germany: *OncoTherm Scientific Papers;* 1993.

39. Bull J. An update on the anticancer effects of a combination of chemotherapy and hyperthermia. *Cancer Res.* 1984;44(Suppl.):4853-4856.

40. Hahn G. Potential for therapy of drugs and hyperthermia. *Cancer Res.* 1979;39:2264-2268.

41. Meyn R. Thermal enhancement of DNA strand breakage in mammalian cells treated with bleomycin. *Int J Radit Oncol Biol Phys.* 1979;5:1487-1489.

42. Dynlacht J. Hyperthermia can reduce cytotoxicity from Etoposide without a corresponding reduction in the number of topoisomerase II-DNA cleavable complexes. *Cancer Res.* 1994;54:4129-4137.

43. Herman T. Reversal of methotrexate resistance by hyperthermia. *Cancer Res.* 1981;41:3840-3843.

44. Wallner K. Hyperthermic enhancement of cell killing by Mitomycin C in Mitomycin C resistant Chinese hamster ovary cells. *Cancer Res.* 1987;47:1308-1312.

45. Kakehi M. Multi-institutional clinical studies on hyperthermia combined with radiotherapy or chemotherapy in advanced cancer of deep-seated organs. *Intl J Hypertherm.* 1990;6:719-740.

46. Boik J. *Cancer and Natural Medicine.* Princeton, Minn: Oregon Medical Press; 1996:54-56.

47. Elia G. Regulation of heat shock protein synthesis by quercetin in human erythroleukaemia cells. *Biochem J.* 1994;15(Pt 1):201-209.

48. Wei Y. Induction of apoptosis by quercetin: involvement of heat shock protein. *Cancer Res.* 1994;54:4952-4957.

49. Agullo G. Quercetin exerts a preferential cytotoxic effect on active dividing colon carcinoma HT29 and caco-2 cells. *Cancer Lett.* 1994;87:55-63.

50. Kim J. Quercetin: an inhibitor of lactate transport and hyperthermic sensitizer of hela cells. *Cancer Res.* 1984;44:102-106.

51. Kaltsas H. Too hot for cancer—hyperthermia and electrotherapy. *Altern Med Digest.* September 2000:42-52.

52. *Electro Cancer Therapy* (brochure). Bad Aibling, Germany: Oncotherm GmbH; 1998.

53. Mir L. Introduction of definite amounts of non-permeant molecules into living cells after electropermeabilization: direct access to the cytosol. *Exper Cell Res.* 1988;175:15-25.

54. Okino M. Electrical impulse chemotherapy for rat solid tumors. *Proc Jpn Cancer Congress.* 1987;46:420.

55. Okino M. Optimal electric conditions in electrical impulse chemotherapy. *Jpn J Cancer Res.* 1992;83:1095-1101.

56. Okino, M. The effects of a single high-voltage electrical stimulation with anticancer drug on in vivo growing malignant tumors. *Jpn J Surgery.* 1990;20:197-204.

57. Kanesada H. Anticancer effect of high voltage pulses combined with concentration dependent anticancer drugs on Lewis lung carcinoma, in vivo. *J Jpn Soc Cancer Ther.* 1990;25:2640-2648.

58. Orlowski S. Transient electropermeabilization of cells in culture: increase of the cytotoxicity of anticancer drugs. *Biochem Pharmacol.* 1988;37:4727-4733.

59. Mir L. Electrochemotherapy potentiation of antitumour effect of bleomycin by local electric pulses. *Europ J Cancer.* 1991;27:68-72.

60. Belehradek J. Electrochemotherapy of spontaneous mammary tumors in mice. *Europ J Cancer.* 1991;27:73-76.

61. Mir L. Electrochemotherapy tumor treatment is improved by interleukin-2 stimulation of the host's defenses. *Eur Cytokine Netw.* 1992;3:331-334.

62. Sersa G. Potentiation of bleomycin anti-tumor effectiveness by electrotherapy. *Cancer Lett.* 1993;69:81-84.

63. Dev S. Electrochemotherapy—a novel method of cancer treatment. *Cancer Treat Rev.* 1994;20:105-115.

64. Salford L. Electrochemotherapy—a possible treatment for malignant brain tumors. Paper presented at: Annual Meeting of the European Association Neurosurgical Society; Feb. 18-20, 1993; Rome, Italy.

65. Mir L. Electrochemotherapy, a novel anti-tumor treatment: first clinical trial. *C R Acad Sci Paris.* 1991;313:613-618.

66. Belehradek M. Electrochemotherapy: a new anti-tumor treatment. *Cancer.* 1993;72:3694-3700.

67. Questionable methods of cancer management: hydrogen peroxide and other "hyperoxygenation" therapies. *CA Cancer J Clin.* 1993;43:47-56.

68. Altman N. *Oxygen Healing Therapies.* Rochester, Vt: Healing Arts Press; 1998.

69. Gray L. The concentration of oxygen dissolved in tissues at the time of irradiation as a factor in radiotherapy. *Br J Radiol.* 1953;26:638-648.

70. Hollcroft J. Factors modifying the effect of x-irradiation on regression of a transplanted lymphosarcoma. *J Natl Cancer Inst.* 1952;12:751-763.

71. Gray L. The influence of oxygen on the radiosensitivity of cells and tissues. In: *Proceedings of the Second Australisian Conference on Radiation Biology,* Melbourne, Australia: 1958. London: Butterworth, Inc.; 1958:152-168.

72. Bacq Z. *Fundamentals of Radiobiology,* rev 2nd ed. New York, NY: Pergamon Press; 1961.

73. Churchill-Davidson I. Oxygenation in radiotherapy. *Br J Radiol.* 1957:406-422.

74. Krementz E. The effect of increased oxygen tension on the tumoricidal effect of nitrogen mustard. *Surgery.* 1961;50:266-271.

75. Krementz, E. The enhancement of chemotherapy by increased tissue oxygen tension. *Cancer Chemother Report.* 1960;10:125

76. Smith A. Effects of increased oxygen tension on tumor response to an alkylating agent. 135-136.

77. Kaibara N. Experimental studies on enhancing the therapeutic effect of Mitomycin-C with hydrogen peroxide. *Jp J Exp Med.* 1971;41:323-329.

78. Faber M. Lipid peroxidation products and vitamin and trace element status in patients with cancer before and after chemotherapy including Adriamycin: a preliminary study. *Biol Trace Elem Res.* 1995;47:117-123.

79. Subramaniam S. Oxidant and antioxidant levels in the erythrocytes of breast cancer patients treated with CMF. *Med Sci Res.* 1993;21:79-80.

80. Lamson D. Antioxidants and cancer therapy II: quick reference guide. *Altern Med Rev.* 2000;5:152-163.

81. Conklin K. Dietary antioxidants during cancer chemotherapy: impact on chemotherapeutic effectiveness and development of side effects. *Nutr Cancer.* 2000;37:1-18.

82. Scambia G. Inhibitory effect of quercetin on primary ovarian and endometrial cancers and synergistic activity with cis-diamminedichloroplatinum (II). *Gyn Oncol.* 1992;45:13-19.

83. Seifter E. Vitamin A and beta-carotene as adjunctive therapy to tumor excision, radiation therapy, and chemotherapy. In: Prasad K, ed. *Vitamins, Nutrition and Cancer.* Basel, Switzerland: Karger; 1984:1-19.

84. Bohm S. A feasibility study of cisplatin administration with low-volume hydration and glutathione protection in the treatment of ovarian carcinoma. *Anticancer Res.* 1991;11:1613-1616.

85. Di Re F. Efficacy and safety of high-dose cisplatin and cyclophosphamide with glutathione protection in the treatment of bulky advanced epithelial ovarian cancer. *Cancer Chemother Pharmacol.* 1990;25:355-360.

86. Oriana S. A preliminary clinical experienced with reduced glutathione as protector against cisplatin toxicity. *Tumori.* 1987;73:337-340.

87. Cascinu S. Neuroprotective effect of reduced glutathione on cisplatin-based chemotherapy in advanced gastric cancer: a randomized double-blind placebo-controlled trial. *J Clin Oncol.* 1995;13:26-32.

88. Vadgama J. Synergistic effects of selenium and anticancer drugs. *Anticancer Res.* 2000;20:1391-1414.

88. Sweet, F., Ming-Shian Kao, and Song-Chiau D. Lee. Ozone selectively inhibits growth of human cancer cells. *Science* 980 Vol. 209: 931-933

CHAPTER 23
ESTRADIOL: THE NEMESIS OF FEMALE CANCERS

1. Murphy G, Lawrence W, Lenhard R, eds. *American Cancer Society Textbook of Clinical Oncology.* 2nd ed. Atlanta, Ga: American Cancer Society; 1995.

2. Doll R. Health and the environment in the 1990s. *Am J Public Health.* 1993;82:933-941.

3. Williams G, Weisburger J. Chemical carcinogenesis. In: Amdur M, Doull J, Klaassen C, eds. *Casarett and Doull's Toxicology: The Basic Science of Poisons.* 4th ed. New York, NY: Pergamon Press; 1991:127-200.

4. Murray M. A comprehensive evaluation of premenstrual syndrome. *Am J Nat Med.* 1997;4:6-22.

5. Mayo J. Premenstrual syndrome: a natural approach to management. *Clin Nutr Insights.* 1997;5:1-8.

6. Curtis M. *Glass's Office Gynecology.* Baltimore, Md: Williams & Wilkins; 1999:62-69.

7. Hacker N. *Essentials of Obstetrics and Gynecology.* Philadelphia, Pa: W.B. Saunders; 1986.

8. Barnhart K. A clinician's guide to the premenstrual syndrome. *Med Clin North Am.* 1995;79:1457-1472.

9. Facchinetti F. Estradiol/progesterone imbalance and the premenstrual syndrome. Lancet. 1983;2:1302.

10. Munday M. Correlations between progesterone, estradiol, and aldosterone levels in the premenstrual syndrome. *Clin Endocrinol.* 1981;14:1-9.

11. Brinker F. A comparative review of eclectic female regulators. *J Naturopathic Med.* 1997;7:11-25.

12. Hoffman D. Phytoestrogens, receptors, and the phytotherapist. *Protocol J Botan Med.* 1996;1: 8-10.

13. Abraham G. Nutritional factors in the etiology of the premenstrual tension syndromes. *J Reprod Med.* 1983;28:446-463.

14. Abraham G. Nutrition and the premenstrual tension syndromes. *J Appl Nutr.* 1984;36:103-117.

15. Hargrove J. Effect of vitamin B6 on infertility in women with the premenstrual tension syndrome. *Infertility.* 1979;2:315.

16. Clarke A. Premenstrual syndrome: single or multiple causes? *Can J Psych.* 1985;30:474-482.

17. Head K. Premenstrual syndrome: nutritional and alternative approaches. *Altern Med Rev.* 1997;2:12-25.

18. Sliutz G. Inhibit pituitary production of prolactin in cases of slight hyperprolactinemia. *Hormone Metab Res.* 1993;5:253-255.

19. Snow J. Vitex *agnus-castus. Protocol J Botanic Med.* 1996;1:2-7.

20. Brown D. *Herbal Prescriptions for Better Health.* Rocklin, Calif: Prima Publishing; 1996.

21. Milewicz A. *Vitex agnus-castus* extract in the treatment of luteal phase defects due to latent hyperprolactinemia: results of a randomized placebo-controlled double-blind study. *Arzneim-Forsch Drug Res.* 1993;43:752-756.

22. Bohnert K. The use of *Vitex agnus-castus* for hyperprolactinemia. *Quar Rev Nat Med.* 1997;Spring:19-21.

23. Mayo J. Black cohosh and chasteberry: herbs valued by women for centuries. *Clin Nutr Insights.* 1998;7:1-4.

24. Canavan T. Managing endometriosis. *Postgrad Med.* 2000;107:213-224.

25. Koninckx P. Suggestive evidence that pelvic endometriosis is a progressive disease, whereas deeply infiltrating endometriosis is associated with pelvic pain. *Fertil Steril.* 1991;55:759.

26. DeGroot L, ed. *Endocrinology.* Vol 3. Philadelphia, Pa: W.B. Saunders; 1995:2086-2088.

27. American Fertility Society. Classification of endometriosis. *Fertil Steril.* 1979(revised 1985);32:633.

28. Waller K. Gonadotropin-releasing hormone analogues for the treatment of endometriosis: long-term follow-up. *Fertil Steril.* 1993;59:511-515.

29. The Nafarelin European Endometriosis Trial Group. Nafarelin for endometriosis: a large-scale, danazol-controlled trial of efficacy and safety, with 1-year follow-up. *Fertil Steril.* 1992;57:514-522.

30. Bontis J. Etiopathology of endometriosis. *Ann NY Acad Sci.* 1997;816:305-309.

31. Schmidt C. Endometriosis: a reappraisal of pathogenesis and treatment. *Fertil Steril.* 1985;44:157-173.

32. Wheeler J. Recurrent endometriosis: incidence, management, and prognosis. *Am J Obstet Gynecol.* 1983;146:247-253.

33. Canavan T. Managing endometriosis. *Postgrad Med.* 2000;107:213-224.

34. Schenken R. *Endometriosis: Contemporary Concepts in Clinical Management.* Philadelphia, Pa: J.B. Lippincott; 1989.

35. Goldberg B. Fibroids: an alternative approach. *Townsend Lett Doctors Patients.* 2000;January:84-97.

36. Bartisch E. Leiomyosarcoma of the uterus: a 50-year review. *Obstet Gynecol.* 1968;32:101.

37. Miller N. Original introduction and critical review of a chronic pain condition. *Pain.* 2000;86:3-10.

38. Leiomyofibroma of the uterus and endometrial cancer. *Am J Obstet Gynecol.* 1947;53:846.

39. *Women's Alternative Medicine Report.* Larchmont, NY: Mary Ann Liebert, publishers; 1999:1:3-5.

40. Abou-Issa H. Relative efficacy of glucurate on the initiation and promotion phases of rat mammary carcinogenesis. *Anticancer Res.* 1995;15:805-810.

41. Odell W. The menopause and hormonal replacement. In: Degroot L, ed. *Endocrinology.* 3rd ed. Philadelphia, Pa: W.B. Saunders; 1995:2128-2139.

42. Ashley L. Testosterone in the postmenopausal woman. *Townsend Lett Doctors Patients.* 1996; June:161-163.

43. Werbach M. *Textbook of Nutritional Medicine.* Tarzana, Calif: Third Line Press; 1999:521-525.

44. Langdon S, ed. *Biology of Female Cancers.* Boca Raton, Fla: CRC Press; 1997.

45. Brinkley D, Haybittle JL. Long-term survival of women with breast cancer. *Lancet.* 1984;1:1118.

46. Adair F. Long-term follow-up of breast cancer patients: the thirty-year report. *Cancer.* 1974;33:1145.

47. Le M.D. Long-term survival of women with breast cancer: a study of the curability of the disease. *Lancet.* 1984;2:922.

48. Korenman SG. Reproductive endocrinology and breast cancer in women. In: Pike MC, Siiteri PK, Wesch CW, eds. *Hormones and Breast Cancer.* New York, NY: CSH Publishing; 1981:71-82.

49. Pike M. Breast cancer in young women and use of oral contraceptives: possible modifying effect of formulation and age at use. *Lancet.* 1983;2:926.

50. McPherson K. Early oral contraceptive use and breast cancer: results of another case-control study. *Br J Cancer.* 1987;56:653.

51. Bulbrook R. Relation between risk of breast cancer and bioavailability of estradiol in blood: prospective study in Guernsey. In: Angelli A, Bradlow HL, Dogliotto L, eds. *Endocrinology of the Breast: Basic and Clinical Aspects. Ann NY Acad Sci.* 1986;373:464.

52. Lemon H. Reduced estriol excretion in patients with breast cancer prior to endocrine therapy. *JAMA.* 1966;196:112-136.

53. Prentice R. Dietary fat reduction and plasma oestradiol concentration in healthy post-menopausal women. *J Natl Cancer Inst.* 1990;129:82.

54. Rose D. High-fiber diet reduces serum estrogen concentrations in premenopausal women. *Am J Clin Nutr.* 1991;54:520-525.

55. Zimmerman K. Frequency anatomical distribution and management of local recurrences after definitive therapy for breast cancer. *Cancer.* 1966;19:672-672.

56. Rubin P, ed. *Clinical Oncology for Medical Students and Physicians.* 3rd ed. Atlanta, Ga: American Cancer Society; 1970:90-104.

57. Haagensen C. *Diseases of the Breast.* Philadelphia, Pa: W.B. Saunders; 1956.

58. Henderson I. Breast cancer. In: Murphy G, Lawrence W, Lenhard R, eds. *American Cancer Society Textbook of Clinical Oncology.* 2nd ed. Atlanta, Ga: American Cancer Society; 1995:198-219.

59. Bonadonna G. Ten-year experience with CMF-based adjuvant chemotherapy in resectable breast cancer. *Breast Cancer Res Treat.* 1985;5:95-115.

60. Fisher B. Significance of ipsilateral breast tumour recurrence after lumpectomy. *Lancet.* 1991;338:327-331.

61. Fisher B. Eight-year results of a randomized clinical trial comparing total mastectomy and lumpectomy with or without irradiation in the treatment of breast cancer. *N Eng J Med.* 1989;320:822-828.

62. Singer S, Grismaijer S. *Dressed to Kill.* Garden City, NY: Avery Publishing Group; 1995.

63. Bair F. *Cancer Sourcebook.* Detroit, Mich: Omnigraphics, Inc.; 1992:305.

64. Lee H. Dietary effects on breast-cancer risk in Singapore. *Lancet.* 1991;337:1197-1200.

65. Adelercreutz H. Urinary excretion of lignans and isoflavonoid phytoestrogens in Japanese men and women consuming a traditional Japanese diet. *Am J Clin Nutr.* 1991;54:1093-110.

66. Boik J. *Cancer and Natural Medicine.* Princeton, Minn: Oregon Medical Press; 1996.

67. Heerdt A. Calcium glucarate as a chemopreventive agent in breast cancer. *Isr J Med Sci.* 1995;31:101-105.

68. Zheng W. Urinary excretion of isoflavonoids and the risk of breast cancer. *Cancer Epidemiol Biomarkers Prev.* 1999;8:35-40.

69. Hsieh C. Estrogenic effects of genistein on the growth of estrogen receptor-positive human breast cancer cells in vitro and in vivo. *Cancer Res.* 1998;58:3833-3838.

70. McMichael-Phillips D. Effects of soy-protein supplementation on epithelial proliferation in the histologically normal human breast. *Am J Clin Nutr.* 1998;68:1431S-1436S.

71. Kuiper G. Interaction of estrogenic chemicals and phytoestrogens with estrogen receptor beta. *Endocrinology.* 1998;139:4252-4263.

72. Lu L. Decreased ovarian hormones during a soya diet: implications for breast cancer prevention. *Cancer Res.* 2000;60:4112-4121.

73. Newcomb P. Lactation and a reduced risk of premenopausal breast cancer. *N Engl J Med.* 1994;330:81-87.

74. Brind J. Reading the data: defining a link between abortion and breast cancer. *Focus on the Family Phys Mag.* July/August 2000:4-7.

75. Brind J. Induced abortion as an independent risk factor for breast cancer: a comprehensive review and meta-analysis. *J Epidemiol Com Health.* 1996;50:481-496.

76. Dao T. Effect of estrogen and progesterone on cellular replication of human breast tumors. *Cancer Res.* 1982;42:359-362.

77. Podhajcer O. In vitro analysis of the cellular proliferative response to 17-b-estradiol of human breast cancer. *Cancer.* 1988;61:1807-1812.

78. Whitaker P. Serum equilin, estrone, and estradiol levels in postmenopausal women receiving conjugated equine estrogens (Premarin). *Lancet.* 1980;5:14-18.

79. Fishman J. Effect of thyroid on hydroxylation of estrogen in man. *J Clin Endocrinol Metab.* 1965;213:365-372.

80. Zumoff B. The role of endogenous estrogen excess in human breast cancer. *Anticancer Res.* 1981;1:39-44.

81. Zumoff B. Hormone profiles and the epidemiology of breast cancer. In: Stoll BA, ed. *Endocrine Relationships in Breast Cancer.* London, UK: William Heinemann Medical Books; 1982.

82. Bradlow H. 16a-Hydroxylation of estradiol: a possible risk marker for breast cancer. *Ann NY Acad Sci.* 1986;464:138-151.

83. Bradlow H. Effects of dietary indole-3-carbinol on estradiol metabolism and spontaneous mammary tumors in mice. *Carcinogenesis.* 1991;12:1571-1574.

84. Schneider J. Effect of obesity on estradiol metabolism: decreased formation of nonuterotrpic metabolites. *J Clin Endocrinol Metab.* 1983;56:973-978.

85. Hershcopf R. Obesity, diet, endogenous estrogens, and the risk of hormone sensitive cancers. *Am J Clin Nutr.* 1987;45:283-289.

86. Santisteban G. *Biochem Biophys Res Comm.* 1983;132:1174-1180.

87. *Carcinogenesis.* 1998;19:1631-1639.

88. *Anticancer Drugs.* 1998;9:141-148.

89. *Pro Soc Experi Bio Med.* 1997;216:246-252.

90. Induction of estradiol metabolism by dietary indole-3-carbinol in humans. *J Natl Cancer Inst.* 82:947-949.

91. Altered estrogen metabolism and excretion in humans following consumption of indole-3-carbinol. *Nutr Cancer.* 16:59-66.

92. Changes in levels of urinary estrogen metabolites after oral indole-3-carbinol treatment in humans. *J Natl Cancer Inst.* 1997;89:718-723.

93. Wright J. Cabbages, broccoli, et al. versus sex hormone related cancers. *Nutr Healing.* February 2000:1-8.

94. Sharma S. Screening of potential chemopreventive agents using biochemical markers of carcinogenesis. *Cancer Res.* 1994;54:5848-5855.

95. Chen I. Indole-3-carbinol and diindolylmethane as aryl hydrocarbon receptor agonists and antagonists in T47D human breast cancer cells. *Biochem Pharmacol.* 1996;51:1069-1076.

96. Indole-3-carbinol: the tamoxifen substitute. *Life Exten.* October 1999:28-34.

97. Christensen J. Reversal of multidrug resistance in vivo by dietary administration of the phytochemical indole-3-carbinol. *Cancer Res.* 1996;56:574-581.

98. Bell M. Placebo-controlled trial of indole-3-carbinol in the treatment of CIN. *Gynecol Oncol.* 2000;78:123-129.

99. Vermeulen A. Sex hormone concentrations in postmenopausal women: relation to obesity, fat mass, age, and years post-menopause. *Clin Endocrinol.* 1978;9:59-67.

100. James V. Studies of estrogen metabolism in postmenopausal women with cancer. *J Steroid Biochem.* 1981;15:235-243.

101. Miller W. The relevance of local oestrogen metabolism with the breast. *Proc R Soc Edinburgh.* 1989;95:203-211.

102. Walaszek Z. Metabolism, uptake and excretion of a D-glucuric acid salt and its potential use in cancer prevention. *Cancer Detec Prev.* 1997;21:178-190.

103. Simone C. The role of glucarate in cancer treatment. *Intl J Integ Med.* 2000;2:42-47.

104. Wong M. Insulin binding by normal and neoplastic colon tissue. *Int. J Cancer.* 1985;35:335-341.

105. Mountjoy K. Insulin receptor regulation in cultured human tumor cells. *Cancer Res.* 1983;43:4537-4542.

106. Gross G. Perturbation by insulin of human breast cancer cell kinetics. *Cancer Res.* 1984;44:3570-3575.

107. Holdaway I. Hormone binding by human mammary carcinoma. *Cancer Res.* 1977;37:1946-1952.

108 Laslo J. Oncology introduction. In: *Cecil's Textbook of Medicine.* 18th ed. Philadelphia, Pa: W.B. Saunders; 19XX:1082-1089.

109. Bontenbal M. Effect of hormonal manipulation and doxorubicin administration on cell cycle kinetics of human breast cancer cells. *Br J Cancer.* 1989;60:688-692.

110. Murray M. Breast cancer: update on a growing epidemic. *Nat Med J.* 1999;2:1-6.

111. Axelson M. Origin of lignans in mammals and identification of a precursor from plants. *Nature.* 1982; 298: 659-660.

112. Borriello S. Production and metabolism of lignans by the human faecal flora. *J Appl Bacteriol.* 1985; 58: 37-43.

113. Serraino M. The effect of flax seed supplementation on early risk markers for mammary carcinogenesis. *Cancer Lett.* 1991; 60: 135-142.

114. Jenab M. The influence of flax seed and lignans on colon carcinogenesis and B-glucosidase activity. *Carcinogenesis* (Lond.). 1996; 17: 153-159.

115. Hutchins, A. Flax seed influences urinary lignan excretion in a dose-dependent manner in postmenopausal women. *Cancer Epidemiology, Biomarkers & Prevention.* 2000; 9: 1113-1118.

116. Adlercreutz, H. Dietary phytoestrogens and cancer: in vitro and in vivo studies. *Journal of Steroid Biochemistry and Molecular Biology.* 1992; 41: 331-337.

117. Adlecreutz, H. Inhibition of human aromatase by mammalian lignans and isoflavonoid phytoestrogens. *Journal of Steroid Biochemistry and Molecular Biology.* 1993; 44: 147-153.

118. Johnston, P. Flax seed oil and cancer: α-linolenic acid and carcinogenesis. *In Flax Seed in Human Nutrition,* S.C. Cunnane and L.U. Thompson (eds). Champaign, IL: Am Oil Chem Soc, 1995, 207-218.

119. Fishman J. Oxidative metabolism of estradiol. J *Biol Chem.* 1960; 235: 3104-3107.

120. Fishman, J. the role of estrogen in mammary carcinogenesis. *Ann NY Acad Sci.* 1995; 768: 91-100.

121. Bradlow H. 2-Hydroxyestrone: The "good" estrogen. *J Endocrinol.* 1996; 150: S259-S265.

122. Kabat G. Urinary estrogen metabolites and breast cancer: a case-control study. *Cancer Epidemiol Biomarkers Prev.* 1997; 6: 505-509.

123. Ho, G. Urinary 2/16α-hydroxyestrone ratio: correlation with serum insulin-like growth factor binding protein-3 and a potential marker of breast cancer risk. *Ann Acad Med* Singapore. 1998; 27: 294-299.

124. Zheng W. Urinary estrogen metabolites and breast cancer: a case-control study. *Cancer Epidemiol Biomarkers Prev* 1997; 6: 505-509, Cancer Epidemiol Biomarkers Prev 1998; 7: 85-86.

125. Anderson K. The influence of dietary protein and carbohydrate on the principal oxidative biotransformations of estradiol in normal subjects. *J Clin Endocrinolo Metab.* 1984; 59: 103-107.

126. Longcope C. The effect of a low fat diet on estrogen metabolism. *J Clin Endocrinol Metab.* 1987; 64: 1246-1250.

127. Bradlow H. Long-term responses of women to indole-3-carbinol or a high fiber diet. *Cancer Epidemiol Biomarkers Prev.* 1994; 3: 591-594.

128. Haggans C. Effect of flax seed consumption on urinary estrogen metabolites in postmenopausal women. *Nutrition and Cancer.* 1999; 33: 188-195.

129. Haggans C. The effect of flax seed and wheat bran consumption on urinary estrogen metabolites in premenopausal women. *Cancer Epidemiology, Biomarkers & Prevention.* 2000; 9: 719-725.

CHAPTER 26
UNDERSTANDING CANCER PHYSIOLOGY: THE KEY TO SUCCESS

1. Issels J. *Cancer: A Second Opinion.* New York, NY: Avery Publishing Group.
2. Prehn R.T. *Am J Pathol.* 1974;77:119-122.
3. Bucher N. *Regeneration of the Liver and Kidney.* Boston, Mass: Little, Brown; 1971.
4. Pierce G. Differentiation of malignant to benign cells. *Cancer Res.* 19XX;31:127-134.
5. Sachs L. Regulation of normal development and tumor suppression. *Int J Dev Biol.* 1993; 37:51-59.
6. Lennon S. Dose-dependent induction of apoptosis in human tumour cell lines by widely divergent stimuli. *Cell Proliferation.* 19XX;24:203-214.
7. Goel S. Role of cell death in the morphogenesis of thell amniote limbs. In: Fallon JF, Caplan AL, eds. *Limb Development and Regeneration. Part A.* New York, NY: Alan R. Liss; 19XX:175-182.
8. Pierce G. The cancer cell and is control by the embryo. *Am J Pathol.* 1983;113:117-124.
9. Pierce G. Mechanisms of programmed cell death in the blastocyst. *Proc Natl Acad Sci USA.* 19XX;86:3654-3658.
10. Parchment R. The implications of a unified theory of programmed cell death, polyamines, oxyradicals, and histogenesis in the embryo. *Int J Dev Biol.* 1993;37:75-83.
11. Bastida E. The metastatic cascade: potential approaches for the inhibition of metastasis. *Semin Thromb Hemost.* 1988;14:66-72.
12. Stracke M. Multi-step cascade of tumor cell metastasis. *In Vivo.* 1992;6:309-316.
13. Sinha A. Localization of Type IV collagen in the basement membranes of human prostate and lymph nodes by immunoperoxidase and immunoalkaline phosphatase. *Prostate.* 1991;18:93-104.
14. Shields S. Degradation of basement membrane collagens by metalloproteases released by human, murine, and amphibian tumours. *J Pathol.* 1984;143:193-197.
15. Alvarez O. Inhibition of collagenolytic activity and metastasis by a recombinant human tissue inhibitor of metalloproteinases. *J Natl Cancer Inst.* 1990;82:589-595.

16. Seppanen E. Temperature-dependent dissociation of Lucke renal adenocarcinoma cells. *Differentiation.* 1984;26:227-230.
17. McCutcheon M. Studies on invasiveness of cancer: adhesiveness of malignant cells in various human adenocarcinomas. *Cancer.* 1948;1:460-467.
18. Coman D. Decreased mutual adhesiveness, a property of cells from squamous cell carcinoma. *Cancer Res.* 1944;4:625-629.
19. Coman D. Mechanisms responsible for origin and distribution of blood-borne tumor metastases; review. *Cancer Res.* 1953;13:397-404.
20. Seppanen E. Temperature-dependent dissociation of Lucke renal adenocarcinoma cells. *Differentiation.* 1984;26:227-230.
21. McKinnell R. The Lucke renal adenocarcinoma, an anuran neoplasm: studies at the interface of pathology, virology, and differentiation competence. *J Cell Physiol.* 1997;173:115-118.
22. Epner D. Association of glycer-aldehyde-3-phosphate dehydrogenase expression with cell motility and metastatic potential of rat prostatic adenocarcinoma. *Cancer Res.* 1993;53:1995-1997.
23. Repesh L. Adriamycin-induced inhibition of melanoma cell invasion is correlated with decreases in tumor cell motility and increases in focal contact formation. *Clin Exp Metast.* 1993;11:91-102.
24. Tarin D. Correlation of collagenase secretion with metastatic-colonization potential in naturally occurring murine mammary tumors. *Br J Cancer.* 1982;46:266-278.
25. Michaels L. Cancer incidence and mortality in patients having anticoagulant therapy. *Lancet.* 1964;2:832-835.
26. Ryan J. Warfarin treatment of mice bearing autochthonous tumors: effect of spontaneous metastases. *Science.* 1968;162:1493-1494.
27. Zacharski L. Effect of warfarin on survival in small cell carcinoma of the lung. *J Am Med Assoc.* 1981;245:831-835.
28. D'Amore P. Antiangiogenesis as a strategy for antimetastasis. *Semin Thromb Hemost.* 1988;14:73-78.
29. Pierce G. Neoplasms, differentiations, and mutations. *Am J Pathol.* 1974;77:103-118.
30. Weber G. Enzymology of cancer cells. *N Engl J Med.* 1977;296:486-493.
31. Tubiana M. The role of local treatment in the cure of cancer. *Europ J Cancer.* 1992;28A:2061-2069.

32. Boik J. *Cancer and Natural Medicine.* Princeton, Minn: Oregon Medical Press; 1996:8-30.

33. Pierce G. Differentiation of normal and malignant cells. *Fed Proc.* 1970;29:1248-1254.

34. Yoshida M. The effect of quercetin on cell cycle progression and growth of human gastric cancer cells. *FEBS Lett.* 1990;260:10-13.

35. Mousavi Y. Genistein is an effective stimulator of sex hormone-binding globulin production in hepatocarcinoma human liver cancer cells and suppresses proliferation of these cells in culture. *Steroids.* 1993;58:301-304.

36. Aaronson S. Growth factors and cancer. *Science.* 1991;254:1146-1153.

37. Pardee A. *Science.* 1989;246:603-612.

38. Resnicoff M. Correlation between apoptosis, tumorigenesis, and levels of insulin-like growth factor 1 receptors. *Cancer Res.* 1995;55:3739-3741.

39. Resnicoff M. Rat glioblastoma cells expressing an antisense RNA to the insulin-like growth factor-1 receptor are nontumorigenic and induce regression of wild-type tumors. *Cancer Res.* 1994;54:5531-5534.

40. Resnicoff M. Growth inhibition of human melanoma cells in nude mice by antisense strategies to the type 1 insulin-like growth factor receptor. *Cancer Res.* 1994;54:4848-4850.

41. Mitter C. Plasma levels of d-dimer: a crosslinked fibrin-degradation product in female breast cancer. *J Cancer Res Clin Oncol.* 1991;117:259-262.

42. Bu L. The role of proteases in the growth, invasion, and spread of cancer cells. *Tidsskr Nor Laegeforen.* 1990;110:3753-3756.

43. Honn K. The role of platelets in metastasis. *Biorrheology.* 1987;24:127-137.

44. Nagy J. Pathogenesis of tumor stroma generation: a critical role for leaky blood vessels and fibrin deposition. *Biochem Biophys Acta.* 1989;948:305-326.

45. Brown L. Leaky vessels, fibrin deposition, and fibrosis: a sequence of events common to solid tumors and to many other types of diseases. *Am Rev Respir Dis.* 1989;140:1104-1107.

46. Zacharski L. Effect of warfarin on survival in small cell carcinoma of the lung. *JAMA.* 1981;245:831-835.

47. Chlebowski R. Inhibition of human tumor growth and DNA biosynthetic activity by vitamin K and warfarin: in vitro and clinical results. *AACR Abstracts.* March 1983:165.

48. Zacharski L. Anticoagulation in the treatment of cancer in man. In: Donati M, Davidson J, Garattini, S, eds. *Malignancy and the Hemostatic System.* New York, NY: Raven Press; 1981.

49. Martin, W. Anticancer effect of dipyridamole. *Townsend Lett Doctors Patients.* May 2000:114-115.

50. Egyud L. Resistance of cancer cells to immune recognition and killing. *Med Hypoth.* 2000;54:456-460.

51. Folkman J. Growth and metastasis of tumor in organ culture. *Cancer.* 1963;16:453-467.

52. Folkman J. Induction of angiogenesis during the transition from hyperplasia to neoplasia. *Nature.* 1989;339:58-63.

53. Thompson W. Tumours acquire their vasculature by vessel incorporation, not vessel ingrowth. *J Pathol.* 1987;151:323-333.

54. Skinner S. Microvascular architecture of experimental colon tumors in the rat. *Cancer Res.* 1990;50:2411-2419.

55. Folkman J. What is the evidence that tumors are angiogenesis dependent? *J Natl Cancer Inst.* 1990;82:4-10.

56. Williams C. Host cyclooxygenase-2 modulates carcinoma growth. *J Clin Invest.* 2000;105:1589-1594.

57. Tsujii M. Cyclooxygenase regulates angiogenesis induced by colon cancer cells. *Cell.* 1998;93:705-716.

CHAPTER 27
THE CANCER CLOTTING COAT

1. Murray R. *Harper's Biochemistry.* 24th ed. Stamford, Conn: Appleton and Lange; 1996:671-673.

2. Aggeler J. An irreversible tissue inhibitor of collagenase in human amniotic fluid: characterization and separation from fibronectin. *Biochem Biophys Res Comm.* 1981;100:1195-1201.

3. Alitalo K. Extracellular matrix proteins characterize human tumor cell lines. *Intl J Cancer.* 1981;27:755-761.

4. Kwann H. Fibrinolysis and cancer. *Semin Thromb Haemost.* 1990;16:230-235.

5. Kondera-Anasz Z. Selected parameters of coagulation, fibrinolysis, and antibodies to fibrinogen in lung cancer. *Pneumolo Alergol Pol.* 1993;61:461-466.

6. Kaufman P. The fibrinoids of human placenta: origin, composition, and functional relevance. *Ann Anat.* 1996;178:485-501.

7. Uszynski M. Isolation of peptides with anti-urokinase activity from the human placenta. *Thrombos Haemost.* 1980;42:1411-1416.

8. Dvorak H. Fibrin gel investment associated with line 1 and line 10 solid tumor growth, angiogenesis, and fibroplasia in guinea pigs. *JNCI.* 1979;62:1459-1472.

9. Brown L. Leaky vessels, fibrin deposition, and fibrosis: a sequence of events common to solid tumors and to many other types of disease. *Am Rev Respir Dis.* 1989;140:1104-1107.

10. Nagy J. Pathogenesis of tumor stroma generation: a critical role of leaky blood vessels and fibrin deposition. *Biochem Biophys Acta.* 1989;948:305-326.

11. Liu H. Interactions between fibrin, collagen, and endothelial cells in angiogenesis. *Adv Exp Med Biol.* 1990;281:19-31.

12. Sack G. Trousseau's syndrome and other manifestations of chronic disseminated coagulopathy in patients with neoplasms: clinical, pathophysiologic, and therapeutic features. *Medicine.* 1977;56:1-37.

13. Hu T. Synthesis of tissue factor messenger RNA and procoagulant activity in breast cancer cells in response to serum stimulation. *Thromb Res.* 1993;72:155-168.

14. Goodnough L. Increased incidence of thromboembolism in stage IV breast cancer patients treated with a five-drug chemotherapy regimen. *Cancer.* 1984;54:1264-1268.

15. Mitter C. Plasma levels of d-dimer: a cross-linked fibrin-degradation product in female breast cancer. *J Cancer Res Clin Oncol.* 1991;117:259-262.

16. Bu L. The role of proteases in the growth, invasion, and spread of cancer cells. *Tidsskr Nor Laegeforen.* 1990;110:3753-3756.

17. Honn K. The role of platelets in metastasis. *Biorheology.* 1987;24:127-137.

18. Hamilton P. Disseminated intravascular coagulation: a review. *J Clin Pathol.* 1978;31:609-619.

19. Miller S. Coagulation disorders in cancer: I. clinical and laboratory studies. *Cancer.* 1967;20:1452-1462.

20. Cosgriff S. Thromboembolic complications associated with ACTH and cortisone therapy. *JAMA.* 1951;147:924-931.

21. Gabazza E. Alteration of coagulation and fibrinolysis systems after multidrug anticancer therapy for lung cancer. *Europ J Cancer.* 1994;30A:1276-1281.

22. Rickles F. Hemostatic alterations in cancer patients. *Cancer Metas Rev.* 1992;11:237-248.

23. Spillert C. Altered coagulability: an aid to selective breast biopsy. *JAMA.* 1993;85:273-277.

24. Boik J. *Cancer and Natural Medicine.* Princeton, Minn: Oregon Medical Press; 1996:26-28.

25. Chlebowski R. Inhibition of human tumor growth and DNA biosynthetic activity by vitamin K and warfarin: in vitro and clinical results. *AACR Abstracts.* March 1983:165.

26. Zacharski L. Effect of warfarin on survival in small cell carcinoma of the lung. *JAMA.* 1981;245:831-835.

27. Martin P. Anticancer fffect of dipyridamole. *Townsend Lett Doctors Patients.* May 2000:114-115.

28. Harris R. Breast cancer and NSAID use: heterogeneity of effect in a case-control study. *Prev Med.* 1995;24:119-120.

29. Harris R. Epidemiologic study of nonsteroidal anti-inflammatory drugs and breast cancer. *Oncol Reports.* 1995;2:591-592.

30. Prescott S. Is cyclooxygenase-2 the alpha and the omega in cancer? *J Clin Invest.* 2000;105:1511-1513.

31. Kwann, H. Disorders of fibrinolysis. *Med Clin N Amer.* 1972; 56: 163-172.

32. Duchesne, J. A unifying biochemical theory of cancer, senescence and maximal life span. *J Ther Biol.* 1977; 66: 137-145.

33. Egyud, L. Significance of fibrin formation and dissolution in the pathogenesis and treatment of cancer. *Medical Hypothesis.* 1991; 36: 336-340.

34. Goodwin C. Increased expression of procoagulant activity on the surface of human platelets exposed to heavy-metal compounds. *Biochem J.* 1995;308:15-21.

CHAPTER 28
WARNING: HERBS ARE NO SUBSTITUTE FOR AN IPT PHYSICIAN

1. Prehn R. *Immunomodulation of Tumor Growth.* Am J Pathol. 1974;77:119-122.

2. Thomas L. In: Lawrence HS, ed. *Cellular and Humoral Aspects of Hypersensitivity States.* New York, NY: Hoeber;1959.

3. Filipovich A, Spector B. *Malignancies in the Immunocompromised Human.* New York, NY: Elsevier North Holland;1980.

4. Prehn R. Perspectives on oncogenesis: does immunity stimulate or inhibit neoplasia? *J Reticulo Soc.* 1971;10:1-16.

5. Prehn R. An immunostimulation theory of tumor development. *Transplant Rev.* 1971;7:26-54.

6. Medina D. Cell mediated "immunostimulation" induced by mammary tumor virus-free Balb/c mammary tumors. *Nature.* 1973;242:329-330.

7. Fidler I. In vitro studies of cellular-mediated immunostimulation of tumor growth. *J Natl Cancer Inst.* 1973;50:1307-1312.

8. Prehn R. The immune reaction as a stimulator of tumor growth. *Science.* 1972;176:170-171.

9. Jeejeebhoy H. Stimulation of tumor growth by the immune response. *Intl J Cancer.* 1974.

10. Herberman R. Principles of tumor immunology. In: Murphy G, ed. *American Cancer Society Textbook of Clinical Oncology.* 2nd ed. Atlanta, Ga.: American Cancer Society; 1995:135-145.

11. Klein G. Rejectability of virus induced tumors and nonrejectability of spontaneous tumors—a lesson in contrasts. *Transplant Proc.* 1977;9:1095-1104.

12. Bakemeier R. Basic principles of tumor immunology and immunotherapy. In: Rubin P, ed. *Clinical Oncology for Medical Students and Physicians.* 3rd ed. Rochester, NY: American Cancer Society; 1970:423-430.

13. Fidler I. Molecular biology of cancer: invasion and metastasis. In: DeVita VT Jr, Hellman S, Rosenberg SA, eds. *Cancer Principles and Practice of Oncology.* 5th ed. Philadelpha, Pa.: Lippincott-Raven; 1997:135-152.

14. Albino A. Heterogeneity in surface antigen and glycoprotein expression of cell lines derived from different melanoma metastases of the same patient. *J Exp Med.* 1981;154:1764-1771.

15. Bystryn J. Immunophenotype of human melanoma cells in different metastases. *Cancer Res.* 1985;45:5603-5610.

16. Albertini M. Tumor immunology and immunotherapy. In: Abeloff M, ed. *Clinical Oncology.* 2nd ed. New York, NY: Churchill Livingstone; 2000:214-241.

17. Filipovich A. Immunodeficiency and cancer. In: Abeloff M, ed. *Clinical Oncology.* 2nd ed. New York, NY: Churchill Livingstone; 2000:210.

18. Sibinga N. Opioid peptides and opioid receptors in cells of the immune system. *Ann Rev Immunol.* 1988;6:219-249.

19. Bryant H. Role of adrenal cortical activation in the immunosuppressive effects of chronic morphine treatment. *Endocrinology.* 1991;128:3253-3258.

20, Pellis N. Suppression of the induction of delayed hypersensitivity in rats by repetitive morphine treatments. *Exper Neurol.* 1986;93:92-97.

21. Lopez M. Spleen and thymus cells subsets modified by long-term morphine administration and murine AIDS. *Intl J Immunopharmacol.* 1993;15:909-918.

22. Sei Y. Morphine-induced thymic hypoplasia is glucocorticoid-dependent. *J Immunol.* 1991;146:194-198.

23. Bryant H. Immunosuppressive effects of chronic morphine treatment in mice. *Life Sci.* 1987;41:1731-1738.

24. Bussiere J. Differential effects of morphine and naltrexone on the antibody response in various mouse strains. *Immunopharmacol Immunotoxicol.* 1992;14:657-673.

25. Hung C. Proc. Soc. Exp. Biol. Med. 1973;142:106-111.

26. Nair M. Decreased natural and antibody-dependent cellular cytotoxic activities in intravenous drug abusers. *Clin Immunol Immunopathol.* 1986;38:68-78.

27. Eisenstein T. Opioid modulation of immune responses: effects on phagocyte and lymphoid cell populations. *J Neuroimmunol.* 1998; 83:36-44.

28. Gilman A. *The Pharmacological Basis of Therapeutics.* Elmsford, NY: Pergamon Press; 1990:486.

29. García D.P., García y Bellón DP. *Cellular Cancer Therapy.*

30. Tsai Y-C. Effects of tramadol on T lymphocyte proliferation and natural killer cell activity in rats with sciatic constriction injury. *Pain.* 2001;92:63-69.

31. Maibach H. Aspirin and nonsteroidal anti-inflammatory drug use and the risk of subsequent colorectal cancer. *Arch Int Med.* 1994;154:394-402.

32. Schreinemachers D. Aspirin use and lung, colon, and breast cancer incidence in a prospective study. *Epidemiology.* 1994;5:138-148.

33. Quillin P. *Beating Cancer with Nutrition.* Tulsa, Okla.: Nutrition Times Press; 1994.

34. Yance D. *Herbal Medicine: Healing and Cancer.* Chicago, Ill.: Keats Publishing; 1999.

35. Greer S. Mental attitudes to cancer: an additional prognostic factor. *Lancet.* 1985:750-755.

36. Reynolds P. Social connections and cancer: a prospective study of Alameda County residents. Paper presented at: Meeting of the Society of Behavioral Medicine; March 5-7, 1986; San Francisco.

37. Levy S. Survival hazards analysis in first recurrent breast cancer patients: seven-year follow-up. *Psychosom Med.* 1988;50:520-528.

38. Dhabhar F. Effects of stress on immune cell distribution. *J Immunol.* 1995;154:5511-5527.

39. Solomon G. Emotions, stress, the central nervous system, and immunity. *Ann NY Acad Sci.* 1970;335-343.

40. Khansari D. Effects of stress on the immune system. *Immunol Today.* 1990;11:170-175.

41. Cohen S. Psychologic stress, immunity, and cancer. *J Natl Cancer Inst.* 1998;90:3-4.

42. Bartrop R. Depressed lymphocyte function after bereavement. *Lancet.* April 16, 1977:834-836.

43. Girard V. *There's No Place Like Hope.* Lynwood, Wash.: Compendium; 2001.

CHAPTER 29
LEARN TO STARVE TUMORS—BECAUSE CANCERS CRAVE SUGAR!

1. Jackson D. Sugar tolerance in cancer with reference to degree of malignancy. *Texas State J Med.* 1934;30:197-203.

2. Sturrock W. The reaction of the blood serum as an aid to the diagnosis of cancer. *Br Med J.* September 27, 1913:780-782.

3. Cori, C. The carbohydrate metabolism of tumors. II. changes in the serum lactic acid, and CO2-combining power of the blood passing through a tumor. *J Biol Chem.* 1925;6:397-405.

4. Warburg O. *Uber den stoffwechsel der tumoren.* Berlin, Germany: Springer; 1926.

5. Harde E. Sur la reaction acide des tumeurs. *Compt Rend Soc Biol.* 1926;95:1489-1490.

6. Warburg O. *The Metabolism of Tumors.* Dickerts F, trans. London, UK: Constable; 1930:5-47.

7. Goldfeder A. Theoretical basis for the acidotic treatment of neoplasia. *Am J Surg.* February 1933:307-312.

8. Kahler H. Hydrogen-ion concentration of normal liver and hepatic tumors. *J Natl Cancer Inst.* 1943;3:495-501.

9. Gatenby R. Potential role of FDG-PET imaging in understanding tumor-host interaction. *J Nuclear Med.* 1995;36:893-899.

10. *Positron Emission Tomography: An Advanced Imaging Technique to Detect Disease* (brochure). Topeka, Kan.: Midwest Imaging; 2000.

11. Mauriac P. Lactacidemie comparee artere-veine de tumeurs epitheliomateuses. Chez la femme. *Compt Rend Soc Biol.* 1931;108:971-972.

12. Bierich R. Uber den milchsauregehalt von normalen und von krebsgeweben. *Z Physiol Chem.* 1933;214:271-280.

13. Holm E. *Substrate Balances Across Colonic Carcinomas in Humans.* Mannheim, Germany: University of Heidelberg; 1996

14. Mayes P. Glycolysis and the oxidation of pyruvate. In: Murray R, ed. *Harper's Biochemistry.* 24th ed. Stamford, Conn.: Appleton & Lange; 1996:176-184.

15. Sauer L. Ketone body, glucose, lactic acid, and amino acid utilization by tumors in vivo in fasted rats. *Cancer Res.* 1983;43:3497-3503.

16. Gullino P. Glucose consumption by transplanted tumors in vivo. *Cancer Res.* 1967;27:1031-1040.

17. Di Chiro G. Glucose utilization of cerebral gliomas measured by (18F) fluorodeoxyglucose and positron emission tomography. *Neurology.* 1982;32:1323-1329.

18. Rhodes C. In vivo disturbance of the oxidative metabolism of glucose in human cerebral gliomas. *Ann Neurol.* 1982;14:614-626.

19. Kallinowski F. Tumor blood flow: the principal modulator of oxidative and glycolytic metabolism, and of the metabolic micromilieu of human tumor xenografts in vivo. *Intl J Cancer.* 1989;44:266-272.

20. Demetrakopoulos G. *Cancer Res.* 1982;42:756S.

21. Di Chiro G. Issues in the in vivo measurement of glucose metabolism of human central nervous system tumors. *Ann Neurol.* 1984;15S:S138-S146.

22. Kern K. Metabolic imaging of human extremity musculoskeletal tumors by PET. *J Nuclear Med.* 1988;29:181-186.

23. LePage G. Phosphorylated intermediates in tumor glycolysis. *Cancer Res.* 1948;8:193-196.

24. Black J. Metabolic abnormalities of lactic acid in Burkitt-type lymphoma with malignant effusions. *Ann Internal Med.* 1966;65:101-108.

25. Field M. The significance of elevations of blood lactate in patients with neoplastic and other proliferative disorders. *Am J Med.* 1966;40:528-547.

26. Roth G. Chronic lactic acidosis and acute leukemia. *Arch Internal Med.* 1970;125:317-321.

27. Holroyde C. Altered glucose metabolism in metastatic carcinoma. *Cancer Res.* 1975;35:3710-3719.

28. Russell D. Effects of total parenteral nutrition and chemotherapy on the metabolic derangements in small cell lung cancer. *Cancer Res.* 1984;44:1706-1712.

30. Vaupel L. Blood flow, oxygen and nutrient supply, and metabolic microenvironment of human tumors: a review. *Cancer Res.* 1989;49:6449-6465.

30. Kallinowski F. Glucose, lactate, and ketone body utilization by human mammary carcinomas in vivo. *Adv Exp Med Biol.* 1985;191:965-970.

31. Kallinowski F. Glucose uptake, lactate release, ketone body turnover, metabolic micromilieu, and pH distribution in human breast cancer xenografts in nude mice. *Cancer Res.* 1988;48:7264-7272.

32. Kallinowski F. Blood flox, metabolism, cellular microenvironment, and growth rate of human tumor xenografts. *Cancer Res.* 1989;49:3759-3764.

33. Busch H. Metabolic patterns for glucose-1-C[14] in tissues of tumor-bearing rats. *Cancer Res.* 1960;20:50-57.

34. Busch, H. Suppression of growth of the walker tumor by dichloropyruvic acid. *Acid Fed Proc.* 1959;18:1474-1481.

35. Busch H. Inhibition of lactic acid dehydrogenase by fluoropyruvic acid. *J Biol Chem.* 1957;229:377-387.

36. Steckel R. The carbohydrate metabolism of the Brown-Pearce carcinoma of the rabbit in normal and hypoglycemic serum. *Cancer Res.* 1951:330-334.

37. Eskey C. Role of oxygen vs. glucose in energy metabolism in a mammary carcinoma perfused ex vivo: Direct measurement by ^{31}P NMR.

38. Cascino A. Plasma amino acids in human cancer: individual role of tumor, malnutrition, and glucose tolerance. *Clin Nutr.* 1988;7:213-218.

39. Rossi-Fanelli F. Abnormal substrate metabolism and nutritional strategies in cancer management. *J Paren Enteral Nutr.* 1991;15:680-683.

40. Freund *E. Wien Med.* 1885;8:268.

41. Glicksman A. *Med Clin North Am.* 1956:887-900.

42. Repert R. Breast carcinoma study: relation to thyroid disease and diabetes. *JMSMS.* October 1952:1315-1317.

43. Vecchia C. A case-control study of diabetes mellitus and cancer risk. *Br J Cancer.* 1994;70:950-953.

44. Muck B. Cancer of the breast, diabetes, and pathological glucose tolerance. *Arch Gynak.* 1975;220:73-81.

45. Muck B. Altered carbohydrate metabolism in breast cancer and benign breast affections. *Arch Gynak.* 1976;221:83-91.

46. Lenhard R, ed. *Clinical Oncology.* Atlanta, Ga.: American Cancer Society; 2001.

47. Carter A. Metabolic parameters in women with metastatic breast cancer. *Clin Endocrin Metab.* 1975;40:260-264.

48. Seely S. Diet and breast cancer: the possible connection with sugar consumption. *Med Hypoth.* 1983;11:319-327.

49. Forsyth I. Human prolactin: evidence obtained by the bioassay of human plasma. *J Endocrin.* 1971;51:157-163.

50. Shafie S. Cyclic adenosine monophosphate and protein kinase activity in insulin-dependent and independent mammary tumors. *Cancer Res.* 1979;39:2501-2505.

51. Santisteban G. Glycemic modulation of tumor tolerance in a mouse model of breast cancer. *Biochem Biophys Res Comm.* 1985;132:1174-1179.

52. Goldfeder A. Theoretical basis for the acidotic treatment of neoplasia. *Am J Surg.* February 1933:307-312.

53. *Stedman's Medical Dictionary.* 26th ed. Baltimore, Md.: Williams & Wilkins; 1995.

54. Guyton A, ed. *Textbook of Medical Physiology.* 9th ed. Philadelphia, Pa.: W.B. Saunders; 1996:857-862.

55. International Food Information Council Foundation. Diabetes: a growing concern. *Food Insight*, March/April 2001. Available at www.ific.org.

56. International Food Information Council Foundation. Childhood "globesity." *Food Insight*, Jan/Feb 2001. Available at www.ific.org.

57. Ran A. Mitogenic factors accelerate later-age diseases: insulin as a paradigm. *Mech Aging Develop.* 1998;102:95-113.

58. Josefson D. High insulin levels linked to deaths from breast cancer. *Br Med J.* June 3, 2000:1496.

59. Papa V. Elevated insulin receptor content in human breast cancer. Am Soc Clin Invest. 1990;86:1503-1510.

60. Heuson J. Cell proliferation induced by insulin in organ culture of rat mammary carcinoma. Exper Cell Res. 1967;45:351-360.

61. Holdaway I. Hormone binding by human mammary carcinoma. *Cancer Res.* 1977;37:1946-1952.

62. Mountjoy K. Insulin receptor regulation in cultured human tumor cells. *Cancer Res.* 1983;43:4537-4542.

63. Hilf R. Regulatory interrelationships for insulin and estrogen action in mammary tumors. *Cancer Res.* 1978;38:4076-4083.

64. Pearson O. Serum Growth Hormone and insulin levels in patients with breast cancer. This study was supported in part by grants from the USPHS Nos. CA-05197-07 and FR-80-04, the American Cancer Society No. T-46-H, and the Health Fund of Greater Cleveland.

65. Seely S. Diet and breast cancer: the possible connection with sugar consumption. *Med Hypoth.* 1983;11:319-327.

66. Seay H. Effects of several forms of transplantable rat leukemias on the carbohydrate metabolism of the host. *Cancer Res.* 1965;25:1823-1827.

67. Brand-Miller J. *The Glucose Revolution.* New York, N.Y.: Marlow & Company; 1999.

68. Lee B. Effect of glucose, sucrose, and fructose on plasma glucose and insulin responses in normal humans: comparison with white bread. *Eur J Clin Nutr.* 1998;52:924-928.

69. Appleton N. Fructose is no answer for a sweetener. *Health Freedom News.* 1996:16-20.

70. Gandini S. Meta-analysis of studies on breast cancer risk and diet: the role of fruit and vegetable consumption and the intake of associated micronutrients. *Eur J Cancer.* March 2000.

71. Laine D. Comparison of predictive capabilities of diabetic exchange lists and glycemic index of foods. *Diabetes Care.* 1987;10:387-394.

72. Coulston A. Effect of source of dietary carbohydrate on plasma glucose and insulin responses to mixed meals in subjects with NIDDM. *Diabetes Care.* 1987;10:395-400.

73. Coulston A. Metabolic effects of added dietary sucrose in individuals with noninsulin-dependent diabetes mellitus (NIDDM). *Metabolism.* 1985;34:962-966.

74. Hollenbeck C. The effects of variations in percent of naturally occurring complex and simple carbohydrates on plasma glucose and insulin response in individuals with noninsulin-dependent diabetes mellitus. *Diabetes.* 1985;34:151-155.

75. Kraft J. Detection of diabetes mellitus in situ. *Lab Med.* 1975;6:10-22.

76. Keane M. *What to Eat If You Have Cancer.* Chicago, Ill.: Contemporary Books; 1996.

77. McMichael-Phillips D. Effects of soy-protein supplementation on epithelial proliferation in the histologically normal human breast. *Am J Clin Nutr.* 1998;68(suppl):S1431-S1436.

78. Shu X. Soyfood intake during adolescence and subsequent risk of breast cancer among Chinese women. *Cancer Epidem Biomarkers Prevent.* 2001;10:483-488.

79. Setchell K. Nonsteroidal estrogens of dietary origin: possible roles in hormone-dependent disease. *Am J Clin Nutr.* 1984;40:569-578.

80. Lee H. Dietary effects on breast-cancer risk in Singapore. *Lancet.* 1991;337:1197-1200.

81. Nagata C. Effect of soymilk consumption on serum estrogen concentrations in premenopausal Japanese women. *J Natl Cancer Inst.* 1998;90:1830-1835.

82. Lu L. Effects of soya consumption for one month on steroid hormones in premenopausal women: implications for breast cancer risk reduction. *Cancer Epidem Biomarkers Prevent.* 1996;5:63-70.

83. Cassidy A. Biological effects of a diet of soy protein rich in isoflavones on the menstrual cycle of premenopausal women. *Am J Clin Nutr.* 1994;60:333-340.

84. Duncan A. Soy isoflavones exert modest hormonal effects in premenopausal women. *J Clin Endocrin Metab.* 1999;84:192-197.

85. Lee-Jane L. Decreased ovarian hormones during a soya diet: implications for breast cancer prevention. *Cancer Res.* 2000;60:4112-4121.

86. Baer A. Breast cancer. In: *Life Extension Disease Prevention and Treatment.* 3rd ed. Hollywood, Fla.: Life Extension Foundation; 2000:106-121.

87. Hsieh C. Estrogenic effects of genistein on the growth of estrogen receptor-positive human breast cancer (MCF-7) cells in vitro and in vivo. *Cancer Res.* 1998;58:3833-3838.

88. Barnes S. Soybeans inhibit mammary tumors in models of breast cancer. *Prog Clin Biol Res.* 1990;347:239-253.

89. Adlercreutz H. Western diet and western diseases: some hormonal and biochemical mechanisms and dissociations. *Scand J Clin Lab Investig.* 1990;50:3-23.

90. Lamartiniere C. Genistein suppresses mammary cancer in rats. *Carcinogenesis* (Lond.). 1995;16:2833-2840.

91. Wang T. Molecular effects of genistein on estrogen receptor mediated pathways. *Carcinogenesis* (Lond.). 1996;17:271-275.

92. Santell R. Dietary genistein exerts estrogenic effects upon the uterus, mammary gland, and the hypothalamic/pituitary axis in rats. *J Nutr.* 1997;127:263-269.

93. Hoffman E. *Cancer and the Search for Selective Biochemical Inhibitors.* Boca Raton, Fla.: CRC Press; 2000.

94. National Toxicology Program. Toxicology and Carcinogenesis Studies of Quercetin in F344/N rats. Technical Report No. 409. NIH Publication No. 91-3140. Research Triangle Park, N.C.: U.S. Department of Health and Human Services, Public Health Service, National Toxicology Program; 1991.

95. Suolinna E. The effect of flavonoids on aerobic glycolysis and growth of tumor cells. *Cancer Res.* 1975;35:1865-1872.

96. Kim J. Quercetin, an inhibitor of lactate transport and a hyperthermic sensitizer of HeLa cells. *Cancer Res.* 1984;44:102-106.

97. Agullo G. Quercetin exerts a preferential cytotoxic effect on active diving colon carcinoma HT29 and Caco-2 cells. *Cancer Lett.* 1994;87:55-63.

98. Lamson D. Antioxidants and cancer III: quercetin. *Altern Med Rev.* 2000;5:196-207.

99. Hugo F. In vitro effect of extracellular AMP on MCF-7 breast cancer cells: inhibition of glycolysis and cell proliferation. *J Cell Physiol.* 1992;153:539-549.

100. Parsons P. Differential effects of NAD, nicotinamide, and related compounds upon growth and nucleoside incorporation in human cells. *Biochem Pharmacol.* 1983;32:871-876.

101. Manz R. Relationship between size and oxygenation status of malignant tumors. *Adv Exp Med Biol.* 1983;159:391-398.

102. Vaupel P. Intracapillary HbO2 saturation in malignant tumors during normoxia and hyperoxia. *Microvasc Res.* 1979;17:181-191.

103. Muller-Klieser W. Intracapillary oxygemoglobin saturation in malignant tumours with central or peripheral blood supply. *Eur J Cancer.* 1980;16:195-207.

104. Kallinowski F. Growth-related changes of oxygen consumption rates of tumor cells grown in vitro and in vivo. *J Cell Physiol.* 1989;138:183-191.

105. Suzuki N. Cell cycle dependency of metastatic lung colony formation. *Cancer Res.* 1977;37:3690-3693.

106. Fidler I. Tumor heterogeneity and the biology of cancer invasion and metastasis. *Cancer Res.* 1978;38:2651-2660.

107. Fugi H. Selection for high immunogenicity in drug resistant sublines of murine lymphomas demonstrated by plaque assay. *Cancer Res.* 1975;35:946-952.

108. Greene H. The relationship between the dissemination of tumor cells and the distribution of metastases. *Cancer Res.* 1964;24:799-811.

109. Sugarbaker E. Mechanisms and prevention of cancer dissemination: an overview. *Sem Oncol.* 1977;4:19-32.

110. Weiss L. A pathobiologic overview of metastasis. *Sem Oncol.* 1977;4:5-17.

111. Willis R. *The Spread of Tumors in the Human Body.* London, UK: Butterworths; 1972.

112. Hockel M. Association between tumor hypoxia and malignant progression in advanced cancer of the uterine cervix. *Cancer Res.* 1996;56:4509-4515.

113. Song C. Increase in tumor oxygenation and radiosensitivity caused by pentoxifylline. *Radiat Res.* 1992;130:205-210.

114. Lee I. Changes in tumour blood flow, oxygenation, and interstitial fluid pressure induced by pentoxifylline. *Br J Cancer.* 1994;69:492-496.

115. Bicher H. Effects of hyperthermia on normal and tumour microenvironment. *Radiology.* 1980;137:523-530.

116. Steiger E. Effect of nutrition on tumor growth and tolerance to chemotherapy. *J Surg Res.* 1975;18:455-461.

117. Torosian M. Nutritional support in the cancer-bearing host: effects on host and tumor. *Cancer.* 1986;58:1378-1386.

118. Torosian M. Stimulation of tumor growth by nutrition support. *J Paren Enteral Nutr.* 1992;16:72S-75S.

CHAPTER 30
WARNING: ADJUNCTIVE THERAPIES ARE NO SUBSTITUTE FOR AN IPT PHYSICIAN!

1. *Merriam Webster's Collegiate Dictionary.* 10th ed. Springfield, Mass.: Merriam-Webster, Inc.; 1993.
2. Lamson D. Antioxidants in cancer therapy: their actions and interactions with oncologic therapies. *Altern Med Rev.* 1999;4:304-323.
3. Lamson D. Antioxidants and cancer therapy II: quick reference guide. *Altern Med Rev.* 2000;5:152-163.
4. Lamson D. Antioxidants and cancer III: quercetin. *Altern Med Rev.* 2000;5:196-207.
5. Conklin K. Dietary antioxidants during cancer chemotherapy: impact on chemotherapeutic effectiveness and development of side effects. *Nutr Cancer.* 2000;37:1-18.
6. Yance D. *Herbal Medicine, Healing & Cancer.* Chicago, Illl.: Keats Publishing; 1999.
7. García D, García y Bellón D. *Cellular Cancer Therapy Through Modification of Blood Physico-Chemical Constants (Donatian Therapy).* Dillinger M, trans.; 1978. Available at: www.IPTQ.org.
8. Goldfeder A. Theoretical basis for the acidotic treatment of neoplasia. *Am J Surg.* 1933;19:307-312.
9. Fischer-Wasels B. Die behandlung der bosartigen geschwulste mit sauerstoff-kohlensauergemisch. *Frankfurt Ztschr F Path.* 1930;39:1-8.
10. Moore, Wilson. *Biochem J.* 1906;1:297-300.
11. Sturrock W. The reaction of the blood serum as an aid to the diagnosis of cancer. *Br Med J.* September 27, 1913:780-782.
12. McDonald E. A theory of cancer causation. *M J & Rec.* 1927;125:795-798.
13. Reding R. L'equilibre acide-base et l'equilibre ionique dans le cancer et le precancer. *Cancer.* 1928;5:97-100.
14. Woodward G. The hydrogen-ion concentration of the blood in untreated cancer cases and its relation to prognosis. *J Lab Clin Med.* 1932:704-712.
15. Meyer K. pH studies of malignant tissues in human beings. *Cancer Res.* 1948;8:513-518.
16. Kahler H. Hydrogenion concentration of normal liver and hepatic tumors. *J Natl Cancer Inst.* 1943;3:495-501.

17. Gullino P. Modifications of the acid-base status of the internal milieu of tumors. *J Natl Cancer Inst.* 1965;34:857-869.
18. Volk T. pH in human tumour xenografts: effect of intravenous administration of glucose. 1994:492-500.
19. Leeper D. Effect of I.V. glucose versus combined I.V. plus oral glucose on human extracellular pH for potential sensitization to thermotherapy. *Intl J Hypertherm.* 1998;14:257-269.
20. Jahde E. Tumor-selective modification of cellular microenvironment in vivo: effect of glucose infusion on the pH in normal and malignant rat tissues. *Cancer Res.* 1982;42:1505-1512.
21. Wolf R. Growth hormone and insulin reverse net whole body and skeletal muscle protein catabolism in cancer patients. *Ann Surg.* 1992;216:280-288.
22. Huntsman W. *Three Years of HCl Therapy.* Portyage, Mich.: The Torrance Company; 1935.
23. Sakurai Y. Insulin-like growth factor-I and insulin reduce leucine flux and oxidation in conscious TNF-infused dogs. *Surgery.* 1995;117:305-313.
24. Davis A. *Magnetism and Its Effects on the Living System.* Metaire, La.: Acres, U.S.A.; 1974.
25. Davis A. *The Magnetic Blueprint of Life.* Metaire, La.: Acres, U.S.A.; 1993.
26. Philpott W. *Magnetic Therapy.* Tiburon, Calif.: Alternative Medicine.com Books; 2000.
27. Jerabck J. *Magnetic Therapy in Eastern Europe: a Review of 30 Years of Research.* 1998.
28. Lyu B. Influence of magnetic field on the oxygen tension, radiosensitivity, and growth of some experimental tumors. *Radiobiologija.* 1981;21:255-260.
29. Batkin S. Effects of alternating magnetic fields on transplanted neuroblastoma. *Res Comm Chem Pathol Pharmacol.* 1977;16:351-362.
30. Piruzian L. Influence of a constant magnetic field on the ascitic tumor sarcoma 37. *Izvestija Akademiinauk SSR Ser Biol.* 1969;6:893-898.
31. Ukolova M. Energy metabolism of the hypothalamo-hypophyseal division of the rat brain following the anti-tumor effect of magnetic field. *Voprosy Onkologii* 1969;15:60-64.
32. MacLean K. The effect of intense and mild permanent magnetic fields on C3H strain mice: a preliminary report. *Obstet Gynecol.* 1959;14:597-599.
33. Weber T. Inhibition of tumor growth by the use of nonhomogeneous magnetic fields. *Cancer.* 1971;28:340-343.

34. Dilman V, Dean W. *The Neuroendocrine Therapy of Aging.* Pensacola, Fla.: The Center for Bio-Gerontology; 1992.

35. Parsons P. Differential effects of NAD, nicotinamide, and related compounds upon growth and nucleoside incorporation in human cells. *Biochem Pharmacol.* 1983;32:871-876.

36. Rapaport E. Treatment of human tumor cells with ADP or ATP yields arrest of growth in the S phase of the cell cycle. *J Cell Physiol.* 1983;114:279-283.

37. Rapaport E. Experimental cancer therapy in mice by adenine nucleotides. *Europ J Cancer Clin Oncol.* 1988;24:1491-1497.

38. Hugo F. In vitro effect of extracellular AMP on MCF-7 breast cancer cells: inhibition of glycolysis and cell proliferation. *J Cell Physiol.* 1992;153:539-549.

39. Adenosine monophosphate injectable (package insert). Scottsdale, Az.: Legere Pharmaceuticals; 1998.

40. Asai K. *Miracle Cure: Organic Germanium.* Tokyo: Japan Publications; 1980.

41. Brewer K. The mechanism of carcinogenesis: comments on therapy. *J Int Acad Prev Med.* 1979;5:29-53.

42. Messiha F. Cesium: a bibliography update. *Pharmacol Biochem Behavior.* 1984;21:113-129.

43. Brewer K. The high pH therapy for cancer tests on mice and humans. *Pharmacol Biochem Behavior.* 1984;21:1-5.

44. Manner H. *The Death of Cancer.* Evanston, Ill.: Advanced Century Publishing; 1978.

45. Pelton R. *Alternatives in Cancer Therapy.* New York, N.Y.: Simon & Schuster; 1994.

46. Walters R. *Options: the Alternative Cancer Therapy Book.* Honesdale, Pa.: Avery; 1993.

47. Yance D. *Herbal Medicine, Healing and Cancer.* Chicago, Ill.: Keats Publishing; 1999.

APPENDIX A
THE HAUSER DIET

1. Quillin P. *Beating Cancer with Nutrition.* Tulsa, Okla.: Nutrition Times Press; 2001:97.

2. Simopoulos A. Omega-3 fatty acids in health and disease and in growth and development. *American Journal of Clinical Nutrition.* 1991; 54: 438-463.

3. Pepping J. Omega-3 essential fatty acids. *American Journal of Health-System Pharmacy.* 1999; 56: 719-724.

4. Caygill, C. Fat, Fish, Fish Oil and Cancer. *British Journal of Cancer.* 1996; 74: 159-164.

5. Quillin P. Beating Cancer with Nutrition. Tulsa, Okla.: *Nutrition Times Press;* 2001:276.

6. Quillin P. Beating Cancer with Nutrition. Tulsa, Okla.: *Nutrition Times Press;* 2001:304.

7. Kellas W. *Thriving in a Toxic World.* Shaklee; 1999.

8. *Shaklee Newsletter Fall Issue,*1999.

9. Diamond W, et al. *Definitive Guide to Cancer.* Tiburon, Calif.: Future Medicine Publishing, Inc.; 1997:591.

10. Block G. Fruit, vegetables, and cancer prevention: A review of the epidemiological evidence. *Nutri Cancer.* 1992; 18: 1-29.

11. Steinmetz, K. Vegetables, fruit, and cancer prevention: a review. *Journal of the American Dietetic Association.* 1996; 96: 1027-1036.

12. Quillin P. Beating Cancer with Nutrition. Tulsa, Okla.: *Nutrition Times Press;* 2001:287.

13. Cree M, et al. Altered urinary excretion of 2-hydroxyestrone in women after soya isoflavone consumption. *Proc Am Assoc Cancer Res.* 1999;40:302.

14. Keane M. *What to Eat If You Have Cancer.* Lincolnwood, Ill.: Contemporary Books; 1996:114.

15. McMichael-Phillips D, et al. Effects of soy-protein supplementation on epithelial proliferation in the histologically normal human breast. *Am J Clin Nutr.* 1998;1431S-1436S.

16. Wright J. Smart Publications Update. 106: *Smart Publications,* Petaluma CA. 2000. Pp. 1-12.

17. Veggies may cut by half risk of prostate cancer. *Seattle Times,* January 4, 2000.

18. Haggans C. Effect of flax seed consumption on urinary estrogen metabolites in postmenopausal women. *Nutr Cancer.* 1999;33:188-195.

19. Rose D. High-fiber diet reduces serum estrogen concentrations in premenopausal women. *Am J Clin Nutr.* 1991;54:520-525.

20. Quillin P. Beating Cancer with Nutrition. Tulsa, Okla.: *Nutrition Times Press;* 2001:34-36.

21. Santisteban G. *Biochem and Biophys Res Comm.* 1985;132:1174.

22. Brand-Miller J, et al. *The Glucose Revolution.* New York, NY: Marlowe and Company; 1999:13.

23. Cataldo C. *Nutrition and Diet Therapy: Principles and Practice.* New York, NY: West Publishing Company; 1986:325-331.

24. Yance D. *Herbal Medicine, Healing, and Cancer.* Chicago, Ill.: Keats Publishing; 1999:307.

25. Kappas A., Anderson K. Nutrition-endocrine interactions: Induction of reciprocal changes in the 5α-reduction of testosterone and the cytochrome P-450-dependent oxidation of estradiol by dietary macronutrients in man. *Proceedings of the National Academy of Sciences.* 1983; 80: 7646-7649.

APPENDIX D
IPT AND INSURANCE

1. Theodosakis J. *Don't Let Your HMO Kill You.* New York, NY: Routledge Press; 2000.

A

Abel, Ulrich: 94
Abortion: 197–198
N-Acetylcysteine: 304
Acne: 41
Adenocarcinomas: 227, 355
Adenosine monophosphate (AMP): 315, 316, 317
Adenosine triphosphate (ATP): 315
Adipose tissue: 73
Adjunctive therapies: 303–319
Adriamycin: 110, 152, 153, 161, 172
Aerobic metabolism: 230–231, 269–270, 298, 315, 332–333
Aging: effects of, 313
Air: 203, 334
Aldosterone: 176, 179
Aldren, Hayle T.: 12, 70
Alkylating agents: 92, 113
Alkylosis: 308–310
Allergens: 41
Allergies: 41, 137, 144
Allopathic medicine: 137, 144, 215
Aloe Master: 351
Alpha fetoprotein: 218
Alternative medicine: 47, 214–216
Alternative Medicine Digest and Cancer Diagnosis: What to Do Next: 111
Alwa, Ratha: 166
AMAS (antimalignin antibody) test: 48, 218, 219, 221
American Cancer Society: 4, 5, 166, 167, 280
American Cancer Society Textbook of Clinical Oncology: 193
American Cancer Society's Guide to Complementary and Alternative Cancer Methods: 158
American Medical Association (AMA): 71
Amino acids: 40, 73, 74
Amygdaline: 352
Anabolic hormones: 311
Androstenedione: 186
Anemia: 344
Anerobic metabolism: 298, 332
Angiogenesis: 231, 236–239, 245, 294, 300
Anorexia: 128
Anthocyanidins: 334
Anthracenedione: 153
Antibiotics: 86, 113, 133, 149–150, 338–340
Anticoagulants: 231, 243–245, 244, 331
Antimetabolites: 91–92, 113
Antineoplastic drugs: 112

Antinuclear antibodies (ANA): 144
Antioxidant assay (AOA), 322
Antioxidants: 334
Antiviral cytokines: 252
Antivirals: 149–150
Apoptosis: 44, 229, 235–236, 236
Appetite loss: 51, 84
Arimidex: 205
Arthritis: 137
Arthritis Can Be Cured, 146
Asai, Kazuhiko: 316, 318
Ascorbic acid: 125
Asthma: 137, 139
Astrocytomas: 128
Atherosclerosis: 32, 75
Austin State Hospital: 63
Autoantibodies: 144
Autoimmune diseases allergic reactions and: 41
  Causes of, 139
  Detection, 143
  IPT and, 125, 133
  Mechanisms of action, 142–144
  Natural medicine approach, 145–146
  Symptoms of, 143–144
  Targets of, 143
Ayre, Steven G.:
  Background, 17
  At Caring Medical, 63
  Contact information, 373
Contemporary Medicine Center and: 8
  Dedications, 2
  With Donato2 and Donato3, 65
  ICT research, 65
  Introduction to IPT, 19–20
  Photo, 70
  Sana Institute and, 11–12
  SCR scores, 111
  Thanks to, 3
  Theory of positive thinking, 260–262
Azidothymidine (AZT): 87

B

B complex vitamins: 125, 333
Baird, Nicole: 3
Barberry tea: 334
Basement membrane: 230
Beating Cancers with Nutrition: 259
Bee venom: 46–47
Berries: 337
Besson, Philippe-Gaston: 70
Beta-carotene: 171, 304, 334